Medicine

Diagnosis and Treatment

Medicine

Diagnosis and Treatment

Edited by
Robert W. Schrier, M.D.
Professor and Chairman,
Department of Medicine,
University of Colorado School of Medicine,
Denver

Little, Brown and Company
Boston/Toronto

Library of Congress Catalog Card No. 88-2240

ISBN 0-316-77484-7

Printed in the United States of America

DON (H)

Contents

Contributing Authors

David Collier, M.D.
Assistant Professor of Medicine, Division of Rheumatology, University of Colorado School of Medicine, Denver; Chief of Rheumatology, Denver General Hospital, Denver

John M. Douglas, M.D.
Assistant Professor of Medicine, Division of Infectious Diseases, University of Colorado School of Medicine, Denver; Assistant Director, Disease Control Service, Denver General Hospital, Denver

Steven L. Dubovsky, M.D.
Associate Professor of Psychiatry and Medicine, University of Colorado School of Medicine, Denver; Director of Clinical Services, Colorado Psychiatric Hospital, Denver

Michael P. Earnest, M.D.
Associate Professor of Neurology and Preventive Medicine, University of Colorado School of Medicine, Denver; Director of Neurology, Denver General Hospital, Denver

William F. Ehni, M.D.
Attending Physician, Department of Medicine, Stevens Memorial Hospital, Edmonds, Washington

Richard T. Ellison, M.D.
Assistant Professor of Medicine, Division of Infectious Diseases, University of Colorado School of Medicine, Denver; Acting Chief, Infectious Disease Service, Denver Veterans Administration Medical Center, Denver

Karl E. Hammermeister, M.D.
Professor of Medicine, Division of Cardiology, University of Colorado School of Medicine, Denver; Chief of Cardiology, Denver Veterans Administration Medical Center, Denver

Fred D. Hofeldt, M.D.
Professor of Medicine, Division of Endocrinology, University of Colorado School of Medicine, Denver; Chief of Endocrine Service, Department of Medicine, Denver General Hospital, Denver

J. Fred Kolhouse, M.D.
Associate Professor of Medicine, Division of Hematology, University of Colorado School of Medicine, Denver

JoAnn Lindenfeld, M.D.
Associate Professor of Medicine, Division of Cardiology, University of Colorado School of Medicine, Denver; Director, Coronary Care Unit, University Hospital, Denver

Andrew Mallory, M.D.
Associate Clinical Professor, Division of Gastroenterology, University of Colorado School of Medicine, Denver; Staff Physician, Rose Medical Center, Denver

J. Joseph Marr, M.D.
Professor of Medicine and Biochemistry, Head, Division of Infectious Diseases, University of Colorado School of Medicine, Denver

Laurel A. Miller, M.D.
Instructor of Medicine, Division of Infectious Diseases, University of Colorado School of Medicine, Denver; Staff Physician, Disease Control Division, Denver General Hospital, Denver

E. Chester Ridgway, M.D.
Professor of Medicine and Head, Division of Endocrinology, University of Colorado School of Medicine, Denver

John Schaefer, M.D.
Professor of Medicine, University of Colorado School of Medicine, Denver; Chief of Gastroenterology, Denver General Hospital, Denver

Robert W. Schrier, M.D.
Professor and Chairman, Department of Medicine, University of Colorado School of Medicine, Denver

Marvin I. Schwarz, M.D.
Professor of Medicine and Head, Division of Pulmonary Sciences, University of Colorado School of Medicine, Denver

James H. Scully, M.D.
Associate Professor of Psychiatry, University of Colorado School of Medicine, Denver; Director of Residency Training in Psychiatry, University of Colorado Affiliated Hospitals, Denver

Scot M. Sedlacek, M.D.
Assistant Professor of Medicine, Division of Medical Oncology, University of Colorado School of Medicine, Denver

Joseph I. Shapiro, M.D.
Assistant Professor of Medicine, Division of Renal Diseases, University of Colorado School of Medicine, Denver; Director of Chronic Dialysis, University Service, Rocky Mountain Kidney Center, Denver

Steven Shoemaker, M.D.
Assistant Professor of Medicine, Division of Pulmonary Sciences, University of Colorado School of Medicine, Denver

James Steigerwald, M.D.
Professor of Medicine and Head, Division of Rheumatology, Medical College of Ohio, Toledo; Attending Physician, University Hospital, Toledo

William L. Weston, M.D.
Professor of Medicine and Chairman, Department of Dermatology, University of Colorado School of Medicine, Denver

Norman E. Wikner, M.D.
Assistant Professor of Medicine, Department of Dermatology, University of Colorado School of Medicine, Denver; Staff Physician, National Jewish Center for Immunology and Respiratory Medicine, Denver

Preface

The initial exposure to internal medicine may be overwhelming to the medical student whose major source of study is one of the larger textbooks of internal medicine. The present book is written as an introduction to internal medicine, which can be read by the medical student during an 8- to 12-week clerkship. The text, *Medicine: Diagnosis and Treatment,* is organized in a manner similar to the approach in which the physician routinely evaluates the patient. Specifically, the important characteristics of the patient's history, physical examination and laboratory findings are presented for the major diseases in each of the subspecialties of internal medicine. The natural history, acute and chronic management, and prognosis are then discussed. Each section is written by physician-educators who have considerable experience and commitment to medical student teaching.

It is our hope that this introductory text will provide medical students with a foundation in internal medicine that will stimulate their interest to seek further in-depth knowledge as they care for their patients. Sir William Osler wrote "To study the phenomena of disease without books is to sail an uncharted sea, while to study books without patients is not to go to sea at all." It is our hope that this introductory text will assist the medical student in launching an exciting life-long voyage in internal medicine.

I would like to acknowledge the excellent support of Jennifer Graves during the course of editing this book.

R.W.S.

Notice

The indications and dosages of all drugs in this book have been recommended in the medical literature and conform to the practices of the general medical community. The medications described do not necessarily have specific approval by the Food and Drug Administration for use in the diseases and dosages for which they are recommended. The package insert for each drug should be consulted for use and dosage as approved by the FDA. Because standards for usage change, it is advisable to keep abreast of revised recommendations, particularly those concerning new drugs.

Medicine

Diagnosis and Treatment

Cardiovascular Diseases

1

JoAnn Lindenfeld and
Karl E. Hammermeister

Coronary Artery Disease

Importance

Although there has been a 25 percent drop in mortality from coronary artery disease in the United States over the past 15 years, it is still the leading cause of death among adults [106]. Of the half million deaths per year attributed to coronary artery disease, over half are sudden and occur outside the hospital. In only about a third of the sudden out-of-hospital deaths is there evidence of acute myocardial infarction; the remainder are presumably the result of an acute arrhythmia—usually ventricular fibrillation, which is often triggered by a premature ventricular beat or ventricular tachycardia. This latter group of acute "electrical" deaths is thought to be particularly amenable to prevention with a better understanding of the pathophysiology of sudden cardiac death.

Pathogenesis of Atherosclerosis

Coronary artery disease manifests itself as six clinical syndromes: acute myocardial infarction, stable angina pectoris, unstable angina pectoris, variant angina, silent myocardial ischemia, and sudden cardiac death. In the vast majority of patients with one of these syndromes, the pathologic substrate is severe atherosclerosis of one or more coronary arteries producing occlusion or partial obstruction. Even after more than 40 years of intense investigation, the pathogenesis of atherosclerosis is incompletely understood. The response to injury hypothesis of Ross explains much of the known epidemiologic and biochemical data [139]. The first step in the genesis of the atherosclerotic plaque is injury to the arterial endothelium; possible culprits are mechanical injury such as abnormal shear stresses associated with hypertension, biochemical injury as is known to occur with homocysteine and might occur with low-density lipoproteins, damage through immunologic mechanisms as yet undefined, viruses (hypothetical at present), or other toxins such as might occur in cigarette smoke. The damaged endothelium has an altered permeability that allows for the transudation of lipids and cellular elements such as macrophages. Platelets adhere to the damaged endothelium and release a mitogenic substance known as platelet growth factor. There is migration and proliferation of smooth-muscle cells in the subintimal region. All this results in the formation of a lipid-laden mass between the intima and media known as the atherosclerotic plaque. With removal of the inciting noxious stimulus, the plaque may heal to leave only a minimal scar; however, often there is progression until there is obstruction of the lumen in medium-sized arteries (coronary arteries and cerebral arteries) or destruction of the media in large arteries to produce aneurysms (aorta).

Risk Factors for Coronary Artery Disease

Beginning with the observation of a reduced coronary heart disease mortality rate in Norway during World War II (attributed to the austere diet of that period), a number of risk factors for coronary artery disease have been identified [95]. These can be classified according to reversibility and the strength of the relationship to coronary events (Table 1-1). By these criteria, the two most important reversible risk factors are hypertension and cigarette smoking—both public health problems of enormous proportions in the United States. Both these risk factors have a strong relationship to risk for coronary heart disease. Strong evidence suggests that elimination of these risk factors reduces the risk of a coronary event; both are controllable through effective public health measures and education.

Table 1-1. *Risk Factors for the Development of Coronary Artery Disease*

Risk factor	Reversibility	Strength
Male sex	No	+ + + +
Age	No	+ + + +
Hypertension	Completely	+ + + +
Smoking	Completely	+ + + +
Renal failure	No	+ + + +
Hyperlipidemia	Partially	+ + +
Family history	No	+ + +
Diabetes	Questionable	+ + +
Premature menopause	Possibly	+ +
Sedentary lifestyle	Possibly	+ +
Obesity	Possibly	+
Oral contraceptives	Yes	+
Hyperuricemia	No	+
Type A personality	Questionable	+

Acute Myocardial Infarction

PATHOPHYSIOLOGY

Acute myocardial infarction is irreversible myocardial cell death due to ischemia. Acute myocardial infarction is classified into two types according to the electrocardiogram: Q-wave infarction and non-Q-wave infarction. Q-wave infarctions are almost always the result of total occlusion of a proximal coronary artery by a recently formed thrombus superimposed on a severe atherosclerotic lesion [41]. In non-Q-wave infarctions the coronary artery is still partially patent, but it is severely obstructed by an atherosclerotic plaque with or without superimposed thrombus. Further classification of myocardial infarction can be made according to location in the left ventricle, which can be determined from the electrocardiogram (Table 1-2).

DIAGNOSIS

Symptoms

The clinical presentation is usually that of severe, oppressive chest discomfort accompanied by diaphoresis lasting from 20 minutes to several hours. Other common presenting symptoms are dizziness and weakness from low cardiac output, dyspnea from a high pulmonary venous pressure, and marked anxiety or fear of death (angor animi). The pain can sometimes be epigastric in location and accompanied by a desire to belch. Occasionally, the pain may be in the back between the scapulae, or confined to the arms, or only in the mandible. Population surveys indicate that 25 percent of patients with electrocardiographic evidence of old myocardial infarction can recall no symptoms.

Despite the relatively typical and severe symptoms in most cases, the average delay from onset of symptoms to arrival at a hospital is 1 to 3 hours. This is the period of time when the acutely ischemic myocardium is most unstable electrically and ventricular fibrillation is most likely to occur. Further patient and public education is needed to make patients at risk more knowledgeable of the symptoms and aware of the dangers of delay in seeking attention. Physicians also must be prepared to deal with many false alarms in emergency rooms and the clinic as well as some ultimately unnecessary hospital admissions.

Table 1–2. Classification, Pathophysiology, and Electrocardiographic Criteria of Acute Myocardial Infarction

Classification	Coronary artery	Pathophysiology	Electrocardiogram
Q-wave infarction:			
Anterior	Left or anterior descending	Complete thrombosis	Q waves in V_2 to V_4
Inferior	right or posterior descending	Complete thrombosis	Q waves II, III, and AVF
Posterior	Circumflex	Complete thrombosis	Broad R waves in V_1 and V_2
Non-Q-wave infarction	Any	Severe stenosis	ST-segment depression and/or T-wave inversion

Table 1–3. Classic Electrocardiographic Findings of Acute Q-wave Myocardial Infarction

ECG finding	ST segment	T wave	QRS complex
Vector*	Toward the infarct	Away from the infarct	Away from the infarct
Time of onset	Earliest (minutes to hours)	Second (2 to 12 hours)	Last (6 to 48 hours)
Persistence	Days	Days to weeks	Generally permanent

*A line depicting the magnitude and direction of the average electrical force for the specified portion of the electrocardiogram.

Physical Signs

The presenting physical signs may be surprisingly few. Diaphoresis, while nonspecific, often means a marked autonomic response to a potentially life-threatening illness. Either hypotension from low cardiac output or hypertension from sympathetic discharge may be present. Similarly, either bradycardia from vagal discharge (more common in inferior infarction) or heart block or tachycardia from reduced stroke volume or sympathetic stimulation may be seen. In a minority of patients, pulmonary congestion may be manifested by tachypnea, dyspnea, rales, or even frank pulmonary edema with frothy sputum. Examination of the heart is often normal; however, some patients may have a gallop rhythm indicating increased diastolic pressure in the ventricle, a murmur of mitral regurgitation due to papillary muscle dysfunction, or a precordial bulge reflecting dyskinetic myocardium (left ventricular wall moving outward with systole).

Electrocardiographic Findings

Although the electrocardiogram rarely may be normal in the early phases of acute myocardial infarction, generally the electrocardiogram is the most useful and cost-effective diagnostic tool after the history. The typical electrocardiographic changes and their sequence are shown in Table 1-3. An example of an acute anterior myocardial infarction with Q waves and ST-segment elevation in leads V_2 to V_5 is shown in Fig. 1-1. Figure 1-2 shows an example of an acute inferior myocardial infarction with Q waves and ST-segment elevation in leads II, III, and AVF. The ST-segment and T-wave changes alone are not specific for acute myocardial infarction; these are the typical changes of a non-Q-wave infarction, but they must be accompanied by other corroborating evidence, such as serum enzyme changes, to make a definite diagnosis of infarction. The abnormal Q wave is relatively specific for myocardial infarction and is a sign of dead or scarred myocardium that is unable to generate an electric field. The Q wave forms the basis for the diagnosis of a remote myocardial infarction from the electrocardiogram.

Serum Enzymes

The dying myocardial cell releases some of its enzymatic contents into the bloodstream because of loss of cell membrane integrity; thus the detection

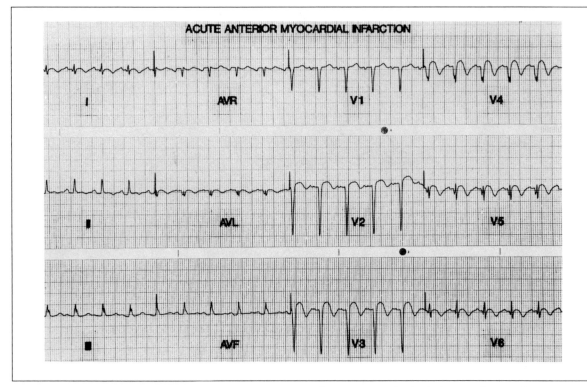

Figure 1–1. Twelve-lead electrocardiogram showing an acute anterior myocardial infarction. Note especially the ST-segment elevation in leads V_2 to V_5 resulting in a ST vector pointing toward the infarction, the T-wave inversion in leads V_3 to V_6 producing a T vector pointing away from the infarct, and the Q waves in leads V_1 to V_5 resulting in an initial 0.04-second QRS vector pointing away from the infarct.

of an increase in myocardial enzymes in serum is useful in diagnosis. Creatine kinase is usually detectable within a few hours of the onset of symptoms, peaks at 12 to 24 hours, and returns to normal levels within 48 to 72 hours. It is the most specific of the commonly used enzymes, but it is found also in substantial quantities in skeletal muscle, vascular smooth muscle, and brain. Trauma or necrosis of one of these organs, such as intramuscular injection of analgesics, can produce creatine kinase elevation that mimics that of acute myocardial infarction. The peak value of serum creatine kinase following an acute infarction correlates in a very rough fashion with infarct size and with prognosis; more accurate estimates of infarct size can be obtained by estimating the area under the plot of creatine kinase versus time.

Serum lactic dehydrogenase is also commonly used diagnostically; it is first detectable in abnormal levels 24 to 48 hours after the onset of symp-toms, peaks at 3 to 6 days, with elevated levels persisting as long as 8 to 14 days. It is this latter characteristic that makes serum lactic dehydrogenase levels useful in the diagnosis of patients who do not seek medical care for several days after the onset of symptoms. However, lactic dehydrogenase is also found in large quantities in red blood cells, liver, kidney, and skeletal muscle. It may be elevated in skeletal muscle trauma, in hemolysis of red cells, in liver disease, and in up to 30 percent of patients with congestive heart failure.

Separation into isoenzymes greatly increases

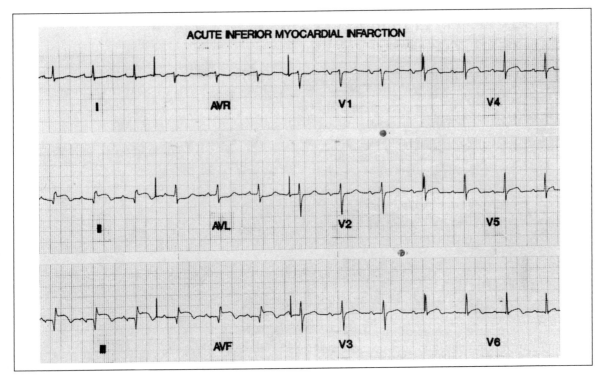

Figure 1–2. Twelve-lead electrocardiogram showing an acute inferior myocardial infarction. Note especially the ST-segment elevation in leads II, III, and AVF resulting in a ST-vector pointing inferiorly toward the infarction, the T-wave inversion in leads II, III, and AVF producing a T vector pointing away from the infarct, and the Q waves in leads II, III, AVF resulting in an initial 0.04-second QRS vector pointing away from the infarction.

the specificity of both creatine kinase and lactic dehydrogenase for the diagnosis of myocardial infarction. Creatine kinase has three isoenzyme fractions: MM, MB, and BB. The MB fraction is nearly specific for myocardial necrosis. Lactic dehydrogenase has five isoenzymes: usually numbered 1 to 5. The pattern of elevation of isoenzyme 1 greater than 2 is relatively specific for myocardial infarction, but it is also seen with hemolysis of red cells. The isoenzyme assays are expensive and overused, because the diagnosis is usually clear from the history, electrocardiogram, and standard enzyme measurement. Situations where isoenzyme measurement would be useful include out-of-hospital cardiac arrest (where high levels of skeletal muscle enzymes are released by the ischemia and trauma of resuscitation), pericarditis, and recent surgical procedures.

TREATMENT

Reperfusion

Treatment of acute myocardial infarction is rapidly evolving from a passive, supportive role aimed primarily at prevention and treatment of lethal ventricular fibrillation to an aggressive, interventional stance aimed at reestablishing myocardial perfusion and minimizing myocardial necrosis. The primary reason for this evolution in treatment is the recognition once again that most cases of myocardial infarction are the result of coronary thrombosis [41], after having ignored for many years the first description of acute myocardial infarction by James Herrick in 1912 as being the result of coronary thrombosis [81]. Animal studies suggest that if perfusion is restored to acutely ischemic myocardium within 3 to 6 hours of coronary occlusion, some of the myocardium supplied by the occluded artery can be salvaged. Three approaches have been tried in humans to promptly restore myocardial blood flow: emergent aortocoronary bypass surgery, thrombolytic therapy, and percutaneous transluminal coronary angioplasty. The latter two forms of therapy singly and in combination seem to offer the most promise and are currently undergoing clinical evaluation in carefully designed randomized trials. Currently available thrombolytic agents (streptokinase and urokinase) administered directly into the coronary artery via a catheter can restore blood flow in about 70 percent of occluded arteries and have reduced early mortality in one randomized trial [99]. However, intracoronary administration of streptokinase is impractical for widespread use because of the enormous demands it places on expensive cardiac catheterization resources. Streptokinase given intravenously is much more practical, but it opens occluded arteries in only 30 to 60 percent of patients. In a very large, unblinded, randomized trial of 12,000 patients in Italy, there was a modest (17 percent) reduction in mortality with thrombolytic therapy, which was statistically significant [71]. The thrombin-specific tissue plasminogen activator is somewhat more effective in reestablishing flow by the intravenous route than streptokinase. A major unresolved problem following the reestablishment of flow by thrombolysis is that there is usually a severe residual atherosclerotic stenosis with abnormal intima that results in a substantial reocclusion rate. Both coronary angioplasty and bypass surgery have been used in attempts to maintain myocardial blood flow; however, there are no controlled trials completed at this time on which to base therapeutic decision making. Nevertheless, it appears likely that some form of thrombolysis and/or angioplasty will become commonplace in the treatment of acute myocardial infarction in the near future.

Table 1–4. *Determinants of Myocardial Oxygen Demand and Delivery*

Myocardial oxygen demand	Myocardial oxygen delivery
Heart rate	Coronary blood flow: Transcoronary pressure gradient
Contractility	Aortic diastolic pressure Left ventricular diastolic pressure Coronary vascular resistance
Left ventricular wall stress: Left ventricular systolic pressure Left ventricular size (radius)	Oxygen extraction: Arterial saturation Arterial–coronary sinus oxygen difference

Standard Therapy

Therapy includes hospitalization in a coronary care unit with continuous electrocardiographic monitoring, treatment of pain with narcotic analgesics, the administration of supplemental oxygen, and attempts to minimize myocardial oxygen demand through attention to the determinants of myocardial oxygen demand (Table 1-4). Hypertension that persists after adequate pain relief should be treated aggressively with short-acting, parenteral antihypertensive agents such as intravenous nitroglycerin or nitroprusside. Tachycardia may be minimized by treating pain and anxiety; morphine sulfate given intravenously in 2- to 4-mg increments is the preferred analgesic agent, since it has minimal hemodynamic effects in the supine position. Nitroglycerin has no analgesic properties; while it is very effective in relieving the pain of unstable angina by relieving coronary spasm and reducing peripheral resistance, it is generally ineffective in relieving the pain of acute myocardial infarction. Similarly, there is no convincing evidence that nitroglycerin can reduce infarct size. It is worthwhile remembering that none of these time-honored forms of therapy has been rigorously tested for efficacy in controlled, randomized trials.

Risk Assessment

Patients with uncomplicated acute myocardial infarction are usually hospitalized for 7 to 10 days. Careful attention should be given to signs of additional myocardial ischemia during this period that might suggest that additional myocardium is in jeopardy. The occurrence of spontaneous angina, angina on minimal exertion, or angina or ST-segment depression on a low-level exercise test performed near the end of the hospitalization have been shown to be predictors of subsequent coronary events [167]. Patients who exhibit additional myocardial ischemia and who are otherwise reasonable candidates for coronary bypass surgery should undergo coronary arteriography. If the angiogram reveals a substantial amount of viable myocardium in jeopardy (that is, ≥ 70 percent stenosis of all three major coronary arteries and/or ≥ 50 percent stenosis of the left main coronary artery), coronary bypass surgery or angioplasty should be considered.

Beta-Adrenergic Blockade

Three large, well-designed, randomized trials have demonstrated that administration of 180 to 240 mg per day propranolol in divided doses, 100 mg metroprolol twice daily, or 10 mg timolol twice daily beginning 7 to 10 days after the infarction and continuing for up to 3 years after the infarction significantly reduces subsequent mortality [83,128,10]. Patients who have severe congestive heart failure due to systolic left ventricular dysfunction (ejection fraction < 0.30), insulin-dependent diabetes, or advanced heart block without a pacemaker should be excluded from this therapy. In patients with severe bronchoconstriction or fixed airway obstruction, a cardioselective beta-adrenergic blocking agent, such as metoprolol, may be tried. However, caution is necessary because in higher doses even cardioselective agents can exacerbate airway obstruction.

Anticoagulation

The use of anticoagulants following acute myocardial infarction is still subject to debate and investigation. One large randomized trial, the VA Cooperative Study, showed no difference in mortality between acute myocardial infarction patients anticoagulated for 30 days and similar patients receiving standard therapy; however, there was a marked reduction in systemic embolism (usually manifested as stroke) and pulmonary embolism with anticoagulation [3]. Subsequent to this study we have learned with two-dimensional echocardiography that intraventricular thrombus occurs in about 30 percent of patients with anterior, apical, or septal infarctions, but rarely in patients with inferior or posterior infarctions. Thus it seems reasonable to anticoagulate all patients with anterior, apical, or septal infarctions for about 30 days, if there is no contraindication. If clot is evident on the echocardiogram, anticoagulation may be continued for 3 to 6 months.

COMPLICATIONS OF ACUTE MYOCARDIAL INFARCTION

Ventricular Arrhythmia

The most common complication is ventricular arrhythmia—occurring in some form in over 90 percent of patients in the first 72 hours following onset of symptoms. Premature ventricular beats are almost universal; more complex forms such as couplets, triplets, and nonsustained ventricular tachycardia are also commonly seen early after myocardial infarction. Because of the concern that a ventricular premature beat falling in the partially refractory period of the preceding beat (downslope of the T wave) might trigger ventricular fibrillation, frequent premature ventricular beats and more complex forms are treated with intravenous lidocaine. This can be given as a 50- to 100-mg bolus followed by a maintenance drip of 1 to 4 mg per minute titrated to therapeutic blood levels of 2 to 4 µg/ml. Some recommend that lidocaine be given to all patients admitted with myocardial infarction, because a randomized trial conducted by Lie and colleagues in Amsterdam showed a significant reduction in the occurrence of ventricular fibrillation in the treated group [108]. However, there was no difference in mortality.

Accelerated idioventricular rhythm is also relatively common in acute myocardial infarction. It can be distinguished from other ventricular rhythms by its rate of 50 to 110 beats per minute. It is generally benign and usually does not warrant therapy.

Atrioventricular Block

First-degree atrioventricular (AV) block, defined as a PR interval of more than 0.20 seconds, occurs in about 10 percent of patients, is almost always intranodal, and is almost always benign. Mobitz I second-degree AV block (see section entitled Arrhythmias) occurs in 4 to 10 percent of patients, is more common in inferior infarction, is associated with a narrow QRS complex, is usually transient (up to 72 hours), is presumed to be due to ischemia of the AV node, rarely progresses to complete AV block, and generally does not require pacing. Mobitz II second-degree AV block is rare in acute myocardial infarction (less than 1 percent of all cases), is due to disease below the bundle of His, is usually associated with a wide QRS complex, often progresses to complete AV block, is more often associated with anterior infarction, and generally requires pacing.

When complete AV block occurs in patients with inferior infarction, it is due to relatively well-localized ischemia of the AV node; the escape rhythm is most often junctional, with a rate of 40 to 60 beats per minute, and generally well tolerated. Pacing is indicated only if the bradycardia produces hemodynamic compromise. This contrasts with the situation when complete AV block complicates anterior infarction. Then the block is due to interruption of each of the three major conduction fascicles below the bundle of His; this means that a large mass of myocardium has infarcted. The escape rhythm is idioventricular, slow (<40), and subject to asystole. The mortality from anterior infarction complicated by complete AV block is very high (70 to 80 percent) because of the severe left ventricular dysfunction. While it is not clear that pacing improves outcome in this disastrous circumstance, it is generally recommended.

Cardiogenic Shock

The other major complication of acute myocardial infarction is cardiogenic shock, occurring in 10 to 15 percent of hospitalized patients. Cardiogenic shock is defined as a cardiac output insufficient to meet the needs of vital organs despite an adequate intravascular volume and ventricular filling pressures. The hemodynamic findings in cardiogenic shock are hypotension (systolic pressure < 80 mmHg), left ventricular filling pressure ≥ 18 mmHg, and cardiac index < 1.8 liters/min/m². Signs of inadequate perfusion of vital organs are oliguria, cool, diaphoretic skin, and altered mental status. When due to left ventricular dysfunction, cardiogenic shock carries a mortality of over 90 percent and is the most common cause of death in hospitalized patients with acute myocardial infarction. When presented with a patient with signs of shock, it is essential for one to exclude hypovolemia, since this is easily treatable. Because physical signs such as jugular venous pressure and pulmonary rales and radiographic findings such as Kerley B lines correlate poorly with left ventricular filling pressure, there is no substitute for direct, invasive measurement of left and right ventricular filling pressures in patients with suspected cardiogenic shock. The Swan-Ganz catheter can generally be passed percutaneously at the bedside without fluoroscopic guidance through a vein (the internal jugular is the safest) and through the right side of the heart to the pulmonary artery to measure the pulmonary artery wedge pressure, a good approximation of left atrial pressure and left ventricular diastolic pressure. Another correctable cause of cardiogenic shock is right ventricular infarction, which often requires volume overexpansion to right atrial pressures of 10 mmHg or more to achieve an adequate cardiac output.

Ventricular septal rupture and papillary muscle rupture each occur in 1 to 3 percent of hospitalized patients with acute infarction and generally result in cardiogenic shock. They can be corrected surgically, albeit at a high operative mortality; however, the mortality rate is close to 100 percent when they are not corrected surgically.

When hypovolemia, right ventricular infarction, and rupture of the septum or papillary muscle have been excluded, acute left ventricular dysfunction involving 40 percent or more of the left ventricle is the likely cause of the shock. Temporary improvement in hemodynamic status can be obtained with a mechanical support device such as the intraaortic balloon; by inflating in diastole and deflating in systole, this balloon can reduce left ventricular afterload and increase coronary perfusion pressure. However, the intraaortic balloon alone will rarely result in long-term survival. In a few highly selected patients, coronary angiography followed by coronary artery bypass surgery has been attempted, with a 30 to 50 percent survival rate [124] compared to the 10 percent survival rate with medically treated cardiogenic shock.

Stable Angina Pectoris

PATHOPHYSIOLOGY

Stable angina pectoris occurs when the myocardial oxygen demand transiently exceeds the myocardial oxygen delivery, generally because of an increase in one of the determinants of myocardial oxygen demand (see Table 1-4). The pathologic substrate in the vast majority of patients is a significant coronary artery obstruction due to an atheromatous plaque. The clinical syndrome of angina pectoris also may occur in patients who have exertional coronary spasm in anatomically normal coronary arteries, in patients with severe aortic valve disease (see below), in patients with hypertrophic cardiomyopathy, and in a small subset of patients without identifiable heart disease in whom the pathophysiology is unknown. It is generally felt that coronary blood flow and myocardial oxygen delivery are either unchanged or fail to rise sufficiently to meet the increased demands. An external precipitating factor increasing myocardial oxygen demand, such as exercise producing tachycardia, is generally identifiable.

DEFINITION

The typical presenting findings are contained in the definition of angina pectoris: chest, arm, or jaw pain or discomfort of a visceral nature precipitated by exercise or emotion and relieved by rest or nitroglycerin. For a useful working definition it is difficult to improve on the first description of angina by William Heberden [15] over 200 years ago [79]:

They who are afflicted with it, are seized while they are walking (more especially if it be up hill, and soon after eating) with a painful and most disagreeable sensation in the breast, which seems as if it would extinguish life, if it were to increase or to continue; but the moment they stand still, all this uneasiness vanishes.

Note particularly that Heberden emphasized the precipitating factor (exercise), what relieves the pain (standing still), and the fear of death that this symptom often induces (angor animi). Unfortunately, Heberden did not recognize the source of the discomfort as being the heart; in fact, controversy persisted regarding the ischemic myocardium as the source of the pain for over 150 years until transient changes in the ST segment of the electrocardiogram were observed in association with angina [177].

DIAGNOSIS

History

In the vast majority of patients the diagnosis can be made from the history alone, providing that proper history-taking skills are combined with a knowledge of the wide variation in symptoms that can occur. Anginal discomfort is by its very nature vague, diffuse, and ill-defined—hence the "visceral nature." Many patients find it difficult to describe such vague symptoms; this is the setting in which directed "yes" or "no" questions can easily lead to an incorrect data base. The importance of initiating the history taking with nondirected questions cannot be overemphasized. Questions such as "Tell me about what brings you to see me today" or "Tell me about what troubles you" are examples of nondirected questions. Give the patient a chance to talk in a nondirected fashion initially, even if it turns out to be totally irrelevant.

The most important pieces of data to elicit from the history regarding angina are the factors that precipitate the attack and what the patient does to relieve it. Typical precipitating factors are exertion, emotion, cold exposure, and large meals. Isometric exertion, such as lifting over the head, is more likely to precipitate angina than isotonic exertion because of the marked increase in blood pressure that occurs with sustained isometric muscle contraction. Exertion performed after a large meal, during times of emotional distress, or on cold exposure is more likely to precipitate angina than exertion under other circumstances. Angina tends to occur more frequently and with less provocation in the first hours after awakening. Stable angina is relieved within minutes by stopping or alleviating the precipitating factor or by sublingual nitroglycerin. Although the pain of esophageal spasm also may be relieved by nitroglycerin, this is a rare phenomenon in the authors' experience.

It is useful to quantify the amount of exertion required to precipitate angina, although this will often be variable within the same patient. Nevertheless, a classification of angina based on the level of the precipitating activity is useful in assessing the effect of therapy, in classifying patients, and in following the progression of disease. The classification of the Canadian Cardiovascular Society [22] is particularly useful because it was designed specifically for angina:

Class 1. Angina with strenuous or rapid or prolonged exertion at work or recreation. Ordinary physical activity such as walking or climbing stairs does not cause angina.

Class 2. Angina results in slight limitation of ordinary activity. It may be produced by walking or climbing stairs rapidly, walking uphill, walking or stair climbing after meals, exercise in cold or during emotional distress, or exercise in the first hours after awakening.

Class 3. Angina results in marked limitation of ordinary physical activity. It may be produced by walking one to two blocks on the level or climbing one flight of stairs in normal conditions and at a normal pace.

Class 4. Angina results in the inability to carry on any physical activity without discomfort. Angina may be present at rest.

The nature and location of angina also provide useful diagnostic clues. Angina is diffuse and vague; many patients refuse to use the word *pain* in describing it and will correct the physician who uses this word in questioning the patient. It is often described as a pressure sensation, a weight on the chest, or a constricting feeling in the chest. A clenched fist is often used by the patient to illustrate the constricting nature of the discomfort. Angina is not pleuritic and usually does not change with change in posture, as does pericardial pain. Angina is not fleeting; brief, stabbing pains in the chest lasting only seconds are probably neuritic in origin. The duration of angina is generally 5 to 15 minutes. While angina may occur virtually anywhere between the diaphragm and the mandible, it is typically retrosternal with radiation into one or both arms or the neck. Occasionally, it may occur only in the arms, only in the mandible, or only in the interscapular region. Sometimes the pain may occur in the epigastrium and may be mistaken by the physician or patient for gastrointestinal pain such as esophagitis or peptic ulcer. Because of its visceral nature, it generally encompasses a substantial area and is deep-seated; pain that is localized to a small area on the chest wall (e.g., less than 1 to 2 inches in diameter) or is superficial is generally not angina. Pain localized by the patient with a single finger is not likely to be angina. Some of the historical characteristics of angina are summarized in Table 1-5.

Table 1–5. *Useful Diagnostic Clues of Angina Pectoris from the History*

Definitely angina	Possibly angina	Not angina
Precipitated by exertion or emotion	Pain at rest	Pleuritic or positional pain
Relieved within minutes by rest or nitroglycerin	Not promptly relieved by rest or nitroglycerin	Not relieved by nitroglycerin
Visceral or vague in nature	Dyspnea	Brief, fleeting, stabbing pain
Diffusely located	Well localized but to a substantial area	Pain sharply localized to a small area (<3 cm diameter)
Worse in cold, after meals, or upon arising	Not worse in cold, after meals, or upon arising	Pain reproduced by palpation over area of involvement

Physical Examination

The physical examination is the least useful of the diagnostic modalities, yet there are useful pieces of data to be obtained. Particular attention to the major controllable determinants of myocardial oxygen consumption, i.e., heart rate and systolic pressure, is essential. Other causes of angina or angina-like pain, such as aortic valve disease, idiopathic hypertrophic subaortic stenosis, or mitral valve prolapse can be excluded by careful examination for the appropriate murmurs or midsystolic click (see below). Reproduction of the pain by firm palpation of the chest or pressing the ribs suggests that the chest wall is the source of the pain. Costochondritis, a specific but uncommon inflammation of the costochondral junction, is best diagnosed by eliciting exquisite pain by light pressure over the costochondral junction about 1 to 2 inches lateral to the sternum. Symptoms and signs of congestive heart failure, such as elevated jugular venous pressure, pulmonary rales, or gallop rhythm, should be sought. Treatment of heart failure also may reduce angina by lowering left ventricular diastolic pressure, thereby improving the perfusion gradient for coronary flow (see Table 1-4).

Routine Laboratory Tests

The resting electrocardiogram is often normal in the absence of an attack of angina. During an attack, there may be either ST-segment depression or elevation. The chest roentgenogram is useful in providing additional assessment for cardiomegaly and congestive heart failure. Severe anemia (hematocrit below 30 percent) needs to be excluded as a precipitating factor. Risk factors for atherosclerosis need to be sought, such as hyperlipidemia and diabetes, but they provide little direct help in assessing the presenting complaints.

Exercise Testing

The exercise stress electrocardiogram is a valuable noninvasive tool for the evaluation of angina pectoris, as well as other presentations of coronary artery disease [19]. Unfortunately, the exercise test is often misused, because its value in relation to other information in the patient data base is not considered. The use of the exercise test should be considered in two principal categories: (1) to diagnose the presence or absence of coronary artery disease, and (2) to assess prognosis in patients with known coronary artery disease. In males with a history of typical angina pectoris (see Table 1-5), there is a 90 percent probability that significant atherosclerotic obstruction will be present in one or more coronary arteries when studied by angiography [171]. The exercise test adds virtually nothing to arriving at a correct diagnosis in this situation. Similarly, patients whose history, physical examination, and routine laboratory studies indicate a very low probability of coronary artery disease will not have a more accurate diagnosis with an exercise test. An example of such a patient would be a 30-year-old female with no coronary artery disease risk factors but who has chest pain that is not typical of angina pectoris.

The data base already indicates a very low probability of coronary artery disease. A negative exercise test does not significantly change this probability, while a positive test has a high likelihood of being a false-positive. A positive test is usually defined as one that shows ST-segment depression of 1 mm or more during or after exercise in one or more leads. Bayes' theorem has been useful in deciding which patients are most likely to have the benefit of greater assuredness of diagnosis with the addition of exercise test information to the existing data base [72]. We have already considered examples where the data base prior to the exercise test indicated a high or low probability of disease; the exercise test adds little here. However, for patients whose pretest probability of disease is in the intermediate range, the exercise test has considerable diagnostic value. An example of such a patient might be a middle-aged male with several risk factors for coronary artery disease who presents with atypical chest pain.

The diagnostic value of exercise testing should not be confused with its other uses: assessment of prognosis or severity of disease, assessment of therapy, and assessment of progression of disease. Many patients whose diagnosis is established from the history should have exercise testing to assess the severity of coronary artery disease to determine if further diagnostic testing, such as coronary arteriography, is indicated or if a revascularization procedure needs to be considered. The ST-segment criteria used for diagnostic purposes are not as useful for assessing severity or prognosis. The duration of exercise or maximum workload achieved and the maximum heart rate and systolic blood pressure achieved are the most powerful prognostic indicators [74]. The maximum duration of exercise attained by normal subjects decreases with increasing age, beginning at about age 20 years, and is also related to sex and activity status (active versus sedentary). The Bruce exercise test protocol was designed so that the duration of exercise is linearly related to oxygen consumption. A patient's maximal exercise capacity or oxygen consumption can be related to normal values using the functional aerobic impairment (FAI), which is the percent decrement from predicted maximal oxygen consumption for age, sex, and activity status. An FAI of 0 percent means that the patient achieved a normal duration or maximal workload for age, sex, and activity status; an FAI of 50 percent means that the patient was able to exercise to only 50 percent of the predicted normal maximal oxygen consumption, i.e., severe impairment. Systolic blood pressure measured in the arm by a cuff normally increases by 40 mmHg or more at maximal exercise in the absence of vasodilating or negative inotropic drugs. A systolic blood pressure increase of less than 20 mmHg, and particularly a drop in systolic blood pressure during exercise (exertional hypotension), is a powerful indicator of impaired prognosis. Marked ST-segment depression (≥ 2 mm) is also a useful prognostic indicator.

Radionuclide Imaging

Radionuclide imaging of the heart or its contained blood is also useful in establishing the diagnosis and assessing prognosis [8]. Two techniques are in common clinical use: (1) imaging of the myocardium with thallium-201, and (2) imaging of the cardiac chambers—particularly the ventricles—with technetium-99m tagged to red blood cells. Thallium is similar to potassium in that it is an intracellular ion; it is avidly taken up by viable myocardial cells. Areas of scar from old myocardial infarctions do not take up thallium; similarly, viable myocardium which becomes transiently ischemic in response to a stress, such as exercise, because it is supplied by a stenotic coronary artery, also does not take up thallium in a normal fashion. When the ischemic episode is over, the affected myocardial cells regain their ability to take up thallium. These pathophysiologic characteristics are used to advantage in rest-exercise thallium myocardial imaging. Thallium is injected at maximal exercise. Nonischemic, viable myocardial cells take up thallium and provide an image of the heart with gamma-camera imaging immediately after the exercise test. However, neither myocardial scar nor areas of myocardium with exercise-induced ischemia are able to take up thallium and can be seen as defects on the gamma-camera image. With recovery from exercise, blood flow through the stenotic coronary artery is sufficient to meet the demands of the myocardium at rest, and the ischemia is relieved. The myocardial cells previously unable to take up thallium begin to transfer thallium from the blood into the intracellular space. Thus, on a gamma-camera image taken several hours after the exercise test, the defects caused by the exercise-induced ischemia have filled in; any defects remaining are due to scar of myocardial infarction.

To summarize, the two principles of thallium myocardial imaging are (1) areas of myocardial infarction do not take up thallium under any physiologic condition, and (2) myocardium supplied by a significantly stenotic artery can be made relatively ischemic by the stress of exercise and will fail to take up thallium at that time, but it recovers and takes up thallium several hours later. Thallium myocardial imaging has proven more useful in assessing the relative amount of myocardium that can be made ischemic, and thereby, prognosis, than in establishing the presence or absence of coronary artery disease. When examined in the context of the history, resting electrocardiogram, and exercise electrocardiogram, thallium imaging increases the ability to establish the correct diagnosis only slightly [137].

Imaging of the blood pool in the cardiac chambers with technetium-99m tagged to red blood cells has proven to be a very useful noninvasive technique to assess ventricular function. This technique, sometimes known by the acronym MUGA (for multiple gated acquisition), divides the cardiac cycle into 20 to 30 short segments or gates. The image information from several hundred cardiac cycles is summed for each gate, reducing the noise due to statistical variation in photon release. The resultant series of frames can be played back as a single cardiac cycle in a continuous loop or analyzed mathematically in a number of ways. Among the most useful data are the ejection fraction and the assessment of segmental wall motion. The ejection fraction, the proportion of end-diastolic volume ejected with

each beat, is easily calculated (without having to make any assumptions about the geometry of the ventricle) by subtracting the end-systolic counts from the end-diastolic counts and dividing by the end-diastolic counts. The ejection fraction is one of the most useful measures of ventricular function. It is a powerful predictor of survival in patients with coronary artery disease [74]. Ejection fractions of less than 0.30 correlate well with clinical congestive heart failure in patients without significant valvular disease. In subjects with normal cardiac function, the ejection fraction increases with exercise as the peripheral vascular resistance drops, and the cardiac output rises. In a variety of heart diseases, but particularly coronary artery disease, the ejection fraction may decrease with exercise. Furthermore, new segmental wall-motion abnormalities will develop in areas of myocardium that become relatively ischemic with exercise.

CORONARY ARTERIOGRAPHY
The final diagnostic technique in common clinical usage in the evaluation of patients with angina is coronary arteriography. Despite major advances in sophisticated noninvasive diagnostic modalities, coronary angiography is the only technique that can reliably determine the location, number, and severity of coronary artery obstructions. It can be performed with relatively low morbidity and mortality (0.2 percent)—even in acutely ill patients, such as those with acute myocardial infarction. However, it is expensive, uses ionizing radiation, and carries a small risk. Generally accepted indications for coronary arteriography are listed in Table 1-6.

TREATMENT
Medical Therapy
Following diagnosis and assessment of prognosis, the first step in the therapy of stable angina should be to eliminate reversible risk factors and to treat associated medical conditions that aggravate angina. Cigarette smoking and hypertension are the two major controllable risk factors (see Table 1-1). Pipe and cigar smoking also have been

Table 1–6. Indications for Coronary Arteriography

I. Patients with angina:
   A. Patients with angina refractory to medical therapy who are being considered for coronary bypass surgery
   B. Patients with medically controllable angina, but who exhibit evidence of high risk for a coronary event on noninvasive testing:
      1. ST-segment depression ≥ 2 mm
      2. Drop or inadequate increase in blood pressure during exercise
      3. Angina or ST-segment depression at a very low workload
   C. Patients with angina or other evidence of coronary heart disease who have high-risk occupations (e.g., airline pilots)
   D. Patients with unstable angina who are otherwise acceptable candidates for coronary artery bypass surgery
II. Patients with acute myocardial infarction:
   A. Patients with acute anterior myocardial infarction seen within 4 hours of onset of symptoms, who may be candidates for streptokinase infusion
   B. Patients experiencing spontaneous angina early following an acute myocardial infarction
   C. Patients with angina or ST-segment depression on a low-level exercise test 7 to 10 days after an acute myocardial infarction
III. Other:
   A. Patients over the age of 40 undergoing cardiac catheterization in consideration of valve replacement
   B. Patients with incapacitating chest pain syndromes that cannot be diagnosed using noninvasive techniques

associated with increased risk of myocardial infarction or death, but to a lesser degree than cigarette smoking—probably because the dose of toxic pollutants is lower due to less inhalation of the smoke. Weight reduction in obese patients, control of hyperglycemia in diabetics, correction of arterial hypoxemia in patients with pulmonary disease, control of tachycardia (particularly that caused by beta agonists used as bronchodilators), and a program of moderate isotonic exercise such as walking are also appropriate first steps. Other medical conditions that aggravate angina, such as severe anemia, thyrotoxicosis, or congestive heart failure, should be diagnosed and treated.

Sublingual nitroglycerin has been the mainstay of treatment of angina ever since the descriptions of the effects of nitrates by Brunton [20] in 1867

and by Murrell [126] in 1879. Nitroglycerin also can be used prophylactically prior to performing exercise likely to precipitate angina, such as climbing stairs. If complete relief is not attained with a single tablet, a second may be used in 5 to 10 minutes. Ischemic myocardial pain not responding to three nitroglycerin tablets within 15 to 20 minutes generally requires medical attention. Nitroglycerin is relatively unstable and will lose its potency over several months—particularly if kept at room temperature. Patients can often tell when this occurs, because the tablets no longer produce a stinging sensation under the tongue or give a feeling of fullness in the head. Most patients will have headaches when initially taking any form of nitrate; however, tolerance usually develops to this side effect, but not usually to the angina-relieving properties. The mechanism of action of nitroglycerin is still the subject of some debate. It probably both reduces myocardial oxygen demand through reducing left ventricular wall stress by causing arterial and venous dilation and increases myocardial oxygen delivery by increasing coronary blood flow to ischemic myocardium through dilatation of coronary stenoses (Table 1-7).

The duration of action of sublingual nitroglycerin is brief—usually 15 to 30 minutes; therefore, it is not practical as a long-term prophylactic drug. A number of long-acting nitrate preparations with a mechanism of action similar to sublingual nitroglycerin are available. Among the most commonly used are the oral organic nitrate isosorbide dinitrate and the various types of topical nitrates. Isosorbide can be begun at a dose of 10 mg four times daily and increased every several days in 10-mg increments to 40 mg of the sustained-release form four times daily. Nitroglycerin ointment is probably the most effective nonparenteral form of nitroglycerin for patients with severe angina. When applied to the skin, it is slowly absorbed over a period of several hours. It comes in tubes that supply a dose of 15 mg per inch of paste as it is squeezed out of the tube. Doses of 7.5 mg (0.5 inch) to 30 mg (2 inches) applied to several square inches of nonhairy skin

Table 1-7. *Mechanism of Action of Antianginal Drugs*

Determinant of oxygen supply-demand balance	Antianginal drug		
	Nitrates	Beta blocker	Calcium-channel blocker
Myocardial oxygen demand:			
Heart rate	Increase moderately	Decrease moderately	Variable, but usually little change
Contractility	No change	Decrease moderately	Variable degree of decrease
Left ventricular wall stress	Decrease moderately	No change unless induced by congestive heart failure	Variable degree of decrease
Myocardial oxygen delivery:			
Aortic diastolic pressure	Decrease moderately	Decrease slightly	Decrease moderately
Left ventricular diastolic pressure	Decrease moderately	No change unless induced by congestive heart failure	Variable, but usually no change
Coronary vascular resistance	Decrease moderately	No change or increase slightly	Decrease moderately
Arterial saturation	Decrease slightly	No change	No change

and covered with a plastic film four times per day are generally quite effective in relieving angina refractory to oral nitrates. It is particularly useful when applied just before sleep for patients having frequent nocturnal angina. Because nitroglycerin paste often soils underclothes, several pharmaceutical firms have developed sustained-release patches with the nitroglycerin impregnated in a polymer. Although these do result in sustained low blood levels, tolerance appears to develop very rapidly; serious questions as to the efficacy of nitroglycerin patches are currently under investigation.

Beta-adrenergic blocking drugs are very effective in reducing the frequency and severity of anginal attacks and improving exercise tolerance in patients with stable exertional angina. The primary mechanism of action is reduction in myocardial oxygen demand through reducing resting and exercise heart rate and, to a lesser extent, systolic pressure (see Table 1-7). The most common side effects are fatigue, mental depression, and exacerbation of congestive heart failure in patients with severe left ventricular dysfunction or a history of heart failure. Nonselective beta-adrenergic blocking drugs are relatively contraindicated in patients with severe obstructive airway disease

because they may increase bronchoconstriction through blocking of the beta$_2$-adrenergic bronchodilating receptors in the lungs. Selective beta$_1$-adrenergic blocking drugs have been developed (e.g., metoprolol) to minimize the bronchoconstriction side effect; however, at the higher doses often required for control of angina (150 to 200 mg per day) they lose their selectivity and can cause bronchospasm. These drugs are also relatively contraindicated in insulin-dependent diabetics because they block the sympathetic response to hypoglycemia, thereby prolonging the episode and impairing its recognition.

More recently, a group of drugs that causes vascular smooth muscle to relax by blocking the calcium channel in the cell membrane has been introduced in the United States. Although the mechanism of action at the cellular or organ level is similar to that of the nitrates (see Table 1-7), the biochemical site of action is different; therefore, these agents may be synergistic with nitrates in the treatment of angina. In contrast to the nitrates, these agents are also myocardial depressants, verapamil having a more potent negative inotropic effect than diltiazem, which in turn is more potent than nifedipine. Verapamil should be used very cautiously or not at all in patients with severe left ventricular dysfunction or congestive heart failure. Nifedipine and diltiazem rarely exacerbate congestive heart failure. Both verapamil and diltiazem slow atrioventricular conduction and should not be used in patients with second- or third-degree atrioventricular block. Nifedipine commonly causes minor degrees of ankle edema, which can usually be controlled with a diuretic. Because these are potent vasodilators, headache and orthostatic hypotension are common side effects—particularly when these agents are used in combination with large doses of nitrates.

The history is useful in the choice of the first antianginal agent to initiate. In patients whose angina is primarily exertional or provoked by other stresses that increase myocardial oxygen demand, the beta-adrenergic blocking agents are highly effective, as are the nitrates and calcium-channel blocking drugs. In patients with angina at rest, where the mechanism may be a spontaneous reduction in coronary blood flow due to vasospasm, nitrates or calcium-channel blocking drugs are preferable, because of their antispasmodic, vasodilating properties. Theoretically, beta-adrenergic blocking drugs could exacerbate coronary spasm by leaving the alpha-adrenergic vasoconstrictor activity unopposed. These three classes of antianginal drugs are useful in combination in patients with severe angina. Medical therapy is often not considered to have been maximal until the patient is receiving a drug from all three classes in therapeutic doses (unless specifically contraindicated).

Surgical Therapy

A variety of surgical procedures have been tried for relief of severe angina since the 1930s. However, none had been demonstrated to be more effective than a placebo or sham operation [27] until the aortocoronary bypass operation. With the development of this procedure by Favalaro [47] in 1967, a truly effective way of improving myocardial blood flow became available at an acceptable operative risk. This operation is based on the angiographic observation that in the earlier phases of symptomatic coronary artery disease, the atherosclerotic obstructions are in the proximal portions of the coronary arteries, leaving the distal portions of the vessels relatively free of disease. Direct surgical attack on the obstructive lesions was unsuccessful because of the small size of the arteries. However, the construction of a bypass conduit of saphenous vein from the ascending aorta to the coronary artery distal to the obstruction has been shown in randomized trials to be more effective than medical therapy in relieving symptoms and improving exercise tolerance. The operation, which requires the use of cardiopulmonary bypass to allow the delicate anastomoses to be made on the arrested heart, can now be performed at an operative mortality rate of 2 to 3 percent. The probability of early graft patency is high (90 percent), as is the relief of symptoms (80 percent). However, as the atherosclerotic process progresses in the native coronary arteries and develops in the saphenous veins, symptoms return at a rate of 3 to 4 percent of operated patients each year after the operation. By the end of 5 years after surgery, about 30 percent of patients will have angina. The internal thoracic artery is now frequently used as the bypass conduit to coronary arteries on the anterior surface of the heart because it does not appear to develop atherosclerotic obstruction, resulting in better late patency rates than venous conduits.

While the beneficial symptomatic results of coronary bypass surgery in patients who are severely symptomatic preoperatively are quite clear, the effect of surgery on survival has been more controversial. With the publication of three large randomized trials comparing survival of surgically and medically treated patients [164,46,26], it is now accepted that survival is improved with surgical therapy in patients with significant obstruction of the left main coronary artery [164] and in patients with three-vessel coronary artery disease and left ventricular dysfunction [26]. No study has shown improved survival with surgical therapy in patients with single-vessel disease. The European randomized trial showed substantially improved survival rates in symptomatic patients with three-vessel disease and normal left ventricular function [46]. However, the Coronary Artery Surgery Study (CASS) conducted in the United States and Canada showed no survival benefit for minimally symptomatic patients with three-vessel disease and normal left ventricular function [26]. While neither the VA Cooperative Study nor the Coronary Artery Surgery Study showed improved survival in patients with two-vessel disease, some of the data from the European study suggest that if one of the two involved vessels is the left anterior descending coronary artery, survival might be prolonged with surgical therapy [46]. These and other data relating to the effects of coronary artery bypass surgery on survival have been reviewed in greater detail by one of the authors [73].

The indications for coronary bypass surgery may be viewed in two categories: relief of symptoms and prolongation of life (Table 1-8). Patients who are significantly limited by angina despite adequate medical therapy, who have one or more coronary arteries that could be bypassed, and whose left ventricular function and general medical condition make the risk of surgery acceptable should be offered surgery for relief of symptoms. Patients who have a 50 percent or greater stenosis of the left main coronary artery, or three-vessel disease with left ventricular dysfunction (ejection fraction < 0.50), or possibly three-vessel disease and normal left ventricular function, or two-vessel disease involving the left anterior descending should be offered bypass surgery for prolongation of survival.

In the last several years percutaneous transluminal coronary angioplasty (PTCA) has been introduced as an alternative to coronary bypass surgery in selected patients. This is a procedure that can be performed in the cardiac catheterization laboratory under local anesthetic. A small balloon is inflated within the coronary stenosis to dilate the obstruction. In skilled hands, significant reduction of the coronary obstruction can be obtained in about 90 percent of attempts. However, in up to 5 percent of attempts emergency surgery is required because the attempted angioplasty oc-

Table 1–8. Indications for Coronary Bypass Surgery

I. Generally accepted indications:
   A. Relief of symptoms: Patients meeting all the following criteria:
      1. Unacceptable angina despite adequate medical therapy
      2. One or more major coronary vessels obstructed and bypassable
      3. Age, general condition, and left ventricular function make risk of surgery reasonable
   B. Prolongation of survival:
      1. Patients with left main coronary obstruction ≥ 50 percent
      2. Patients with three-vessel disease and left ventricular dysfunction
II. Possible indications:
   A. Patients with three-vessel disease and normal left ventricular function (for prolongation of survival)
   B. Patients with two-vessel disease, one of which is the anterior descending coronary artery (for prolongation of survival)
   C. Patients requiring valve replacement, who also have coronary artery disease
   D. Patients in cardiogenic shock due to acute myocardial infarction

cluded the obstructed vessel. The most disturbing aspect of coronary angioplasty is that the stenosis recurs at the dilated site in about a third of patients within 6 months; however, this recurrent stenosis is often amenable to a second angioplasty. In patients with single-vessel disease, coronary angioplasty is often the procedure of choice; also, it is being increasingly applied to patients with multivessel disease and in acute myocardial infarction following reperfusion with a thrombolytic agent. The efficacy of angioplasty in these last two groups of patients is still the subject of study.

Unstable Angina

DEFINITION

Unstable angina is angina which occurs with little or no provocation, such as angina occurring at rest or angina awakening a patient from sleep. Previously, patients with new-onset angina and patients with a crescendo pattern to their exertional angina were included in the unstable angina group. However, these latter two subgroups probably have a different pathophysiology and definitely a different prognosis.

PATHOPHYSIOLOGY
Patients with unstable angina usually have a very severe stenosis(es) (≥90 percent) in one or more major coronary arteries, but the vessel(s) is(are) still patent. The angina occurs without any change in the determinants of myocardial oxygen demand; therefore, it must be the result of a reduction in coronary blood flow due to an increase in coronary vascular resistance (see Table 1-4). The increase in resistance occurs primarily at the severe atherosclerotic stenosis either as a result of partial occlusion by a platelet thrombus, an increase in vasomotor tone producing a small reduction in lumen area which can effect a large increase in resistance, or a combination of both these mechanisms. Rarely, an unstable angina pattern may occur in patients with arteriographically normal coronary arteries; in these patients, coronary spasm must be the primary mechanism.

DIAGNOSIS
History
As with stable angina, the history provides most of the information required for the diagnosis of unstable angina. The pain is similar to that of stable exertional angina; within the same patient, the pain pattern is usually the same as that he or she experiences with exercise. The major difference from stable angina is that the discomfort comes on at rest, with little or no change in heart rate or blood pressure preceding the onset. The pain may be more severe than that of the stable exertional angina and may last 30 minutes or longer. Unstable angina is often poorly responsive or unresponsive to the usual doses of sublingual nitroglycerin. In patients without previous objective evidence of coronary heart disease, such as prior myocardial infarction or typical exertional angina, the presenting complaint of chest pain at rest may be difficult to distinguish from noncardiac pain on the basis of history alone.

Physical Examination
The physical examination is often unrevealing, just as in stable angina. Nevertheless, it is necessary to look for evidence of congestive heart failure, aortic valve disease, uncontrolled hypertension, tachycardia, fever, severe anemia, marked anxiety, and other signs that might indicate impaired oxygen delivery to the heart or increased myocardial oxygen demand.

Electrocardiogram
Most patients with unstable angina will have transient ST-segment depression or elevation or T-wave inversion with the anginal episode. However, the absence of electrocardiographic changes with the pain does not exclude the diagnosis of unstable angina.

Laboratory Studies
Frequently, unstable angina can be differentiated from a non-Q-wave infarction only by the absence of serum enzyme rises. The pain pattern and electrocardiographic changes alone do not distinguish unstable angina from a non-Q-wave infarction. Thallium myocardial imaging during an episode of unstable angina will reveal a perfusion deficit that returns to normal following relief of pain. This observation forms the basis for understanding the pathophysiology (i.e., transient reduction in coronary blood flow). However, thallium imaging is generally not required to establish the diagnosis. Exercise testing is generally contraindicated in patients while they are unstable. In patients for whom immediate coronary arteriography is not appropriate, exercise testing may be performed after a period of stability of several weeks.

TREATMENT
Medical Therapy
Patients with unstable angina should be admitted to the hospital and placed at bed rest in a quiet, anxiety-free environment. Continuous monitoring of the electrocardiogram for arrhythmia and ST-segment shifts is generally advisable. If arterial

hypoxemia is present, oxygen should be administered. Factors that increase myocardial oxygen demand or coronary artery resistance should be vigorously treated; most important of these are hypertension and cigarette smoking. Nitrates are the primary mode of medical therapy. If oral or topical nitrates are unsuccessful in providing prompt pain relief within a short time, nitroglycerin should be given intravenously starting at 10 μg per minute, increasing by 10 μg per minute every 10 minutes until a minimum dose of 50 μg per minute or pain relief is achieved. If the pain persists or recurs, nitroglycerin may be titrated upward to a maximal dose of 300 μg per minute providing that the systolic arterial blood pressure does not fall below a level of approximately 100 mmHg. Calcium-channel blocking drugs are useful adjuncts to nitroglycerin therapy. The use of beta-adrenergic blocking agents in unstable angina is more controversial because of the theoretical possibility of increasing coronary vascular resistance by withdrawing the beta$_1$ vasodilator effect, leaving alpha-adrenergic vasoconstrictor tone unopposed. However, there is little or no evidence to document a deleterious effect of these drugs in unstable angina aside from the usual side effects discussed for stable angina. If the patient was on a beta-adrenergic blocking drug at the time of admission, it should be continued unless congestive heart failure, marked bradycardia (rate less than 50 beats per minute), or bronchospasm is present. Sudden withdrawal of beta-adrenergic blocking drugs has been associated with a rebound phenomenon, resulting in more severe angina or myocardial infarction.

Two recent randomized trials conducted in patients with unstable angina have shown a marked beneficial effect of aspirin in the prevention of myocardial infarction and death over the subsequent several months [107,21]. However, many surgeons feel that aspirin increases the risk of bleeding at the time of coronary bypass surgery. If the patient appears to be a poor candidate for coronary bypass surgery (e.g., advanced age, poor general medical condition, or previous coronary bypass surgery) and has no contraindication to its use, aspirin should be instituted at a dose of 325 mg per day. If the patient appears to be a potential candidate for surgical revascularization, coronary arteriography might be performed first and a decision regarding medical versus surgical therapy then made on the basis of coronary anatomy and clinical status before deciding to initiate aspirin.

Surgical Therapy
Revascularization by coronary bypass surgery or percutaneous transluminal angioplasty is the therapy of choice for patients whose angina cannot be controlled by oral and/or topical antianginal agents and for those in whom surgery prolongs life (e.g., left main coronary artery stenosis or three-vessel disease with left ventricular dysfunction; see Table 1-7). The intraaortic balloon is highly effective in temporarily controlling pain and probably preventing infarction in those patients whose pain cannot be controlled by intravenous nitroglycerin. However, this mechanical device is only a temporizing therapy until coronary arteriography and coronary bypass surgery or angioplasty can be accomplished. The mechanism of myocardial protection by the intraaortic balloon is through augmentation of diastolic aortic pressure, which increases coronary blood flow, and through reduction of systolic pressure, which reduces myocardial oxygen demand.

Sudden Cardiac Death
EPIDEMIOLOGY
Sudden cardiac death can be defined as unexpected death occurring without symptoms or preceded by symptoms of no more than 1 hour's duration. The incidence of sudden cardiac death in the United States is approximately 400,000 per year—80 percent of which are due to coronary artery disease. Conversely, of all deaths due to coronary artery disease, one-half to two-thirds are sudden. There is a strong male predominance, with an average age of approximately 60 years. In three-fourths of patients dying suddenly, some

clinical manifestation of heart disease has been present prior to demise—most commonly angina or previous myocardial infarction. However, in 20 to 25 percent of cases, sudden death is the first manifestation of heart disease. Because atherosclerotic coronary artery disease is the most common cause of sudden cardiac death, the risk factors for coronary heart disease are also associated with sudden death: smoking, hypertension, and hyperlipidemia. In patients with heart disease, frequent and/or complex ventricular premature beats, such as nonsustained ventricular tachycardia, have been demonstrated to be associated with an increased risk for sudden death [141]. If there is associated ventricular dysfunction, the risk of sudden death becomes very substantial—as much as 40 percent in a 2-year period. However, asymptomatic complex ventricular premature beats appear to carry very little risk of sudden death in patients without demonstrable heart disease.

PATHOPHYSIOLOGY

Nearly all patients in whom an electrocardiogram has been recorded during sudden cardiac death have had ventricular fibrillation, usually triggered by premature ventricular beats and/or ventricular tachycardia. Studies in patients resuscitated from out-of-hospital sudden cardiac death in Seattle have shown that only about a third have evidence of myocardial necrosis; in other words, sudden death is the result of pure electrical instability in about two-thirds of instances [28]. It is in this latter group of patients that preventive measures would offer the most hope. The mechanism by which a patient with coronary heart disease progresses from his or her stable, nonacutely ill state to ventricular fibrillation and sudden death is incompletely understood. The mechanism(s) and prevention of sudden death constitute an area of intense investigation at this time. There has been considerable speculation that the autonomic nervous system may play a major role in triggering sudden death.

A large variety of cardiovascular diseases make up the underlying pathologic substrate in the 20 percent of patients in whom atherosclerotic coronary artery disease does not seem to be causative. These include aortic stenosis, hypertrophic cardiomyopathy (both the obstructive and nonobstructive forms), dilated cardiomyopathy, congenital anomalies of the coronary arteries, other forms of complex congenital heart disease, primary pulmonary hypertension, Marfan's syndrome, and dissecting hematoma of the aorta. It is rare that a careful autopsy will not reveal a significant cardiovascular lesion.

TREATMENT

Treatment should be considered in two broad areas: (1) resuscitation from the acute event, and (2) prevention of recurrent ventricular fibrillation. Most episodes occur outside of the hospital, well away from any medical care facility. It has been known for many years that primary ventricular fibrillation (i.e., that occurring as the result of electrical instability and not cardiogenic shock) in the intensive care unit could be easily treated by prompt defibrillation; patients experiencing such an event often had a relatively good prognosis upon leaving the hospital. Beginning in the early 1970s, the intensive care unit experience was transferred to the community setting by the development of "mobile coronary care units." The system developed in Seattle by Cobb et al. has been extraordinarily successful and has served as a model for many other communities [28,6]. They reasoned that one or several mobile coronary care units (as had been tried in other communities) could not arrive at the scene of sudden death within 4 minutes of onset (the time at which irreversible cerebral damage begins) in a sufficient number of patients to be cost-effective. Instead, they developed a tiered response system. The first tier consists of the general public trained in cardiopulmonary resuscitation. The second tier consists of firefighters—most of whom have received an intermediate level of training and give cardiopulmonary resuscitation but no drugs or defibrillation. The final tier is the mobile coronary care unit manned by highly trained and skilled paramedics who are capable of tracheal intubation, drug administration under physician orders via radio, and defibrillation. The first tier, the general public trained in cardiopulmonary resuscitation, has proven to be a particularly vital link in the success of this system. Over half the adult population in Seattle has received training in cardiopulmonary resuscitation—generally through the fire department. The long-term survival rate for patients with out-of-hospital ventricular fibrillation is almost twice as high for victims in whom resuscitation is initiated by a bystander than if it was initiated by the firefighters, because of the shorter response time. Presently, about 30 percent of victims of out-of-hospital ventricular fibrillation in Seattle survive to hospital discharge—most in their previous state of health. Permanent cerebral dysfunction from anoxia has been surprisingly uncommon.

Even with the highly successful, innovative tiered emergency response system in Seattle (now being copied in many communities), over two-thirds of patients experiencing out-of-hospital ventricular fibrillation will not be long-term survivors. Thus prevention is vital. Unfortunately, we neither know how to sensitively and specifically identify patients at risk, nor do we know how to prevent these episodes of lethal electrical instability. Many of the treatment modalities discussed above and shown to prolong survival in patients with angina or following a myocardial infarction do so by reducing the incidence of sudden death. Beta-adrenergic blocking agents administered for several years following acute myocardial infarction reduce the chances of sudden death and recurrent infarction. Coronary bypass surgery prolongs survival in certain subsets of patients with severe coronary artery disease by preventing sudden death. However, these studies represent only a very small proportion of the population at risk for sudden death. Since two-thirds of patients with sudden cardiac death appear to have "pure" electrical instability (often occurring in the setting of asymptomatic, frequent, or complex ventricular premature beats), the role of antiarrhythmic agents needs to be considered. There are no controlled clinical trials showing pro-

longed survival with treatment with an antiarrhythmic agent; however, this is an area of intense interest at this time.

Other Myocardial Ischemic Syndromes
VARIANT ANGINA
Clinical Description
Variant angina, or Prinzmetal's angina, was described by Prinzmetal as patients with angina at rest accompanied by ST-segment elevation in the absence of exertional angina. He postulated that it might be due to spasm of the proximal coronary arteries. Unfortunately, subsequent investigation by coronary arteriography of patients fitting this definition has shown findings varying from normal coronary arteries to severe atherosclerotic coronary artery obstruction in multiple vessels. Thus it is not a single disease entity. Patients with arteriographically normal coronary arteries have pure spasm, while patients with severe atherosclerotic obstruction can have marked changes in coronary resistance with modest changes in diameter due to physiologic vasomotion. This latter group overlaps with unstable angina. Nevertheless, there appears to be a small group of patients who have predominantly unprovoked rest angina with dramatic ST-segment changes and sometimes malignant ventricular arrhythmias in whom spasm of the coronary arteries is the primary pathophysiologic mechanism. Many of these patients are premenopausal females who smoke cigarettes. Anginal attacks are most frequent in the morning hours. There is marked variability over time in the disease activity. The mechanism of the spasm is unknown, although in about a quarter of patients there is evidence of a more generalized vasospastic syndrome, such as Raynaud's phenomenon or migraine headaches.

Diagnosis
The diagnosis is best made by demonstrating the marked ST-segment shifts during episodes of unprovoked angina in a patient who otherwise has normal exercise tolerance. Coronary arteriography during an anginal episode will usually

show spasm in the coronary artery predicted by the electrocardiogram. However, since anginal episodes occur unpredictably, such an episode is unlikely to occur spontaneously during coronary arteriography. Ergonovine maleate, an ergot alkaloid, has been used to provoke coronary artery spasm during coronary arteriography; there seems to be a good relationship between provokable spasm with ergonovine and the clinical syndrome. In patients with significant atherosclerotic obstruction of one or more coronary arteries, ergonovine has produced total occlusion and even acute myocardial infarction. For this reason, ergonovine testing is now done only in the cardiac catheterization laboratory after the coronary arteries have been demonstrated to be free of severe obstructions and where there is an opportunity to give intracoronary nitroglycerin if severe obstruction ensues.

Treatment

Both nitrates and calcium-channel blocking drugs are generally effective in these patients either separately or in combination. Of course, cessation of smoking should be mandatory. The prognosis in patients with arteriographically normal coronary arteries is good, although acute myocardial infarction may occur rarely.

SILENT MYOCARDIAL ISCHEMIA

Silent myocardial ischemia is the occurrence of unprovoked ST-segment shifts consistent with myocardial ischemia but in the absence of pain or other discomfort. It is most commonly detected by ambulatory electrocardiographic monitoring. Many patients with more typical exertional angina also will have episodes of silent myocardial ischemia; some patients will have no symptoms whatever. Most patients with silent ischemia probably have significant atherosclerotic coronary artery disease. It is unknown whether this represents relatively small areas of ischemia that do not reach the pain threshold or whether these patients have a defect in visceral pain perception. Conflicting evidence supports both mechanisms. The clinical and prognostic significance of silent myocardial ischemia is unknown at this time. Since, by definition, there are no symptoms, the only reason for treatment would be to prevent myocardial infarction or death. The relation of silent ischemia to sudden death or subsequent myocardial infarction is unknown; therefore, treatment of silent ischemia alone at this time is premature.

Valvular Heart Disease

Normal Physiology

The cardiac valves function to direct the blood in a forward direction only. They open and close in response to pressure differences between the two cardiac chambers they separate. When open with blood flowing across them, basic physical principles require that the pressure in the upstream chamber be higher than that in the downstream chamber; however, this pressure difference is of sufficiently small magnitude to not be readily measurable with the standard pressure measuring and recording techniques used in the cardiac catheterization laboratory. Thus, when a pressure gradient is reported across a cardiac valve, some degree of functional stenosis is present.

The normal valve leaflets have such small mass that there is very little inertia to closing. Thus they close very rapidly with no detectable leak using angiographic techniques. The same is not true of mechanical prosthetic valves where the poppet has appreciable mass, and inertia to closing may result in detectable leak (regurgitation) early in the closing cycle. Doppler ultrasound appears to be very sensitive in the detection of regurgitation, with regurgitant signals being reported in substantial proportions of apparently normal native valves—particularly the tricuspid valve.

The atrioventricular valves (mitral and tricuspid) are much more complex in their anatomy and normal physiology than the semilunar valves (pulmonic and aortic). The atrioventricular valve apparatus must be thought of as not only the leaflets, but also all the supporting structures: the valve ring to which the leaflets are attached, the chordae tendineae, the papillary muscles, and the ventricular wall to which the papillary muscles are attached. An abnormality in structure or function of any one of these components can result in abnormal valve function. In contrast, abnormal function of the semilunar valves must be the result of an abnormality in either the valve cusps or the supporting valve ring (the base of the aorta or pulmonary artery).

Pathophysiology

Abnormal valve function can be expressed in only three ways: obstruction, leak, or a combination of the two. Obstruction is always reflected as a measurable pressure gradient across the valve; the measurement of this pressure gradient is one way of assessing the severity of the obstruction. However, the gradient across a valve is dependent on the flow across the valve. Clinical conditions are encountered in aortic stenosis where the flow across the valve is markedly reduced as a result of myocardial failure from severe long-standing stenosis, yet, because of the very low flow, the gradient is relatively small. Similarly, conditions of high flow, such as occurs with exercise or fever, may produce a high gradient across a mildly obstructed valve. Bernoulli first described the relation between flow and pressure gradient across a stenotic orifice. Gorlin and Gorlin [66] applied this concept to valvular heart disease and showed that the valve orifice area (A) could be estimated as the ratio between flow across the valve (F) and the square root of the pressure gradient ($grad$) times a constant (k):

$$A = \frac{F}{(k\sqrt{grad})}$$

This formula is used in the cardiac catheterization laboratory to estimate the area of stenotic valves.

Normal atrioventricular valves have an orifice area of approximately 4 to 5 cm², while normal semilunar valves have an orifice area of about 3 cm². Significant symptoms and functional disability begin when the estimated orifice area falls to about a third of normal.

When a cardiac valve leaks, the regurgitating blood either is ejected into the upstream chamber in ventricular systole (atrioventricular valves) or falls back into the ejecting ventricle in diastole (semilunar valves). In an attempt to maintain normal forward flow to the tissues, the ventricle increases its stroke volume by increasing its end-diastolic volume through the Starling mechanism. Initially, the ejection fraction (the fraction of end-diastolic volume ejected on each beat) is maintained at its normal value of two-thirds of the end-diastolic volume. As myocardial failure develops, the end-systolic volume rises and the ejection fraction falls. The pathophysiologic response to significant valvular regurgitation is ventricular dilatation; the ventricular end-diastolic volume is a measure of both the severity of regurgitation and myocardial function, while the end-systolic volume and ejection fraction reflect the integrity of myocardial function.

Techniques have been developed for estimating ventricular volumes from contrast cineangiograms, radionuclide ventriculograms, and two-dimensional echocardiograms. The difference between the end-diastolic volume and the end-systolic volume is the total ventricular stroke volume, which is the sum of both the net forward flow and the regurgitant flow. The Fick and indicator dilution techniques for measuring cardiac output measure only net forward flow. The difference between the total ventricular output and the net forward output is an estimate of the regurgitant volume. Table 1-9 is an illustration of the use of this technique to estimate regurgitant volume and myocardial function in a patient with severe regurgitation and preserved ventricular function (A) and another patient with moderate regurgitation and myocardial failure (B). The examples in this table illustrate the value of ventricular volume measurements in estimating both the severity of regurgitation and myocardial function [42].

Table 1–9. *Illustrations of the Use of Ventricular Volumes to Evaluate the Severity of Regurgitation and Myocardial Function.*

	A. Severe regurgitation and normal myocardial function	B. Moderate regurgitation and myocardial failure
End-diastolic volume	300 ml	300 ml
End-systolic volume	− 100 ml	− 200 ml
Total stroke volume	200 ml	100 ml
Heart rate	× 80/min	× 80/min
Total ventricular output	16,000 ml/min	8,000 ml/min
Net forward output (Fick)	− 5,000 ml/min	− 4,000 ml/min
Regurgitant flow	11,000 ml/min	4,000 ml/min
Ejection fraction	0.67	0.33

An Approach to the Patient with Valvular Disease

Cardiac valve lesions may be divided into acute and chronic. Acute lesions, such as occur with endocarditis, may result in significant valve regurgitation within a matter of days or weeks, leaving little time for the heart to adapt to the sudden volume overload. Symptoms of congestive heart failure may be seen with only moderate regurgitation.

Chronic heart valve dysfunction frequently has a very long asymptomatic period, lasting up to several decades or more. The heart can successfully adapt to remarkable degrees of valve dysfunction—particularly aortic regurgitation. Resting cardiac output is maintained, and few or no symptoms are present at rest. However, even moderate degrees of chronic valve dysfunction can result in symptoms of excessive dyspnea or fatigue that limit maximal exercise performance.

If significant pressure overload from semilunar valve stenosis or volume overload from regurgitation of any valve persists for a sufficiently long period, the affected ventricle will ultimately fail. Such failure is manifested by a rising end-diastolic pressure and a falling ejection fraction. Ventricular failure is often irreversible—particularly when it is the result of regurgitant lesions.

Surgical repair or replacement of the dysfunctional valve relieves resting symptoms, improves exercise tolerance, and prevents the development of further ventricular dysfunction. Thus an algorithm defining the timing of surgical intervention must make use of symptoms, exercise tolerance, and ventricular performance. Figure 1-3 illustrates an algorithm for the evaluation of patients with valvular heart disease in consideration of valve repair or replacement. The first step is to evaluate symptoms and degree of functional disability from the patient history. The New York Heart Association Functional Classification is a useful way to classify the degree of disability due to valvular heart disease based on the patient's history:

Class I: Cardiac abnormality, but no symptoms at any level of exercise

Class II: Symptoms on more than ordinary activity, such as running, climbing stairs rapidly, or heavy lifting

Class III: Symptoms on activities of daily living, such as walking or performing routine household chores

Class IV: Symptoms at rest

In patients with moderate or severe symptoms (class III or IV), the primary task is to ascertain whether the symptoms are the result of valvular heart disease or other organ system dysfunction. This is accomplished by noninvasive evaluation of valve dysfunction and careful examination of the patient for other organ system dysfunction. Present noninvasive techniques making use of physical examination, electrocardiogram, chest film, and particularly cardiac ultrasound (both echocardiography and Doppler) are sufficiently precise

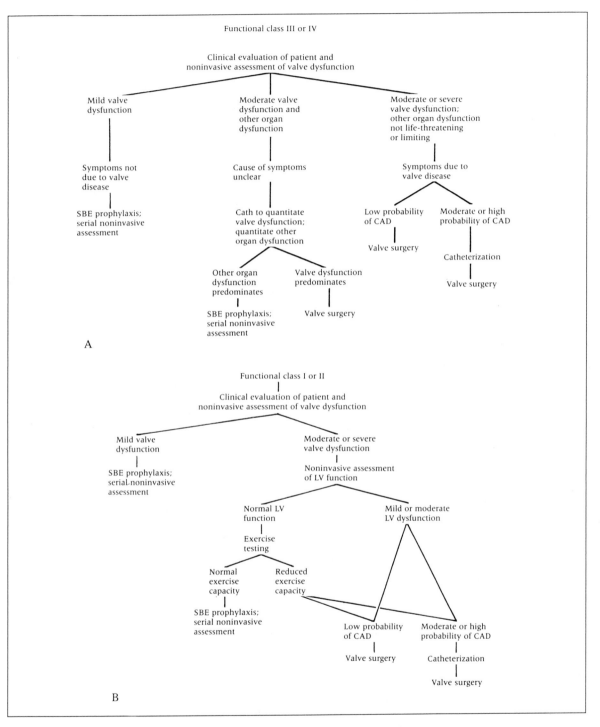

Figure 1–3. Decision trees for the evaluation of patients with valvular heart disease leading to consideration of valve replacement or other mechanical intervention. (A) Patients with significant symptoms in New York Heart Association functional class III or IV. (B) Patients with few or no symptoms in functional class I or II. See text for discussion. (CAD, coronary artery disease; SBE, subacute bacterial endocarditis; LV, left ventricular.)

to allow accurate assessment of the severity of valve dysfunction in most cases. Patients who have unequivocal findings of severe valve dysfunction of a single valve on noninvasive examination and who are at low risk for concomitant coronary artery disease may undergo valve repair or replacement without cardiac catheterization. Patients for whom the noninvasive findings are ambiguous, who have evidence of multivalve disease, or who are likely to have coronary artery disease should undergo cardiac catheterization. Patients who have both significant valvular dysfunction and other organ system dysfunction (e.g., obstructive airway disease) require accurate quantitative assessment of the heart by cardiac catheterization and appropriate studies of the other involved organ system. In patients with only mild valve dysfunction, the significant symptoms must be due to other organ system dysfunction. The severity of the valve lesion can be followed noninvasively (particularly by cardiac ultrasound), and the patient can be instructed in bacterial endocarditis prophylaxis (see below).

Patients with mild or no symptoms (functional class I or II) and noninvasive evidence of moderate or severe valve dysfunction present a more difficult therapeutic decision. Their symptoms cannot be improved by surgical intervention, yet persistent, untreated valve dysfunction may result in irreversible myocardial failure, permanent functional disability, and even premature death. The algorithm for timing of intervention (Figure 1-3) makes use of assessment of maximal exercise performance and noninvasive assessment of ventricular function (e.g., radionuclide angiography).

Treatment of Valvular Disease

GENERAL PRINCIPLES

The treatment of valvular disease will be discussed in more detail under each specific valve lesion. However, a few general principles pertain to all lesions. Most severe, symptomatic valve lesions are now treated by valve replacement; exceptions occur in some patients with mitral stenosis and a few with mitral regurgitation, in whom reparative operations are successful. Be-

cause the perfect prosthetic valve has not yet been found (and likely never will), prosthetic valve replacement trades native valve disease for prosthetic valve disease. Two types of prosthetic valves are currently in common use: the totally prosthetic, mechanical valve and the bioprosthetic valve. The mechanical valves are either of the tilting-disk variety or the ball-in-a-cage variety. The bioprosthetic valve is a porcine aortic valve mounted on a stent for easier placement in either the aortic, mitral, or tricuspid position of the recipient. Because the porcine valve is avascular, and perhaps because of its sterilization and treatment with glutaraldehyde, it is nonantigenic. Nevertheless, it is a nonliving biologic structure; the stresses imposed by millions of openings and closings under pressure result in gradual disintegration of the collagen and elastic fibers in the valve. Biologic valves are expected to have a finite functional lifespan—perhaps in the range of 10 years. On the other hand, they are relatively nonthrombogenic; patients with these valves generally do not require anticoagulation for prevention of thromboembolism. Mechanical prostheses are durable, but they are thrombogenic and require anticoagulation with warfarin.

Bleeding is the most frequent valve-related complication after mechanical valve replacement, occurring at a rate of up to 7 percent per year [76]. Valve-related complications that occur less frequently are endocarditis, systemic embolism, valve thrombosis, and primary valve failure (bioprosthetic valves). Most prosthetic valves have some degree of obstruction to them.

ENDOCARDITIS PROPHYLAXIS

Diseased native valves and prosthetic valves are susceptible to developing endocarditis if there is bacteremia from any cause. Therefore, the administration of prophylactic antibiotics is generally recommended prior to any procedures that are likely to produce bacteremia, such as any dental procedure, instrumentation of the urinary tract, colon surgery, colonoscopy, etc. [150]. For dental procedures, most patients should receive 2.0 gm penicillin V orally 1 hour prior to the procedure and 1.0 gm 6 hours after the initial dose. For patients allergic to penicillin, 1.0 gm erythromycin orally 1 hour prior to the procedure and 500 mg 6 hours after the initial dose should be used. For patients in whom endocarditis presents a greater threat, such as patients with prosthetic valves, 1.0 to 2.0 gm ampicillin plus 1.5 mg/kg gentamicin IM or IV both given 30 minutes before the procedure and 1.0 gm penicillin V orally 6 hours after the initial dose should be given. For these higher-risk patients allergic to penicillin, 1 gm vancomycin IV over 60 minutes begun 60 minutes before the procedure is recommended. For all patients with valvular heart disease or prosthetic valves undergoing gastrointestinal or genitourinary tract surgery or instrumentation, the same regimen described above for high-risk patients is recommended.

Aortic Stenosis

PATHOPHYSIOLOGY

There are three causes of aortic stenosis in the adult. The most common cause of severe, isolated aortic stenosis is a congenitally abnormal valve. The valve may have been initially bicuspid, one of the most common congenital cardiac anomalies, or there may have been three unequal-sized cusps. The valve functions with little or no hemodynamic derangement for the first three or four decades of life. However, the abnormal anatomy predisposes to fibrotic thickening and deposition of calcium until the valve becomes severely stenotic in middle life. This is a disease predominantly of males. A second pathologic picture is seen in the elderly, in whom gradual wear and tear produces thickening of the three originally normal cusps. This process is a common cause of systolic ejection murmurs in the elderly and mildly thickened leaflets seen on echocardiography, but most often this age-related degenerative process does not result in severe stenosis requiring valve replacement. The third pathologic picture is that created by the late sequelae of rheumatic fever. The inflammatory process of rheumatic fever produces thickening and shortening of the leaflets

and commissural fusion; this usually results in the hemodynamic findings of mixed aortic stenosis and regurgitation. Nearly always the mitral valve is also affected by the rheumatic process, resulting in mitral stenosis or mixed mitral stenosis and regurgitation.

The thickening and calcification of the aortic valve leaflets produce obstruction to ejection of blood from the left ventricle. The left ventricle hypertrophies (increases wall thickness) in response to this "pressure overload" and is able to maintain a normal stroke volume only by markedly increasing the intraventricular systolic pressure from the normal 120 mmHg to over 200 mmHg in severe cases. In severe aortic stenosis, the pressure gradient between the left ventricle and aorta may be 100 mmHg or more (Fig. 1-4). The left ventricle may be able to compensate for this marked pressure overload for many years; however, eventually, myocardial failure will develop. The left ventricle increases its preload (diastolic pressure) to maintain the falling stroke volume. With increasing preload comes ventricular dilatation and a decreased ejection fraction. The rising diastolic pressure required to maintain cardiac output results in pulmonary venous hypertension, which in turn creates decreased pulmonary compliance because of the transudation of fluid across the capillary membrane. The decreased pulmonary compliance results in increased work of breathing and the sensation of dyspnea. Once the full syndrome of congestive heart failure ensues, the prognosis of untreated aortic stenosis is poor; half of such patients will die within 2 years without valve replacement. Furthermore, patients with congestive heart failure have a poorer outcome following valve replacement than those without; therefore, valve replacement should be undertaken before congestive heart failure occurs.

DIAGNOSIS

Symptoms

The most common clinical presentation is that of a relatively asymptomatic middle-aged male with a systolic ejection murmur and possible evidence of left ventricular hypertrophy on the electrocar-

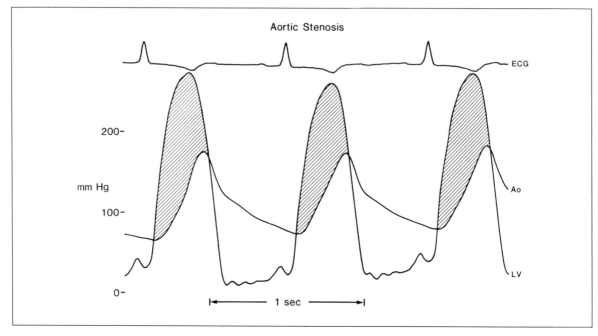

Figure 1–4. *A recording of aortic and left ventricular pressures from a patient with aortic stenosis. The cross-hatched area represents the abnormal gradient across the stenotic aortic valve (ECG, electrocardiogram; Ao, aortic pressure; LV, left ventricular pressure).*

diogram. Although the symptoms of angina, congestive heart failure, and syncope have been emphasized in the past, the most common early symptom is dyspnea on exertion. If the diagnosis is delayed until congestive heart failure or angina have intervened, it is likely that irreversible myocardial failure also will have occurred. In other words, aortic stenosis must be diagnosed and treated before left ventricular dilatation and heart failure occur.

Physical Examination

The physical signs are very useful in suspecting that aortic stenosis is present, but they are less useful in assessing the severity of the lesion. The characteristic finding is a systolic ejection murmur in the aortic area with radiation to both carotid arteries. Often, however, the ejection murmur is well heard—or even loudest—at the apex. In severe stenosis, the peripheral pulses may have reduced amplitude and slowed upstroke—pulsus parvus et tardus. However, these signs are often modulated by the compliance of the vascular sys-

tem and have not been consistently useful in judging severity. The left ventricular impulse is often sustained, a sign of hypertrophy, but it is in the normal location if dilatation has not occurred. A thrill palpable over the upper sternum is uncommon, but when present, it means severe stenosis. Because the thickened, calcified leaflets are relatively immobile, they do not make a sound when closing; thus splitting of the second sound is not heard in adult aortic stenosis. Likewise, a systolic ejection click is almost never heard in adults.

Electrocardiogram

The electrocardiogram provides important clues to the presence of left ventricular hypertrophy, which in the absence of systemic hypertension may mean significant aortic valve stenosis. Left

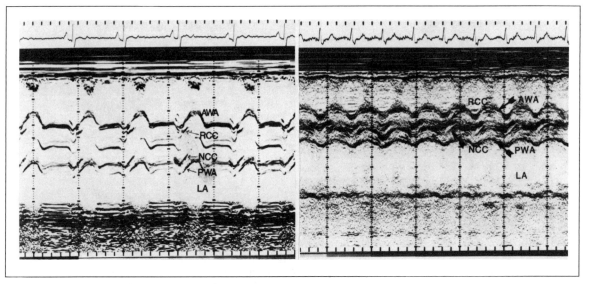

Figure 1–5. *A M-mode echocardiogram of the aortic root and valve from a patient with aortic stenosis (*right*) with a similar view from a normal patient (*left*) for comparison. Note particularly the marked thickening and immobility of the valve leaflets, represented by the very dense echoes within the aortic root (AWA, anterior wall of aorta; RCC, right coronary cusp of aortic valve; NCC, noncoronary cusp of aortic valve; PWA, posterior wall of aorta; LA, left atrium).*

ventricular hypertrophy can be diagnosed by increased QRS voltage—particularly in the precordial leads (S in V_1 or V_2 plus R in V_5 or $V_6 \geq 35$ mm). Even more useful in the assessment of aortic stenosis is evidence of left ventricular "strain" or repolarization abnormalities (T-wave inversion and ST-segment depression most commonly seen in the lateral precordial leads).

Chest Roentgenogram

The chest roentgenogram is generally of little help in assessing the severity of the stenosis. It is useful in evaluating for left ventricular dilatation and pulmonary vascular congestion—both signs of myocardial failure. Rarely, one may see evidence of calcification of the aortic valve on the chest roentgenogram. However, since calcification is universally present in the valves of adults with significant stenosis, more sensitive techniques to detect the calcification must be used, such as fluoroscopy. The absence of valve calcification in the adult means that the stenosis is not severe; obviously, this is not the case in children with congenital aortic stenosis.

Cardiac Ultrasound

The M-mode and two-dimensional echocardiograms provide useful anatomic information, such as valve thickening and immobility (Fig. 1-5). However, precise information regarding the severity of the stenosis cannot be obtained from these noninvasive tests. The one useful finding is that valve leaflet separation of 15 mm or more reliably excludes hemodynamically significant stenosis. More recently, the measurement of blood velocity by the Doppler principle has proven to be very useful in the noninvasive assessment of the severity of the stenosis. To maintain a normal stroke volume, the blood passing through the narrowed aortic orifice must do so at an increased velocity. Using a modification of the Bernoulli equation, which relates pressure drop

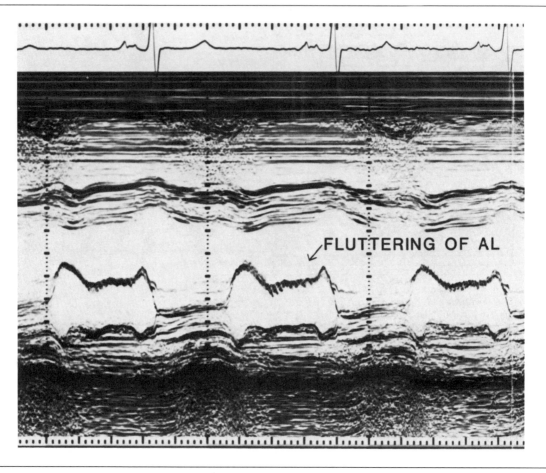

FLUTTERING OF AL

Figure 1–6. A M-mode echocardiogram from a patient with aortic regurgitation showing the high-frequency diastolic fluttering of the anterior leaflet of the mitral valve (AL) caused by the regurgitant jet striking the leaflet.

drop across a stenosis to velocity (V), one can estimate the instantaneous aortic valve gradient:

$$\text{Instantaneous gradient} = 4V^2$$

Comparison of the estimated gradient from the Doppler examination with a simultaneously measured pressure gradient at cardiac catheterization shows an excellent correlation [36].

Cardiac Catheterization

Cardiac catheterization has been very useful in defining the severity of the aortic stenosis, assessing ventricular function, and determining whether there is associated coronary artery disease. The pressure drop across the stenotic valve can be measured directly by simultaneously recording pressures from the left ventricle and the ascending aorta (see Fig. 1-4). Now, with accurate Doppler ultrasound techniques for quantitating the severity of aortic stenosis and radionuclide or echocardiographic techniques for assessing ventricular function, some younger patients with aortic stenosis may undergo valve replacement without prior cardiac catheterization. However, cardiac catheterization is still the preferred diagnostic study in older patients with a substantial risk of concomitant coronary artery disease, because it is the only technique for identifying and localizing coronary artery obstructions.

PROGNOSIS

Patients with aortic stenosis who are asymptomatic and maintain normal exercise tolerance probably have a good prognosis. However, the prognosis changes precipitously with the onset of symptoms. Patients with angina or syncope have a median survival of 3 to 4 years, while half of those with congestive heart failure will be dead in 1 to 2 years. The presence of concomitant coronary artery disease also significantly increases the risk of death.

TREATMENT

Valve Replacement

The primary therapeutic issue in aortic stenosis patients is the timing of valve replacement (see Fig. 1-3). Medical therapy has little to offer symptomatic patients other than to minimize the risks of valve replacement by optimizing the preoperative hemodynamic status. Certainly, all patients with angina, syncope, or congestive heart failure due to aortic stenosis should be offered valve replacement if their general medical condition makes the risk of surgery acceptable and allows a meaningful life following valve replacement. In patients with symptomatic aortic stenosis, cardiac catheterization will show a mean aortic valve gradient of 40 mmHg or more (there is no measurable gradient across normally functioning valves) and an estimated valve orifice area of 1.0 cm^2 or less (normal $\geq$ 3.0 cm^2). It is still controversial whether asymptomatic patients with severe aortic stenosis and preserved left ventricular function also should be offered valve replacement. However, if there is evidence of left ventricular dysfunction, valve replacement needs to be considered to preserve ventricular function.

Aortic valve replacement can be accomplished at an operative mortality rate of 5 to 10 percent [130]. Reparative procedures on the aortic valve have been tried, but they are not very effective because of failure to relieve the stenosis or rapid recurrence of the stenosis.

Balloon Valvuloplasty

Recently, percutaneous balloon valvuloplasty has been attempted as a palliative therapy in elderly patients with severe stenosis who are high-risk operative candidates. A guide wire is passed across the stenotic valve, and a balloon catheter is placed over the wire. By inflating the balloon to a diameter of approximately 23 mm, dilatation of the stenotic valve can be achieved. However, as would be expected from the pathology of the valve, the gains are modest, with the mean orifice area increasing from about 0.5 cm^2 to about 0.9 cm^2, which is approximately half the orifice area of a prosthetic valve [119,129]. Many of these patients, who were desperately ill and high-risk operative candidates because of their age, have been significantly improved symptomatically. However, it is too early to tell what the long-term results of this procedure will be or its risk-benefit ratio.

Aortic Regurgitation

PATHOPHYSIOLOGY

Aortic regurgitation may occur either if the aortic root supporting the cusps dilates such that the cusps can no longer coapt in diastole or if the cusps themselves are damaged. Table 1-10 lists some of the causes of aortic regurgitation classified according to acute (developing in days to weeks) and chronic (developing in months to years). The most common causes of aortic regurgitation are rheumatic heart disease, congenitally bicuspid valve, and infective endocarditis (often occurring on a previously diseased valve).

The amount of regurgitation is dependent on the regurgitant valve area (the area of incompetence), the diastolic pressure gradient between the aorta and the left ventricle, and the amount of diastolic time per minute. The latter two determinants are of particular importance because they can be altered by medical therapy. For ex-

Table 1–10. Causes of Aortic Regurgitation

Chronic		Acute	
Disease of aortic root	Disease of valve cusps	Disease of aortic root	Disease of valve cusps
Syphilis	Rheumatic heart disease	Acute aortic dissection	Acute rheumatic fever
Takayasu's aortitis	Bicuspid aortic valve	Rupture of sinus of Valsalva aneurysm	Infective endocarditis
Marfan's syndrome	Atherosclerosis		
Ehlers-Danlos syndrome	Myxomatous degeneration	Blunt chest trauma	
Osteogenesis imperfecta	Infective endocarditis		
Ventricular septal defect			
Sinus of Valsalva aneurysm			
Ankylosing spondylitis			
Reiter's syndrome			
Rheumatoid arthritis			
Systemic lupus erythematosus			
Hypertension			

ample, a patient with severe hypertension and aortic regurgitation will have a smaller regurgitant volume when his or her blood pressure has been controlled with antihypertensive medication. The effect of heart rate on the amount of aortic regurgitation is an important concept. As the heart rate increases, diastole shortens, while the duration of systole remains approximately the same; therefore, the amount of diastolic time per minute decreases as the heart rate increases. This explains why many patients with aortic regurgitation have preserved exercise tolerance for so long; as they exercise, their heart rate increases and the regurgitant volume decreases. In a similar vein, patients with significant aortic regurgitation should not be treated with agents that slow the heart rate, such as beta-adrenergic receptor blocking agents.

With the volume overload due to blood leaking back into the left ventricle, the left ventricle dilates. If the aortic regurgitation develops slowly so that the ventricle can adapt, systolic function (ejection fraction) is preserved and the patient may remain asymptomatic. The left ventricle may gradually dilate to a larger volume than in virtually any other disease process; left ventricular

volumes four to five times normal (70 ± 20 ml/m^2) and total left ventricular outputs of 20 liters per minute (normal is about 5 liters per minute) at rest have been reported (see Table 1-9). However, if severe aortic regurgitation persists long enough, eventually myocardial failure will ensue, the end-systolic volume will increase out of proportion to the end-diastolic volume, the ejection fraction will fall, the left ventricular end-diastolic pressure will rise, and symptoms of congestive heart failure will appear.

DIAGNOSIS
Symptoms
Patients with aortic regurgitation usually have a very long asymptomatic period if the regurgitation develops slowly, allowing the left ventricle to compensate for the volume overload. The symptoms of aortic regurgitation are nonspecific. Initially, the symptoms reflect the inability to appropriately increase cardiac output during exercise (fatigue and dyspnea), and subsequently, they reflect the development of congestive heart failure (orthopnea, paroxysmal nocturnal dyspnea, etc.). Angina occurs somewhat less frequently in patients with aortic regurgitation than in patients

with aortic stenosis, but it still may not be the result of coronary artery disease.

Physical Examination

Aortic regurgitation is generally easily diagnosed by the characteristic high-pitched, blowing, decrescendo diastolic murmur best heard along the left sternal border. The murmur may be difficult to hear in mild degrees of regurgitation or in severe heart failure, but it can be brought out by having the patient lean forward and hold his or her breath in exhalation. Pulmonic regurgitation may produce a similar murmur in the same location; however, it is far less common than aortic regurgitation.

The physical signs are also useful in assessing the severity of the regurgitation. The low-resistance runoff back into the left ventricle lowers the diastolic pressure, while the increased total left ventricular stroke volume increases the systolic pressure and pulse pressure (the difference between systolic and diastolic pressure). A diastolic pressure of less than 70 mmHg in males and less than 60 mmHg in females generally indicates severe aortic regurgitation. The very large systolic stroke volume creates bounding pulses. The reversed diastolic flow in the peripheral vessels can be detected by partially compressing the femoral artery with the edge of the diaphragm of the stethoscope and hearing the diastolic murmur created by blood flowing back toward the heart (Duroziez's sign).

The most useful physical signs in regard to severity of the regurgitation are those reflecting the size of the left ventricle. When systolic function is yet preserved, the left ventricular end-diastolic volume is directly proportional to the regurgitant volume. Therefore, a left ventricular impulse markedly displaced leftward and inferiorly and a generalized precordial heave over the left ventricle are signs of severe regurgitation.

Electrocardiogram

The electrocardiogram may show increased QRS voltage as a result of left ventricular hypertrophy. The development of ST-segment depression and T-wave inversion (left ventricular strain) usually signals severe chronic regurgitation. Sinus rhythm usually is present, unless heart failure has been present for some time.

Chest Roentgenogram

The chest roentgenogram is useful as a more accurate indicator of cardiac enlargement than the physical examination. Evidence of pulmonary vascular congestion and heart failure also can be detected. It can also give clues of primary aortic disease as the cause of the regurgitation, such as dissection of the ascending aorta or an aortic aneurysm.

Cardiac Ultrasound

As in other types of valvular heart disease, the cardiac ultrasound examination is the most useful noninvasive diagnostic tool after the physical examination. The dimensions (and volume in the absence of segmental wall-motion abnormalities) of the left ventricle can be easily measured and give an accurate assessment of left ventricular dilatation and systolic function. The regurgitant jet of blood falling back into the left ventricular outflow tract strikes the anterior leaflet of the mitral valve and causes it to vibrate. This is the genesis of the Austin-Flint murmur of relative mitral stenosis. The high-frequency diastolic fluttering of the anterior leaflet is a relatively sensitive and highly specific sign of aortic regurgitation (see Fig. 1-6, p. 30). The Doppler examination reveals a turbulent signal in the left ventricular outflow tract in diastole; this is a very sensitive sign for aortic regurgitation. The area of the left ventricle in which this diastolic turbulence can be mapped provides a very rough estimation of the severity of the regurgitation.

Cardiac Catheterization

Cardiac catheterization and angiography provide the most accurate way to estimate left ventricular volume and quantitate the severity of the regurgitation (see Table 1-9). A subjective visual estimation of the severity of aortic regurgitation can be obtained by injecting radiographic contrast material into the aortic root and observing it re-gurgitate into the left ventricle. However, patients with a low risk of coronary artery disease and good-quality cardiac ultrasound studies docu-menting marked left ventricular dilatation and se-vere aortic regurgitation do not require catheter-ization prior to undertaking valve replacement.

TREATMENT

Patients who have significant symptoms or re-striction of exercise capacity due to aortic regur-gitation should undergo aortic valve replacement, provided that their general medical condition and age allow an acceptable operative mortality rate. The average operative mortality rate for aortic valve replacement is approximately 7 percent [130]. However, as indicated earlier, patients with aortic regurgitation may remain asymptomatic until myocardial failure occurs. The decision-making process in patients with significant re-gurgitation and no or few symptoms is more dif-ficult—particularly since the valve should be replaced before severe, irreversible myocardial failure has occurred. Useful clues as to the need for valve replacement in these patients include the appearance of repolarization abnormalities (ST-segment depression and T-wave inversion) on the electrocardiogram, an end-systolic dimen-sion on echocardiography of 5.5 cm or more, an ejection fraction of less than 0.50 on radionuclide angiography, or marked left ventricular dilatation (end-diastolic volume $\geq$ 200 ml/m^2) on angiog-raphy.

Patients with any degree of aortic regurgitation are at increased risk for endocarditis when bac-teremia occurs and should receive endocarditis prophylaxis for dental and other procedures that produce bacteremia [150].

Mitral Stenosis

PATHOPHYSIOLOGY

The vast majority of cases of mitral stenosis in adults are the result of chronic rheumatic heart disease, even though a history of acute rheumatic fever is present in only about 50 percent. Congen-ital mitral stenosis is a rare cause of mitral valve obstruction in the newborn. In the elderly, marked calcification beginning in the mitral an-nulus and extending into the base of the leaflets may rarely result in obstruction to blood flow. Atrial myxoma is another rare cause of mitral valve obstruction.

Rheumatic fever produces scarring of the valve leaflets and chordae tendineae. The anterior and posterior leaflets become thickened, immobile, reduced in surface area, and fused at the commis-sures. The chordae tendineae also become thick-ened, shortened, and fused. The mitral valve ap-paratus becomes funnel-shaped, with the apex of the funnel being formed by the fused and thick-ened chordae. Calcification of the leaflets occurs late in the disease process. The time from the bout(s) of acute rheumatic fever to advanced mi-tral stenosis may be 20 years or more. The orifice area is reduced from the normal of approximately 4 cm^2 to less than 1 cm^2 in severe cases.

The obstruction at the mitral valve results in in-creased left atrial pressure, which in turn results in left atrial dilatation. Left ventricular pressures and size remain normal (see Fig. 1-8, p. 38). The increased left atrial pressure is reflected backward into the pulmonary veins and pulmonary capil-laries. When the increased pulmonary capillary pressure exceeds the forces opposing transudation of fluid across the capillary alveolar membranes (plasma oncotic pressure and tissue hydrostatic pressure), edema occurs in the alveolar wall and space. This is pulmonary edema. With time, com-pensatory mechanisms allow increased drainage of this edema fluid through dilated pulmonary lymphatics, which can be seen on the chest roent-genogram as Kerley B lines. The pulmonary ar-tery pressure is increased not only in direct pro-portion to the increase in pulmonary capillary pressure, but also by a reflex vasoconstriction. In advanced cases of mitral stenosis, the pulmonary artery pressure may be increased to five times normal or equal to the systemic arterial pressure. The right ventricle, normally a relatively thin-walled structure, hypertrophies in response to the gradual increase in pulmonary artery pressure and ultimately is unable to handle this pressure overload. It then dilates, resulting in a decreased ejection fraction not dissimilar to the left ventricular failure of advanced aortic stenosis. With dilatation of the right ventricle, the tricuspid valve annulus also dilates, such that the tricuspid valve becomes incompetent; this in turn results in right atrial dilatation and an increase in systemic venous pressure. The increased systemic venous pressure accounts for most of the signs of right-sided heart failure: peripheral edema, increased jugular venous pressure, enlarged, congested liver, and ascites. The resting cardiac output becomes reduced relatively early in mitral stenosis, resulting in fatigue as a prominent symptom.

As a result of the increased atrial pressure and dilatation of the left atrium, atrial fibrillation is seen in about half the patients with significant mitral stenosis. The combination of this arrhythmia, the dilated chamber, and the low cardiac output results in stasis of blood in the left atrium and thrombus formation; thrombus is most likely to form in the left atrial appendage. Systemic embolism is a not uncommon complication in patients with mitral stenosis and atrial fibrillation and is particularly devastating when it results in a debilitating stroke in a young person.

DIAGNOSIS

With careful attention to the history, physical examination, and chest roentgenogram, the diagnosis should not be missed. Yet, it often is missed—probably because the murmur is sometimes difficult to hear.

Symptoms

The most common symptoms in patients with mitral stenosis are dyspnea and fatigue. Because the stenosis develops gradually over decades, the symptoms develop insidiously and may not be recognized by the patient until an acute event such as atrial fibrillation or systemic embolism occurs. With loss of atrial contraction due to the onset of atrial fibrillation, there is a sudden decrease in cardiac output, which accelerates compensatory mechanisms such as the renin aldosterone system leading to rapid fluid retention and possible acute pulmonary edema. Pulmonary edema is readily recognized by the marked air hunger, pulmonary rales, and sometimes blood-tinged frothy sputum.

Physical Examination

The characteristic physical sign of mitral stenosis is the low-pitched, rumbling diastolic murmur heard best at the apex. In patients with mild stenosis, in patients with rapid atrial fibrillation, or in patients with very severe heart failure, the diastolic murmur is particularly difficult to hear. However, it can nearly always be brought out by examining the patient in the left lateral decubitus position with the bell of the stethoscope placed lightly at the point of maximum pulse. Also, the murmur will be missed rarely if one remembers the context in which it occurs: loud first heart sound, an opening snap following the second heart sound by approximately 0.1 second, and an irregular rhythm due to atrial fibrillation. Other useful signs relate primarily to the effect of the pressure overload on the right ventricle. These include a parasternal lift due to pulmonary hypertension and tricuspid regurgitation, large systolic pulsations in the jugular veins due to tricuspid regurgitation, and the murmur of tricuspid regurgitation which increases with inspiration. It is important to remember that tricuspid regurgitation is often present in the absence of a murmur.

Chest Roentgenogram

The chest roentgenogram of the patient with mitral stenosis is relatively characteristic; the left ventricle is normal-sized or even small, but the left atrium is dilated. There are four important radiographic features of left atrial enlargement: (1) straightening of the left border of the heart due to the dilated left atrial appendage, (2) widening of the angle between the main-stem bronchi (normally an acute angle), (3) a smoothly curving double density in the right midportion of the heart formed by the right inferior border of the left atrium, and (4) the posterior displacement of the cardiac silhouette seen on the lateral film.

Electrocardiogram

The electrocardiogram may be normal in many patients with mild mitral stenosis. One of the first abnormalities is the broad, bifid P wave in lead 2 and the biphasic P wave in lead V_1, indicating left atrial enlargement. As indicated earlier, atrial fibrillation is commonly present. The electrocardiogram is relatively insensitive in detecting right ventricular hypertrophy; if present, it may be manifested by rightward deviation of the mean QRS axis and large R waves in V_1 and V_2.

Cardiac Ultrasound

The echocardiogram is the most useful noninvasive diagnostic tool after the physical examination. Rheumatic mitral stenosis produces typical changes in the mitral valve echocardiogram (Fig. 1-7). The leaflets are thickened and have reduced amplitude of diastolic motion. The diastolic closure rate (EF slope) is markedly reduced due to the pressure gradient keeping the valve maximally open throughout diastole. The posterior leaflet often moves anteriorly in diastole; this is probably the result of commissural fusion, so that the posterior leaflet follows the motion of the larger anterior leaflet. The stenotic orifice often can be accurately visualized and measured in the two-dimensional short-axis view. As in aortic stenosis, the Doppler can be used to detect the increased velocity of blood across the mitral valve; the modified Bernoulli equation can be used to estimate the peak instantaneous gradient (see the section entitled Aortic Stenosis). There is a useful empiric inverse relationship between the time it takes for the pressure gradient across the valve to fall by half (pressure half-time or *PHT*) and the mitral orifice area (*MVA*):

$$MVA = \frac{220}{PHT}$$

The time at which the pressure gradient has fallen to half its maximal value can be easily determined by finding the point on the Doppler velocity tracing where the velocity is $1/1.414$ of the peak velocity.

Cardiac Catheterization

For patients who have good-quality echo-Doppler studies and are at low risk for coronary disease (e.g., females or males without risk factors under the age of 40), cardiac catheterization is not necessary to make a decision regarding need for cardiac surgery. Cardiac catheterization is generally recommended for patients with known coronary artery disease or at increased risk for coronary artery disease, for patients with multivalvular disease, and for patients for whom the noninvasive data are ambiguous.

TREATMENT

Medical Therapy

Medical therapy of mitral stenosis can do nothing about the valve obstruction, but it can be effective in controlling symptoms of congestive heart failure, maintaining sinus rhythm or controlling the ventricular rate of atrial fibrillation, and preventing systemic embolism and endocarditis. Congestive heart failure in mild to moderate stenosis will respond to the use of diuretics and digoxin. Vasodilating agents, such as captopril, are ineffective and even dangerous because the valve obstruction prevents an increase in cardiac output in response to the reduced peripheral resistance. In more severe cases of stenosis, only relief of the obstruction will aid the congestive heart failure. In patients who have had transient or brief episodes of atrial fibrillation, an antiarrhythmic agent, such as quinidine, can be effective in maintaining sinus rhythm. However, established atrial fibrillation due to significant mitral stenosis usually can be returned to sinus rhythm only by relieving the valve obstruction first. As indicated earlier, the combination of mitral stenosis and atrial fibrillation creates a high risk for left atrial clot and systemic embolism; we believe these pa-

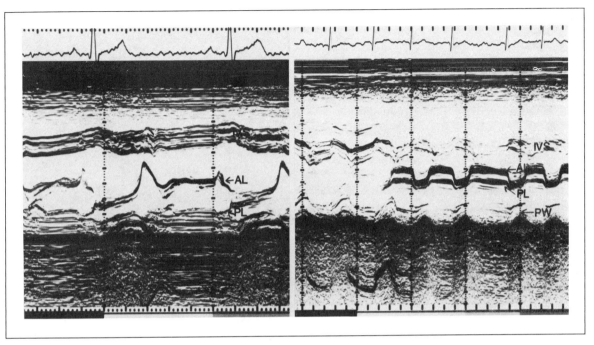

Figure 1–7. *A M-mode echocardiogram of the mitral valve from a patient with mitral stenosis (right). An echocardiogram of a normal mitral valve is shown on the left for comparison. Note the marked thickening and immobility of both leaflets and the anterior motion of the posterior leaflet (IVS, interventricular septum; AL, anterior leaflet of the mitral valve; PL, posterior leaflet of the mitral valve; PW, posterior wall of the left ventricle).*

tients should be anticoagulated with warfarin. Finally, like all damaged valves, the rheumatic mitral valve is at increased risk for endocarditis. Bacterial endocarditis prophylaxis should be provided for all procedures likely to produce bacteremia [150].

Surgical Therapy
The mechanical obstruction of significant mitral stenosis responds only to mechanical relief. One of the very first intracardiac operations attempted in humans was an attempt to relieve mitral stenosis either by blindly incising the commissures or by attempting to separate the fused commissures by finger dilatation. The latter procedure,

known as closed mitral commissurotomy, was first successfully performed by Henry Souttar in London in 1928 by inserting his finger into the stenotic mitral orifice via the left atrial appendage. However, this procedure was not repeated again for approximately 20 years, when it became widely and successfully used. Mitral stenosis in its earlier phases is particularly amenable to commissurotomy, because much of the obstruction is caused by fusion of the commissures. However, in more advanced disease, fusion of the chordae contribute to the stenosis; the leaflets also become calcified and incompetent. The function of such a valve will no longer be improved by commissurotomy, and the valve must be replaced. The first successful valve replacement was a mitral valve replacement performed by Albert Starr in Portland, Oregon, in 1960. Currently, the average operative mortality rate for mitral valve replacement is 5 to 10 percent.

Mitral valve surgery is indicated when the symptoms cannot be controlled by medical ther-

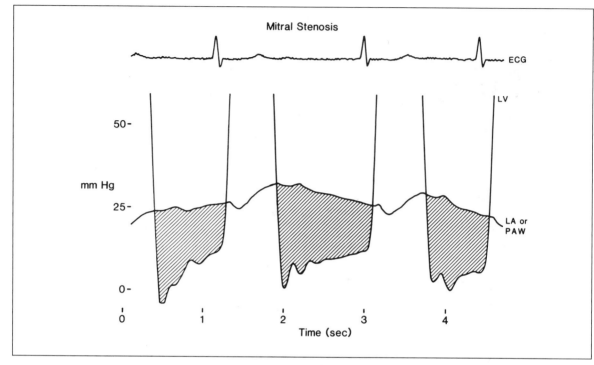

Figure 1–8. *A recording of left atrial and left ventricular pressures from a patient with mitral stenosis. The pressures are recorded at high gain, so that the left ventricular pressure goes off the top of the recording. The cross-hatched area represents the abnormal gradient across the mitral valve (LA or PAW, left atrial or pulmonary artery wedge pressure; LV, left ventricular pressure).*

apy or when significant pulmonary hypertension has occurred. The valve obstruction should be relieved before the pulmonary hypertension results in irreversible right ventricular failure. Because the operative risk is lower and postoperative valve-related complications are uncommon, mitral commissurotomy may be performed at an earlier phase of the disease than valve replacement. However, in a significant proportion of patients, restenosis will occur in several years, necessitating valve replacement. It takes a greater than 50 percent reduction in orifice area from the normal value of 3 to 4 cm^2 to result in symptoms and/or significant limitation of exercise. Most patients undergoing mitral valve surgery have mitral valve orifices of = < 1.0 cm^2, a reduced cardiac index (normal 3.0 ± 0.5 liters/min/m^2), a widened arteriovenous oxygen difference (normal 4.5 ± 0.5 ml/dl), and an increased pulmonary artery pressure (normal mean ≤ 20 mmHg).

Balloon Valvuloplasty
In 1986 a new form of nonoperative therapy was introduced for mitral stenosis, balloon valvuloplasty. In this procedure, a balloon catheter is placed across the mitral valve via puncture of the interatrial septum, and the stenotic valve is dilated by inflation of the balloon. Mechanically, the effect on the mitral valve is essentially the same as the closed commissurotomy performed by Souttar in 1928; inflation of the balloon separates the valve at the fused commissures. As long as commissural fusion is the principal cause of the obstruction (as it is in the earlier stages of mitral stenosis), any procedure to separate this fusion

will be effective. This is likely to be a very useful procedure in areas where rheumatic heart disease is still prevalent at a young age, such as many developing countries. In the United States, most rheumatic mitral valve disease is seen in older persons with more advanced pathology, such as fusion of the chordae. In these patients, balloon valvuloplasty is unlikely to be as effective.

Mitral Regurgitation

PATHOPHYSIOLOGY

The normal physiology by which the mitral valve maintains its competence when closing is very complex. The free edges of the leaflets would prolapse far back into the left atrium if it were not for the supporting structures: chordae tendineae, papillary muscles, and ventricular wall. The leaflets and chordae are of relatively fixed length; therefore, as the distance between the apex of the left ventricle and the mitral valve ring decreases during systole, the papillary muscles also must shorten to prevent the leaflets from prolapsing and becoming incompetent. Similarly, if the ventricle dilates significantly, the distance relationships of the mitral apparatus are disturbed, making incompetence likely. Thus abnormal structure or function of any of the four major components of the mitral apparatus may lead to mitral regurgitation (Table 1-11).

With ejection of a portion of its stroke volume into the left atrium through the incompetent mitral valve, the left ventricle dilates to maintain a normal forward stroke volume. Because the pressure in the left atrium is low compared to that in the aorta, the impedance to left ventricular ejection falls. With the decreased impedance to ejection, the left ventricle is able to empty more completely, and the left ventricular ejection fraction may rise initially. If the mitral regurgitation is severe, myocardial failure will ultimately ensue, and the ejection fraction will begin to fall, as in volume overload due to aortic insufficiency. This accounts for the seeming paradox in severe mitral regurgitation of significant myocardial dysfunc-

Table 1–11. *Causes of Mitral Regurgitation*

I. Disturbances of mitral annulus structure or function:
   A. Mitral annular calcification
II. Disturbances of leaflet structure or function:
   A. Rheumatic valvular disease
   B. Bacterial endocarditis
   C. Myxomatous degeneration
   D. Ostium primum atrial septal defect
   E. Inherited connective-tissue disorders:
      1. Marfan's syndrome
      2. Ehlers-Danlos syndrome
      3. Osteogenesis imperfecta
III. Disturbances of chordal structure or function:
   A. Rheumatic valvular disease
   B. Bacterial endocarditis
   C. Myxomatous degeneration
   D. Inherited connective-tissue disorders:
      1. Marfan's syndrome
      2. Ehlers-Danlos syndrome
      3. Osteogenesis imperfecta
   E. Blunt chest trauma
IV. Disturbances of papillary muscle structure or function:
   A. Papillary muscle ischemia
   B. Papillary muscle infarction without rupture
   C. Papillary muscle rupture (usually the result of acute infarction)
V. Disturbances of left ventricular wall function:
   A. Myocardial ischemia
   B. Myocardial infarction
   C. Dilated cardiomyopathy from any cause

tion despite apparently normal left ventricular emptying as reflected in the ejection fraction. With the drop in ejection fraction, forward cardiac output also begins to fall, resulting in symptoms of fatigue.

The regurgitating blood into the left atrium increases intraatrial pressure in systole. In severe regurgitation there may be peak systolic pressures in the left atrium of 60 mmHg or more; this pressure wave is known as a giant V wave. The increased pressure in the left atrium causes it to dilate; in severe regurgitation it becomes the largest chamber in the heart and may form portions of both the left and right borders of the heart on the chest film. As in mitral stenosis, the increased pressure and volume of the left atrium predisposes to atrial fibrillation. The increased pressure is reflected back into the pulmonary veins and capillaries resulting in pulmonary congestion or edema. As in mitral stenosis, the pulmonary artery pressure may be increased out of proportion to the increase in pulmonary capillary pressure because of reflex vasoconstriction. With long-standing pulmonary hypertension, right ventricular hypertrophy and dilatation occur; functional tricuspid regurgitation is common as a result of the right ventricular dilatation.

DIAGNOSIS

Symptoms

As in other types of valvular heart disease, the symptoms are nonspecific. The most common is impairment of maximal exercise tolerance by dyspnea and/or fatigue. With more severe hemodynamic impairment, symptoms of congestive heart failure will appear.

Physical Examination

The murmur of mitral regurgitation can be varied in quality and location depending on the cause of mitral regurgitation and the direction of the regurgitant jet. However, the classic mitral regurgitation murmur, as commonly heard in rheumatic disease, is a high-pitched, pansystolic murmur encompassing the second heart sound that is heard best at the apex with radiation to the axilla. If the regurgitation is due to mitral valve prolapse (see below), it may be limited to mid and late systole. In unusual cases of ruptured chordae, the regurgitant jet may be directed toward the aorta, causing the murmur to be heard in the aortic area, or directed posteriorly toward the spine, causing the murmur to be heard along the thoracic and cervical spine and at the top of the head. The distinction between murmurs of mitral regurgitation and aortic stenosis is better made by the quality of the murmurs (pansystolic for mitral regurgitation and ejection for aortic stenosis) than by location. The murmur of aortic stenosis is often well heard at the apex, while the murmur of mitral regurgitation can sometimes be heard at the base of the heart. As in aortic insufficiency, the size of the left ventricle provides an important clue to the severity of the volume overload. The point of maximum impulse is shifted to the left

and inferiorly. In addition, there may be a parasternal lift indicating either systolic expansion of the left atrium or a dilated right ventricle due to pulmonary hypertension.

Electrocardiogram

The electrocardiogram may show evidence of left ventricular hypertrophy and left atrial enlargement. Atrial fibrillation is common in patients with long-standing, severe mitral regurgitation, just as it is with any lesion that results in marked increases in left atrial size and pressure.

Chest Roentgenogram

The chest roentgenogram can be quite helpful in arriving at the correct diagnosis and assessing its severity. In significant mitral regurgitation, both the left atrium and the left ventricle are enlarged—the ventricle in proportion to the severity of the regurgitation. Also, examination of the pulmonary vasculature is useful in assessing for the presence and severity of pulmonary congestion and edema.

Cardiac Ultrasound

The cardiac ultrasound study is most helpful in quantitating the degree of left ventricular dilatation and in evaluating left ventricular systolic function. In many patients with nonrheumatic mitral regurgitation, the mitral leaflets and chordae tendineae may appear normal on M-mode and two-dimensional echocardiography. However, characteristic findings are seen in patients with mitral valve prolapse (see below) and in patients with ruptured chordae or a ruptured papillary muscle. An infarcted papillary muscle can often be identified by the very bright echoes representing scar tissue. Mitral annular calcification is common in the elderly, frequently is associated with mitral regurgitation, and is easily detected by echocardiography. Doppler ultrasound is a very sensitive technique for the qualitative detection of mitral regurgitation. A very rough estimate of the severity of the regurgitation can be obtained by mapping the area of the left atrium in which the regurgitant jet can be detected.

Cardiac Catheterization

Cardiac catheterization is useful in directly visualizing the mitral regurgitation and assessing its effects on hemodynamics. However, cardiac catheterization is not always necessary prior to valve replacement or repair if the ultrasound studies are of good quality and the patient is at low risk for coronary artery disease. By injecting radiographic contrast material into the left ventricle, it is possible to visualize the contrast regurgitating into the left atrium, to measure left ventricular volumes, and to assess left ventricular systolic performance. By subtracting the net forward cardiac output measured by the Fick or thermodilution techniques from the total left ventricular output measured from the angiographic volumes, the amount of regurgitation can be quantitated as illustrated in Table 1-9. By measuring the oxygen content in the mixed venous (pulmonary artery) and arterial blood, the arteriovenous oxygen difference can be calculated (normal = 4.5 ± 0.5 ml/dl). A widened arteriovenous oxygen difference indicates that cardiac output is inadequate for the oxygen needs of the body, which compensates by extracting more oxygen from the blood. An abnormal arteriovenous oxygen difference is also a strong predictor of impaired prognosis, unless valve replacement is undertaken [75]. As in aortic regurgitation, the degree of left ventricular dilatation is a good measure of the severity of the mitral regurgitation if sufficient time has elapsed for compensatory dilatation to occur and systolic function is preserved. Left ventricular volumes of three to four times normal (70 ± 20 ml/m^2) can be seen in patients with severe regurgitation. Calculated regurgitant volumes may be as high as 15 liters per minute.

TREATMENT

Medical Therapy

Asymptomatic patients with mitral regurgitation require bacterial endocarditis prophylaxis for pro-

cedures likely to cause bacteremia [150]. If the patient is under age 30 and the regurgitation is the result of rheumatic heart disease, rheumatic fever prophylaxis also needs to be given. The recommended rheumatic fever prophylaxis regimens are 1.2 million units benzathine penicillin IM every 4 weeks, or 1.0 gm sulfadiazine orally daily, or 250,000 units oral penicillin daily. If signs or symptoms of congestive heart failure are present, digoxin and diuretics should be administered. The distribution of blood ejected from the left ventricle between the aorta and the left atrium is dependent on the comparative impedances at the two orifices. The aortic impedance can be reduced and the proportion of left ventricular stroke volume ejected out through the aortic valve can be increased by vasodilator therapy; in some cases, effective vasodilator therapy can virtually eliminate the mitral regurgitation. Angiotensin-converting enzyme inhibitors such as captopril and enalopril seem to be particularly effective in this regard.

Surgical Therapy

Patients whose symptoms due to mitral regurgitation persist despite medical therapy need to be considered for surgical therapy. Also, patients who exhibit deteriorating left ventricular function need to be considered as well, regardless of symptoms. However, the substantial proportion of patients with dilated cardiomyopathy, who also have mitral regurgitation because of the ventricular dilatation, do not benefit from mitral valve surgery because the primary problem is severe myocardial dysfunction. Two types of surgical procedures can be offered. If the leaflets and chordae are relatively intact, a reparative procedure can sometimes restore competence to the mitral valve. This is often accomplished by reducing the circumference of the mitral annulus either by placing sutures through the commissures (annuloplasty) or by sewing the entire annulus to a fixed ring (Carpentier ring). However, the majority of patients with severe mitral regurgitation require valve replacement. The overall operative mortality rate is between 5 and 10 percent in patients whose regurgitation is not the result of coronary artery disease and between 10 and 20 percent in patients with regurgitation due to coronary artery disease. Either mechanical prostheses or bioprostheses may be used, with the relative advantages and disadvantages of each as discussed earlier.

Mitral Valve Prolapse
PATHOPHYSIOLOGY
Mitral valve prolapse may occur as a result of any pathologic process that interferes with the structure or function of the valve leaflets, chordae tendineae, or papillary muscles; however, by far the most common cause is myxomatous degeneration. This poorly understood condition is manifested by large, redundant leaflets and elongated chordae, resulting in prolapse of either or both leaflets into the left atrium. Typically, the prolapse occurs after the ventricle has begun to shorten—often in midsystole. In some patients the prolapse is severe enough to result in mitral regurgitation; in a small minority the regurgitation is sufficiently severe as to require operative therapy. The etiology of the myxomatous degeneration is unknown, as is the pathogenesis of the other major features of this syndrome, which are chest pain and ventricular arrhythmias. There is some evidence that this is a genetic disorder, at least in some patients. However, the high reported incidence of 10 percent in females and 1 to 2 percent in males raises the question as to whether minor degrees of mitral valve prolapse might be a normal variant. Although sudden cardiac death has been reported in a few patients with mitral valve prolapse and ventricular arrhythmias, in the vast majority of patients mitral valve prolapse is a benign condition.

DIAGNOSIS
Symptoms
In most patients in whom mitral valve prolapse is diagnosed by the characteristic physical examination findings or cardiac ultrasound findings,

there are no symptoms. Some patients have an atypical type of chest pain. The pathogenesis of the chest pain is unknown, but it is probably not the result of myocardial ischemia. A few patients will have symptoms from the associated ventricular arrhythmias: palpitations, dizziness, and rarely, syncope.

Physical Examination
The onset of prolapse is often marked by a snapping sound, known as a midsystolic click. This click is thought to be the result of the leaflet tensing at its maximal prolapsed position, much as a sail snaps in the wind. The click may or may not be followed by a regurgitant murmur. Other features of this mitral valve prolapse syndrome are an asthenic body habitus, chest-wall deformity, and psychiatric disturbances (particularly anxiety syndromes).

Electrocardiogram and Chest Roentgenogram
There are no characteristic findings of mitral valve prolapse on these studies. If the resultant mitral regurgitation is significant, then findings of left ventricular hypertrophy and dilatation will be found, as discussed for mitral regurgitation above.

Cardiac Ultrasound
The echo-Doppler study is the most useful diagnostic study after the physical examination. However, if the physical examination reveals the typical midsystolic click and late systolic murmur, further diagnostic studies are not necessary if there are no symptoms or cardiac enlargement. Prolapse of the mitral valve can be readily demonstrated on the M-mode echocardiogram (Fig. 1-9). A Doppler study can confirm the presence or absence of mitral regurgitation.

TREATMENT
For most patients who have either the midsystolic click–late systolic murmur or echocardiographic findings of mitral valve prolapse (see Fig. 1-9), no treatment is necessary. If a murmur is present

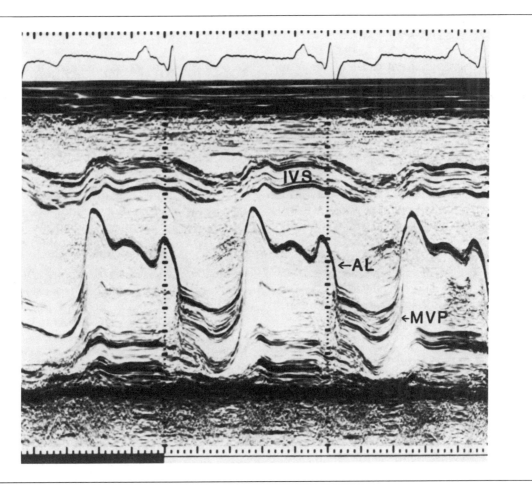

Figure 1–9. *A M-mode echocardiogram of the mitral valve in a patient with mitral valve prolapse. (See Fig. 1-7 for a M-mode echocardiogram of a normal mitral valve.) Note the posterior motion of the valve leaflets in systole in contrast to the anterior motion in systole of the normal valve (AL, anterior leaflet of mitral valve; MVP, prolapsing mitral valve).*

suggesting mitral regurgitation, or if there is Doppler evidence of regurgitation, bacterial endocarditis prophylaxis is generally recommended. The criteria for other medical or surgical therapy is the same as that described earlier for mitral regurgitation. The chest pain is said to respond to propranolol, but well-controlled studies of efficacy have not been done. In patients with symptoms from ventricular arrhythmia, therapy with an antiarrhythmic agent may be helpful.

Hypertensive Cardiovascular Disease

Hypertension is a significant cause of death and disability in adults in developed countries. Although hypertension itself is often asymptomatic, it results in complications due to hypertension itself as well as to accelerated atherosclerosis. Complications of the hypertension include left ventricular hypertrophy, heart failure, renal failure, hemorrhagic stroke, and aortic dissection, while acceleration of the atherosclerotic process in the coronary, cerebral, and peripheral vascular beds may culminate in angina, myocardial infarction, thrombotic stroke, and peripheral vascular insufficiency. Coronary artery disease and aortic and peripheral vascular disease are discussed separately. This section will focus on the left ventricular hypertrophy associated with hypertension.

Pathophysiology

Left ventricular hypertrophy develops in response to an increase in myocardial wall stress [117]. Myocardial wall stress, as defined by the LaPlace relationship, is a function of the left ventricular intracavitary pressure (P) times the left ventricular radius (R) divided by the left ventricular wall thickness (h):

$$\text{Wall stress} = \frac{PR}{2h}$$

Wall stress is increased by an increase in pressure generated by the ventricle such as occurs in systemic hypertension (pressure overload) or by an increase in blood volume presented to the ventricle such as results from aortic insufficiency (volume overload). Wall stress may also increase when a portion of the myocardium is damaged and hypertrophy is stimulated in the remaining normal myocardium. Thus any single factor or combination of these factors may result in hypertrophy. In addition, ventricular hypertrophy may be provoked by such things as chronically increased levels of catecholamines and probably other, as yet unknown, stimuli. When hypertrophy is caused by a pressure overload, concentric hypertrophy occurs. Concentric hypertrophy refers to hypertrophy with a decreased ventricular volume to wall thickness ratio. When increased left ventricular volume is the stimulus for hypertrophy, eccentric hypertrophy results and is characterized by a normal or increased ventricular volume to wall thickness ratio. Long-standing systemic hypertension most often results in concentric hypertrophy, although various patterns of hypertrophy may be seen [2].

Initially, myocardial hypertrophy is a compensatory response to systemic hypertension. Thus, if systemic blood pressure increases, the increase in myocardial wall thickness prevents a large increase in wall stress by the LaPlace relationship. In both animal and human models of left ventricular hypertrophy, the hypertrophy minimizes left ventricular dysfunction brought about by high systemic pressures. However, despite these improvements, evidence exists that the hypertrophied myocardium may not be entirely normal [67]. Increased amounts of fibrous tissue may be present, and biochemical abnormalities in hypertrophied myocardial cells have been described [117]. In addition, there is a decrease in coronary flow reserve, i.e., the maximum possible increase in coronary blood flow over resting flow [114].

Left ventricular hypertrophy begins much earlier in the course of hypertension than was once thought [35]. However, symptoms of hypertrophy and myocardial dysfunction are rarely noted until hypertension has been long-standing. Probably the earliest manifestations are subtle changes in diastolic performance of the ventricle detected as decreased diastolic filling rates using echocardiography [52]. These changes usually precede abnormalities in systolic function. If hypertension remains uncontrolled, overt diastolic and systolic dysfunction may occur, resulting in symptoms of congestive heart failure [93]. In fact, hypertension is one of the most common predisposing factors to heart failure. However, significant individual variation occurs in the myocardial response to long-standing hypertension. While the ambulatory mean systolic blood pressure over 24 hours is most closely correlated to the presence of left ventricular hypertrophy, other factors such as age, sex, race, and therapy all combine to influence the development of left ventricular hypertrophy [140,59,122].

Diagnosis

The physical examination in patients with left ventricular hypertrophy reveals a sustained left ventricular apical impulse and a fourth heart sound. The sustained apical impulse is more sensitive for the diagnosis of left ventricular hypertrophy than is the electrocardiogram (ECG). Physical findings of congestive heart failure also may be present.

While the ECG has been the standard tool for the diagnosis of left ventricular hypertrophy, the echocardiogram is much more sensitive [40,144]. M-mode echocardiograms can define left ventricular wall thickness, and both M-mode and two-dimensional echocardiograms can be used to estimate myocardial mass.

The chest x-ray is not helpful in detecting left ventricular hypertrophy because an increase in wall thickness of 1 to 3 mm, which is significant hypertrophy, cannot be easily detected on the chest film.

Treatment

Although left ventricular hypertrophy may initially be an adaptive response to systemic hypertension, data from the Framingham Study suggest a poor long-term prognosis. In subjects with ECG-defined left ventricular hypertrophy, the risk of any cardiac event (coronary disease, stroke, heart failure, and peripheral vascular disease) is increased severalfold [91]. When one corrects

these data for the level of blood pressure, left ventricular hypertrophy by voltage criteria does not confer additional risk over the hypertension alone. However, left ventricular hypertrophy with repolarization abnormalities, i.e., ST-segment and T-wave abnormalities, also known as left ventricular hypertrophy with strain, predicts a substantially increased risk of future cardiac events. Echocardiography is likely to be even better at assessing risk in patients with hypertension because of its increased sensitivity in the diagnosis of left ventricular hypertrophy [25].

Recent animal and human studies show that left ventricular hypertrophy associated with systemic hypertension is indeed at least partially reversible [165]. These data are complemented by studies demonstrating decreased cardiovascular risk in treated hypertensive subjects. However, there is marked individual variability in the reversal of hypertrophy even in individuals treated with the same drug. The type of antihypertensive therapy also influences the regression of hypertrophy. Treatment of hypertension with sympatholytic agents such as reserpine and methyldopa, angiotensin-converting enzyme inhibitors, calcium-entry blockers, and probably beta-adrenergic receptor blockers results in regression of left ventricular hypertrophy. Vasodilators such as hydralazine or diuretics alone may not lead to regression of hypertrophy. At present, it would seem wise to choose an antihypertensive regimen which results in regression of left ventricular hypertrophy, but medical therapy also must be individualized according to associated problems as diabetes, peripheral vascular disease, angina, or heart failure.

Finally, one must be concerned as to whether regression of left ventricular hypertrophy is always an appropriate goal [166]. If sudden elevations in arterial pressure occur, will ventricular function be adequate? Is myocardial function restored to normal with reversal of hypertrophy? While these questions cannot be answered with certainty, the poor prognosis associated with left ventricular hypertrophy and the improvement in outcome in patients with treated hypertension suggest that hypertension should be treated aggressively. A therapeutic regimen designed to induce regression of left ventricular hypertrophy is probably most appropriate. It is important to remember that our understanding of the control of myocardial hypertrophy is incomplete. Better understanding will improve treatment regimens [166].

Because of the increased risk of atherosclerosis in patients with hypertension, attention must be given to other risk factors, such as hyperlipidemia and cigarette smoking.

Cardiomyopathies

Cardiomyopathies are diseases involving the heart muscle. The term is generally used to refer to myocardial diseases not associated with hypertension, valvular, congenital, pericardial, or ischemic heart disease. Cardiomyopathies are often divided into three categories based primarily on myocardial structure and function; these categories are dilated (congestive), hypertrophic, and restrictive [146]. The basic differentiating features are outlined in Table 1-12.

Dilated (Congestive) Cardiomyopathy

PATHOPHYSIOLOGY

Presumably, dilated cardiomyopathy begins with injury to myocardial cells by an infectious, toxic, or metabolic process. Systolic function (contractility) is primarily affected, resulting in ventricular dilation with increases in both end-diastolic and end-systolic volume and a decrease in ejection fraction. Cardiac output may be maintained early because of the increased volumes and tachycardia. Diastolic function may or may not be affected [69].

Often the dysfunction involves all four myocardial chambers, although occasionally one chamber or one side of the heart may be predominately affected. As systolic dysfunction progresses, end-diastolic pressures rise, ejection fraction falls more, and cardiac output is progressively compromised, particularly with exercise. Pathologic examination either postmortem or by cardiac biopsy shows varying degrees of myocardial cell hypertrophy and degeneration, as well as interstitial and perivascular fibrosis [54]. Inflammatory cell infiltrates or biopsy may indicate myocarditis

[37]. Mural thrombi, especially in the ventricular apex, are often noted at postmortem examination.

Most often no specific etiology is discovered. These cases are often presumed to be of viral origin; however, it is not clear if all or even most cases of idiopathic dilated cardiomyopathy are a result of a viral myocarditis. Many other causes of dilated cardiomyopathy have been described. Although most of these are rare, dilated cardiomyopathy associated with pregnancy, heavy alcohol use, or adriamycin therapy does occur with some frequency [88].

DIAGNOSIS

Unfortunately, symptoms are usually not present until late in the course of the cardiomyopathy. Symptoms of congestive heart failure are the most common presenting complaints, but chest pain may be present [131]. Atrial or ventricular arrhythmias or, less commonly, systemic emboli may first draw attention to the underlying cardiac disease.

The physical examination demonstrates an enlarged displaced apex impulse. A third heart sound is usually heard over either or both ventricles, and a fourth heart sound may be present. Murmurs of mitral or tricuspid regurgitation result from ventricular dilation, which in turn causes distortion of the subvulvular structures and dilatation of the valve ring. Other physical findings depend on the relative involvement of the right and left sides of the heart, as well as the severity of heart failure. Low arterial blood pressure, a narrow pulse pressure, and pulsus alternans reflect low cardiac output. Signs of left-sided

Table 1–12. *Features of the Cardiomyopathies*

	Dilated (congestive)	Hypertrophic	Restrictive
Systolic function	Decreased	Mildly increased or decreased	Normal or decreased
Ventricular cavity size	Increased	Slightly decreased	Slightly decreased
Diastolic function	Normal or slightly decreased	Decreased	Decreased
End-diastolic pressures	Increased	Increased	Increased
Myocardial mass	Increased	Increased	Normal or increased
Myocardial wall thickness	Normal	Increased	Normal or increased
Ventricular outflow gradient	None	Often present/provokable	None

Source: Adapted from C. M. Oakley, Clinical decisions in the cardiomyopathies, *Hosp. Pract.* 20: 47–49, Oct., 1985.

heart failure such as rales and of right-sided heart failure such as edema, ascites, and hepatomegaly are often present.

The chest x-ray demonstrates cardiac enlargement and pulmonary vascular redistribution. Interstitial and alveolar edema and pleural effusions may be present depending on the severity of the heart failure.

The electrocardiogram is usually abnormal but not specific. Sinus tachycardia, conduction defects such as left bundle-branch block or intramyocardial conduction delay, and nonspecific ST-segment and T-wave changes are all common. Atrial and ventricular arrhythmias are frequent, especially as the cardiomyopathy worsens.

Echocardiography is useful to exclude significant valvular disease and to define the size of the cardiac chambers, ventricular function, and myocardial wall thickness [38]. Four-chamber dilatation with globally diminished ventricular function is most often found. Radionuclide ventriculography can be used to assess ventricular function, but it is less accurate than echocardiography in defining chamber size. Cardiac catheterization with coronary angiography can be used to measure intracardiac pressures and cardiac output, to perform ventriculography, and to detect significant coronary artery disease; however, cardiac catheterization is often not necessary because similar information may be obtained noninvasively from radionuclide angiography and echocardiography. End-diastolic pressures in both ventricles are usually increased, and pulmonary hypertension is

often present. Resting cardiac output may be normal or depressed. Ventriculography shows a globally hypokinetic left ventricle often with mild to moderate mitral regurgitation.

A cardiac biopsy may be done at the time of right-sided heart catheterization. A bioptome is inserted percutaneously into the right ventricle through the internal jugular vein, and four or five biopsies are taken from the interventricular septum. Biopsy results are usually nonspecific in dilated cardiomyopathy; however, certain diseases such as myocarditis, sarcoidosis, hemochromotosis, and others can be detected by biopsy [54].

When a patient presents with dilated cardiomyopathy, careful evaluation is necessary [88]. Patients should be asked about travel to regions endemic for Chagas' disease, treatment with anthracyclines, and alcohol intake. Normal blood urea nitrogen and creatinine, phosphorus, and calcium levels exclude uremia, hypophosphatemia, and hypocalcemia, respectively, as causes. Serum iron levels may exclude hemochromatosis. Echocardiography can detect unsuspected valvular disease such as aortic stenosis and determine wall thickness and ventricular size and function. Tests for sarcoidosis may be necessary if there are other suggestive findings, and levels of antinuclear antibodies and rheumatoid factor may be helpful. If the illness has been recent, especially if associated with fever, antistreptolysin O, enterovirus, *Toxoplasma,* and *Mycoplasma* titers are warranted.

At present, the need for cardiac biopsy in every

case of dilated cardiomyopathy is controversial. Although inflammatory cell infiltrates may occasionally be found and may be presumptive evidence of myocarditis, the absolute pathologic criteria for this diagnosis vary, and it is not yet clear whether immunosuppressive therapy is beneficial.

TREATMENT

Therapy for dilated cardiomyopathy is directed at the underlying cause, the exacerbating factors, and the symptoms of congestive heart failure. With some diseases, such as hemochromotosis, specific treatment is available. When anthracyclines or alcohol are the precipitating factor, they should be scrupulously avoided. Most often, since the underlying cause is not known, there is no specific therapy. Factors that might increase the workload of the heart, such as anemia and thyrotoxicosis, should be corrected, and myocardial depressants, such as alcohol, beta-adrenergic blockers, some calcium blockers, and disopyramide, should be avoided. Hypertension should be controlled, and some restriction of physical activity is probably wise. While evidence suggests that prolonged bed rest may lead to improvement in myocardial function, this is not universally accepted; few patients are able to tolerate prolonged strict bed rest. When left ventricular dysfunction is marked, anticoagulation may decrease the incidence of systemic embolization from mural thrombus [60]. Antiarrhythmic drugs are indicated for sustained or symptomatic arrhythmias. The place of these drugs in patients with dilated cardiomyopathy and nonsustained ventricular tachycardia is not yet clear. Diuretics, vasodilators, and inotropic drugs may ameliorate symptoms of congestive heart failure and are discussed in more detail in that section.

The prognosis of patients with dilated cardiomyopathy is poor. Usually there is progressive deterioration, with half the patients dying suddenly and the other half dying of worsening heart failure. More than half are dead within 5 years [60]. A better prognosis is found in young patients and patients with low intracardiac filling pressures, a cardiac index greater than 3 liters/min/m² and few ventricular arrhythmias [60,56,33]. Only recently has drug therapy with hydralazine and isosorbide dinitrate (Isordil) or with enalapril been shown to provide some improvement in survival [33,30]. Cardiac transplantation offers prolonged survival in those most critically ill, although the economic and emotional costs are great [53].

Prognosis may be better in some situations. In patients with alcoholic cardiomyopathy, complete abstinence may reverse or at least halt the cardiomyopathic process [135]. In some women with peripartum cardiomyopathy, heart size may improve or return to normal within 6 months. However, the syndrome may occur in subsequent pregnancies, particularly in those women with persistent cardiomegaly [84]. Finally, cardiomyopathy associated with chemotherapeutic agents such as doxorubicin, is dose-related and probably can be minimized [96].

Hypertrophic Cardiomyopathy

PATHOPHYSIOLOGY

Hypertrophic cardiomyopathy reflects a spectrum of abnormalities of the myocardium in which the primary problem is myocardial hypertrophy without an obvious cause for the hypertrophy such as hypertension or aortic stenosis. The hypertrophy most commonly occurs in the ventricular septum, accounting for the term *asymmetric septal hypertrophy*. However, hypertrophy may involve the left ventricle symmetrically or occasionally involve only localized portions of the ventricle such as the left ventricular apex or the posterior septum [115]. In as many as 15 percent of cases, the right ventricular outflow tract may be involved. Hypertrophy may range from mild to massive. Microscopic inspection of the hypertrophic myocardium shows significant myocardial fiber disarray—the cells are wider and shorter than normal and often have bizarre shapes and disorganized orientation. Small areas of these bizarre cells are interspersed among normal-appearing myocardial cells in a patchy pattern. While this pattern of myocardial fiber disarray was once felt to be specific for hypertrophic cardiomyopathy, it is now known to occur in many disease states such as congenital heart disease, concentric left ventricular hypertrophy due to a pressure overload, and coronary artery disease. However, the amount of disorganization and disarray appears to be quantitatively different in that it involves much more of the myocardium in hypertrophic cardiomyopathy.

In patients with hypertrophic cardiomyopathy, ventricular filling is impeded by the stiffness and abnormal relaxation of the ventricle. Thus end-diastolic pressure increases, atrial pressure increases, and dyspnea, the most common presenting symptom, results. In many cases of hypertrophic cardiomyopathy, the left ventricular outflow tract is narrowed by the hypertrophied septum and the anterior leaflet of the mitral valve which abuts the septum in systole. This results in obstruction to left ventricular outflow and a gradient between the left ventricular cavity and the aortic subvalvular region. This obstruction led to such initial terminology for this disease as idiopathic hypertrophic subaortic stenosis (IHSS) and hypertrophic obstructive cardiomyopathy (HOCM). While significant controversy still exists concerning the importance of the obstruction in the pathophysiology, several factors suggest that the abnormal diastolic function and not the obstruction is most important [125,147]. The degree of obstruction does not clearly predict either symptoms or prognosis, and most of the blood is ejected from the ventricle more rapidly than normal in hypertrophic cardiomyopathy irrespective of the presence or degree of measurable obstruction.

The cause of hypertrophic cardiomyopathy is unknown. It has been suggested that abnormal ventricular geometry or abnormal sympathetic stimulation may lead to increased wall stress with resulting hypertrophy. The disease is inherited as an autosomal-dominant trait, but as in Marfan's syndrome, there is marked variation in its actual expression.

DIAGNOSIS
Patients with hypertrophic cardiomyopathy may be asymptomatic or may have severe, incapacitating symptoms. The most common symptom is dyspnea, but fatigue, angina pectoris, and syncope or near syncope are common [58]. Exertion exacerbates most of these symptoms. Angina occurs in the absence of atherosclerotic coronary disease, although in the older patient coronary disease is not uncommon. Syncope may occur particularly with cessation of exercise when sympathetic stimulation is still high, but venous return falls as muscular action is no longer pumping blood back to the heart. While hypertrophic cardiomyopathy is most often a disease of young people, as many as one-third of patients referred for cardiac catheterization are over age 60 [174]. In the elderly, the symptoms are often attributed to aortic valve disease or coronary artery disease.

Ventricular arrhythmias are quite common in hypertrophic cardiomyopathy, with as many as 50 percent of patients having multiform or coupled ventricular extrasystoles and 25 percent having nonsustained ventricular tachycardia [120]. Ventricular arrhythmias may predict those patients at highest risk of sudden death [120]. Sudden death is a particular problem in the young patient with hypertrophic cardiomyopathy who may be otherwise asymptomatic. Hypertrophic cardiomyopathy is the most common definable cause of unexpected sudden death in young, competitive athletes [116].

Physical examination is helpful in the diagnosis of hypertrophic cardiomyopathy [58]. The carotid upstroke is usually brisk, reflecting the rapid ejection of blood. This is in contrast to the slowly rising carotid pulse of aortic stenosis. In addition, the carotid upstroke may demonstrate a double systolic impulse due to the systolic gradient. A prominent *a* wave is seen in the jugular veins due to the hypertrophied, poorly compliant septum. A presystolic impulse is often palpable over the left ventricular apex as the noncompliant ventricle provokes a forceful atrial systole. The apical impulse may be displaced and is usually sustained and forceful. A double systolic impulse, again reflecting the systolic gradient, may be palpated over the ventricular apex. Combined with the presystolic impulse, this may give a characteristic triple apical beat [34]. A fourth heart sound is frequent, and a systolic ejection click is rare. The second heart sound is usually normal, but with severe obstruction it may be paradoxically split. A third heart sound is a variable finding. The typical murmur is systolic, harsh, crescendo-decrescendo, and best heard between the lower left sternal border and the apex. The murmur radiates toward the base of the heart but not into the neck, a feature that helps distinguish it from the murmur of aortic stenosis. The murmur is due to turbulence of blood as it is forcefully ejected through the narrowed left ventricular outflow tract. The murmur may be more holosystolic and blowing at the apex due to the mitral regurgitation which is often present. The murmur often increases with maneuvers that decrease the size of the ventricle (Valsalva, amyl nitrite inhalation) or increase myocardial contractility (isoproterenol, post-premature ventricular contraction). Maneuvers that increase ventricular size or decrease ventricular contractility have the opposite effect [34]. These maneuvers may help distinguish the most common systolic murmurs heard in adults, as shown in Table 1-13.

The electrocardiogram is usually abnormal, with the most common findings being ST-segment and T-wave abnormalities. Evidence of ventricular hypertrophy is common, and pathologic Q waves may occur, particularly in the inferior, right, or lateral precordial leads, simulating myocardial infarction [58]. Both ventricular and supraventricular arrhythmias are common.

The chest x-ray is nonspecific and may show a normal or enlarged left ventricle. Signs of pulmonary vascular redistribution may be present. Signs of valvular aortic stenosis such as a dilated proximal aorta or calcium in the aortic valve are helpful by their absence.

The echocardiogram is particularly useful in the diagnosis of hypertrophic cardiomyopathy [48]. There is hypertrophy of the septum, often with relative sparing of the left ventricular posterior wall. However, as already discussed, there is marked variation in the patterns of hypertrophy in individual patients [115]. A ratio of at least 1.3:1 of the septal thickness to posterior wall thickness is often found, reflecting the predominant involvement of the septum. In fact, this asymmetric septal hypertrophy (ASH) is often seen in asymptomatic first-degree relatives of patients with hypertrophic cardiomyopathy, reflecting the autosomal-dominant genetic transmission in many patients. However, asymmetric septal hypertrophy may occur in patients undergoing hemodialysis and in patients with hypertrophy due to aortic stenosis or hypertension, and hypertrophic cardiomyopathy may occur without asymmetric septal hypertrophy. Septal motion and thickening are usually both decreased, and signs of diminished left ventricular compliance are present. The cross-sectional echocardiogram is especially useful for identifying unusual areas or patterns of hypertrophy. During systole, the mitral anterior leaflet may move toward and even touch the interventricular septum—the so-called systolic anterior motion (SAM) of the mitral valve. The role of obstruction in the pathophysiology of this disease is still being debated. There is a relationship between the degree of systolic anterior motion and the pressure gradient measured at catheterization between the body of the left ventricle and the left ventricular outflow tract just below the aortic valve. Just as the Valsalva maneuver or administration of amyl nitrite may increase the systolic murmur, the degree of systolic anterior motion and pressure gradient may be provoked or increased with these maneuvers. However, even systolic anterior motion is not specific for hypertrophic cardiomyopathy and may occur in other situations.

Cardiac catheterization is not necessary in the diagnosis of hypertrophic cardiomyopathy, because the echocardiographic and Doppler ultrasound features are diagnostic. However, some rel-

Table 1-13. *Effects of Several Maneuvers on Systolic Murmurs*

	Valsalva	Post-PVC	Handgrip	Amyl nitrite
Aortic stenosis	↓	↑	↓	↑
Hypertrophic cardiomyopathy	↑	↑	↓	↑
Mitral regurgitation	↓	—	↑	↓

↑ = increase, ↓ = decrease, — = no change

atively specific hemodynamic features may be noted at catheterization, and if angina is a significant symptom, coronary angiography may be necessary. Owing to diastolic dysfunction, an elevated left ventricular end-diastolic pressure is generally present. A pressure gradient between the left ventricular cavity and the aortic subvalvular region may be present or absent at rest but is often provokable by the same maneuvers which increase the murmur. The lability of the obstruction is peculiar to hypertrophic cardiomyopathy. A characteristic response is a marked increase in the pressure gradient and a fall in aortic pulse pressure that occurs following a premature ventricular beat. (The fall in aortic pulse pressure is referred to as the Brockenbrough response.) The decrease in aortic systolic pressure after a premature beat is the reverse of the normal post-premature ventricular contraction (post-PVC) response in aortic pressure. Left ventriculography may demonstrate hypertrophy, particularly of the papillary muscles, left ventricular cavity obliteration, and a peculiar appearance of the left ventricular cavity in end-systole. It should be noted that some patients with hypertrophic cardiomyopathy have neither a resting nor a provokable gradient [148].

TREATMENT

Therapy is generally directed toward improving diastolic function and decreasing contractility and increasing ventricular volume, the latter in an attempt to decrease the subvalvular pressure gradient. Most experience has been gained with beta-adrenergic blocking drugs, which decrease contractility and may improve diastolic function. Angina responds better than dyspnea, but symptomatic improvement is not always sustained

[148]. Calcium-channel blocking drugs may improve diastolic function and reduce contractility [110]. Most experience has been gained with verapamil, although nifedipine has been used with some success. Long-term symptomatic benefit may occur; however, serious adverse effects also may result. Other drugs, such as the antiarrhythmic agent disopyramide, which depress left ventricular function, may occasionally play a role in therapy. Amiodarone is perhaps the most promising new form of therapy [121]. In addition to its other effects, its antiarrhythmic actions may decrease the risk of sudden death. Because of the serious side effects associated with amiodarone, further study will be necessary to define its role.

Several other therapeutic measures are important. Patients should be instructed in endocarditis prophylaxis [58]. Strenuous exercise should be specifically avoided because of the risk of sudden death. When atrial fibrillation occurs, it often leads to marked hemodynamic deterioration because of the stiff ventricle; electrical cardioversion is usually necessary. Vasodilators are relatively contraindicated because they may decrease filling and lead to a reflex increase in sympathetic activity. Positive inotropic drugs such as digoxin are contraindicated except for rate control in atrial fibrillation. Occasionally, surgical therapy is recommended because of severe and refractory symptoms. The most common operation is resection of a portion of the septum, which does result in improved symptoms in some patients [163].

The prognosis in hypertrophic cardiomyopathy is quite variable. Most patients' symptoms remain stable, but progression often occurs. While the elderly are the most symptomatic, sudden death is a particular problem in the younger patient. Patients with a family history of sudden death, syncope, severe dyspnea, or significant ventricular arrhythmias seem to be at highest risk of sudden death [120]. To date, neither medical nor surgical therapy has been demonstrated to improve survival, although there is some hope that therapy with amiodarone, especially in high-risk patients, may improve prognosis. Rarely, hypertrophic cardiomyopathy progresses to a dilated cardiomyopathy. This seems to occur most often following septal resection or myocardial infarction.

Restrictive Cardiomyopathy

PATHOPHYSIOLOGY

Restrictive cardiomyopathy is a descriptive term for a group of diseases all of which result in a similar clinical and hemodynamic pattern. These diseases cause thickening of the ventricular walls due to infiltration or fibrosis and may involve the endocardium. The basic abnormality is increased ventricular stiffness resulting in a restriction to filling. The disease is often idiopathic, but a secondary identifiable cause such as amyloidosis, scleroderma, sarcoidosis, hemochromatosis, carcinoid, Fabry's disease, or endomyocardial fibrosis may be found. Usually the ventricles are normal in size or only slightly enlarged with infiltration and scarring of the myocardium. Specific microscopic features of the causative diseases can be found with myocardial biopsy or at postmortem examination. Because of the increased ventricular stiffness, the ventricular end-diastolic pressure is usually increased with resulting increases in atrial pressures. Systolic ventricular function may be normal early but often decreases as the disease progresses.

DIAGNOSIS

Most patients present with symptoms and signs of left- or right-sided heart failure or both. Dyspnea, especially with exertion, is a prominent feature, since the exercise-induced tachycardia accentuates the limitation in diastolic filling. Weakness is often present, but chest pain is not common [180]. The jugular veins are usually elevated with prominent *x* and *y* descents. The apical impulse is most often normal or only slightly displaced. An S_4 and S_3 are common, and the murmurs of tricuspid and mitral regurgitation are often present. Signs of pulmonary and/or systemic venous congestion are present depending on the severity of the disease. The chest x-ray is not specific, often revealing pulmonary venous congestion and/or mild cardiomegaly. The ECG is also nonspecific and may show low voltage, nonspecific ST-T-wave changes, conduction disturbances, and atrial and ventricular arrhythmias. The low voltage is particularly suggestive of an infiltrative (as opposed to a hypertrophic) process when the echocardiogram detects an increased left ventricular wall thickness and mass [24].

Typical echocardiographic features include thickened ventricular walls with little increase in chamber size. The atria are usually dilated, and systolic ventricular function is normal or reduced. The echocardiogram may be useful in excluding a pericardial effusion and cardiac tamponade. Some of the diseases may have specific echocardiographic features such as bright speckled myocardial echoes in amyloidosis [24].

Cardiac catheterization demonstrates elevated right and left ventricular end-diastolic pressures—usually with the left-sided pressures higher. The ventricular diastolic pressure shows an early dip with a rise to a plateau—the square root sign. The right atrial pressure shows the prominent *x* and *y* descents (the M sign) as described in the jugular veins. Myocardial biopsy is often indicated and may be done at the time of catheterization.

It is often difficult to differentiate restrictive cardiomyopathy from constrictive pericarditis. In restrictive disease, the left-sided pressures are usually a little higher than the right-sided pressures—especially with exercise or volume loading—whereas with constrictive pericarditis they are equal. Other hemodynamic features may help differentiate the two processes, and biopsy may help in the diagnosis of a specific restrictive process [9]. On occasion, surgical exploration may be necessary, especially since constrictive pericarditis is a reversible problem.

TREATMENT

The therapy of restrictive cardiomyopathy is usually frustrating. Occasionally, processes such as sarcoidosis or hemochromatosis may be arrested or reversed medically. Surgery may be helpful in endomyocardial fibrosis, but in general, supportive therapy is all that is available. A low-salt diet and diuretics improve pulmonary and systemic venous congestion. Cardiac glycosides may be helpful in some patients, but patients with amyloidosis may be particularly prone to toxicity. Vasodilators are not usually beneficial, but specific venous vasodilators such as nitroglycerin may decrease pulmonary congestion. Anticoagulation may be of benefit in preventing pulmonary emboli and left ventricular thrombi in some of these patients [180].

In general, most of the diseases causing restrictive cardiomyopathy have a poor prognosis. However, those patients with idiopathic restrictive cardiomyopathy may have a better overall prognosis, with some patients actually demonstrating clinical improvement over time [9].

Myocarditis

Pathophysiology

Myocarditis is an inflammatory process involving the myocardium. It may be associated with infections resulting from direct involvement by the infectious agent, by toxins, or by an autoimmune process initiated by the infection. In addition, radiation, physical toxins, and other agents may cause myocarditis [180]. The process may be acute or chronic and mild or severe, resulting in various degrees of myocardial dysfunction.

Diagnosis

The diagnosis of myocarditis is made only rarely, although it probably occurs much more frequently, since autopsy studies show evidence of healed myocarditis in 4 to 10 percent of routine postmortem examinations. The symptoms of the causative infection or toxin often predominate, and the symptoms of myocarditis such as palpitations, fatigue, or mild dyspnea may be attributed to the underlying infection. Thus, unless the myocarditis is severe and significant symptoms of heart failure develop, myocarditis is often not detected.

Sinus tachycardia is frequent and often out of proportion to any fever. Heart sounds may be muffled, and a third heart sound may be noted.

The ECG often shows nonspecific ST-T-wave abnormalities; atrial and ventricular arrhythmias and conduction defects also may be seen [1]. The diagnosis is usually made by identifying the underlying disease along with subtle evidence of myocardial dysfunction. The latter may be detected with echocardiography or radionuclide studies. Endomyocardial biopsy may document the myocardial inflammation, but it does not usually elucidate the underlying cause [50].

Treatment

Treatment is supportive and directed at the underlying illness. Strenuous exertion should be avoided during the acute illness, and known myocardial toxins should be avoided. Rarely, serious arrhythmias or conduction defects will require therapy. If heart failure develops, routine management is useful. The role of steroids and immunosuppressive therapy is not yet clear.

Congestive Heart Failure

There are 2 to 3 million people in the United States with heart failure, and 200,000 to 300,000 new cases are diagnosed each year [154]. The costs of treatment as well as disability are enormous. Understanding of the pathophysiology of this syndrome has significantly improved in the last 10 years, and with this understanding have come therapeutic gains. However, much remains to be learned if we are to alter the grim prognosis associated with congestive heart failure.

Pathophysiology

Heart failure is often defined as the inability of the heart (due to a cardiac abnormality) to pump enough blood to meet the metabolic needs of the body. However, at times, oxygen delivery is adequate, but symptoms of pulmonary or systemic venous congestion limit the patient. Thus it is probably most accurate to define heart failure as the heart's inability to pump enough blood to prevent symptoms of either inadequate oxygen delivery or pulmonary or systemic venous congestion.

Heart failure is not a specific disease, but rather a symptom complex or syndrome. There are a large number of disease processes which result in heart failure due to myocardial disease, mechanical obstruction, electrical abnormalities, or a combination of these factors (Table 1-14).

The initiating event in heart failure is a decrease in cardiac output due to any of the causes listed in Table 1-14. This is demonstrated in Fig. 1-10a with a typical set of ventricular function curves. These curves are drawn with a measure of cardiac output (cardiac output, cardiac index, stroke volume, stroke volume index) on the y axis, plotted against a measure of ventricular filling pressure on the x axis. Ventricular filling pressure may be represented as the left ventricular end-diastolic pressure (LVEDP), the left atrial pressure (LAP), or the pulmonary capillary wedge pressure (PCWP). As shown in Fig. 1-10a, in heart failure, the ventricular function curve is shifted downward and

Table 1–14. *Causes of Heart Failure*

I. Myocardial:
  A. Primary:
    1. Idiopathic cardiomyopathy:
      a. Dilated
      b. Hypertrophic
      c. Restrictive
  B. Secondary:
    1. Ischemic heart disease (e.g., myocardial infarction)
    2. Pressure overload (e.g., aortic stenosis, hypertension)
    3. Volume overload (e.g., valvular regurgitation, atrial septal defect)
    4. Connective-tissue diseases (e.g., scleroderma, polymyositis)
    5. Metabolic diseases (e.g., hemochromatosis)
    6. Infections (e.g., Chagas' disease)
    7. Inherited diseases (e.g., Fabry's disease)
    8. Metals (e.g., cobalt)
    9. Miscellaneous (e.g., sarcoid)
II. Mechanical:
  A. Obstruction to ventricular filling (e.g., mitral stenosis, pericardial constriction or tamponade)
  B. Miscellaneous (e.g., ventricular aneurysm, left atrial myxoma)

to the right; thus, at any given ventricular filling pressure, cardiac output is less than normal. An understanding of the four major determinants of myocardial performance are necessary if one is to understand the pathophysiology of heart failure: (1) the length-force relationship, (2) afterload, (3) contractility, and (4) heart rate. Shortening and force of contraction are improved as muscle fiber length is increased—the Frank-Starling effect. The change in fiber length, or preload, is represented by ventricular end-diastolic volume in the intact heart or organism. Because end-diastolic volume is difficult to measure, a measure of end-diastolic pressure is substituted. The effect of an increase in preload on cardiac output is shown in Fig. 1-10b. Afterload, or the load against which the ventricle must eject blood, is best defined as wall stress, that is,

$$\text{Wall stress} = \frac{PR}{2h}$$

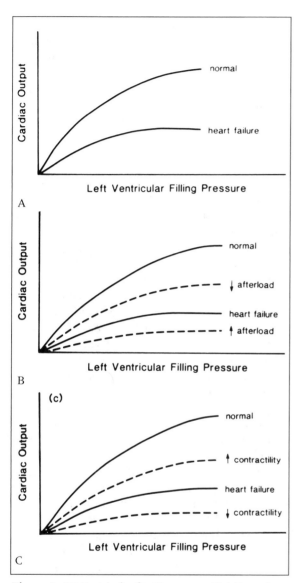

Figure 1–10. *Ventricular function curves. (A) Normal and heart failure. (B) Effect of increasing and decreasing afterload. (C) Effects of increasing and decreasing contractility.*

where P = ventricular systolic pressure, R = ventricular radius, and h = ventricular wall thickness. With increased afterload, the ventricular function curve shifts downward and to the right, while the opposite occurs with a decrease in afterload (see Fig. 1-10b). A primary change in the force or velocity of contraction is referred to as a change in contractility. An increase in contractility shifts the ventricular function curve upward and to the left (Fig. 1-10c), while a decrease in contractility shifts the curve downward and to the right [18]. Finally, if other factors are stable, the cardiac output will vary with the heart rate.

Once a fall in cardiac output occurs, compensatory mechanisms, both acute and chronic, are useful in supporting cardiac output [182,57]. Initially, when cardiac output falls, there is increased activity of the sympathetic nervous system leading to increased heart rate and myocardial contractility. Increased arteriolar tone in muscle and splanchnic beds allows for adequate perfusion of vital organs such as the brain and heart. Increased venous tone may increase venous return. Although in general these are beneficial processes, the increase in systemic vascular resistance may further reduce cardiac output. In fact, this is the basis for the beneficial effect of vasodilator therapy in heart failure. In addition to increased sympathetic activity, there may be increased activity of the renin-angiotensin-aldosterone axis promoting both salt and water retention as well as vasoconstriction [44]. Other neurohumoral mechanisms mediated by vasopressin or atrial natriuretic peptide also may be important [161,45,15]. A second compensatory mechanism which occurs is the Frank-Starling mechanism already discussed. As the ventricle dilates and salt and water retention occur, end-diastolic volume increases resulting in increased stroke volume and cardiac output. The enlarged end-diastolic volume may allow maintenance of stroke volume despite the overall decrease in myocardial function. For example, a normal ventricle with an end-diastolic volume of 100 ml and an ejection function of 60 percent has a stroke volume of 60 ml. A dilated ventricle with an end-diastolic volume of 200 ml and an ejection fraction of only 30 percent still has a stroke volume of 60 ml. However, there may be a negative side to the increased end-diastolic volume—an increase in myocardial wall stress. If the ventricle dilates without an accompanying increase in ventricular wall thickness, wall stress is increased, further compromising ventricular function. If myocardial hypertrophy is enough to increase wall thickness as volumes are increasing, wall-stress changes may be less severe. Thus ventricular hypertrophy may be an additional beneficial compensatory mechanism.

Understanding of the pathophysiology of heart failure would be incomplete without attention to the balance between myocardial oxygen supply and demand (see Table 1-4). Coronary perfusion pressure may be limited by low aortic diastolic pressure, by high ventricular diastolic pressure, or by both. Myocardial oxygen consumption may be increased by such factors as tachycardia, high sympathetic activity, and increased ventricular size and afterload. This balance may assume particular importance in the patient with coronary artery disease, in whom coronary perfusion pressure is critical.

While compensatory mechanisms provide significant benefit in patients with heart failure, detrimental effects also may occur. Increases in left ventricular end-diastolic pressure are reflected by increased left atrial and pulmonary venous pressures. These increases lead to movement of fluid into the interstitial space of the lung resulting in decreased pulmonary compliance. As more fluid collects, gas exchange is affected—especially in the lower lobes of the lungs where capillary pressure is the highest. Local hypoxia results in vasoconstriction of the pulmonary vessels to the lower portions of the lungs, redirecting pulmonary arterial blood flow to the upper portions of the lungs. As pulmonary venous pressure rises even higher, fluid may move into the alveolar spaces resulting in pulmonary edema. Increases in right atrial pressure lead to systemic venous congestion and edema, particularly noticeable in dependent portions of the body where pressures are the

highest. Congestion of the liver, spleen, and bowel may occur and may be severe enough to alter absorption and metabolism of drugs because of hepatic congestion and bowel edema. Fluid may accumulate in the pleural and abdominal cavities. Peripheral arterioles in organ beds are vasoconstricted. High levels of sympathetic activity and angiotensin, as well as other factors, lead to vasoconstriction allowing redistribution of blood flow to vital organs by diverting flow from the exercising muscle bed. In addition, excess salt and water retention or pressure from extravascular fluid may increase vascular stiffness and diminish vasodilatory capacity [182].

Different terms have been used to classify heart failure. These are low-output versus high-output and forward versus backward failure. Heart failure most often occurs when there is low cardiac output; however, some patients will have symptoms of heart failure when the cardiac output is unexpectedly high. This high-output heart failure is usually due to either an arteriovenous shunt or a markedly increased requirement for blood. High-output failure may be associated with anemia, beriberi, thyrotoxicosis, Paget's disease (arteriovenous fistulas in bone), and sepsis. High-output failure is extremely rare if the heart is entirely normal. It usually occurs when there is an increased requirement for blood and mild to moderate myocardial dysfunction. Thus, while cardiac output is higher than usual in patients with heart failure, it is not as high as might be expected with a completely normal heart. In general, patients with high-output failure have warm extremities with bounding peripheral pulses and a widened pulse pressure, in contrast to the patients with low-output failure, who have cool extremities and diminished peripheral pulses.

Forward failure refers to the inability to provide adequate blood supply to peripheral organs. This leads to signs and symptoms of poor cerebral, renal, and skeletal muscle perfusion along with vasoconstriction. Backward failure is said to result when the heart is unable to pump all the blood it receives leading to pulmonary and/or systemic venous congestion. In general, these two are in-

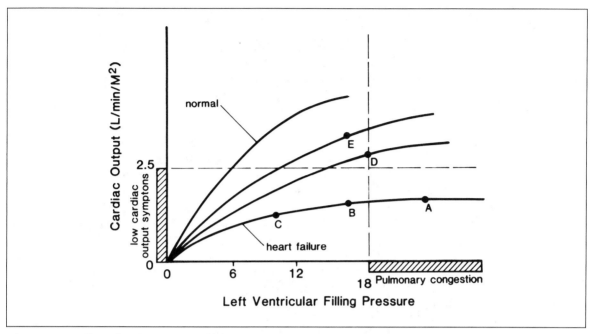

Figure 1–11. *Effects of various interventions in subjects with heart failure on the ventricular function curve. (Adapted from D. T. Mason (Ed.),* Congestive Heart Failure. *New York, Yorke Medical Books, 1976. Reproduced by permission.)*

tricately interrelated, and most patients have symptoms of both forward and backward failure, although one or the other may predominate based on the underlying disease, compensatory mechanisms, and therapy.

Diagnosis

When the left ventricle fails, the major clinical symptoms are varying degrees of dyspnea and signs of poor organ perfusion (Fig. 1-11). Dyspnea is a sense of breathlessness or difficulty breathing. When due to heart failure, it occurs when the lungs are stiffened by interstitial edema. Early in the course of heart failure dyspnea may be present only with exertion. As heart failure worsens, less and less exertion provokes dyspnea, until with severe heart failure dyspnea may occur at rest. Orthopnea is dyspnea occurring in the re-

cumbent position that is relieved by sitting or standing. With recumbency, fluid moves from the extremities and abdomen to the heart, which may not be able to pump the additional blood, resulting in increased pulmonary venous pressure. The severity of orthopnea is often measured by the number of pillows the patient requires to sleep comfortably. Paroxysmal nocturnal dyspnea (PND) usually occurs suddenly. The patient awakes from sleep with a feeling of extreme dyspnea and must sit or stand for several minutes. This occurs when fluid is reabsorbed from the extremities but cannot be accepted by the heart, leading to a sudden increase in pulmonary venous congestion.

Reduced cardiac output may result in symptoms of poor organ perfusion: muscle weakness and fatigue from poor skeletal muscle flow, confusion and somnolence from poor cerebral blood flow, and oliguria and nocturia from poor renal perfusion. Nocturia (increased frequency of urination at night) results when renal vasoconstriction brought on by upright posture and activity is reduced at night, by the increase in cardiac output in the supine position, and by the mobilization of fluid from the lower extremities. Several classifications have been used to grade patients on the degree of symptoms. The most commonly used is the New York Heart Association functional classification (page 24) [63]. The signs of failure of the right ventricle are those resulting from systemic venous hypertension such as elevated jugular venous pressure, dependent edema, and pain over the liver due to hepatic engorgement and stretching of the hepatic capsule. Congestion of the intestine may lead to bloating and abdominal distension, although the latter also may be due to ascites.

The physical findings depend on the cause of heart failure and its severity. The signs may vary from patients who appear normal at rest to those who have severe anxiety and dyspnea requiring them to sit upright. Respirations are often shallow and increased in frequency (tachypnea). If cardiac output is severely limited, the extremities may be cool with low amplitude pulses. The blood pressure is often low with a narrow pulse pressure. Pulsus alternans is alternating strong and weak arterial pulses and occurs when there is very severe left ventricular dysfunction resulting in low cardiac output. Abnormalities of the jugular venous pulse depend on the state of the right ventricle. With right ventricular failure, the mean jugular venous pressure is elevated. Kussmaul's sign, a paradoxical increase in venous pressure with inspiration, may be present. The hepatojugular reflux also may be present—this is best observed when sustained pressure is applied over the abdomen for 30 to 60 seconds while examining at the neck veins. A positive test is a rise in jugular venous pressure reflecting the inability of the right side of the heart to accept additional volume. Palpation of the precordium may reveal an enlarged, dyskinetic, or sustained left ventricular apical impulse depending on the underlying disease.

Auscultation may reveal clues to the specific underlying disease such as the murmur of aortic stenosis, but there are several findings which are

appreciated in most cases. A third heart sound (protodiastolic or ventricular gallop or S_3) is a low-frequency sound heard about 0.13 to 0.16 seconds after S_2. It occurs at the end of the rapid phase of ventricular filling and is due to the sharp deceleration of blood. A left ventricular S_3 is best heard over the apex immediately after inspiration, while a right ventricular S_3 is best heard along the lower left sternal border or over the epigastrium during inspiration. A fourth heart sound (presystolic or atrial gallop) is heard when the ventricle is poorly compliant and there is vigorous atrial contraction.

When there is significant enlargement of either ventricle, supporting structures of either atrioventricular valve may be distorted with resultant murmurs of mitral or tricuspid regurgitation. Rales may be heard at the lung bases in patients with mild heart failure. With worsening failure rales may be heard over more of the lung fields. With pulmonary edema rales are heard over most of the lungs, and the patient often produces blood-tinged, frothy sputum. Occasionally, irritation or congestion of the bronchioles may result in wheezing—referred to as cardiac asthma. Dullness over one or both bases may indicate a pleural effusion.

There are no specific electrocardiographic findings in heart failure, but the ECG may provide a clue to the underlying illness such as Q waves (suggesting a myocardial infarction) or evidence of left ventricular hypertrophy.

The chest x-ray is quite helpful in patients with heart failure. The size of the cardiac silhouette can be evaluated. Specific findings of underlying causes of heart failure such as valvular or pericardial calcification may be noted. Changes in the appearance of the lung fields associated with pulmonary venous congestion can be detected [14]. When pulmonary venous pressures are normal in an upright subject, blood flow is greatest to the lower lobes and these vessels are larger than those to the upper lobes. As pulmonary venous and capillary pressures increase, pulmonary blood flow is diverted to the upper lobes and these upper-lobe vessels appear more prominent. Interstitial edema in the interlobular septa may produce Kerley B lines—sharp, thin, horizontal lines at the periphery of the lungs. Perivascular edema results in haziness of the central and peripheral vessels. Finally, with very high pulmonary capillary pressures, alveolar edema results with infiltrates in the perihilar regions—the "butterfly" appearance. Pleural effusions may appear in either right- or left-sided failure or both.

Once the diagnosis of heart failure is made, additional tests may be necessary to determine the underlying cause of heart failure. The echocardiogram and Doppler studies can be useful in excluding valvular and congenital heart disease, can identify the specific chambers involved, and can be used to estimate the severity of ventricular dysfunction or valve disease. Radionuclide ventriculography can define right and left ventricular ejection fractions. Both techniques are useful in identifying regional wall-motion abnormalities such as occur with myocardial infarction. Cardiac catheterization may be necessary to assess coronary artery disease and can precisely define intracardiac pressures and cardiac output at rest and with exercise.

Blood chemistry studies are not usually abnormal in the untreated patient with mild to moderate heart failure. In more severe heart failure, bilirubin and liver enzyme levels may be elevated if there is hepatic congestion and reduced hepatic blood flow. The specific gravity of the urine is high, and the urinary sodium level is low; however, these change as diuretic therapy is instituted. If renal blood flow and glomerular filtration rate are significantly compromised, the blood urea nitrogen level may rise.

Treatment

It is usually important to define the etiology of heart failure. If there is specific medical or surgical therapy for the disease causing the heart failure, it should be undertaken. Even if no specific therapy is available, knowledge of the underlying disease, its physiology, and its severity is important in assessing prognosis and in applying standard

Table 1–15. *Congestive Heart Failure: Potential Exacerbating Factors*

Increased sodium intake
Medication noncompliance
Medication interactions
Concurrent infections
Anemia
Thyroid disease
Increased cardiac workload
Pulmonary embolism
Arrhythmias
Drug effects:
    Negative inotropic (beta-adrenergic blockers, calcium-channel blockers, disopyramide, alcohol, etc.)
    Sodium retention (steroids, estrogens, nonsteroidal anti-inflammatory drugs, etc.)

medical therapy. If there is no specific therapy for the underlying disease, palliative therapy has five basic goals:

1. Remove precipitating factors
2. Apply standard preventative health measures
3. Reduce the workload of the heart
4. Control salt and water retention
5. Improve myocardial contractility.

Quite frequently, the onset or worsening of heart failure is due to a clear precipitating factor (Table 1-15). It is important to determine if any of these factors are present, since correction or removal of the factor may obviate the need for additional medical therapy. As heart failure progresses, the likelihood of medication interactions or side effects, infections, arrhythmias, and pulmonary emboli all increase. In addition, there may be recurrence of the underlying disease such as new myocardial ischemia or restenosis of the mitral valve after commissurotomy. The myocardial depressant effects of alcohol should be discussed with every patient [155].

Reducing the workload of the heart may be accomplished in several ways. Both physical and emotional stress should be decreased, although this may be difficult, especially in the face of a serious illness. Emotional stress is often improved by giving the patient as much information and control as he or she desires and can handle. The patient should lose weight if he or she is obese. Medical therapy with vasodilators will reduce the workload of the heart, but usually this is reserved for patients with moderate or severe heart failure.

Patients with heart failure should be especially careful about their general medical care. Influenza and pneumococcal pneumonia vaccines should be given to most patients. Good dental care is mandatory in patients with valvular or congenital disease. Infections and other illnesses may exacerbate heart failure and should be treated early and vigorously. Smoking should be stopped.

The control of salt and water retention is begun by avoiding added salt and foods with a very high salt content. More strict sodium restriction is necessary if symptoms are severe. If these measures fail to resolve symptoms of heart failure, pharmacologic therapy, which includes diuretics, digitalis glycosides, and vasodilators, may be instituted.

If symptoms of heart failure are mild, a diuretic such as a thiazide is often combined with sodium restriction. If heart failure is more severe, loop diuretics such as furosemide are used. Digoxin is often added at this stage to improve contractility. As heart failure worsens, diuretic doses are increased, sodium restriction is tightened, and vasodilators are added. The actual order by which each of these pharmacologic measures should be applied—particularly digoxin—remains controversial. The effects of various types of drug therapy on the ventricular function curve are shown in Fig. 1-11. Current studies to determine the value of instituting vasodilator therapy earlier in the course of therapy are in progress. A strong case can be made for using vasodilators prior to digoxin in patients with heart failure who do not have atrial arrhythmias.

Several types of diuretics may be used to treat the salt and water retention which occurs in congestive heart failure [151]. In general, diuretics tend to improve symptoms of pulmonary congestion (see Fig. 1-11, A to B). However, if diuresis is excessive and preload falls too low,

symptoms and signs of low cardiac output may worsen (Fig. 1-11, B to C). If a mild diuretic is needed, thiazides may be valuable; however, if more diuresis is needed, or if there is impaired renal function, loop diuretics (furosemide, ethacrynic acid, bumetanide) are often necessary. Metolazone is a sulfonamide like the thiazides which acts primarily in the distal tubule to inhibit sodium reabsorption. Unlike the thiazides, however, metolazone remains active in the face of poor renal function. If large doses of loop diuretics are not enough, a thiazide or metolazone may be added. However, careful observation is necessary, since hypovolemia and hypokalemia may result. Complications of the loop diuretics are hypovolemia, hypokalemia, metabolic alkalosis, hyponatremia, glucose intolerance, and hyperuricemia. Side effects of the thiazide diuretics include hypokalemia, hypouricemia, hypercalcemia, and glucose intolerance. Many patients require potassium replacement, which is probably best given as the chloride salt. Potassium-sparing diuretics also may be used in patients who cannot tolerate potassium replacement and who do not have renal dysfunction.

Digitalis glycosides have a number of both direct and indirect cardiac effects [152]. The inotropic effects are primarily mediated by inhibition of Na-K ATPase in the sarcolemmal membrane. This inhibition results in increased intracellular sodium, which in turn increases intracellular calcium via the sodium-calcium exchange mechanism. The increased intracellular calcium results in activation of the contractile apparatus. Even though many digitalis preparations are available, digoxin is now used almost exclusively. It is about 80 percent absorbed, and it is excreted by the kidney in proportion to the glomerular filtration rate. Some renal tubular secretion of digoxin also may occur. The total loading dose is related to lean body mass, while the daily maintenance dose must be adjusted according to renal function. The effect of digoxin in heart failure is to move the ventricular function curve upward and to the left (Fig. 1-11, A to D). In the normal ventricle, digoxin may increase oxygen demands because of increased contractility; however, in the failing ventricle, improved function may result in decreased heart size and wall stress with no overall increase in myocardial oxygen demands. While some studies have suggested that digoxin has no long-term benefit in patients with heart failure and sinus rhythm, most carefully done studies indicate a sustained, although modest, symptomatic benefit if patients are correctly selected. The patients most likely to benefit from digoxin are those with myocardial systolic dysfunction [4]. Those with valvular obstruction or diastolic dysfunction are unlikely to benefit from digoxin therapy unless there are concomitant atrial arrhythmias. Patients with the obstructive form of hypertrophic cardiomyopathy may have an adverse response to digoxin. A number of conditions increase sensitivity to the development of digitalis toxicity, including electrolyte disturbances (particularly hypokalemia and hypomagnesmia), hypothyroidism, advanced age, renal insufficiency, amyloid heart disease, and hypoxia. The margin of therapeutic to toxic effects of digoxin is narrow. If there is a question about the correct maintenance dose, digoxin levels may be obtained. The use of digoxin levels is discussed in detail elsewhere [152]. Digoxin toxicity occurs with some frequency. Cardiac manifestations include arrhythmias of every variety, but particularly ventricular arrhythmias and nonparoxysmal junctional tachycardia. Paroxysmal atrial tachycardia with block is particularly suggestive of digoxin toxicity, but it is less common. Conduction abnormalities, particularly in the sinus or atrioventricular nodes, should prompt investigation in a patient on digoxin. Digoxin toxicity may be life-threatening—the patient in whom it is suspected should be hospitalized in a monitored unit and appropriate therapy should be administered [152]. Interactions between digoxin and other drugs (particularly quinidine, verapamil, and amiodarone) may raise digoxin blood levels and result in digoxin toxicity. A thorough knowledge of these interactions is mandatory [4].

Vasodilators represent important therapeutic agents in the patient with congestive heart failure [30]. This group of drugs has either potent venodilating effects (nitrates) or arteriolar dilating effects (hydralazine) or has effects on both systems (prazosin, angiotensin-converting enzyme inhibitors, nitroprusside). The mechanism of action of vasodilation varies among the drugs. Some act directly on vascular smooth muscle (nitrates, hydralazine), while others cause vasodilation by blocking a specific mechanism of vasoconstriction. Thus sympathetic nervous system blockade with prazosin or angiotensin-converting enzyme inhibition with captopril or enalapril all result in vasodilation in the patient with heart failure. Nitrates reduce preload, causing movement to the left on the ventricular function curve (Fig. 1-11, *A* to *B*), thus reducing symptoms of pulmonary venous congestion. In addition, nitrates may decrease wall stress if ventricular size decreases. Arteriolar vasodilators shift the ventricular function curve upward and to the left, resulting in improved cardiac output (Fig. 1-11, *A* to *E*). In general, hydralazine has been most successfully used in combination with long-acting nitrates in patients with heart failure and has been shown to improve life expectancy in these patients [30]. Balanced vasodilation (arteriolar and venous) can be achieved with prazosin and angiotensin-converting enzyme inhibitors. Prazocin is now used less frequently because of tachyphylaxis and because it does not improve survival [30]. Both captopril and enalapril result in long-term improvement in exercise capacity [23]. One study demonstrates improved survival in patients with severe heart failure treated with enalapril [33]. In patients with severe heart failure, particularly those with hyponatremia, the angiotensin-converting enzyme inhibitors should be started at very low doses to avoid severe hypotension. Nitroprusside can be given intravenously to provide balanced vasodilation [31]. All vasodilators can cause significant hypotension, particularly where there is concomitant volume depletion.

A number of potent inotropic agents are available for intravenous use [32]. The sympathomimetic drugs isoproterenol, dopamine, and dobutamine have been available for some time.

Dobutamine is the intravenous inotropic agent of choice in the patient with high ventricular filling pressures and low cardiac output [103]. Dopamine in low doses leads to renal and mesenteric vasodilation via specific dopaminergic receptors. At higher doses, dopamine causes significant vasoconstriction, which is detrimental unless symptomatic hypotension is present [62]. Amrinone is a new nonsympathomimetic inotropic drug approved for intravenous use in patients with heart failure [100].

When the patient continues to have severe symptoms despite medical therapy and has a very limited life expectancy, cardiac transplantation may be considered [53].

The prognosis in patients with heart failure is grim. The average mortality of those in New York Heart Association (NYHA) class II to III is 50 percent over 5 years, while those in NYHA class IV have a 50 percent 1-year mortality [55,56]. Once loss of a significant amount of myocardium has occurred, heart failure appears to be a progressive disease. Hopefully, new insights will lead to significant improvements in prognosis.

Pulmonary Edema

Cardiogenic pulmonary edema results when there is a relatively sudden severe increase in pulmonary capillary pressure. Interstitial edema develops rapidly, creating sufficient pressure to push fluid through the alveolar membranes resulting in alveolar edema. The edema may fill the airways, and the patient may have copious amounts of blood-tinged, foamy sputum. The patient presents with severe respiratory distress—usually sitting upright using the accessory muscles of respiration. Tachycardia, pallor due to peripheral vasoconstriction, cyanosis, and diaphoresis are often present. Rales are heard throughout the lower lung fields and may be heard even at the apices. Rhonchi and wheezes are common, as are ventricular gallop sounds. Other cardiac findings depend on the underlying cause. Pulmonary edema is a life-threatening situation. The patient should be allowed to sit upright and should receive supplemental oxygen. Morphine sulfate given intravenously in 2- to 4-mg doses is very effective because it decreases both the patient's anxiety and sympathetic tone, thus reducing both venous and arteriolar vasoconstriction. Morphine is contraindicated if there is disturbed consciousness or a marked reduction in ventilation as reflected by hypercapnia. Morphine antagonists and/or endotracheal intubation should be available should respiratory depression occur. Furosemide, 40 mg IV over 2 minutes, results in some improvement even prior to the onset of diuresis, probably as a result of venodilation. Digoxin is not usually necessary in the acute stage of pulmonary edema, although it may be valuable if there are associated atrial tachyarrhythmias. Nitroglycerin sublingually may be given to reduce cardiac preload and pulmonary congestion if the patient is not hypotensive. Occasionally, intravenous aminophylline is used, especially if there is doubt about whether the dyspnea may be due to bronchial asthma.

If there is confusion as to whether pulmonary edema is cardiogenic or noncardiogenic, measurement of the pulmonary capillary wedge pressure with a Swan-Ganz catheter will be helpful.

It is important to determine the cause of pulmonary edema, since specific medical or surgical therapy may be appropriate. Acute myocardial infarction is a relatively common cause of pulmonary edema and should be excluded. The other potential etiologies are the same as those for heart failure (see Table 1-14).

Pulmonary Hypertension

Pathophysiology

Pulmonary hypertension exists when the pulmonary artery systolic pressure is greater than 30 mmHg or when the pulmonary artery mean pressure is greater than 20 mmHg. There are a myriad of causes of pulmonary hypertension, but they fall into five basic etiologic categories [70]:

1. Passive pulmonary hypertension due to elevated pulmonary venous pressures
2. Reactive pulmonary hypertension often due to hypoxia
3. Obstructive pulmonary hypertension such as occurs in primary pulmonary hypertension or chronic obstructive lung disease
4. Increased pulmonary blood flow due to left-to-right shunts
5. Increased blood viscosity

Acute elevations in pulmonary venous pressures are accompanied by similar elevations in pulmonary artery pressure. In these acute situations, pulmonary edema often occurs before pressures become high enough to precipitate right ventricular failure. When elevations in pulmonary venous pressures are chronic, the pulmonary vasculature and lymphatic system undergo changes which protect the lungs from pulmonary edema. These include smooth-muscle hypertrophy, thickening of the capillary walls, and increased lymph flow resulting in dilated lymphatics. Over time, the pressure gradient between the pulmonary arteries and veins increases. The reactive component of the pulmonary hypertension may reverse over time if the pulmonary venous pressure returns to normal [16]. Chronic alveolar hypoxia also may lead to reactive pulmonary hypertension. Obstructive pulmonary hypertension is complex and involves a number of factors, including hypoxic vasoconstriction, actual destruction of vessels, edema and inflammation, and loss of vessels due to fibrosis. Long-standing increases in pulmonary blood flow or blood viscosity may

lead to pulmonary hypertension. There are a number of causes for each category of pulmonary hypertension, and there is often more than one potential mechanism in patients with pulmonary hypertension.

Diagnosis

The signs and symptoms of pulmonary hypertension vary with the underlying etiology, but there are a number of common features [70,132]. Dyspnea, fatigue, and dizziness are the most frequent presenting symptoms. Syncope, chest pain, and signs of right ventricular failure also occur. Cyanosis may result from right-to-left shunting in patients with Eisenmenger's syndrome or a patent foramen ovale. The neck veins usually show a prominent *a* wave due to the vigorous contraction of the right atrium against the hypertrophied right ventricle. The mean jugular venous pressure may be elevated. The systolic blood pressure is usually low with a narrow pulse pressure. Tachypnea and tachycardia are frequent. Precordial palpation demonstrates the left parasternal lift of right ventricular hypertrophy. The forceful pulsation of the dilated pulmonary artery may be palpable in the left second intercostal space. The second heart sound is narrowly split with a prominent pulmonary component which may be palpable. Right-sided third and fourth heart sounds may be heard along the lower sternal border in the subxiphoid region. These are identifiable by an increased intensity with inspiration. In severe cases, murmurs of tricuspid and pulmonic regurgitation can be heard and elevated jugular venous pressure, a positive Kussmaul's sign, edema, ascites, and cyanosis may all be present. Patients should be carefully examined for signs of deep venous thrombosis.

The chest x-ray provides some clues to the underlying disease, such as evidence for mitral stenosis or pulmonary parenchymal disease. The pulmonary arteries are enlarged. Cardiomegaly may or may not be present.

The ECG may be normal in cases of mild pulmonary hypertension. As pulmonary hypertension becomes more severe, there is evidence of right ventricular hypertrophy with right-axis deviation and prominent R waves in leads V_1 and V_2. Tall P waves (greater than 2.5 mm) in leads II, III, and aV_F reflect right atrial enlargement.

Echocardiography may help detect valvular or congenital disease. "Contrast" echo studies can detect right-to-left shunts. A bolus of saline is shaken to produce microbubbles and injected intravenously. The bubbles (or "contrast") can be detected by echocardiography as they move through the heart. Doppler studies can sensitively identify tricuspid or pulmonic regurgitation and also may be used to detect intracardiac shunts. A ventilation/perfusion lung scan can occasionally be helpful in excluding thromboembolic disease. Pulmonary function tests to assess lung disease and serologic tests to exclude collagen-vascular disorders affecting the lung are often helpful. Cardiac catheterization may be necessary to directly measure pulmonary pressures and cardiac output unless tricuspid or pulmonic regurgitation is present, in which case pulmonary systolic pressure can be estimated with Doppler studies by application of the Bernoulli relationship. If no cause is found after a careful search, the patient is considered to have primary pulmonary hypertension (PPH) [68]. Primary pulmonary hypertension occurs more often in women than men and often has a progressive downhill course over 2 to 3 years, culminating in death. The cause is unknown.

Treatment

The therapy of pulmonary hypertension is directed at the underlying cause. Chronic oxygen may be necessary if hypoxemia is present. Diuretic therapy is used for fluid retention. Vasodilators probably reduce pulmonary vascular resistance in some patients, but it is not clear if long-term therapy improves prognosis [134]. Heart-lung transplantation has been performed with limited success in some patients with end-stage pulmonary hypertension [136].

Pericardial Diseases

The pericardium consists of a serous membrane which covers the heart (the visceral pericardium) and is reflected back on itself at the great vessels to form the dense, collagenous outer covering (the parietal pericardium). The pericardial sac normally contains up to 50 ml pericardial fluid, which is ultrafiltrate of plasma with a protein content about one-third that of plasma. Removal of the pericardium does not usually lead to any adverse clinical problems. However, the pericardium has several functions, including the prevention of acute cardiac dilation, the distribution of hydrostatic forces equally to all portions of the heart, and the accentuation of the interdependence of the ventricles in diastole [111]. Pericardial disease may present as acute pericarditis, pericardial effusion, cardiac tamponade, or constrictive pericarditis. General causes of pericardial disease are listed in Table 1-16.

Pericarditis

PATHOPHYSIOLOGY

Pericarditis is an acute inflammation of the pericardium characterized by chest pain and a pericardial rub.

DIAGNOSIS

Typical ECG changes and fever are common. The chest pain is usually retrosternal or parasternal. It is aggravated by deep breathing or coughing and usually improves if the patient sits up and leans forward. The pain may radiate to the trapezius ridge or neck. The pericardial friction rub has a superficial and scratchy quality and may be soft

Table 1–16. *Common Causes of Pericardial Disease*

   I. Idiopathic
  II. Infectious:
     A. Viral, bacterial, tuberculous, fungal
 III. Neoplastic:
     A. Primary
     B. Secondary (lung, breast, lymphoma, leukemia, melanoma)
 IV. Trauma
  V. Autoimmune:
     A. Connective-tissue diseases
     B. Post-myocardial infarction/post-pericardotomy syndrome
     C. Drug-Induced
 VI. Aortic or cardiac rupture
VII. Myocardial infarction
VIII. Metabolic:
     A. Uremia, myxedema, etc.
 IX. Radiation
  X. Miscellaneous

or very loud and coarse. The rub is often "three-component," coinciding with cardiac movement with ventricular systole, rapid diastolic filling, and atrial systole. Often the rub will be only "two-component"—the two components occurring with ventricular and atrial systole [157]. Pericardial friction rubs are often evanescent. If a rub is not heard, repeated careful auscultation with the patient leaning forward and in expiration may be helpful. The chest x-ray is not specific, although signs of the underlying disease or enlargement of the cardiac silhouette due to pericardial effusion may be noted. The ECG findings are generalized ST-segment elevation in all leads but AVR and V_1. The ST-segment elevation returns to baseline after several days and may be followed by diffuse T-wave inversion. These changes can usually be separated from the ST-segment elevation associated with acute myocardial infarction [86]. When pericarditis results from an acute myocardial infarction, the classic ECG changes are frequently not present [101]. The echocardiogram is the best test for detecting a pericardial effusion, but there are no specific findings for pericarditis and an effusion may not be present. Acute pericarditis is usually idiopathic or viral in origin, although it is also quite common early following myocardial infarction. Uremia and autoimmune disorders also are frequent causes.

TREATMENT

The pain of acute pericarditis may be treated with aspirin or nonsteroidal anti-inflammatory drugs. Rarely, steroids are necessary, but if so, tuberculous or bacterial etiologies should first be excluded. The underlying cause should be determined, since specific therapy may be necessary.

The prognosis of acute pericarditis depends on the underlying disease. Idiopathic, viral, and post-myocardial infarction pericarditis usually resolve in a few days. Occasionally, patients develop chronic, recurrent episodes of pericarditis.

Pericardial Effusion

Patients may have pericardial effusion with or without evidence of pericarditis. The effusion may develop slowly and may be as large as 1500 ml. Effusions may be serous or bloody or may contain lymph or chyle [111]. Pus will be present if there is bacterial pericarditis. Gross blood is found in cardiac or aortic rupture. If there are no symptoms of pericarditis or tamponade, therapy is directed only at the underlying cause of the pericardial effusion. Even very small effusions can be detected with echocardiography.

Cardiac Tamponade

PATHOPHYSIOLOGY

The most serious complication of pericardial effusion is cardiac tamponade, which occurs when pericardial fluid accumulates causing an increase in intrapericardial pressure that compresses the cardiac chambers and limits filling of the heart. The amount of pericardial fluid required to cause tamponade depends on the rapidity with which the effusion develops, the distensibility of the pericardium, and the compressibility and filling pressure of the cardiac chambers. Thus, if the pericardium is poorly compliant or if fluid develops rapidly, cardiac tamponade may occur with as little as 200 ml. More commonly, there are at least several hundred milliliters of fluid in the pericardial sac. Normally, intrapericardial pressure is subatmospheric. As the effusion accumulates, the intrapericardial pressure rises until ·it impedes diastolic filling of the heart, resulting in decreased cardiac volume and cardiac output. Systolic function is unaffected.

DIAGNOSIS

Patients with cardiac tamponade present with fatigue and dyspnea. Pericardial pain may or may not be present. Systolic blood pressure is often low with a narrow pulse pressure. Pulsus paradoxus is a characteristic finding and consists of a fall in systolic blood pressure during inspiration of greater than 10 mmHg. Less than 10 mmHg fall in systolic blood pressure with inspiration is a normal finding. The mechanism of pulsus paradoxus is complex, with several interrelated factors [145]. The normal inspiratory increase in venous return to the right side of the heart compromises the filling of the left side of the heart, since the total intracardiac blood volume is fixed by the tense pericardium. In addition, blood return to the right side of the heart is augmented with inspiration while blood pools in the lungs, decreasing return to the left side of the heart. Pulsus paradoxus is not specific for cardiac tamponade and is seen in severe obstructive airway disease or bronchial asthma. Pulsus paradoxus may not appear if there is hypotension or volume depletion. Examination of the neck veins demonstrates a high level of mean jugular venous pressure with a prominent *x* descent and an absent *y* descent. Cardiac examination is not specific. There may be a rub, but often the precordium is quiet. The chest x-ray may show cardiomegaly, but this is usually not specific. The ECG often shows sinus tachycardia and low voltage, which are nonspecific. If the effusion is very large, electrical alternans may be present due to the swinging of the heart in the pericardial sac. The echocardiogram is the most important test. Even small effusions are demonstrable, and echocardiographic signs of tamponade may be detectable [49]. Cardiac catheterization may be performed to secure the diagnosis. Equalization of right atrial, right ventricular end-diastolic, pulmonary capillary wedge, left atrial,

and left ventricular end-diastolic pressures is seen in most cases.

TREATMENT

Cardiac tamponade is a life-threatening condition, and pericardial drainage by needle aspiration or surgery is usually necessary. Pericardiocentesis should be performed only by experienced operators under controlled conditions in all but the most extreme circumstances [102]. The pericardial fluid withdrawn should be sent to the laboratory for bacterial, myobacterial, and fungal cultures, for protein and hemoglobin determinations, and for cytologic examination. The prognosis of cardiac tamponade is that of the underlying disease once the tamponade is successfully relieved. The most common diseases resulting in tamponade are neoplasia, uremia, and idiopathic processes. If effusions recur after pericardiocentesis, either intrapericardial instillation of sclerosing drugs or surgery is necessary.

Pericardial Constriction

Pericardial constriction occurs when a thickened and scarred pericardium restricts filling of the heart in diastole. Usually the pericardium is markedly thickened and does not stretch. While the primary problem is limitation of cardiac filling, there are some differences from tamponade [49]. Constriction is usually a slowly developing chronic problem, and subtle differences in physiology lead to different clinical and hemodynamic findings. Cardiac constriction may result from tuberculosis, radiation, uremia, neoplasia, connective-tissue diseases, or be idiopathic. The patient presents with symptoms of heart failure. Complaints of ascites and edema may suggest liver disease. The jugular venous pressure is elevated with prominent *x* and *y* descents. Kussmaul's sign (an inspiratory rise in jugular venous pressure) is present. On auscultation, an early diastolic sound—the pericardial knock—is often heard. It occurs with rapid diastolic filling and may mimic an S_3, although it is usually higher-pitched and earlier. Signs of high systemic venous pressure such as edema, hepatomegaly, and ascites are common. The chest x-ray may not be remarkable, although pericardial calcification is present in some and is best seen on the lateral chest x-ray. The ECG is not usually helpful and the echocardiogram is not specific, but it may be helpful in excluding effusion and some causes of restrictive cardiac disease. The diagnosis is made at cardiac catheterization by the characteristic pressures and waveforms. Cardiac catheterization can usually distinguish restrictive cardiomyopathy from constrictive pericarditis. The treatment of constrictive pericarditis is surgical resection of the pericardium. This is often difficult surgery, and hemodynamic recovery may have a prolonged course [170].

Diseases of the Aorta

The aorta is a remarkably durable vessel. Its strength resides primarily in the media, with sheets of elastic tissue arranged in a spiral fashion to afford great resilience. There is a layer of smooth muscle and collagen between the elastic lamina. The vasa vasorum reside in the adventitia. The elasticity of the aorta allows it to expand in systole as blood is delivered into it. In diastole, if the aortic valve is competent, this stored energy is expended in propelling blood forward. With aging, some of the elasticity of the aorta is lost, which may result in systolic hypertension and elongation of the aorta. The aorta is subject to a number of processes, including aging, cystic medial necrosis, atherosclerosis, inflammation, infection, and trauma, all of which may weaken a portion of its wall ultimately leading to aneurysm formation. An aneurysm is a widening or dilation of the wall of a vessel. Aneurysms may be saccular, involving a small portion of the aortic wall and appearing as an outpouching, or they may be fusiform, involving a larger and more circumferential portion of the aortic wall and appearing globular or fusiform in shape. Aneurysms may occur anywhere along the aorta, although certain diseases often involve a particular location. Aneurysms rarely obstruct the flow of blood through the aorta; thus they are often asymptomatic. Prior to rupture, symptoms usually result only if the aneurysms compress adjacent structures or if they are expanding rapidly. The most serious consequences of aortic aneurysms are rupture and dissection, both of which are sudden and life-threatening. It is not surprising that once the aortic wall is weakened by any process, an aneurysm will gradually increase in size. The law of LaPlace states that wall tension is directly proportional to the product of the pressure in the vessel and its radius. Thus, as the aneurysm enlarges, wall tension progressively increases and the aneurysm expands further.

Abdominal Aortic Aneurysms

The majority of atherosclerotic aortic aneurysms occur in the abdominal aorta, usually between the renal arteries and the aortic bifurcation [143]. The atherosclerotic process weakens the aortic wall by destruction of the elastic elements of the media. Frequently, the aneurysm is asymptomatic and is discovered on routine physical examination as a pulsatile mass. If pain does occur, it is usually in the lower back or abdomen. Acute rupture is usually associated with the sudden onset of pain and hypotension. Rapidly expanding aneurysms may be quite tender when palpated. There is often laminated clot in these aneurysms, and distal embolization may occur. The aneurysms can be sized on abdominal film if there is calcium in the wall. However, not all aneurysms are calcified; thus cross-sectional echocardiography is most commonly used to detect and follow these aneurysms. Angiography is performed if surgery is anticipated to precisely define the aneurysm and evaluate additional disease, including involvement of the renal arteries. The most serious complication of an abdominal aortic aneurysm is rupture, which usually results in death if not treated promptly. The risk of rupture seems to be particularly high in aneurysms larger than 6 cm in diameter, in which case surgical repair is usually recommended. The 5-year mortality rate in unoperated patients with aneurysms larger than 6 cm is about 90 percent, compared to 50 percent for those with resection [162]. In low-risk patients, elective aneurysm resection is sometimes advised if the aneurysms are between 4 and 6 cm [143,159]. The surgical mortality rate is about 5 percent in elective repairs, but it doubles if the aneurysm is expanding and is 30 to 50 percent if the aneurysm has ruptured. It is important to recognize that these patients usually have widespread atherosclerosis, reflected in the high 5-year mortality rate, even in patients undergoing successful aneurysm resection [11]. A careful evaluation for signs or symptoms of coronary or cerebral atherosclerosis is necessary, and risk factors for atherosclerosis, such as smoking, hypercholesterolemia, and hypertension, should be addressed.

Thoracic Aortic Aneurysms

PATHOPHYSIOLOGY

Aneurysms of the thoracic aorta may be seen with atherosclerosis, in patients with Marfan's syndrome or annuloaortic ectasia, in those with causes of aortitis such as syphilis and giant-cell arteritis, and following trauma. Atherosclerotic formation may occur anywhere in the thoracic aorta, but it is the most common in the arch and the descending aorta. Syphilitic aortitis most often affects the ascending aorta. Once the most common cause of aortic aneurysms, luetic aortitis is now rare. Marfan's syndrome is an autosomal-dominant inherited disorder of connective tissue involving the cardiovascular, ocular, and musculoskeletal systems [82]. The patients are tall and have long extremities, arachnodactyly, a high, arched palate, and lax ligaments, including those in the eye, resulting in subluxated lens.

Cardiovascular complications include degeneration of the aortic media, which leads to ascend-

ing aortic aneurysms. There is often dilation of the aortic ring with aortic regurgitation, and mitral valve prolapse is common. Rupture or dissection of the aorta accounts for the majority of deaths in patients with Marfan's syndrome. Annuloaortic ectasia is a process involving the aorta and aortic annulus which results in progressive dilation of the aortic ring and aortic root [104]. As in Marfan's syndrome, cystic medial necrosis is present. Many of these patients represent a forme fruste of the Marfan's syndrome. Arteritis with connective-tissue diseases, such as giant-cell arteritis, Takayasu's arteritis, and others, also may result in aortic aneurysms.

DIAGNOSIS

Thoracic aortic aneurysms are often asymptomatic, although symptoms due to compression of adjacent structures may be present [109]. These include hoarseness (recurrent laryngeal nerve), cough (bronchus), and dysphagia (esophagus). Pain also may result from compression of adjacent structures. Rupture causes sudden severe pain and hemodynamic collapse. Occasionally, the aneurysm may be palpated above the suprasternal notch or eroding through the chest wall. When aortic regurgitation is due to dilation of the aortic root, the murmur of aortic regurgitation is often loudest along the right sternal border rather than the left sternal border, as occurs when the aortic regurgitation is a result of aortic valvular disease [78]. Thoracic aortic aneurysms are usually visible on chest x-ray. Aortic angiography is the definitive technique for documenting the aneurysm, although CT scanning with contrast is also very helpful. The diameter of the proximal ascending aorta also can be assessed by two-dimensional echocardiography.

TREATMENT

Surgery is usually advised for aneurysms of the ascending aorta larger than 7 cm in diameter if there is significant aortic regurgitation, if there are symptoms due to the aneurysm, or if there is evidence of progressive enlargement [159]. In the patient with Marfan's syndrome, prophylactic repair is advised when the aortic root diameter exceeds 5.5 cm [118]. Aneurysms of the descending thoracic aorta are considered for surgical repair when they produce symptoms, are rapidly enlarging, or reach 6 to 7 cm in diameter. Surgery results in paraplegia in 5 percent of patients as a result of interruption of intercostal arteries that perfuse the spinal cord. When aneurysms involve the aortic arch and brachiocephalic vessels, surgical morbidity and mortality are considerably higher.

Aortic Dissection

PATHOPHYSIOLOGY

Aortic dissection occurs when there is a tear in the aortic intima allowing a column of blood to dissect between the intima and adventitia along a variable length of the aorta. Most patients with aortic dissection have evidence of cystic medial necrosis, which is necrosis of the collagen and elastic tissue with cystic changes. Propagation of the dissecting hematoma is accelerated by both the level of blood pressure and the rate of rise of arterial pressure. Most dissecting hematomas arise proximally within a few centimeters of the aortic valve or just distal to the left subclavian artery. Dissecting hematomas are classified as type A (proximal), which includes all dissecting aneurysms arising in the ascending aorta or aortic arch and those distal dissections which have dissected retrograde into the aortic arch, and type B (distal), which includes all dissections that are confined distal to the left subclavian artery. The clinical implications of this classification are discussed below.

DIAGNOSIS

Aortic dissection usually presents dramatically as the sudden onset of severe pain, often described as tearing or ripping [160]. The pain may be in the anterior chest or the interscapular area or both. Other symptoms are related to aortic regurgitation or occlusion of major blood vessels. The physical examination is critical. Blood pressure is usually increased, but hypotension may be present due to rupture of the aneurysm or obstruction of the vessel in which pressure is measured. Major pulses (femoral, brachial, carotid) may be lost by compression from the dissecting hematoma or by obstruction by the intimal flap. Less commonly, myocardial infarction, renal infarction, or mesenteric infarction may result from obstruction of their associated vessels. Aortic regurgitation may occur from dilation of the aortic root supporting the leaflets or from the dissection extending to the base of the leaflets. Signs of heart failure may occur if there is sudden severe aortic regurgitation.

The ECG is not specific for aortic dissection, although left ventricular hypertrophy is often present. The chest x-ray may be suggestive with enlargement of the aortic silhouette, a double density to the aortic shadow, or tracheal deviation to the right. If dissection is suspected, aortic angiography is performed to confirm the diagnosis, localize the intimal tear, document the extent of the false lumen, and determine involvement of vessels distal to the dissection.

TREATMENT

Aortic dissection is an emergency and requires immediate evaluation and therapy [159,109]. Initial therapy should include lowering systolic blood pressure to 100 to 120 mmHg, usually with intravenous nitroprusside. However, nitroprusside may increase the velocity of ventricular ejection, which may worsen the dissection. To counteract this effect, an intravenous beta-adrenergic blocking agent, such as propranolol, is given until a heart rate of 60 to 70 beats per minute is reached. Beta blockers are contraindicated if there is bradycardia, heart failure, or asthma. Trimethaphan, a ganglionic blocker, is also appropriate therapy because it decreases blood pressure and the velocity of blood flow. However, tachyphylaxis and nausea limit its use.

Emergency surgery is usually recommended for patients with type A dissecting aneurysms. Surgery is recommended in patients with type B aneurysms if there is vital organ compromise or continuing pain and dissection. Medical therapy is recommended for all uncomplicated type B dissections and for all uncomplicated type A dissections presenting more than 2 weeks after onset of the dissection. Medical therapy consists of vigor-

ous blood pressure control, usually including a beta-adrenergic blocking agent. In most centers there is now a 70 to 80 percent survival rate for patients with dissecting aortic aneurysms.

Diseases of the Peripheral Arteries

A number of processes involve the peripheral arteries and result in ischemia. These include arteriosclerosis obliterans, thromboangiitis obliterans, and acute occlusion by thrombosis or embolus.

Arteriosclerosis Obliterans
PATHOPHYSIOLOGY
While arteriosclerosis obliterans is the correct term for chronic atherosclerotic occlusion of the aorta and its branches, such other names as peripheral arterial disease or peripheral vascular disease are more commonly used. This is by far the most common etiology of ischemia of the lower extremities. The pathology of these lesions is similar to that of atherosclerotic lesions in other vessels, and in fact, these patients have a significant incidence of atherosclerotic involvement of the coronary and cerebral vessels [90]. Risk factors for arteriosclerosis obliterans are similar to those for coronary disease, although diabetics seem to have a particularly increased risk of atherosclerotic involvement of the peripheral vessels [94]. Cigarette smoking is extremely common in these patients, and continued smoking predicts a poorer outcome with either medical or surgical therapy [90,97].

DIAGNOSIS
The signs and symptoms of peripheral arterial disease are determined by the location of the obstruction, the speed with which the obstruction develops, and the presence of collateral channels [181].

The most common symptom of obstructive arterial disease is claudication [29]. This is pain or

discomfort which comes on with exercise and is relieved by rest. It is the result of ischemia of skeletal muscle distal to the arterial obstruction. Claudication most often occurs in the calf, but it may be noted in the buttocks, hips, thighs, or feet depending on the site of obstruction. Atherosclerotic arterial obstruction does occur in the upper extremities, but it is much less common than in the lower extremities. Impotence together with thigh and buttock claudication is called the LeRiche syndrome and suggests distal aortic disease. As obstruction progresses, resting blood flow may be compromised and rest pain may occur. Rest pain usually occurs in the feet and toes and is relieved by dependency of the leg allowing gravity to aid blood flow.

Physical examination should include palpation of the arterial pulses, including the brachial, radial, femoral, popliteal, dorsalis pedis, and posterior tibial pulses. The dorsalis pedis pulses are congenitally absent in about 10 percent of people. In patients with significant obstructive disease, pallor develops with elevation of the extremity due to the compromised blood flow and rubor develops with dependency due to reactive hyperemia to counteract the ischemia [181]. After the leg is elevated, the patient should be asked to sit up with the leg in a dependent position. Normally, the veins in the dorsum of the feet fill within 15 seconds. If arterial insufficiency is severe, the veins may not fill for 30 seconds or longer. Trophic changes such as hair loss, dry skin, or poor nail growth may reflect arterial insufficiency, although they are not always reliable signs. Ischemic ulcers are a sign of severe arterial insufficiency. They are usually painful and crusted or necrotic and must be distinguished from neurotrophic ulcers in the diabetic, which are painless and often infected.

The diagnosis of arteriosclerosis obliterans is most often made by the history and physical examination, as described. Comparison of blood pressures in the arm and ankle at rest and with exercise may indicate the severity of the obstruction. More extensive evaluation of limb pressures can be made by Doppler examination [98]. If surgery is contemplated, angiography is used to define the precise location and extent of the obstruction.

The differential diagnosis of claudication includes various neurologic disorders, arthritis, venous thrombosis, arteritis, and embolic occlusion. If the systolic blood pressure in the calf is at least 80 percent of that in the brachial artery, the symptoms are probably not due to arterial obstruction.

Over a 5-year period, the symptoms of about three-quarters of patients either remain stable or improve slightly, while one-quarter have progressive symptoms with only a very small percentage developing gangrene [97,87]. In this same period of 5 years, about one-third will suffer a myocardial infarction or stroke [13].

TREATMENT
Because symptoms often stabilize or improve as collateral flow develops, and because of the high risk of the other vascular diseases, medical therapy is undertaken initially [29]. Risk factors for atherosclerosis, especially smoking and hyperlipidemia, should be addressed. A careful evaluation for symptoms of coronary or cerebral atherosclerosis is necessary. The patient should be instructed to avoid any mechanical, thermal, or chemical trauma to the afflicted area. The feet should be kept clean and dry, and nail care is important [133]. Exercise, usually walking, may stimulate collateral blood flow or improve muscular efficiency and increase time to claudication. At present, drug therapy with vasodilators or anticoagulants does not clearly improve symptoms [29]. Early reports suggest promising results with pentoxifylline, a drug that increases red blood cell deformability [142].

Surgery is indicated in patients who are good operative risks when there are signs of resting ischemia or in patients who have had disabling claudication for several months [97]. Percutaneous transluminal angioplasty is complementary to surgery, and indications are similar to those for surgery [138].

Thromboangiitis Obliterans (Buerger's Disease)
Thromboangiitis obliterans is a disease resulting in inflammation of the small arteries and veins [181]. It is much less common than arteriosclerosis obliterans in the United States. The etiology is unknown, but cigarette smoking is somehow critically involved. The pathology is quite distinct from arteriosclerosis obliterans and involves an intense inflammatory reaction in arteries and veins. The disease affects primarily men under the age of 40 years, and a smoking history is always present. Ischemic symptoms usually appear first in either the hands or the feet. Pallor with elevation and dependent rubor occur. Acral ulcers may result with rapid progression of the disease. Phlebitis is often present.

Usually it is not difficult to distinguish Buerger's disease from arteriosclerosis obliterans, however, scleroderma and other connective tissue diseases should be excluded.

Complete abstinence from smoking of any sort is the only effective way to stop progression of this disease. Ischemic extremities or digits should be shielded from trauma and treated as already described. Amputations may be necessary, though are more limited than with arteriosclerosis obliterans.

Acute Arterial Occlusion of the Aorta or Peripheral Vessels
PATHOPHYSIOLOGY
Sudden occlusion of the aorta or a major vessel is a medical emergency which threatens the involved limb as well as the patient's life [65].

Acute occlusion usually occurs from either an embolus or an in situ thrombosis. Emboli most often arise in the heart with mitral valve disease, myocardial infarction with mural thrombus, left ventricular aneurysm, congestive heart failure, atrial fibrillation, prosthetic heart valves, or infective endocarditis as the underlying cause. Occasionally, thrombotic arterial emboli are dislodged from an ulcerated atheroma or aneurysm in the aorta. Less often, an atrial myxoma may be the cause. Paradoxical emboli are uncommon, but they may occur if venous thromboemboli pass through a patent foramen ovale or atrial septal defect. Usually this occurs in the presence of right atrial hypertension. In situ thrombosis often occurs at the site of an atherosclerotic plaque, but it may occur with other types of vascular diseases. Rarely, arterial thrombosis occurs without underlying vascular pathology—although a hypercoaguable state is often present.

DIAGNOSIS

The clinical features are summarized by the five Ps: pulseless, pallor, pain, paresthesias, and paralysis. Most patients report the acute onset of pain, but sudden onset of numbness and paresthesias may occur without pain. The patient should have a careful examination of all the pulses, with note made of the color, temperature, and sensation in the limb. The affected limb is cold and pale with poor capillary filling. A careful cardiac examination is necessary because the heart is often the source of the embolus.

The ECG and chest x-ray do not help with the diagnosis but are necessary in the assessment of cardiac disease. A "silent" myocardial infarction is not uncommon. When acute arterial occlusion occurs, it is important to consider aortic dissection as a possible cause.

TREATMENT

Therapy should be undertaken promptly once the diagnosis is made and includes anticoagulation with heparin, treating the pain with narcotics, keeping the affected limb dependent, and emergency surgical embolectomy. Angiography may be indicated depending on the patient's overall condition.

Sudden arterial occlusion will result in necrosis about half the time without treatment. However, despite techniques which allow embolectomy to be performed simply, the mortality rate remains high at 15 to 30 percent [65]. This high mortality rate is a reflection of the advanced age and underlying cardiovascular disease of most of these patients.

Arrhythmias

The conduction system of the heart is designed to transmit an electric impulse through the heart in an orderly fashion permitting coordinated activity of the various cardiac chambers. The normal impulse is generated in the sinoatrial (SA) node and spreads through the atria and into the atrioventricular (AV) node, where conduction is slowed. This allows completion of atrial systole prior to the onset of ventricular systole. The AV node prevents extremely rapid ventricular rates in situations where the atrial rate is very rapid, such as atrial fibrillation. Once an impulse transverses the AV node, it is conducted through the specialized ventricular conducting system consisting of the bundle of His, the right and left bundle branches, and the Purkinje fibers. This system rapidly conducts the electric impulse to the ventricles, allowing coordinated contraction of these chambers.

The conduction system of the heart includes cells with two different types of action potentials [175]. One type of cell has an action potential that is dependent primarily on transmembrane calcium currents (slow channels). These cells are found in the SA and AV nodes. The other type of cell has a more rapid action potential that is dependent on the movement of sodium ions (fast channels). These types of cells comprise the remainder of the conduction system. Thus drugs which affect transmembrane calcium flux would be expected to have the greatest effect on the SA and AV nodes, while drugs that affect sodium transport have their greatest impact on the conducting tissue of the atria and ventricles.

The normal rhythm of the heart is initiated by depolarization of cells in the SA node. These cells depolarize spontaneously, as do cells in the AV node and the His-Purkinje system. However, the rate is fastest in the SA node; thus cardiac activity is normally initiated from the SA node. If the pacemaker function of the SA node fails, the heart may be driven by cells in the AV node or the His-Purkinje system, although the spontaneous rate gradually decreases as one moves distally in the conduction system [168]. The conduction system is innervated by the autonomic nervous system [183]. Increases in sympathetic activity increase the rate of spontaneous depolarization and conduction velocity throughout the conduction system. Parasympathetic stimulation decreases the rate of spontaneous depolarization in the SA and AV nodes and decreases conduction through the AV node. Thus heart rate responds rapidly to changes in autonomic tone.

Tachyarrhythmias generally result from one of two mechanisms [175,176]. The most common, reentry, occurs when two pathways which normally conduct an impulse become dissociated. An impulse is conducted slowly down one pathway, while conduction in the other pathway is blocked; however, conduction may occur retrograde in the blocked pathway. If this retrograde conduction returns to the unblocked pathway at a time in which it is not refractory, a continuous loop of conduction is formed (Fig. 1-12). Understanding the concept of reentry is important because altering the conduction of either pathway may interrupt the reentry cycle and prevent or stop the reentrant tachycardia. Tachyarrhythmias also may result when cells with pacemaker function increase their rate and take over control of the heart. These are often called automatic or ectopic arrhythmias. Bradyarrhythmias occur when there is either a failure of impulse formation or a failure of impulse propagation.

Interpretation of arrhythmias requires an understanding of the ECG (Fig. 1-13). Depolarization of the sinus node is not seen on the surface electrocardiogram. The P wave represents depolarization of atrial muscle. Depolarization of the AV node and His-Purkinje system also is not seen on the surface electrocardiogram, but it is included in the PR interval. Depolarization of ventricular muscle is represented by the QRS complex. When one is evaluating an abnormality of rhythm or conduction, three basic rules should be followed:

1. Identify atrial activity—atrial rate, regularity, and morphology.
2. Identify ventricular activity. Is the QRS normal or abnormal, regular or irregular?
3. Determine atrioventricular conduction. Is there a QRS complex for each P wave? Is atrioventricular conduction antegrade or retrograde? What is the PR interval, and is it constant or variable?

Multiple leads from the surface ECG are adequate for the diagnosis of most arrhythmias. However, occasionally, other techniques such as recording from an esophageal electrode or intracardiac recording may be necessary to make the correct diagnosis [39,77]. Arrhythmias may be provoked and evaluated with intracardiac electrodes during electrophysiologic testing [39]. Intracardiac leads may be used to terminate or overdrive some arrhythmias. Repeated provocation of arrhythmias by intracardiac electrodes may be used to assess the adequacy of drug therapy.

Finally, when one is confronted with a patient with an arrhythmia or conduction abnormality, one must decide whether intervention is necessary. If blood pressure is inadequate, emergency therapy is necessary. If blood pressure is adequate and there are no signs of poor perfusion to vital organs, treatment will depend on the natural history of the specific arrhythmia, the underlying cause of the arrhythmia, associated drug therapy,

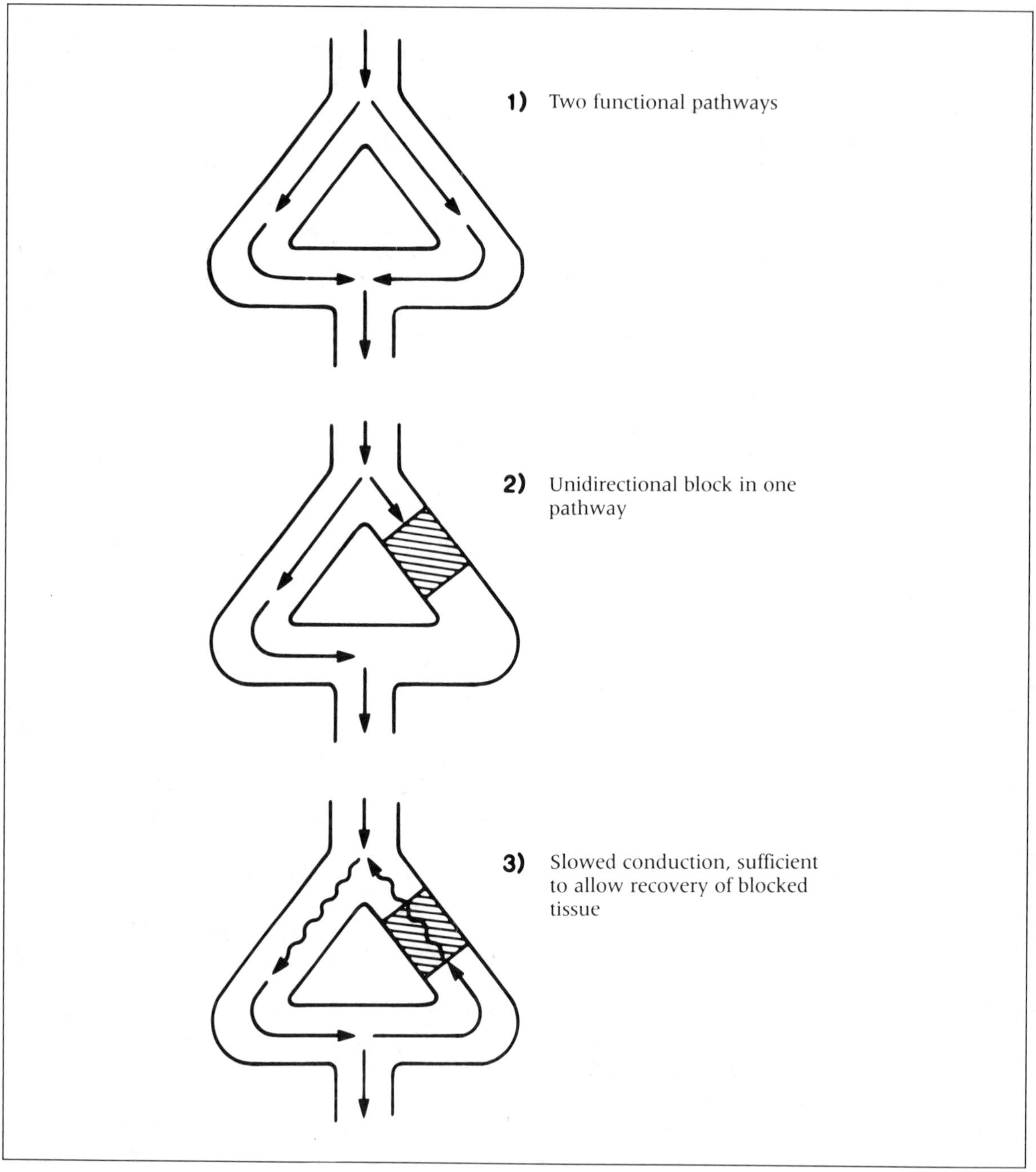

1) Two functional pathways

2) Unidirectional block in one pathway

3) Slowed conduction, sufficient to allow recovery of blocked tissue

Figure 1–12. *Mechanism of reentrant arrhythmias. Reentrant arrhythmias require two distinct functional pathways, transient unidirectional block in one pathway, and slowed conduction enough to allow recovery of blocked tissue. (Courtesy of Dr. Michael J. Reiter.)*

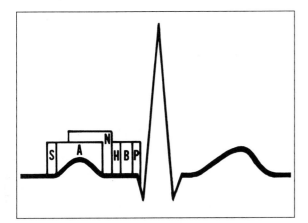

Figure 1–13. Representation of depolarization of various portions of the heart and conduction system on the surface electrocardiogram (S, sinus node; A, atrial activation; N, nodal or AV junction; H, His-bundle; B, bundle branches; P, Purkinje fibers). (Reprinted with permission from H. J. L. Marriott, Workshop in Electrocardiography. *Oldsmar, Fla.: Tampa Tracings, 1972.)*

the presence of precipitating factors, and the risks of therapy.

Normal sinus rhythm, which is not an arrhythmia, is initiated in the sinus node at a rate between 60 and 100 beats per minute. Heart rates slower than 60 beats per minute are called *bradycardias,* while rates over 100 beats per minute are referred to as *tachycardias.*

Sinus arrhythmia is a normal phenomenon consisting of a phasic variation in the sinus rate with respiration caused by alterations in vagal tone. The sinus rate increases with inspiration and decreases with expiration. The P-wave configuration is normal, and the PP interval varies cyclically with respiration. Sinus arrhythmia is usually seen at slow heart rates. No therapy is required.

Sinus tachycardia is the most common tachycardia and is the normal response to a variety of stresses, including exercise, anxiety, fever, myocardial dysfunction, and anemia. The atrial rate is greater than 100 beats per minute, the P-wave configuration is normal, and the PR interval is constant. Each P wave is followed by a QRS complex. The onset or termination of sinus tachycar-

dia usually occurs with a gradual increase or decrease in heart rate. A history of an abrupt change in heart rate within one or two beats suggests another type of tachycardia. The maximum sinus rate can be estimated by subtracting the patient's age from 220, but sinus tachycardia with rates greater than 140 beats per minute are unusual in adults at rest. Since sinus tachycardia is usually due to an underlying condition, therapy is directed at the underlying cause.

Premature atrial contractions (PACs) are premature beats arising in the atria. The P wave is different than the normal P wave because the beat is initiated in an ectopic focus resulting in an abnormal sequence of atrial depolarization. PACs are conducted through the AV node and His-Purkinje system and thus are usually followed by a normal QRS configuration. Occasionally, the QRS complex will be wide due to "aberrant" conduction through part of the bundle-branch system. PACs may be blocked in the AV node, resulting in a pause that is often mistaken for sinus arrest if the ectopic P wave is not noticed. PACs may occur in people with no heart disease and no precipitating factors. Tobacco, caffeine, alcohol, and stimulant drugs may provoke PACs. In patients with underlying heart disease, PACs may precede overt heart failure. Patients with lung disease frequently have PACs. PACs rarely cause hemodynamic problems unless they initiate episodes of supraventricular tachycardia. Elimination of the precipitating factor or treatment of the underlying disease is usually sufficient therapy. In healthy individuals, reassurance may be all that is necessary. Drugs such as digoxin, verapamil, or beta-adrenergic blocking agents may prevent initiation of a supraventricular tachycardia by delaying AV nodal conduction. Quinidine or procainamide also may be used to suppress PACs.

Paroxysmal atrial tachycardia (PAT) is often referred to as paroxysmal supraventricular tachycardia (PSVT) [89]. It is characterized by abrupt onset and termination with a rate of 150 to 250 beats per minute. Paroxysmal supraventricular tachycardia is initiated by a PAC, and 1:1 AV conduction is usually present with normal QRS complexes. Paroxysmal supraventricular tachycardia may occur by several different mechanisms, but the most common are reentry within the AV node and reentry using a concealed bypass tract. In AV nodal reentry, a PAC is not conducted in one pathway of the AV node and conducts slowly through another pathway. After completing the slowly conducting pathway, the impulse is conducted both antegrade to the His-Purkinje system and retrograde over the initially blocked AV nodal pathway to excite the atria. If this reentry circuit continues, the atria and ventricles are excited nearly simultaneously, with ventricular conduction proceeding in the normal fashion and atrial conduction occurring retrograde from the AV node. Thus there are usually normal QRS complexes but P waves, if visible separate from the QRS, are inverted in ECG leads II, III, and AVF. A larger reentry circuit is present in patients with a bypass tract—these bypass tracts are bands of myocardial tissue connecting atria to ventricles, bypassing the AV node and His-Purkinje system. Bypass tracts may be evident on the ECG when there are characteristic findings of ventricular preexcitation (see below). A normal impulse may transverse the AV node and His-Purkinje system in antegrade fashion but be conducted retrograde over the concealed bypass tract to the atria before the next sinus impulse. If the AV node is not refractory, the impulse will be conducted back down the AV node and a reentry circuit is established. Once again, there is usually 1:1 AV conduction; the QRS complexes are normal because the ventricles are activated through the normal pathway. Because there is retrograde conduction through the atria, P waves, if visible, are inverted in ECG leads 2, 3 and AVF. Other types of paroxysmal supraventricular tachycardia also occur, but they are much less common. Careful inspection of the ECG offers a number of clues which help in differentiating the various mechanisms [89,179]. Paroxysmal supraventricular tachycardia often occurs in young, healthy adults and does not affect long-term prognosis. Therapy is directed at termination of the acute event and prevention of recurrence. Termination of the acute

event may be accomplished by prolonging conduction in the AV node with vagal maneuvers such as carotid sinus massage or the Valsalva maneuver. If vagal maneuvers fail, verapamil, 5 to 10 mg IV, is usually successful. Occasional episodes of paroxysmal supraventricular tachycardia may not require any prophylactic therapy; however, if episodes are frequent or symptomatic, digoxin, calcium-channel antagonists, or beta-adrenergic antagonists are usually successful in preventing recurrences.

Paroxysmal atrial tachycardia with block (PAT with block) has an atrial rate of 150 to 250 beats per minute with abnormal P-wave morphology and impaired AV conduction; 2:1 and 4:1 atrioventricular block are most common, resulting in ventricular rates of 50 to 120 beats per minute. Paroxysmal atrial tachycardia with block is often due to digoxin toxicity, but it can occur in patients with underlying heart or lung disease in the absence of digoxin.

Atrial fibrillation is characterized by rapid irregular atrial activity at a rate greater than 400 beats per minute and a ventricular response usually between 140 and 180 beats per minute. The atrial activity may be coarse with irregular, variable *f* waves, or atrial activity may be difficult to define. The ventricular response is irregular. Atrial fibrillation usually occurs when there is underlying disease such as hypertension, mitral valve disease, cardiomyopathy, or thyrotoxicosis [92]. Atrial fibrillation also may be precipitated by hypoxia, acute alcoholism, chest surgery, infection, and other stresses. The hemodynamic response to atrial fibrillation depends on the rapidity of the ventricular response, as well as on the importance of atrial systole in each patient. If the ventricular response is rapid and the patient is hypotensive with signs of diminished cerebral perfusion or is having chest pain, synchronized dc cardioversion is necessary [112]. If the situation is not so acute, rate control can usually be achieved with intermittent doses of IV digoxin. Digoxin is usually given to decrease the resting rate to 100 beats per minute or less; however, it must be remembered that digoxin will not control the resting ventricular response if there is excessive sympathetic stimulation such as occurs with fever, congestive heart failure, or sepsis [64]. Occasionally, verapamil, diltiazem, or beta-adrenergic blocking agents are added to digoxin to control the ventricular response. Beta-adrenergic blockers may be used alone to control the ventricular response in patients with thyrotoxicosis. Many patients revert to normal sinus rhythm without additional therapy. If they do not, the decision to attempt to restore sinus rhythm depends on the underlying disease, the duration of atrial fibrillation, the left atrial size, and the patient's tolerance for type IA antiarrhythmic drugs (Table 1-17). If sinus rhythm is deemed desirable and possible, the patient is usually given a type I antiarrhythmic drug orally until a therapeutic drug level is reached [156]. Many patients will revert with medical therapy alone; those who do not may undergo electrical cardioversion. When quinidine is used, the digoxin dose must be decreased, because quinidine increases serum digoxin levels [153]. Cardioversion restores sinus rhythm initially in most patients, but reversion to atrial fibrillation is distressingly common in the ensuing 6 months, especially if a type I antiarrhythmic drug is not continued. Systemic embolization is a serious risk of either medical or electric cardioversion. Prior to electrical cardioversion, patients at highest risk of systemic embolization, such as those with mitral valve disease, prior systemic emboli, hypertrophic cardiomyopathy, congestive heart failure, atrial fibrillation for more than a few days, or prosthetic heart valves, should be fully anticoagulated [12]. The necessity of anticoagulation in other patient groups undergoing cardioversion is controversial.

Long-term anticoagulation must be considered in patients with chronic atrial fibrillation. It is known that these patients have a higher than expected rate of stroke [178]. In the high-risk groups already mentioned, prophylactic anticoagulation is probably valuable to prevent cerebral emboli. However, in patients with atrial fibrillation who do not have a high risk for systemic embolization, it is not clear that the benefits of long-term anticoagulation outweigh the risks [43].

Atrial flutter is characterized by rapid regular atrial flutter waves usually occurring at a rate of 300 per minute, but with a range of 250 to 350. These flutter waves have a characteristic "sawtooth" appearance in ECG leads 2, 3, and AVF. The flutter waves are too fast to be conducted 1:1 through a normal AV node to the ventricles, and most often 2:1 AV block occurs. Higher degrees of AV block can be elicited transiently with vagal maneuvers such as carotid sinus massage. Carotid sinus massage should be performed only after careful auscultation for carotid bruits. Only one carotid artery should be compressed at a time and for no longer than a few seconds. Continuous ECG monitoring is necessary. Atrial flutter is almost always associated with underlying heart disease, with the etiologies similar to those for atrial fibrillation. Atrial flutter is usually paroxysmal and often reverts to sinus rhythm or atrial fibrillation. Electrical cardioversion is usually the most effective therapy in atrial flutter, since it is difficult to control the ventricular rate with digoxin alone. The prevention of recurrent atrial flutter is similar to that for atrial fibrillation.

Multifocal atrial tachycardia (MAT) is the term used to describe a tachycardia with P waves of at least three configurations and with varying PR and PP intervals [149]. Because of the irregular atrial rhythm and frequent blocked P waves, the ventricular response is often irregular. Multifocal atrial tachycardia is usually associated with severe underlying disease, particularly lung disease, and often seems to be precipitated by excessive theophylline [105]. Treatment is directed at the underlying cause. If the ventricular response must be controlled, verapamil may be effective and may even occasionally suppress the tachycardia.

Wolff-Parkinson-White (WPW) syndrome is a syndrome consisting of paroxysmal supraventricular tachycardia and preexcitation in which there is an anomalous band of myocardial tissue connecting the atria to the ventricles allowing conduction to bypass the AV node [61,172]. These bypass tracts may conduct retrograde as part of a reentry circuit with the AV node resulting in paroxysmal supraventricular tachycardia. The most feared problem

78

Table 1–17. *Classification of Antiarrhythmic Drugs*

Class	Predominant electrophysiologic effects	Conduction/refractoriness	Effects	Drugs
I	Fast channels; all depress phase 0*	—	—	—
IA	Fast channels: Depress phase 0 Prolong repolarization	↓ conduction ↑ refractoriness	↑ QRS ↑ QT	Quinidine, procainamide, disopyramide (pirmenol), imipramine
IB	Fast channels (particularly ischemic tissue): Depress phase 0 Shorten repolarization	— conduction ↓ refractoriness	— QRS ↓ QT	Lidocaine, phenytoin, tocainide, mexilitine
IC	Fast channels: Depress phase 0 Little change in repolarization	↓ conduction — refractoriness	↑ ↑ QRS — QT	Flecainide, encainide, (moricizine), (propafenone)†, (cibenzoline)
II	Beta-adrenergic receptor blockade	↓ conduction (AV node) ↑ refractoriness (AV node)	— QRS — QT	Propranolol, timolol, atenolol, nadolol, metoprolol, (sotolol)†, esmolol
III	Precise effect unknown: Depress phase 0 Prolongs repolarization	↓ conduction ↑ refractoriness	↑ QRS ↑ ↑ QT	Amiodarone†, bretylium†, sotolol†
IV	Slow (calcium) channel blockade	↓ conduction (AV node) ↑ refractoriness (AV node)	— QRS —QT	Verapamil, diltiazem

*Phase 0 is the initial rapid upstroke of the action potential of atrial and ventricular contractile tissue.
†Drugs which have additional electrophysiologic properties important in their antiarrhythmic effects.
‡Drugs listed in parentheses are still experimental.

is antegrade conduction in the presence of atrial fibrillation, where impulses may be conducted to the ventricle very rapidly, resulting in hemodynamic collapse or degeneration to ventricular fibrillation. The characteristic ECG hallmarks of preexcitation are a short PR interval and the delta wave—a slowing of the initial portion of the QRS. Medical or surgical therapy may be indicated. If the bypass tract conducts only retrograde, the characteristic ECG features of preexcitation may not be present.

Premature ventricular contractions (PVCs) are ectopic beats arising within the ventricles. Because these beats do not activate the ventricles via the usual sequence of conduction through the Purkinje system, the QRS complex is wide (≥ 0.12 second) and abnormal. Usually the beats are premature enough that there is no preceding P wave. PVCs are categorized in many ways: by frequency, as multiform or uniform, and by timing (early or R or T). Three or more PVCs in a row are usually termed ventricular tachycardia. The Lown classification is a common way to categorize PVCs, although the classification has little relation to prognosis [113]. PVCs may occur in normal people; however, as the frequency and complexity increase, they are more likely to be associated with underlying heart disease. In patients without underlying heart disease, PVCs do not usually require therapy. In patients following myocardial infarction or with heart failure, PVCs do seem to predict a poorer prognosis; however, it is not yet clear that treatment of PVCs in the absence of sustained ventricular tachycardia improves the prognosis of these patients [80]. If patients are bothered by palpitations, antiarrhythmic therapy may be used to suppress PVCs, but the risks of these drugs must be kept in mind [169].

Ventricular tachycardia (VT) is defined as at least three consecutive PVCs at a rate greater than 100 beats per minute. Ventricular tachycardia is often separated into sustained and nonsustained ventricular tachycardia (NSVT). While definitions of sustained ventricular tachycardia vary, any tachycardia which requires intervention or lasts longer than 15 to 30 seconds is usually considered sustained. The QRS complexes are wide and have a bizarre configuration, occurring at a rate of 120 to 220 beats per minute. At times it may be difficult to differentiate ventricular tachycardia from paroxysmal supraventricular tachycardia with aberrant conduction. Factors which suggest ventricular tachycardia are atrioventricular dissociation, fusion beats, marked left-axis deviation, and a QRS complex wider than 0.14 seconds [173]. Fusion beats occur when ventricular muscle is activated by both supraventricular and ventricular impulses, creating a QRS complex which resembles a fusion of the two beats. However, it may not be possible to differentiate ventricular tachycardia from paroxysmal supraventricular tachycardia with aberrancy without intracardiac recordings. Ventricular tachycardia is usually seen in patients with significant underlying heart disease and ventricular dysfunction. Antiarrhythmic drugs, beta-adrenergic agonists, and digitalis may precipitate ventricular tachycardia and should be considered as a possible cause especially in a patient who had no sustained ventricular tachycardia prior to the use of antiarrhythmic drugs [169].

The therapy of sustained ventricular tachycardia depends on the clinical situation of the patient. If significant hypotension is present, synchronized dc cardioversion is necessary. If the situation is less urgent, intravenous lidocaine is the most commonly used initial drug therapy. Precipitating factors such as electrolyte abnormalities, hypoxia, digitalis toxicity, and antiarrhythmic drugs should be corrected or eliminated as required. Acute myocardial infarction should be excluded. Usually, however, the patient will require long-term antiarrhythmic drugs to prevent further episodes, since ventricular tachycardia recurs in most patients and has a very poor prognosis. The exception is patients in the first 72 hours following an acute myocardial infarction, where ventricular tachycardia or ventricular fibrillation is much less likely to recur after recovery from the infarction. One of the most difficult problems in the therapy of ventricular tachycardia is in assessing the success of antiarrhythmic drug therapy. Episodes of ventricular tachycardia are sporadic, and suppression of PVCs does not always correlate with prevention. The provocation of ventricular tachycardia during electrophysiologic study may be used to assess drug therapy. The inability to provoke ventricular tachycardia on therapy suggests long-term success in a patient with previously provokable ventricular tachycardia [175]. If a patient has frequent PVCs, Holter monitoring may be adequate to assess drug therapy. However, PVCs have a marked spontaneous variation in frequency; thus stringent criteria should be used to assess success of drug therapy [123]. Patients who have only nonsustained ventricular tachycardia may or may not require treatment depending on the degree of risk the nonsustained ventricular tachycardia confers and the risks of therapy [80]. A variety of antiarrhythmic drugs are currently available for use in patients with ventricular tachycardia. Each has its partic-

ular electrophysiologic actions and potentially adverse effects (see Table 1-17).

Ventricular fibrillation (VF) is a chaotic ventricular rhythm. The fibrillation waves are fine or coarse and usually very rapid. The patient with ventricular fibrillation always has cardiovascular collapse. Immediate defibrillation is mandatory. If defibrillation is unsuccessful, cardiopulmonary resuscitation is instituted [158]. Once ventricular fibrillation is terminated, the evaluation and therapy should proceed as with ventricular tachycardia.

Accelerated idioventricular rhythm (AIVR) is a regular ventricular rhythm occurring at a rate of 60 to 120 beats per minute. Accelerated idioventricular rhythm most commonly occurs in the setting of acute myocardial infarction. It is transient, rarely associated with hemodynamic compromise, and rarely requires specific therapy [127].

Bradyarrhythmias

Sinus bradycardia is a sinus rhythm with a rate of less than 60 beats per minute. Sinus bradycardia is common in the physically fit and during sleep and occurs with vagal stimulation. Treatment is usually not necessary. When sinus bradycardia is marked, it may be classified as the sick sinus syndrome.

The *sick-sinus syndrome (SSS)* is a syndrome of sinus node dysfunction often with accompanying AV nodal and atrial abnormalities [7]. The diagnosis is made from the ECG abnormalities and consists of the following:

1. Inappropriate sinus bradycardia
2. Atrial fibrillation with a slow ventricular response (without medical therapy)
3. Sinus arrest or sinus exit block without a junctional escape rhythm
4. Alternating bradycardia and supraventricular tachycardia ("brady-tachy" syndrome)

Most often the cause of sick-sinus syndrome is not known, but it may be associated with older age and a wide variety of underlying cardiac diseases. In addition, drugs such as beta-adrenergic antagonists, calcium-channel antagonists, sympatholytic agents, lithium, digitalis, type I antiarrhythmic drugs, and amiodarone may exacerbate sick-sinus syndrome [7]. If symptoms of dizziness or presyncope can be clearly correlated with episodes of bradycardia, and discontinuation of any of the above drugs is not beneficial, a permanent pacemaker is usually necessary.

Junctional rhythm (also called junctional escape rhythm) occurs when the pacemaker tissue with the fastest rate is in the AV nodal region. The rate is usually 40 to 60 beats per minute, and the QRS complexes are normal because ventricular depolarization proceeds along the normal ventricular conduction system. P waves may not be present or may be associated with a short PR interval and abnormal P-wave configuration due to retrograde conduction from the AV nodal region to the atria. Junctional rhythm usually occurs with excessive vagal stimulation or with failure of the sinus mechanism. If there are symptoms, atropine may restore sinus rhythm, but if not, a temporary (rarely, a permanent) pacemaker may be necessary.

Idioventricular rhythm (ventricular escape rhythm) is a slow (rate 30 to 40 beats per minute) rhythm with wide QRS complexes. It implies failure of both sinus and junctional pacemakers and occurs with serious underlying cardiac disease. Because the rate is so slow, this rhythm is almost always associated with severe symptoms and requires immediate therapy—usually a pacemaker. Intravenous isoproterenol is often used in an attempt to increase the rate while pacing is being instituted.

Abnormalities of Conduction

Abnormalities of conduction may arise anywhere in the conducting tissue of the heart, but the most common areas are the AV node, the His bundle, and the bundle branches. Conduction block in the AV node is often referred to as *nodal* or *proximal block*, while block in the His bundle or bundle branches is called *infranodal* or *distal block*. Atrioventricular block is divided into first-, second-, and third-degree block.

First-degree AV block occurs when the sinus beat is conducted to the ventricles more slowly than normal, reflected by a PR interval longer than 0.20 second. The site of block is most often in the AV node, although it may be in the atria, the His bundle, or the bundle branches. First-degree AV block is often associated with increasing age, heart disease of almost any type, increased vagal tone, digoxin, beta-adrenergic antagonists, and some calcium-channel antagonists. The prognosis is that of the underlying heart disease. By itself, first-degree AV block is of little significance and requires no specific therapy.

Second-degree AV block occurs when some but not all impulses from the atria to the ventricles are blocked. Two types of second-degree AV block are recognized with the distinction helpful for both prognostic and therapeutic reasons. In *Mobitz type I second-degree AV block* (also called Wenckebach rhythm), the PR interval gradually increases until a P wave fails to conduct. The QRS is usually narrow. This type of block is almost always proximal to the His bundle in the AV nodal region. Type I

second-degree block is usually transient and rarely leads to hemodynamic difficulty. If therapy is necessary, intravenous atropine may restore normal AV conduction. Rarely, temporary pacing may be necessary. The most common cause is acute inferior myocardial infarction, but the block may also occur with digoxin toxicity, with acute myocarditis, or following cardiac surgery. Occasionally, healthy young individuals, particularly those who are physically fit, have Mobitz type I AV block at rest or during sleep. *Mobitz type II second-degree AV block* occurs when the PR interval is constant but not all P waves are conducted. Block most often occurs in a constant ratio such as 2:1, 4:1, or 3:2. The site of block is usually below the AV node, and often there is fascicular or bundle-branch block demonstrated by a wide QRS complex. Type II second-degree AV block is associated with more serious underlying heart disease than type I block and often results in hemodynamic problems. Thus pacing is frequently necessary. When 2:1 block is present, it may not be possible initially to determine if it is type I or type II block. However, the clinical setting and the presence of fascicular or bundle-branch block may help. Increases or decreases in the sinus rate may alter the pattern of block, clarifying the type.

Third-degree AV block (complete heart block) is diagnosed when no atrial impulses reach the ventricles. This may be due to block at the AV nodal level, in which case there is usually a narrow (junctional) escape mechanism at a rate of 40 to

60 beats per minute. This type of heart block is usually transient and most often occurs with inferior myocardial infarction or excessive vagal tone. Because the junctional escape rhythm is reliable and not too slow, hemodynamic problems may not occur. However, if the slow rate causes hypotension, atropine, 0.5 to 1 mg IV, is given to improve conduction. If atropine is not successful, temporary pacing may be necessary. When complete heart block is due to infranodal disease, the escape rhythm is ventricular; thus the rate is slower (30 to 40 beats per minute) and the QRS is wide. Ventricular escape rhythms are intrinsically unstable and are usually accompanied by hemodynamic compromise. Temporary and often permanent pacing are required. Infranodal block usually results from extensive disease of the myocardium or the conducting tissue.

Antiarrhythmic Drugs

Antiarrhythmic drugs have recently been classified into four types (see Table 1-17). While this classification groups drugs according to their general effects, there are often significant differences within a group. Before using these drugs, it is important to understand their pharmacologic properties as well as their cardiac effects. In addition, some of these drugs have potent negative inotropic actions, while many may actually precipitate or worsen ventricular arrhythmias. Furthermore, many of these have significant interactions with other drugs. Thus the decision to institute antiarrhythmic therapy must involve a careful evaluation of the potential risks as well as the potential benefits [5,51,85].

References

1. Abelmann, W. H. Viral myocarditis and its sequelae. *Ann. Rev. Med.* 24: 145, 1973.
2. Abi-Samra, F., Fouad, F. M., and Tarazi, R. C. Determinants of left ventricular hypertrophy and function in hypertensive patients: An echocardiographic study. *Am. J. Med.* 75(3A): 26, 1983.
3. Anticoagulants in acute myocardial infarction: Results of a cooperative clinical trial. *J.A.M.A.* 225: 724, 1973.
4. Arnold, S. B., Byrd, R. C., Meister, W., et al. Long-term digitalis therapy improves left ventricular function in heart failure. *N. Engl. J. Med.* 303: 1443, 1980.
5. Arnsdorf, M. F. Basic understanding of the electrophysiologic actions of antiarrhythmic drugs. *Med. Clin. North Am.* 68: 1247, 1984.
6. Baum, R. S., Alvarez, H., III, and Cobb, L. A. Survival after resuscitation from out-of-hospital ventricular fibrillation. *Circulation* 50: 1231, 1974.
7. Belic, N., and Talano, J. V. Current concepts in the sick sinus syndrome. *Arch. Int. Med.* 145: 521, 1985.
8. Beller, G. A. Radionuclide techniques in the evaluation of the patient with chest pain. *Mod. Concepts Cardiovasc. Dis.* 50: 43, 1981.
9. Benotti, J. R., and Grossman, W. Restrictive cardiomyopathy. *Ann. Rev. Med.* 35: 113, 1984.
10. Beta Blocker Heart Attack Study Group. The beta-blocker heart attack trial. *J.A.M.A.* 246: 2073, 1981.
11. Beven, E. G. Routine coronary angiography in patients undergoing surgery for abdominal aortic aneurysm and lower extremity occlusion disease. *J. Vasc. Surg.* 3: 682, 1986.
12. Bjerkelund, C. J., and Orning, O. M. The efficacy of anticoagulant therapy in preventing embolism related to dc electrical conversion of atrial fibrillation. *Am. J. Cardiol.* 23: 208, 1969.
13. Boyd, A. The natural cause of arteriosclerosis of the lower extremities. *Angiology* 11: 10, 1960.

14. Braunwald, E. Clinical Manifestation of Heart Failure. In: E. Braunwald (Ed.), *Heart Disease: A Textbook of Cardiovascular Medicine.* Philadelphia: Saunders, 1984. P. 488.

15. Braunwald, E. *Pathophysiology of Heart Failure.* In: E. Braunwald (Ed.), *Heart Disease: A Textbook of Cardiovascular Medicine.* Philadelphia: Saunders, 1984. Pp. 447–464.

16. Braunwald, E., Braunwald, N. S., Ross, R., Jr., et al. Effects of mitral valve replacement on pulmonary vascular dynamics of patients with pulmonary hypertension. *N. Engl. J. Med.* 273: 509, 1965.

17. Braunwald, E., Lambrew, C. T., Rockoff, S., et al. Idiopathic hypertrophic subaortic stenosis. *Circulation* 29-30(Suppl. 4): 1, 1964.

18. Braunwald, E., Ross, J., Jr., and Sonnenblick, E. *Mechanisms of Contraction in the Normal and Failing Heart,* 2d Ed. Boston: Little, Brown, 1976.

19. Bruce, R. A. Exercise testing of patients with coronary heart disease. *Ann. Clin. Res.* 3: 323, 1971.

20. Brunton, T. L. Use of nitrate of amyl in angina pectoris. *Lancet* 2: 97, 1967.

21. Cairns, J. A., Gent, M., Singer, J., et al. Aspirin, sulfinpyrazone, or both in unstable angina: Results of a Canadian multicenter trial. *N. Engl. J. Med.* 313: 1369, 1985.

22. Campeau, L. Grading of angina pectoris (Letter). *Circulation* 54: 522, 1976.

23. Captopril Multicentre Research Group. A placebo-controlled trial of captopril in refractory heart failure. *J. Am. Coll. Cardiol.* 2: 755, 1983.

24. Carroll, J. D., Gaasch, W. H., and McAdams, K. P. W. J. Amyloid cardiomyopathy: Characterization by a distinct voltage/mass relationship. *Am. J. Cardiol.* 49: 9, 1982.

25. Casale, P. N., Devereux, R. B., Milner, M., et al. Value of echocardiographic measurement of left ventricular mass in predicting cardiovascular morbid events in hypertensive man. *Ann. Intern. Med.* 105: 173, 1986.

26. CASS Principal Investigators and their Associates: Coronary Artery Surgery Study (CASS). A randomized trial of coronary bypass surgery: Survival data. *Circulation* 68: 939, 1983.

27. Cobb, L. A., Thomas, G. I., Dillard, D. H., et al. An evaluation of internal mammary artery ligation by a double-blind technique. *N. Engl. J. Med.* 260: 115, 1959.

28. Cobb, L. A., Werner, J. A., and Trobaugh, G. R. Sudden cardiac death: I. A decade's experience with out-of-hospital resuscitation. *Mod. Concepts Cardiovasc. Dis.* 49: 31, 1980.

29. Coffman, J. Intermittent claudication and rest pain: Physiologic concepts and therapeutic approaches. *Prog. Cardiovasc. Dis.* 22: 53, 1970.

30. Cohn, J. N., Archibald, D. G., Ziesche, S., et al. Effect of vasodilator therapy on mortality in chronic congestive heart failure: Results of a Veterans Administration Cooperative Study. *N. Engl. J. Med.* 314: 1547, 1986.

31. Cohn, J. N., and Burke, L. P. Nitroprusside. *Ann. Intern. Med.* 91: 752, 1979.

32. Colucci, W. S., Wright, R. F., and Braunwald, E. New positive inotropic agents in the treatment of congestive heart failure. *N. Engl. J. Med.* 314: 290, 1986.

33. CONSENSUS Trial Study Group. Effects of enalapril on mortality in severe congestive heart failure: Results of the Cooperative North Scandinavian Enalapril Survival Study (CONSENSUS). *N. Engl. J. Med.* 316: 1429, 1987.

34. Crawford, M., and O'Rourke, R. A. A systematic approach to the bedside differentiation of cardiac murmurs and abnormal sounds. *Curr. Probl. Cardiol.* 1(11): 1, 1977.

35. Culpepper, W. S., Sodt, P. C., Messerli, F. H., et al. Cardiac status in juvenile borderline hypertension. *Ann. Intern. Med.* 98: 1, 1983.

36. Currie, P. J., Seward, J. B., Reeder, G. S., et al. Continuous-wave Doppler echocardiographic assessment of severity of calcific aortic stenosis: A simultaneous Doppler-catheter correlative study in 100 adult patients. *Circulation* 71: 1162, 1985.

37. Dec, G. W., Jr., Palacios, I. F., Fallon, J. T., et al. Active myocarditis in the spectrum of acute dilated cardiomyopathies: Clinical features, histologic correlates, and clinical outcome. *N. Engl. J. Med.* 312: 885, 1985.

38. DeMaria, A. N., Bommer, W., Lee, G., and Mason, D. T. Value and limitations of two-dimensional echocardiography in assessment of cardiomyopathy. *Am. J. Cardiol.* 46: 1225, 1980.

39. Denes, P., and Ezri, M. D. Clinical electrophysiology: A decade of progress. *J. Am. Coll. Cardiol.* 1: 292, 1983.

40. Devereux, R. B., and Reichek, N. B. Echocardiographic determination of left ventricular mass in

man: Anatomic validation of the method. *Circulation* 55: 613, 1977.

41. DeWood, M. A., Spores, J., and Notske, R. Prevalence of total coronary occlusion during the early hours of transmural myocardial infarction. *N. Engl. J. Med.* 303: 897, 1980.

42. Dodge, H. T., and Baxley, W. A. Left ventricular volume and mass and their significance in heart disease. *Am. J. Cardiol.* 23: 528, 1969.

43. Dunn, M. R., Claggett, P. C., and Salzman, E. W. Antithrombotic therapy in atrial fibrillation. *Chest* 89(Suppl.): 68, 1986.

44. Dzau, V. J., Colucci, W. S., Hollenberg, N. K., et al. Relation of the renin-angiotensin-aldosterone system to clinical state in congestive heart failure. *Circulation* 63: 645, 1981.

45. Dzau, V. J., Packer, M., Swartz, S. L., et al. Prostaglandins in heart failure: Relationship to renin-angiotensin system and hypoatremia. *N. Engl. J. Med.* 310: 347, 1984.

46. European Coronary Surgery Study Group. Prospective randomized study of coronary artery bypass surgery in stable angina pectoris. *Lancet* 2: 491, 1980.

47. Favalaro, R. G. Saphenous vein graft in the surgical treatment of coronary artery disease: Operative technique. *J. Thorac. Cardiovasc. Surg.* 58: 178, 1969.

48. Feigenbaum, H. Diseases of the Myocardium. In H. Feigenbaum (Ed.), *Echocardiography.* Philadelphia: Lea and Febiger, 1986. Pp. 514–547.

49. Feigenbaum, H. Pericardial Disease. In: H. Feigenbaum (Ed.), *Echocardiography.* Philadelphia: Lea and Febiger, 1986. Pp. 548–578.

50. Fenoglio, J. J., Ursell, P. C., Kellogg, C. F., et al. Diagnosis and classification of viral myocarditis by endomyocardial biopsy. *N. Engl. J. Med.* 308: 12, 1983.

51. Fenster, P. E. Clinical pharmacology: Clinical uses of pharmacokinetic principles in prescribing cardiac drugs. *Med. Clin. North Am.* 68: 1281, 1984.

52. Fouad, F. M. Left ventricular diastolic function in hypertensive patients. *Circulation* 75(Suppl. 2): 48, 1987.

53. Fowler, M. B., and Schroeder, J. S. Current status of cardiac transplantation. *Mod. Concepts Cardiovasc. Dis.* 55: 37, 1986.

54. Fowles, R. E., and Mason, J. W. Role of cardiac biopsy in the diagnosis and management of cardiac disease. *Prog. Cardiovasc. Dis.* 27: 153, 1984.

55. Franciosa, J. A., Wien, M., Ziesche, S., et al. Survival in men with severe chronic left ventricular failure due to either coronary heart disease or idiopathic dilated cardiomyopathy. *Am. J. Cardiol.* 51: 831, 1983.

56. Francis, G. S. Development of arrhythmias in the patients with congestive heart failure: Pathophysiology, prevalence and prognosis. *Am. J. Cardiol.* 57(Suppl. B): 3, 1986.

57. Francis, G. S., Goldsmith, S. R., Levine, T. B., et al. The neurohumoral axis in congestive heart failure. *Ann. Intern. Med.* 101: 377, 1984.

58. Frank, S., and Braunwald, E. Idiopathic hypertrophic subaortic stenosis: Clinical analysis of 126 patients with emphasis on the natural history. *Circulation* 37: 759, 1968.

59. Frohlich, E. D., and Tarazi, R. C. Is arterial pressure the sole factor responsible for hypertensive cardiac hypertrophy? *Am. J. Cardiol.* 44: 959, 1979.

60. Fuster, V., Gersh, B. J., Giuliani, E. R., et al. The natural history of idiopathic dilated cardiomyopathy. *Am. J. Cardiol.* 47: 525, 1981.

61. Gallagher, J. J., Pritchett, E. L. C., Sealy, W. C., et al. The preexcitation syndromes. *Prog. Cardiovasc. Dis.* 20: 285, 1978.

62. Goldbert, L. I., Hsieh, Y., and Resnelcov, L. Newer catecholamines for treatment of heart failure and shock: An update on dopamine and a first look at dobutamine. *Prog. Cardiovasc. Dis.* 19: 327, 1977.

63. Goldman, L., Hashimoto, B., Cook, E. F., et al. Comparative reproducibility and validity of symptoms for assessing cardiovascular functional class: Advantages of a new specific activity scale. *Circulation* 64: 1227, 1981.

64. Goldman, S., Probst, P., Selzer, A., and Cohn, K. Inefficacy of "therapeutic" serum levels of digoxin in controlling the ventricular rate in atrial fibrillation. *Am. J. Cardiol.* 35: 651, 1975.

65. Gordon, R. D., and Fogarty, T. J. Peripheral Arterial Embolism. In R. B. Rutherford (Ed.), *Vascular Surgery.* New York: McGraw-Hill, 1984. Pp. 449–459.

66. Gorlin, R., and Gorlin, S. G. Hydraulic formula for calculation of the area of the stenotic mitral valve, other cardiac valves, and central circulatory shunts. *Am. Heart J.* 41: 1, 1951.

67. Grossman, W. Cardiac hypertrophy: Useful adaptation or pathologic process. *Am. J. Med.* 69: 576, 1980.
68. Grossman, W., Alpert, J. S., and Braunwald, E. *Pulmonary Hypertension in Heart Disease: A Textbook of Cardiovascular Medicine.* Philadelphia: Saunders, 1984. Pp. 83–844.
69. Grossman, W., McLaurin, L. P., and Rolett, E. L. Alterations in left ventricular relaxation and diastolic compliance in congestive cardiomyopathy. *Cardiovasc. Res.* 13: 514, 1979.
70. Groves, B. M., and Reeves, J. T. Pulmonary Hypertension. In L. D. Horwitz and B. M. Groves (Eds.), *Signs and Symptoms in Cardiology.* Philadelphia: Lippincott, 1985. P. 381.
71. Gruppo Italiano Per Lo Studio Della Streptochinas: Nell'infarto Myocardico (GISSI). Effectiveness of intravenous thrombolytic treatment in acute myocardial infarction. *Lancet* 1: 397, 1986.
72. Hamilton, G. W., Trobaugh, G. B., Ritchie, J. L., et al. Myocardial imaging with 201-thallium: An analysis of clinical usefulness based on Bayes theorem. *Semin. Nucl. Med.* 8: 358, 1978.
73. Hammermeister, K. E. The effect of coronary bypass surgery on survival. *Prog. Cardiovasc. Dis.* 15: 297, 1983.
74. Hammermeister, K. E., DeRouen, T. A., and Dodge, H. T. Variables predictive of survival in patients with coronary disease. Selection by univariate and multivariate analyses from the clinical, electrocardiographic, exercise, arteriographic and quantitative angiographic evaluation. *Circulation* 59: 421, 1979.
75. Hammermeister, K. E., Fisher, L., Kennedy, J. W., et al. Prediction of late survival in patients with mitral valve disease from clinical, hemodynamic, and quantitative angiographic variables. *Circulation* 57: 341, 1978.
76. Hammermeister, K. E., Henderson, W. G., Burchfiel, C. M., et al. Comparison of outcome after valve replacement with a bioprosthetic versus a mechanical prosthesis. Initial five-year results of a randomized trial. *J. Am. Coll. Cardiol. (in press).*
77. Hammill, S. C., and Pritchett, E. L. C. Simplified esophageal electrocardiography using bipolar recording leads. *Ann. Intern. Med.* 95: 14, 1981.
78. Harvey, W., Corrado, M. A., and Perloff, J. K. "Right-sided" murmurs of aortic insufficiency. *Am. J. Med. Sci.* 245: 53, 1963.
79. Heberden, W. Some account of a disorder of the breast. *Med. Trans. Coll. Physicians (Lond.)* 2: 59, 1772.
80. Heger, J. J. Diagnosis and management of cardiac arrhythmias. *Curr. Probl. Cardiol.* 10: 1, 1985.
81. Herrick, J. B. Clinical features of sudden obstruction of the coronary arteries. *J.A.M.A.* 59: 2015, 1912.
82. Hirst, A. E., Jr., and Gore, I. Marfan's syndrome: A review. *Prog. Cardiovasc. Dis.* 16: 187, 1973.
83. Hjalmarson, A., Herlitz, J., Holmberg, S., et al. The Goteborg metoprolol trial. Effects on mortality and morbidity in acute myocardial infarction. *Circulation* 67(Suppl. 1): 26, 1983.
84. Homans, D. C. Peripartum cardiomyopathy. *N. Engl. J. Med.* 312: 1432, 1985.
85. Huang, S. K., and Marcus, F. I. Antiarrhythmic drug therapy of ventricular arrhythmias. *Curr. Probl. Cardiol.* 11: 182, 1986.
86. Hull, E. The electrocardiogram in pericarditis. *Am. J. Cardiol.* 7: 21, 1961.
87. Imparato, A., Geun-Enn, K., Davidson, T., and Browley, J. Intermittent claudication: Its natural cause. *Surgery* 78: 795, 1975.
88. Johnson, R. A., and Palacios, I. Dilated cardiomyopathies of the adult. *N. Engl. J. Med.* 307: 1051, 1982.
89. Josephson, M. E., and Kastor, J. A. Supraventricular tachycardia: Mechanisms and management. *Ann. Intern. Med.* 87: 346, 1977.
90. Juergens, J., Barber, N., and Hines, E. Arteriosclerosis obliterans: Review of 520 cases with special reference to pathogenic and prognostic factors. *Circulation* 21: 188, 1960.
91. Kannel, W. B. Prevalence and natural history of electrocardiographic left ventricular hypertrophy. *Am. J. Med.* 75(3A): 4, 1983.
92. Kannel, W. B., Abbott, R. D., Savage, D. D., and McNaMara, P. M. Epidemiologic features of chronic atrial fibrillation: The Framingham Study. *N. Engl. J. Med.* 306: 1018, 1982.
93. Kannel, W. B., Castelli, W. P., McNamara, P. M., et al. Role of blood pressure in the development of congestive heart failure. *N. Engl. J. Med.* 287: 781, 1972.
94. Kannel, W. B., and McGee, D. Diabetes and cardiovascular disease: The Framingham Study. *J.A.M.A.* 241: 2035, 1979.
95. Kannel, W. B., McGee, D., and Gordon, T. A

general cardiovascular risk profile. The Framingham Study. *Am. J. Cardiol.* 38: 46, 1976.

96. Kantrowitz, N. E., and Bristow, M. R. Cardiotoxicity of antitumor agents. *Prog. Cardiovasc. Dis.* 27: 195, 1984.

97. Kempczinski, R. F., and Bernhard, V. M. The Management of Chronic Ischemia of the Lower Extremities: Introduction and General Considerations. In R. B. Rutherford (Ed.), *Vascular Surgery.* Philadelphia: Saunders, 1984. Pp. 547–558.

98. Kempczinski, R. F., and Rutherford, R. B. Current status of the vascular diagnostic laboratory. *Adv. Surg.* 12: 1, 1978.

99. Kennedy, J. W., Ritchie, J. R., Davis, K. B., et al. Western Washington randomized trial of intracoronary streptokinase in acute myocardial infarction. *N. Engl. J. Med.* 309: 1477, 1983.

100. Klein, N. A., Siskind, S. J., Frishman, W. H., et al. Hemodynamic comparison of intravenous amrinone and dobutamine in patients with chronic congestive heart failure. *Am. J. Cardiol.* 48: 170, 1981.

101. Krainin, F. M., Flessas, A. P., and Spodick, D. H. Infarction-associated pericarditis: Rarity of diagnostic electrocardiogram. *N. Engl. J. Med.* 311: 1211, 1984.

102. Krikorian, J. G., and Hancock, E. W. Pericardiocentesis. *Am. J. Med.* 65: 808, 1978.

103. Leier, C. V., Hebain, P. T., Huss, P., et al. Comparative systemic and regional hemodynamic effects of dopamine and dobutamine in patients with cardiomyopathic heart failure. *Circulation* 58: 466, 1978.

104. Lemon, D. K., and White, C. W. Annuloaortic ectasia: Angiographic, hemodynamic and clinical comparison with aortic valve insufficiency. *Am. J. Cardiol.* 41: 482, 1978.

105. Levine, J. H., Michael, J. R., and Guarnieri, T. Multifocal atrial tachycardia: A toxic effect of theophylline. *Lancet* 1: 12, 1985.

106. Levy, R. I. Declining mortality in coronary artery disease. *Arteriosclerosis* 1: 312, 1981.

107. Lewis, H. D., Jr., Davis, J. W., Archibald, D. G., et al. Protective effects of aspirin against acute myocardial infarction and death in men with unstable angina: Results of a Veterans Administration Cooperative Study. *N. Engl. J. Med.* 309: 396, 1983.

108. Lie, K. I., Wellens, H. J., van Capelle, F. J., et al. Lidocaine in the prevention of primary ven-

tricular fibrillation: A double-blind randomized study of 212 consecutive patients. *N. Engl. J. Med.* 291: 1324, 1974.

109. Lindsay, J., Jr., DeBakey, M. E., and Beall, A. C. Diseases of the Aorta. In: J. W. Hurst (Ed.), *The Heart.* New York: McGraw-Hill, 1982. Pp. 1432–1456.

110. Lorell, B. H. The use of calcium blockers in hypertrophic cardiomyopathy. *Am. J. Cardiol.* 78(2B): 43, 1985.

111. Lorell, B. H., and Braunwald, E. Pericardial Disease. In E. Braunwald (Ed.), *Heart Disease: A Textbook of Cardiovascular Medicine.* Philadelphia: Saunders, 1984. Pp. 1470–1527.

112. Lown, B., and DeSilva, R. A. In J. W. Hurst (Ed.), *The Technique of Cardioversion in the Heart.* New York: McGraw-Hill, 1982. P. 1752.

113. Lown, B., and Wolf, M. Approaches to sudden death from coronary heart disease. *Circulation* 44: 130, 1971.

114. Marcus, M. L., Koyanagi, S., Harrison, D. G., et al. Abnormalities in the coronary circulation that occur as a consequence of cardiac hypertrophy. *Am. J. Med.* 75(3A): 66, 1983.

115. Maron, B. J. Asymmetry in hypertrophic cardiomyopathy: The septal to free wall thickness ratio revisited. *Am. J. Cardiol.* 55: 835, 1985.

116. Maron, B. J., Roberts, W. C., McAllister, H. A., et al. Sudden death in young athletes. *Circulation* 62: 218, 1980.

117. Massie, B. M. Myocardial hypertrophy and cardiac failure: A complex interrelationship. *Am. J. Med.* 75(3A): 67, 1983.

118. McDonald, G. R., Schaff, H. V., Pyeritz, R. E., et al. Surgical management of patients with the Marfan's syndrome and dilation of the ascending aorta. *J. Thorac. Cardiovasc. Surg.* 81: 180, 1981.

119. McKay, R. G., Safian, R. D., Lock, J. E., et al. Assessment of left ventricular and aortic valve function after aortic balloon valvuloplasty in adult patients with critical aortic stenosis. *Circulation* 75: 192, 1987.

120. McKenna, W. J., and Goodwin, J. F. The natural history of hypertrophic cardiomyopathy. *Curr. Probl. Cardiol.* 6(4): 1, 1981.

121. McKenna, W. J., Harris, L., Rowland, E., et al. Amiodarone for long-term management of patients with hypertrophic cardiomyopathy. *Am. J. Cardiol.* 54: 802, 1984.

122. Messerli, F. H. Clinical determinants and conse-

quences of left ventricular hypertrophy. *Am. J. Med.* 75(3A): 51, 1983.

123. Morganroth, J., Michelson, E., Horwitz, L. W., et al. Limitations of routine long-term electrocardiographic monitoring to assess ventricular ectopic frequency. *Circulation* 58: 408, 1978.

124. Mundth, E. D. Surgical treatment of cardiogenic shock and of acute mechanical complications following myocardial infarction. *Cardiovasc. Clin.* 8(3): 241, 1977.

125. Murgo, J. P., Alter, B. R., Dorethy, J. F., et al. Dynamics of left ventricular ejection in obstructive and nonobstructive hypertrophic cardiomyopathy. *J. Clin. Invest.* 66: 1369, 1980.

126. Murrell, W. Nitroglycerine as a remedy for angina pectoris. *Lancet* 1: 80, 1979.

127. Norris, R. M., and Mercer, C. J. Significance of idioventricular rhythms in acute myocardial infarction. *Prog. Cardiovasc. Dis.* 16: 455, 1974.

128. The Norwegian Multicenter Study Group. Timolol-induced reduction in mortality and reinfarction in patients surviving acute myocardial infarction. *N. Engl. J. Med.* 304: 801, 1981.

129. Participants in the VA Cooperative Study on Valvular Heart Disease (report prepared by Khuri, S., Folland, E., Sethi, G., Souchek, J., Oprian, C., Wong, M., Burchfiel, C. M., Henderson, W., and Hammermeister, K. E.). Six-month postoperative hemodynamics of the Hancock heterograft and the Bjork Shiley prosthesis: Results of a Veterans Administration cooperative prospective randomized trial. *J. Am. Coll. Cardiol.* (in press).

130. Participants in the VA Cooperative Study on Valvular Heart Disease (report prepared by Sethi, G. K., Miller, D. C., Souchek, J., Oprian, C., ul Hassan, Z., Folland, E., Khuri, S., Scott, S. M., Burchfiel, C., and Hammermeister, K. E. Clinical, hemodynamic, and angiographic predictors of operative mortality in patients undergoing single valve replacement. *J. Thorac. Cardiovasc. Surg.* 93: 884, 1987.

131. Pasternac, A., Noble, J., Streulens, Y., et al. Pathophysiology of chest pain in patients with cardiomyopathies and normal coronary arteries. *Circulation* 65: 778, 1982.

132. Perloff, J. K. Auscultatory and phonocardiographic manifestations of pulmonary hypertension. *Prog. Cardiovasc. Dis.* 9: 303, 1967.

133. Porter, J., Culter, B., Lee, B., et al. Pentoxifylline efficacy in treatment of intermittent claudication:

Multicenter controlled double-blind trial with objective assessment of chronic, occlusive arterial disease. *Am. Heart J.* 104: 66, 1982.

134. Reeves, J. T., Groves, B. M., and Turkevich, D. The case for treatment of selected patients with primary pulmonary hypertension. *Am. Rev. Respir. Dis.* 134: 342, 1986.

135. Regan, T. J. Alcoholic cardiomyopathy. *Prog. Cardiovasc. Dis.* 27: 141, 1984.

136. Reitz, B. A., Wallwork, J. L., Hunt, S. A., et al. Heart-lung transplantation: Successful therapy for patients with pulmonary vascular disease. *N. Engl. J. Med.* 306: 557, 1982.

137. Ritchie, J., Zaret, B. L., Strauss, H. W., et al. Myocardial imaging with thallium 201: A multicenter study in patients with angina pectoris or acute myocardial infarction. *Am. J. Cardiol.* 42: 345, 1978.

138. Roberts, B., and McLean, G. K. Role of percutaneous angioplasty in the treatment of peripheral arterial disease. *Adv. Surg.* 19: 329, 1986.

139. Ross, R. The pathogenesis of atherosclerosis: An update. *N. Engl. J. Med.* 314: 488, 1986.

140. Rowlands, D. B., Glover, D. R., and Ireland, M. A. Assessment of left ventricular mass and its response to antihypertensive treatment. *Lancet* 1: 467, 1982.

141. Ruberman, W., Weinblatt, E., Goldberg, J. D., et al. Ventricular premature complexes and sudden death after myocardial infarction. *Circulation* 64: 297, 1981.

142. Rutherford, R. B. Nonoperative Management of Chronic Peripheral Arterial Insufficiency. In R. B. Rutherford (Ed.), *Vascular Surgery*. New York: McGraw-Hill, 1984. Pp. 564–565.

143. Rutherford, R. B. (Ed.). *Infrarenal Aortic Aneurysms in Vascular Surgery*. Philadelphia: Saunders, 1984. Pp. 755–771.

144. Savage, D. D., Drayer, J. I. M., Henry, W. L., et al. Echocardiographic assessment of cardiac anatomy and function in hypertensive patients. *Circulation* 59: 623, 1979.

145. Shabetai, R. Cardiac Tamponade and Constriction. In L. D. Horwitz and B. M. Groves (Eds.), *Signs and Symptoms in Cardiology*. Philadelphia: Lippincott, 1985. Pp. 298–331.

146. Shabetai, R. Cardiomyopathy: How far have we come in 25 years, how far yet to go? *J. Am. Coll. Cardiol.* 1: 252, 1983.

147. Shah, P. M. Controversies in hypertrophic car-

diomyopathy. *Curr. Probl. Cardiol.* 11: 566, 1987.

148. Shah, P. M., Adelman, A. G., Wigle, E. D., et al. The natural (and unnatural) history of hypertrophic obstructive cardiomyopathy. *Circ. Res.* 34-35(Suppl. 2): 11, 1974.

149. Shine, K. I., Kastro, J. A., and Yurchak, P. Multifocal atrial tachycardia: Clinical and electrocardiographic features in 32 patients. *N. Engl. J. Med.* 279: 344, 1968.

150. Shulman, S. T., Amren, D. P., Bisno, A. L., et al. Prevention of bacterial endocarditis. *Circulation* 70: 1123A, 1984.

151. Smith, T., and Braunwald, E. The Management of Heart Failure. In E. Braunwald (Ed.), *Heart Disease: A Textbook of Cardiovascular Medicine*. Philadelphia: Saunders, 1984. Pp. 503–550.

152. Smith, T. W. *Digitalis Glycosides*. Orlando, Fla.: Grune and Stratton, 1986.

153. Smith, T. W., Antman, E. M., Friedman, P. L., et al. Digitalis glycosides: Mechanisms and manifestations of toxicity. *Prog. Cardiovasc. Dis.* 26: 413, 1984.

154. Smith, W. F. Epidemiology of congestive heart failure. *Am. J. Cardiol.* 55: 3A, 1985.

155. Sodeman, W. A., and Burch, G. E. The precipitating causes of congestive heart failure. *Am. Heart J.* 15: 22, 1938.

156. Sodermark, T., Edhag, E., Sjorgren, A., et al. Effect of quinidine on maintaining sinus rhythm after conversion of atrial fibrillation of flutter: A multicentre study from Stockholm. *Br. Heart J.* 37: 486, 1975.

157. Spodick, D. H. Pericardial rub: Prospective, multiple observer variation investigation of pericardial friction in 100 patients. *Am. J. Cardiol.* 35: 357, 1975.

158. Standards and guidelines for cardiopulmonary resuscitation and emergency cardiac care. *J.A.M.A.* 255: 2905, 1986.

159. Stater, E. C., and Braunwald, E. Diseases of the Aorta. In E. Braunwald (Ed.), *Heart Disease: A Textbook of Cardiovascular Medicine*. Philadelphia: Saunders, 1984. Pp. 1540–1571.

160. Stater, E. E., and DeSanctis, R. W. The clinical recognition of dissecting aortic aneurysm. *Am. J. Med.* 60: 625, 1976.

161. Szatalowicz, V. L., Arnold, P. E., Chaimovitz, C., et al. Radioimmunoassay of plasma arginine vasopressin in hyponatremic patients with congestive heart failure. *N. Engl. J. Med.* 305: 253, 1981.

162. Szilagyi, D. E., Smith, R. F., DeRusso, F. J., et al. Contribution of abdominal aortic aneurysmectomy to prolongation of life. *Ann. Surg.* 164: 678, 1966.

163. Tajik, A. J., Guiliani, E. R., Weidman, W. H., et al. Idiopathic hypertrophic subaortic stenosis. Long-term surgical follow-up. *Am. J. Cardiol.* 34: 815, 1974.

164. Takaro, T., Hultgren, H. N., Lipton, M. J., et al. The VA Cooperative Randomized Study of surgery for coronary arterial occlusive disease: II. Subgroup with significant left main lesions. *Circulation* 54(suppl. 3): 107, 1976.

165. Tarazi, R. C., and Fouad, F. M. Reversal of cardiac hypertrophy by medical treatment. *Ann. Rev. Med.* 36: 407, 1985.

166. Tarazi, R. C., and Frohlich, E. D. Is reversal of hypertrophy a desirable goal of antihypertensive therapy? *Circulation* 75(suppl. 2): 113, 1987.

167. Theroux, P., Waters, D. D., Halphen, C., et al. Prognostic value of exercise testing soon after myocardial infarction. *N. Engl. J. Med.* 301: 341, 1979.

168. Vasalle, M. Cardiac automaticity and its control. *Am. J. Physiol.* 233: H625, 1977.

169. Velbilt, V., Podrid, P. J., Lown, B., et al. Aggravation and provocation of ventricular arrhythmias by antiarrhythmic drugs. *Circulation* 65: 886, 1982.

170. Viola, A. R. The influence of pericardectomy on the hemodynamics of chronic constrictive pericarditis. *Circulation* 48: 1038, 1973.

171. Weiner, D. A., Ryan, T. J., McCabe, C. H., et al. Correlations among history of angina, ST-segment response and prevalence of coronary artery disease in the Coronary Artery Surgery Study (CASS). *N. Engl. J. Med.* 301: 230, 1979.

172. Wellens, H. J. J. Wolff-Parkinson-White syndrome. *Mod. Concepts Cardiovasc. Dis.* 52: 53, 1983.

173. Wellens, H. J. J., Bar, F. W. H. M., and Lie, K. I. The value of the electrocardiogram in the differential diagnosis of a tachycardia with a widened QRS complex. *Am. J. Med.* 64: 27, 1978.

174. Whiting, R. B., Powell, W. J., Jr., Dinsmore, R. E., and Sanders, C. A. Idiopathic hypertrophic subaortic stenosis in the elderly. *N. Engl. J. Med.* 285: 196, 1971.

175. Wit, A. L., and Rosen, M. R. Cellular electrophysiology of cardiac arrhythmias: I. Arrhythmias caused by abnormal impulse generation. *Mod.*

Concepts Cardiovasc. Dis. 50: 1, 1981.

176. Wit, A. L., and Rose, M. R. Cellular electrophysiology of cardiac arrhythmias: II. Arrhythmias caused by abnormal impulse generation. *Mod. Concepts Cardiovasc. Dis.* 50: 7, 1981.

177. Wood, F. C., and Wolferth, C. C. Angina pectoris: The clinical and electrocardiographic phenomena of the attack and their comparison with the effects of experimental temporary coronary occlusion. *Arch. Intern. Med.* 47: 339, 1931.

178. Wolf, P. A., Dawber, T. R., Thomas, H. E., Jr., et al. Epidemiologic assessment of chronic atrial fibrillation and risk of stroke: The Framingham Study. *Neurology* 28: 973, 1978.

179. Wu, D. Supraventricular tachycardia. *J.A.M.A.* 249: 3357, 1983.

180. Wynne, J., and Braunwald, E. The Cardiomyopathies and Myocarditis. In E. Braunwald (Ed.), *Heart Disease.* Philadelphia: Saunders, 1984. Pp. 1399–1456.

181. Young, J. R., and deWolf, V. G. Diseases of the Peripheral Arteries. In J. W. Hurst (Ed.), *The Heart.* New York: McGraw-Hill, 1982. Pp. 1457–1485.

182. Zelis, R., and Flaim, S. F. Alterations in vasomotor time in congestive heart failure. *Prog. Cardiovasc. Dis.* 24: 437, 1982.

183. Zipes, D. P. Genesis of Cardiac Arrhythmias: Electrophysiologic Considerations. In E. Braunwald (Ed.), *Heart Disease: A Textbook of Cardiovascular Medicine.* Philadelphia: Saunders, 1984. P. 609.

Respiratory Diseases

2

*Steven Shoemaker and
Marvin I. Schwarz*

Chronic Obstructive Pulmonary Disease

Pathophysiology

Chronic obstructive pulmonary disease (COPD) [4,32] consists of two diseases, chronic bronchitis, which has a clinical definition, and emphysema, which has specific pathologic findings [39]. Most patients with chronic obstructive pulmonary disease have a combination of both, while a minority have predominantly emphysema or chronic bronchitis.

Chronic bronchitis is characterized by a daily cough productive of sputum for at least 3 months in a year for 2 successive years. Pathologically, it is characterized by hyperplastic and hypertrophic mucous glands in the large cartilaginous bronchi. The small airways are narrowed by mucus plugging, mural fibrosis accompanied by goblet-cell hyperplasia, and inflammatory cell infiltrates. The cause of chronic bronchitis is airway irritation, usually as a result of cigarette smoke. Other contributing factors include viral and bacterial infections, environmental factors (i.e., occupational exposure), and possible genetic predisposition.

Emphysema is defined pathologically as an abnormal enlargement of the air spaces distal to the nonrespiratory bronchi accompanied by destructive changes of alveolar walls. Mild emphysema is part of the normal aging process. The destructive changes seen in emphysema appear to be the result of an imbalance in the proteolytic system, which is normally involved in remodeling fibrotic processes, and the antiproteolytic system, which normally protects against overly aggressive connective-tissue lysis. As in chronic bronchitis, inflammation appears to play a key etiologic role. Inflammatory cells release proteolytic enzymes. In addition, oxidants found in cigarette smoke and released by activated inflammatory cells may inactivate antiproteolytic enzymes. The result is that proteolysis predominates and alveolar walls are destroyed.

Diagnosis

The most common symptom in chronic obstructive pulmonary disease is dyspnea. In emphysema, dyspnea tends to follow a progressive course, being initially present only on exertion and later at rest. In chronic bronchitis, dyspnea may be episodic. By definition, patients with chronic bronchitis cough. Cough may be absent in emphysema.

On physical examination patients with emphysema tend to be thin, while chronic bronchitics usually are not. Patients with emphysema are often found sitting, leaning forward, using accessory muscles of respiration, and using pursed-lip breathing. In emphysema, the anteroposterior diameter of the chest is often increased, and the chest is hyperresonant to percussion. Other signs of hyperinflation include inferiorly displaced hemidiaphragms with a decreased excursion on respiration. Breath sounds are uniformly decreased. In chronic bronchitis, there is less hyperinflation. Percussion of the chest is often normal. The breath sounds in emphysema are decreased and are often accompanied by inspiratory crackles. In chronic bronchitis, breath sounds are often normal. During an acute bronchitic exacerbation, however, there are coarse rhonchi throughout the respiratory cycle and asthmatic type wheezing also may be heard. Patients who develop pulmonary hypertension and cor pulmonale will be found to have an increased component of the second heart sound, a right-sided S_3, a right ventricular lift, an elevated jugular venous pressure, hepatomegaly, and peripheral edema.

The chest roentgenogram in emphysema (Fig. 2-1) demonstrates decreased lung markings with signs of hyperinflation (flattened or inverted hemidiaphragms, increased retrosternal air space, and a normal or small heart size). In chronic bronchitis, the lung vasculative may be promi-

nent, especially during an exacerbation. If pulmonary hypertension is present, the pulmonary arteries will be enlarged. If cor pulmonale develops, the right ventricle will enlarge, impinging on the retrosternal air space.

The ECG in emphysema is characterized by decreased voltage. When pulmonary hypertension and cor pulmonale develop, the ECG reveals P pulmonale, right-axis deviation, and in severe cases, signs of right ventricular hypertrophy.

Pulmonary function tests in chronic obstructive pulmonary disease are useful for confirming the diagnosis, assessing the severity, following the progression, and monitoring therapeutic responses. Figure 2-2 illustrates the basic parameters obtained from standard spirometry and static lung volume measurements.

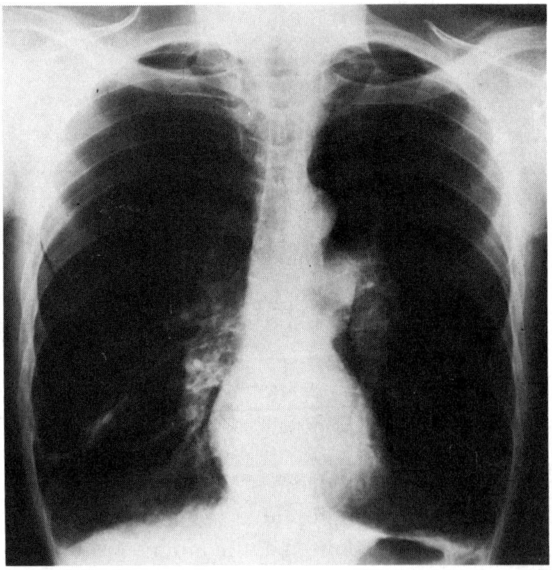

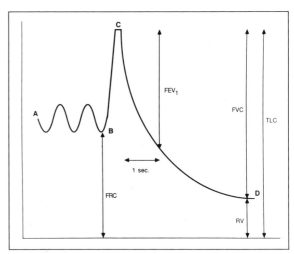

Figure 2–2. Spirometry and static lung volumes. A volume time curve is illustrated above. Time is on the x axis and volume is on the y axis. At point A, the patient begins normal tidal breathing. The volume at end expiration (point B) is the functional residual capacity (FRC). The patient is instructed to inhale maximally. The lung volume at full inspiration (point C) is the total lung capacity (TLC). The patient is next instructed to exhale as rapidly as possible. The minimum volume (point D) is the residual volume (RV). The volume of air exhaled from the maximum volume (TLC) to the minimum value (RV) is the forced vital capacity (FVC). The volume exhaled in the first second is the FEV_1.

Figure 2–1. Chest roentgenogram of a patient with severe bullous emphysema. Hyperinflation is pronounced with flattening of both hemidiaphragms. The size of the pulmonary arteries is increased consistent with pulmonary artery hypertension.

Spirometry can be carried out using relatively simple machines, and some argue that spirometers should be as common as sphygmomanometers in the practice of medicine. The most important parameters measured by spirometry are the forced expiratory volume in 1 second (FEV$_1$), the forced vital capacity (FVC), and the FEV$_1$/FVC ratio.

In obstructive lung diseases such as chronic obstructive pulmonary disease, the FEV$_1$ is decreased. In restrictive diseases, the FVC is decreased. However, neither of these parameters can be interpreted alone. There are times when the FEV$_1$ is decreased in restricted processes (as all lung volumes decrease) and times when the FVC is decreased in obstructive processes (when there is significant air trapping). This is why the first parameter that should be examined when studying spirometry is the FEV$_1$/FVC ratio. If this ratio is less than 70 percent, an obstructive process is present. If this ratio is greater than 70 percent, the spirometry is normal or a restrictive process may be present. The FVC distinguishes between these two possibilities. An FVC greater than 80 percent of predicted is normal, and a figure less than 80 percent of predicted is consistent with a restrictive process. There are times when combined obstructive and restrictive processes are present, which often cannot be sorted out by spirometry. In this situation, static lung volumes may be helpful. Other tests are also available which are beyond the scope of this discussion.

In patients with known chronic obstructive pulmonary disease, the most important parameter to follow the progression of disease is the FEV$_1$. The FEV$_1$ is also the best parameter to diagnose early disease in patients with minimal chronic obstructive pulmonary disease. As mentioned earlier, it is also one of the simplest measurements to make. The utility of the FEV$_1$ in chronic obstructive pulmonary disease cannot be overemphasized.

The static lung volumes, functional residual capacity (FRC), residual volume (RV), and total lung capacity (TLC) (see Fig. 2-1) are important for assessing the degree of hyperinflation and air trapping present in chronic obstructive pulmonary disease. The FRC is the most reliable parameter because it does not depend on patient effort. The FRC is the equilibrium volume reached as the patient relaxes, with the lungs tending to collapse to smaller volumes and the chest wall tending to expand to larger volumes. In emphysema there is a loss of lung elastic recoil so that the lung has a decreased tendency to collapse. The FRC is therefore increased. For the same reason, the TLC is increased. The loss of elastic recoil makes it easier for the muscles of respiration to stretch the lungs to higher volumes.

In contrast, in fibrotic lung disease resulting in restrictive defects, the elastic recoil is increased. The lungs have a greater tendency to collapse, and the FRC is decreased. The lungs are harder to stretch, so the TLC is also decreased. Airways in chronic obstructive pulmonary disease tend to collapse at low lung volumes, resulting in decreased flow and air trapping. The RV increases out of proportion to the TLC. This increases the RV/TLC ratio, a parameter often used to assess air trapping. The FRC also may be increased in obstructive processes, even without the loss of elastic recoil.

In addition to spirometry and static lung volumes, the diffusion capacity for carbon monoxide (DLCO) is often measured as part of routine pulmonary function tests. The diffusion capacity of carbon monoxide measures the amount of carbon monoxide which moves from the alveolar space into the pulmonary circulation. The term *diffusion* is somewhat of a misnomer, since the diffusion of carbon monoxide from the alveolar space to the capillaries is rarely a limiting factor. The diffusion capacity for carbon monoxide more accurately reflects the surface area available at the alveolar-capillary interface. In emphysema, alveolar walls are lost, and this surface area is reduced. This is manifested by a reduction in the diffusion capacity for carbon monoxide. This diffusion capacity is normal in chronic bronchitis.

In both chronic bronchitis and emphysema, spirometry reveals evidence of airflow limitation (or obstruction). The FEV$_1$/FVC ratio and the

FEV_1 are decreased. There is usually more hyper-inflation (increased FRC and TLC) in emphysema secondary to the loss of elastic recoil, as well as more air trapping (increased RV/TLC ratio) compared to chronic bronchitis. These measurements are often made before and after the inhalation of a beta-adrenergic agent. A positive bronchodilator response is defined as a significant increase in airflow parameters (FEV_1/FVC) or a significant decrease in air trapping and hyperinflation. Usually there is no acute bronchodilator response in chronic obstructive pulmonary disease. There are some patients with this disease who demonstrate a partial response (10 to 30 percent improvement), and these are most often patients with chronic bronchitis. In contrast, patients with asthma demonstrate a total correction of airflow abnormalities after adequate bronchodilator therapy.

Gas-exchange problems are usually more severe with chronic bronchitis than with emphysema. The P_{O_2} tends to be lower, and the P_{CO_2} tends to be higher. Often the best way to distinguish chronic bronchitis and emphysema is to examine the diffusion capacity of carbon monoxide. This is decreased in emphysema and is normal in chronic bronchitis.

Treatment

The primary goal in the management of chronic obstructive pulmonary disease should be to prevent disease progression. To accomplish this, patients must be identified early in the course of airway obstruction. Attempts must then be made to remove the irritants causing inflammation. In most cases this involves getting the patient to stop smoking. Once airway obstruction is established, the goal should be to slow the progression of the disease and prevent complications such as cor pulmonale.

Patients with early disease may be identified by utilizing pulmonary function screening to search for reductions in the FEV_1. The next step, getting patients to stop smoking, is much more difficult. New techniques such as use of nicotine gum offer some hope when combined with a group program.

When airway obstruction occurs, it should be treated with bronchodilators. The important question of whether early treatment of airway obstruction in chronic obstructive pulmonary disease can slow the progression of the disease is as yet unanswered, but it is currently being studied. The mainstays of bronchodilator therapy are inhaled beta-adrenergic agents (i.e., metaproterenol, albuterol, and terbutaline) and theophyllines.

The treatment of acute exacerbations of chronic obstructive pulmonary disease requiring hospital admission is similar to that for acute asthmatic attacks. This is outlined later in this chapter. The following is a discussion of the outpatient treatment of chronic obstructive pulmonary disease.

Beta-adrenergic agents may be inhaled or taken orally. Many believe that side effects (i.e., tachycardia and tremulousness) are diminished when these agents are inhaled. For convenience, these agents are often supplied as metered-dose inhalers (MDI). Patients must be carefully instructed if they are to achieve maximal benefit from these inhalers. The goal is to inhale smaller particles generated by metered-dose inhalers which reach the small airways and avoid deposition of the large particles on the oropharyngeal mucosa. The result is decreased systemic absorption of the drug. This can be accomplished by holding the inhaler 4 to 6 inches away from the mouth before discharging. This also can be accomplished by using a spacer device or reservoir device. In reservoir devices, the inhaler is first discharged into a large container and the resulting mist is then inhaled.

Theophyllines are commonly used in chronic obstructive pulmonary disease, often without evidence that they are effective in partially reversing the airway obstruction. There is a subgroup of these patients with a reversible component (FEV_1

Table 2–1. *Theophylline Dose Factors*

Factors that decrease theophylline clearance:
  Hypoxia
  Fever
  Liver disease
  Congestive heart failure
  Viral infections
  Erythromycin
  Troleandomycin
Factors that increase theophylline clearance:
  Cigarettes
  High-protein diet

increased more than 20 percent after inhaled beta agent) who have clearly been shown to improve airflow by adding theophyllines to beta agents.

Theophyllines are available as sustained-release capsules, which is the preferred therapy for outpatients. Initial starting dose is 10 mg/kg per day given two to three times a day. Theophyllines are metabolized by the liver, and many factors must be considered when selecting the dose (see Table 2-1) [34]. Minor side effects include gastrointestinal upset and headaches. Major side effects include cardiac arrhythmias and seizures which may be fatal. Side effects are rare at theophylline levels less than 20 µg/ml. The therapeutic range is 10 to 20 µg/ml.

Anticholinergic agents also may be useful in patients with chronic bronchitis. Until recently, inhaled atropine was the only available anticholinergic drug on the market in the United States. Its use is somewhat limited by systemic side effects. A related compound, ipratropium bromide, is now available and offers the advantage of being poorly absorbed systematically after inhalation. Studies have shown that approximately 50 percent of patients with chronic bronchitis will improve their airflow parameters when inhaled ipratropium bromide is combined with inhaled beta-adrenergic agents.

Recurrent infections are important factors responsible for the progression of airway obstruction in chronic obstructive pulmonary disease.

Bronchitis usually begins as a viral infection. Secondary bacterial infections may develop and are most commonly caused by *S. pneumoniae* and *H. influenzae*. Broad-spectrum antibiotics are used to treat acute episodes of bronchitis. In addition, it is essential that patients with chronic obstructive pulmonary disease receive a one-time polyvalent Pneumovax vaccination and yearly influenza vaccinations.

The use of corticosteroids in chronic obstructive pulmonary disease remains controversial. Long-term use is associated with significant side effects. There are, however, a small subgroup of patients who show a dramatic response to corticosteroids. Patients with chronic bronchitis and reactive airways during acute exacerbations often benefit by the addition of oral or intravenous corticosteroids to their bronchodilator regimen. If corticosteroid treatment is begun in a patient with chronic obstructive pulmonary disease, it is essential to obtain baseline pulmonary function tests so that an objective response can be assessed.

Chronic oxygen therapy has a definite role in the management of chronic obstructive pulmonary disease [31]. Its main goal is to prevent the development of pulmonary hypertension and cor pulmonale. In addition, chronic oxygen therapy has been shown to prolong life and improve the quality of life by reducing the number of hospitalizations, allowing for increased mobility and improving intellectual abilities.

Who should be treated with chronic oxygen therapy? Two factors must be considered. What is the degree of hypoxemia, and what effect is the hypoxemia having on the patient? Patients should be evaluated for chronic therapy after their disease has stabilized on an optimal medical regimen for at least 3 weeks. At least two arterial blood gases should be evaluated. If the P_{O_2} is less than 55 mmHg or between 55 and 59 mmHg accompanied by cor pulmonale and/or polycythemia (hematocrit $\geq$ 55 percent), oxygen therapy should be initiated. Other patients who are able to increase their physical activity with supplemental O_2 also should be considered.

Asthma

Pathophysiology

Asthma is a symptom complex characterized by reversible airway obstruction [26]. It therefore differs from the fixed airway obstruction of emphysema and chronic bronchitis. The airways of an asthmatic patient are, by definition, hyperreactive, and bronchoconstriction is initiated by stimuli which would have little or no effect on a normal airway.

Diagnosis

The diagnosis is usually not difficult. There are instances, however, when asthma is confusesd with congestive heart failure, upper airway obstruction, hysteria syndromes, recurrent aspiration, vasculitis syndromes, industrial bronchitis, and cystic fibrosis.

Early symptoms of asthma include cough, chest tightness, and wheezing, and these may progress to dyspnea in more severe cases. When interviewing an asthmatic patient it is important to determine that individual's trigger factors. Potential trigger factors include (1) exposure to pollens and animal danders in patients with a history of atopic disease, (2) cold air exposure and hyperventilation, (3) exposure to molds and certain bacteria such as thermophilic actinomyces found in cold, damp environments and around humidifiers, (4) ingestion of aspirin (in patients with triad asthma), metabisulfites (food additives used to prevent oxidation), and/or tartrazine (used in certain food dyes), (5) esophageal reflux with or without aspiration, and (6) viral or bacterial upper respiratory tract infections. As with other pulmonary diseases, it is important to obtain a careful occupational history in the asthmatic individual. Exposure to substances in the work environment may initiate respiratory symptoms. These symptoms are often delayed, occurring after the subject leaves the workplace. Similarly, extended periods away from the workplace (weekends or vacations) often relieve symptoms. In patients with chronic asthma, rhinitis and sinusitis are frequently present, and reactivations of these conditions are associated with worsening asthma.

Physical findings in mild asthma include tachypnea, a prolonged expiratory phase, and wheezing. As the asthma worsens, patients develop pulsus paradoxus (blood pressure fall > 15 mmHg on inspiration), tachycardia (>130 heartbeats per minute), use of the accessory muscles of respiration, and the inability to talk in complete sentences. Also, the breath sounds diminish and there are physical findings of chest hyperinflation as a result of severe bronchoconstriction and air trapping. During this phase, wheezing may actually diminish or disappear. The nasal mucosa should be carefully examined for signs of chronic rhinitis and polyps, which are characteristic of triad or aspirin-sensitive asthma.

Laboratory findings include eosinophilia, the presence of which often predicts a favorable response to corticosteroid treatment. Eosinophilia also raises the possibility of allergic bronchopulmonary aspergillosis (ABPA) as an exacerbating factor. In allergic bronchopulmonary aspergillosis, an allergic response to the colonization of *Aspergillus* species in the airway is accompanied by asthma, pulmonary infiltrates, and mucoid impaction of the bronchus.

During an acute asthmatic attack the arterial blood gases reveal hypoxemia and hyperventilation resulting in respiratory alkalosis. A rising P_{CO_2} is a poor prognostic sign and indicates worsening asthma with air trapping and patient fatigue. When this occurs, the patient should be admitted to an intensive care facility and mechanical ventilation considered.

Pulmonary function tests are characterized by decreased flow rates and expiratory lung volumes. The FEV_1/FVC ratio is decreased, and static lung volumes are increased consistent with hyperinflation. The preceding physiologic profile typifies an active asthmatic condition, which is usually completely reversible with treatment and/ or removal of trigger factors. The most common chest radiographic finding is hyperinflation. Routine chest roentgenograms are not indicated in many exacerbations. They are indicated if pneumonia or pneumothorax is suspected. In patients with refractory asthma, sinus films will sometimes indicate persistent infections which may be asymptomatic and making the asthma worse.

In those patients in whom asthma is suspected but not easily diagnosed, bronchoprovocation is indicated. Bronchial challenges with inhaled histamine or the cholinergic agent mecholyl may be used to diagnose hyperreactive airways. Asthmatics develop bronchospasm at much lower doses of inhaled histamine or mecholyl when compared to normal subjects. In addition, specialized centers can perform inhalational challenges with agents suspected of causing industrial asthma. Finally, exercise testing often triggers asthma and may be used to test for hyperreactive airways.

There is a subset of asthmatic patients who develop wheezing because of paradoxical vocal cord motion (i.e., narrowing of laryngeal orifice with inspiration) [5]. This is related to emotional factors and often responds to voice training and psychotherapy. The diagnosis is suspected on examination of inspiration/expiratory flow volume loops with these patients showing evidence of airflow imitation on inspiration and expiration. The most direct way to make this diagnosis is by laryngoscopic observation during an acute episode.

Treatment

When designing a treatment regimen for the asthmatic patient it is important to consider the specific cause of airway obstruction. Considerations include (1) bronchial smooth-muscle contraction, (2) increased mucous secretion (infection), and (3) bronchial mucosal edema.

Acute exacerbations should initially be treated with beta-adrenergic agents and theophyllines. Beta-adrenergic agents may be administered subcutaneously (younger patients) or, alternatively,

Table 2–2. *Intravenous Aminophylline*

Loading dose	5 mg/kg
Maintenance dose:	
1. Normal individuals	0.6 mg/kg/h
2. Severe liver disease, congestive heart failure (CHF), pneumonia	0.2 mg/kg/h
3. Severe bronchial obstruction	0.4 mg/kg/h
4. Drugs: cimetidine, erythromycin	0.3 mg/kg/h

inhaled to reduce systemic effects. If the patient has never taken theophyllines, a loading dose should be given followed by a maintenance dose (Table 2-2). Theophyllines are metabolized by the liver. The maintenance dose should be decreased in older patients and in patients with liver disease, particularly chronic passive congestion of the liver. Additionally, other factors affect theophylline metabolism (see Table 2-1). Theophylline side effects include gastrointestinal upset (nausea), headaches, and seizures which may be fatal. The therapeutic range is 10 to 20 μg/ml.

In more severe asthmatic attacks which do not respond to maximum therapeutic doses of beta-adrenergic agonists and theophylline, corticosteroids are indicated and should initially be given parenterally. In addition, anticholinergic agents may be useful when cough is a predominant symptom. Patients who do not respond to the management outlined above must be monitored in the hospital [37]. As stated before, a rising P_{CO_2} is ominous, and hypoventilation remains a major cause for mortality. If the P_{CO_2} begins to rise and/ or the patient appears to be tiring, the patient should be intubated and mechanical ventilation initiated. At this time it may be necessary to sedate and at times even paralyze the patient so that mechanical ventilation can be delivered. At this point, isoproterenol is often given by constant intravenous infusion. Additional causes of death in asthmatics requiring mechanical ventilation include tension pneumothorax and endotracheal tube malfunctions.

While most patients show significant improvement with the preceding therapy, there are patients with persistent airway obstruction and patients who experience frequent recurrences. This type of asthmatic often requires chronic corticosteroid therapy as well as daily inhaled beta-adrenergic agents and oral theophyllines. Every effort should be made to taper oral corticosteroids and achieve the lowest maintenance dose possible. In order to accomplish this, inhaled corticosteroids and inhaled cromolyn sodium are often added to the treatment regimen. If the oral prednisone cannot be tapered to acceptable daily doses to control symptoms, alternate-day prednisone may be considered.

Patient education also has an important role in asthma therapy. Asthmatics must learn to recognize the early signs of an exacerbation and either titrate their proven therapy or seek medical care immediately. In addition, asthmatics must be aware of and avoid trigger factors: e.g., workplace-related, cold exposure, exercise, and metabisulfite ingestion. Allergic rhinitis, if present, should be vigorously treated, as should sinusitis and gastroesophageal reflux.

Factors that Affect Theophylline Clearance
Decreased clearance (physician should decrease dose):
1. Hypoxia
2. Fever
3. Liver disease
4. Cardiac decompensation
5. Drugs: cimetidine, erythromycin
6. Viral infections
Increased clearance (physician should increase dose):
1. Cigarettes
2. High-protein diet

Interstitial Lung Disease

Interstitial lung disease (ILD) is a broad term encompassing many etiologies which can cause fibrosis of the alveolar walls [9,22,40]. Etiologically, interstitial lung disease can be separated into five categories: (1) pneumoconioses (Table 2-3), (2) drug-induced (Table 2-4), (3) collagen-vascular (a more detailed discussion follows), (4) primary diseases (Table 2-5), and (5) idiopathic pulmonary fibrosis [6,7]. Idiopathic pulmonary fibrosis (IPF) is diagnosed by excluding the first four categories.

Early recognition and initiation of indicated treatment are essential. Therefore, interstitial lung disease should be considered in all patients who have unexplained dyspnea. When interstitial lung disease is suspected, an aggressive approach should be taken in order to establish a diagnosis.

Table 2–4. *Commonly Used Drugs that Cause Interstitial Lung Disease*

Nitrofurantoin
Gold
Bleomycin
Cyclophosphamide
Methotrexate
Busulfan
Carmustine

Table 2–5. *Primary Diseases that Cause Interstitial Lung Disease*

Sarcoidosis (phase 3)
Eosinophilic granuloma (histiocytosis X)
Chronic hypersensitivity pneumonitis
Pulmonary hemorrhage syndromes
Lymphangitic carcinomatosis
Neurofibromatosis
Lymphangioleiomyomatosis
Hereditary
After infection

Table 2–3. *Pneumoconioses*

Asbestos
Silica
Talc
Fiberglass
Beryllium
Aluminum
Iron

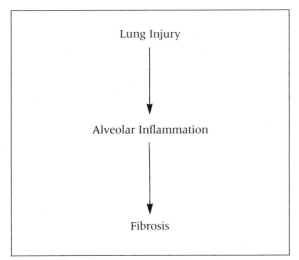

Figure 2–3.

Pathophysiology

The hypothesized pathogenesis of interstitial lung disease is outlined in Fig. 2-3. An initial injury to the epithelial cells of the lung is accompanied by an inflammatory response, characterized by cellular outpouring of pulmonary macrophages, lymphocytes, plasma cells, and occasionally, neutrophils and eosinophils. This is followed by fibroblast proliferation and the laying down of collagen and elastin. As fibrosis progresses, there is also progressive destruction of the normal alveolar architecture, resulting in the development of cystic areas. This end-stage form of interstitial lung disease is often referred to as "honeycomb lung."

Diagnosis

The most common presenting symptom in interstitial lung disease is dyspnea, which is often insidious. The next most common symptom is nonproductive cough. In obtaining the patient's history, special emphasis should be placed on (1) occupational exposures which could be responsible for a pneumoconiosis (i.e., silicosis or asbestosis) or hypersensitivity pneumonitis (farmer's lung), (2) special hobbies and/or pets which could

also lead to hypersensitivity pneumonitis (i.e., pigeon breeders lung), (3) medications, and (4) symptoms of collagen-vascular disease. Characteristic physical findings include digital clubbing and fine inspiratory, or "Velcro," rales in the lower lung zones.

Routine laboratory evaluation should include an antinuclear antibody (ANA) profile and rheumatoid factor to exclude interstitial lung disease associated with collagen-vascular disease. Modest increases in ANA and rheumatoid factor titers are, however, often seen in idiopathic pulmonary fibrosis. In addition, circulating immune complexes also may be increased in idiopathic pulmonary fibrosis.

Pulmonary function tests are characterized by a restrictive defect without airflow limitation. Lung volumes (FVC and TLC), pulmonary compliance, and the diffusing capacity for carbon monoxide are reduced. The most sensitive test indicative of abnormal gas exchange is a widened alveolar-arterial oxygen gradient after exercise.

The chest roentgenogram may be normal in a small percentage of patients, especially early in the course of the disease. Typical abnormalities include bilateral, lower-zone, reticular, and reticular-nodular infiltrates. Lung volumes are decreased in more advanced disease, and evidence of pulmonary hypertension may develop. In end-stage disease, small cystic spaces appear representing honeycombing, discussed above.

A lung biopsy is often required to establish a diagnosis. Certain diseases can be diagnosed by transbronchial biopsies obtained during bronchoscopy, particularly sarcoidosis and lymphangitic carcinomatosis. The relatively small amount of tissue obtained from a transbronchial biopsy, however, is a limiting factor, and most patients require an open lung biopsy.

An important prognostic feature one obtains from biopsy is the degree of cellularity versus fixed fibrosis. Patients with active cellular disease have better responses to treatment. Efforts have been made to develop less invasive ways of determining disease activity, such as bronchoalveolar lavage [42].

The results of bronchoalveolar lavage studies vary. Most authors agree that the presence of increased numbers of lymphocytes by bronchoalveolar lavage indicates underlying alveolar disease and predicts improved therapeutic responsiveness.

Treatment

The treatment of interstitial lung disease involves identifying the etiologic agent and removing it if possible (e.g., drug-induced or hypersensitivity pneumonitis). Treatment in general attempts to suppress ongoing inflammation.

The standard treatment for active disease is the administration of corticosteroids at starting doses of 1 to 2 mg/kg per day. Other drugs include cytotoxic agents such as cyclophosphamide. Patients with predominantly fibrosis on biopsy with little inflammation should have a trial of corticosteroids and/or cyclophosphamide, since a small percentage of these patients will respond. This may occur because biopsies are often performed at the periphery of the lung, which may be the area of greatest fibrosis. Early inflammatory changes may be present more centrally.

The third approach to treatment includes preventing complications. These patients are at increased risk to develop infections and should be given a one-time polyvalent pneumococcocal vaccine in addition to yearly influenza vaccines. Oxygen should be given to severely hypoxic patients to prevent cor pulmonale.

The prognosis in patients with interstitial lung disease is variable. The mean survival is 3 to 4 years. Patients with the most fibrosis on biopsy have the worst prognosis. For this reason, it is extremely important to diagnose these patients as early as possible and begin treatment.

Pleuropulmonary Manifestations of Collagen-Vascular Disease

All the major collagen-vascular diseases have been shown to cause pleural and/or pulmonary disease. Pleuropulmonary disease may be the first manifestation of the collagen-vascular disease and also may be the major cause of morbidity and mortality.

Rheumatoid Arthritis

The pleuropulmonary manifestations of rheumatoid arthritis are listed in Table 2-6 and are more common in men. Pleural disease is the most frequent manifestation; pleuritic pain without effusion occurs in approximately 20 percent and pleural effusions occur in 3 to 5 percent. Presenting symptoms include pleuritic pain and dyspnea, if the effusion is large enough. The fluid is exudative and has a low glucose level (<30 mg/dl) in 80 percent of patients. This may be accompanied by a low pleural fluid pH. If the pleural effusion is chronic, it is often cloudy due to the accumulation of cholesterol, which is released from degenerating inflammatory cells. Rheumatoid arthritis is thus one of the more common causes of chyliform effusions (see the section entitled Pleural Disease). The diagnosis of a rheumatoid pleural effusion in the absence of joint disease is difficult. The presence of a high-titer rheumatoid factor in the effusion is nonspecific and may occur with malignancy and tuberculosis. A pleural biopsy is also nonspecific in most cases.

The effusions often spontaneously resolve, but

Table 2–6. Pleuropulmonary Manifestations of Rheumatoid Arthritis

Pleurisy with or without effusion
Interstitial pneumonitis
Necrobiotic nodule(s)
Caplan's syndrome
Pulmonary hypertension
Small airways disease/bronchiolitis obliterans

they may leave residual pleural thickening. Resolution of the pleural effusion may be enhanced by systemic corticosteroids.

Interstitial pneumonitis, which is clinically and pathologically identical to idiopathic pulmonary fibrosis, is also relatively common in association with rheumatoid arthritis, but the exact incidence has not been established. When pulmonary function tests are performed, up to 40 percent of patients have abnormalities. Most of these patients are asymptomatic, and only 5 to 10 percent have abnormal chest roentgenograms.

Common symptoms include cough and dyspnea. Fine inspiratory crackles are usually heard at the lung bases. Subcutaneous nodules and finger clubbing are frequently found. The evidence to support the therapeutic efficacy of corticosteroid and other immunosuppressive therapy for the treatment of interstitial pneumonitis associated with rheumatoid arthritis is anecdotal with no prospective trials.

Necrobiotic nodules in the lung may be single or multiple, and cavitation is common. Pathologically, these nodules are identical to subcutaneous nodules. They must be distinguished from primary and metastatic carcinomas.

Caplan's syndrome is a combination of a pneumoconiosis (usually coal worker's pneumoconiosis or silicosis) and rheumatoid arthritis. Round densities occur primarily in the upper lobes. Pathologically, inflammatory cells containing the offending mineral are surrounded by palisading epithelial cells, and central necrosis of the nodule often occurs. These densities may be infected with tuberculosis.

Pulmonary hypertension may occur secondary to either interstitial lung disease and hypoxic pulmonary vasoconstriction or a primary plexiform occlusion of small pulmonary vessels. The latter is similar to the syndrome of primary pulmonary hypertension and is not associated with vasculitis or thromboembolic disease.

Up to 30 percent of nonsmoking rheumatoid arthritis patients will have evidence of airway obstructions on pulmonary function testing; pathologically, these obstructions are peribronchiolar mononuclear cell infiltrates. Bronchiolitis obliterans may occur de novo or as a complication of penicillamine therapy.

Systemic Lupus Erythematosus (SLE) (Table 2-7)

Pleuritis is the most common pleuropulmonary manifestation of systemic lupus erythematosus. Pleural effusions, which may or may not be present with pleuritis, tend to be bilateral. Pleural fluid characteristics vary. The fluid may be clear or serosanguineous, and the pleural fluid glucose level is usually normal, as is pH. There are two findings which help differentiate SLE effusions. One is a pleural fluid DNA titer greater than 1:160, and the other is the presence of lupus cells in the pleural fluid.

Two types of acute immunologic pneumonia occur in systemic lupus erythematosus: acute lupus pneumonitis and acute hemorrhagic alveolitis. These patients present with the acute onset of fevers, dyspnea, and nonproductive cough. Hemoptysis may occur in the hemorrhagic alveolitis, but it is not invariably present. The histologic picture of the lung is variable and nonspecific; the findings include significant mononuclear cell infiltrates and alveolitis without vasculitis. Progression to frank respiratory failure may occur. The response to therapy in patients with hemorrhagic pneumonitis is often disappointing, and plasmapheresis has had only minimal success. Acute lupus pneumonitis differs from the hemorrhagic alveolitis in that it is often the presenting mani-

Table 2–7. *Pleuropulmonary Manifestations of Systemic Lupus Erythematosus*

Pleurisy with or without effusion
Acute lupus pneumonitis
Chronic interstitial pneumonitis
Uremic pulmonary edema
Atelectasis due to diaphragmatic dysfunction
Infections

festation of systemic lupus erythematosus. Half the patients with acute lupus pneumonitis clear their infiltrates completely following treatment with corticosteroids and azathiaprine. Pulmonary fibrosis may follow repeated episodes of acute lupus pneumonitis.

Lung volumes are decreased in systemic lupus erythematosus for several reasons. Platelike atelectasis may develop from prolonged pleuritis and splinting. In addition, diaphragmatic dysfunction results in a reduction in transdiaphragmatic pressures.

Other causes for infiltrates in systemic lupus erythematosus include edema secondary to uremia and infection. Infections are common in these patients, and because they are frequently the cause of major morbidity and mortality, they should be excluded in any acute pulmonary process occurring with systemic lupus erythematosus.

Progressive Systemic Sclerosis

Pleuropulmonary involvement occurs in up to 90 percent of patients with progressive systemic sclerosis (PSS) or patients with the CREST syndrome. Skin involvement is often the most prominent manifestation of progressive systemic sclerosis, while clubbing, Raynaud's phenomenon, esophageal dysfunction, sclerodactyly, and telangiectasias characterize the CREST syndrome. The pleuropulmonary manifestations of progressive systemic sclerosis are listed in Table 2-8.

Diffuse interstitial fibrosis is eventually seen in almost all patients with progressive systemic sclerosis. The most common symptoms are dyspnea on exertion and cough. Physical examination is remarkable for basilar inspiratory crackles, and

chest roentgenograms reveal diffuse interstitial infiltrates and honeycombing in end-stage disease.

Treatment of this disease is essentially supportive. The interstitial fibrosis does not respond well to corticosteroids or cytotoxic agents.

Pulmonary hypertension is often present in patients with progressive systemic sclerosis and is due to hypoxic vasoconstriction secondary to the pulmonary fibrosis. A primary pulmonary vascular disease in the absence of pulmonary fibrosis occurs in 10 to 15 percent of CREST syndrome patients.

Pathologically, intimal proliferation is found which leads to virtual obliteration of the vessel lumen. Medium and small pulmonary arteries are the most commonly involved. As with pulmonary fibrosis, there is no evidence that corticosteroids or cytotoxic agents affect the progression of this vascular disease.

Recurrent aspiration pneumonitis secondary to esophageal dysmotility occurs with progressive systemic sclerosis and the CREST syndrome. Pleural disease is less common in progressive systemic sclerosis than in rheumatoid arthritis and systemic lupus erythematosus. Patients with progressive systemic sclerosis and pulmonary fibrosis are at increased risk to develop bronchiolar carcinoma, which should be kept in mind when evaluating changes seen on chest roentgenograms.

Polymyositis and Dermatomyositis

The pleuropulmonary manifestations of these two diseases are listed in Table 2-9. Polymyositis is a degenerative and inflammatory disease of striated muscle which causes symmetric weakness and atrophy, principally of the limb girdles, neck, and

Table 2–8. *Pleuropulmonary Manifestations of Scleroderma*

Diffuse interstitial fibrosis
Pulmonary vascular disease
Pleural disease
Aspiration pneumonitis
Bronchiolar carcinoma

Table 2–9. *Pleuropulmonary Manifestations of Polymyositis and Dermatomyositis*

Interstitial pneumonitis
Aspiration pneumonia
Atelectasis, respiratory failure, pneumonia
Methotrexate pneumonitis

pharynx. When associated with a characteristic rash, the disease is known as dermatomyositis. Both conditions have a female predominance.

Interstitial pneumonitis occurs in 5 percent of these patients; in 40 percent of these patients the pulmonary manifestation precedes the muscle and skin manifestations. Clinical findings are similar to those in other patients with interstitial pneumonitis. Importantly, about half these patients respond to corticosteroids, and this is dependent on the cellularity of the open lung biopsy.

Esophageal involvement results in recurrent aspiration pneumonias. Involvement and eventual weakness of the respiratory muscles result in atelectasis, respiratory failure, and pneumonia. The use of methotrexate for treatment of the muscle disease may result in a hypersensitivity pneumonitis.

Sjögren's Syndrome

Sjögren's syndrome is manifested by keratoconjunctivitis sicca, xerostomia (dry mouth), and parotid enlargement. It may be a primary disease or associated with any of the collagen-vascular diseases: rheumatoid arthritis (50 percent of patients), systemic lupus erythematosus, scleroderma, and dermatomyositis. There is striking predominance of women (90 percent).

Pulmonary manifestations occur frequently, but it is often difficult to determine which are due to Sjögren's syndrome and which are due to the underlying collagen-vascular disease, if present.

With Sjögren's syndrome pleurisy may occur with or without effusion, and interstitial pneumonitis occurs in 15 percent of patients. Involvement of respiratory tract mucous glands may result in inspissated secretions leading to atelectasis and secondary infection. Finally, lymphoid interstitial pneumonia may result in diffuse reticulonodular or coarse nodular infiltrates in patients with Sjögren's syndrome.

Lymphocytic interstitial pneumonia may progress to a B-cell lymphoma. Corticosteroids and/or cytotoxic agents have benefited a limited number of patients.

Sarcoidosis

Sarcoidosis is a multiorgan systemic disease of unknown etiology. It is characterized by noncaseating granulomas composed of chronic inflammatory, epithelioid, and Langerhans' giant cells [28].

Sarcoidosis occurs worldwide. In the United States it is most common in blacks, but in Sweden the incidence is similar to that of black population in the United States. The majority of patients are younger than 40 years on presentation, with a peak incidence in the third and fourth decades. There is a female predominance. Recent evidence suggests that the incidence is decreased in smokers.

Diagnosis

Patients with sarcoidosis often display decreased delayed-type hypersensitivity, skin-test anergy, and a peripheral lymphocytopenia. However, immunoglobulin levels are characteristically increased. In contrast to what is found peripherally, there appears to be an increased cellular immune response at the site of the granulomas [8]. For example, bronchoalveolar lavage of patients with pulmonary sarcoidosis reveals increased numbers of T cells, suggesting that these cells are accumulating in the lung at the expense of the peripheral circulation. It is unclear what the initiating stimulus is for the augmented immune response

Table 2–10. *Staging for Intrathoracic Sarcoidosis*

Stage	Aden-opathy	Parenchymal Infiltrate	Incidence	Percent who Spontaneously Resolve
Type 0	−	−	5–15%	—
Type 1	+	−	50%	50–75%
Type 2	+	+	25–50%	25–75%
Type 3	−	+	10–15%	10–25%

which precedes and leads to granuloma formation. In addition, it is unclear what controls the balance of this inflammatory response, so that progressive disease is found in some patients and spontaneous regression is seen in other patients.

The lungs are the most common organ system affected, being involved in 90 percent of patients. The chest roentgenogram is used to stage intrathoracic disease and is divided into four types. These are outlined in Table 2-10.

Hilar and mediastinal adenopathy are present in types 1 and 2, the most common types, and appear to predict a more favorable outcome. The parenchymal infiltrates in type 2 disease may be reticular, reticulonodular, or alveolar (Fig. 2-4). Type 3 disease (no adenopathy) usually indicates chronic progressive disease and often reveals fibrosis on histologic examination in addition to granuloma formation. As the fibrosis progresses, there is retraction of the hila and formation of dense bands of fibrosis tissue and cysts. These cysts may become colonized with *Aspergillus* species, resulting in the formation of a mycetoma (fungus ball). Uncommon chest roentgenographic findings include pleural thickening and/or effusions, cavitation of alveolar nodules, scattered parenchymal calcifications, and eggshell calcification of the mediastinal nodes. The differential diagnosis of the infiltrates seen in sarcoidosis are listed in Table 2-11.

Dermatologic lesions are common in sarcoidosis. The presence of erythema nodosum associated with fever, arthralgias, and hilar adenopathy is classic for sarcoidosis and carries an excellent

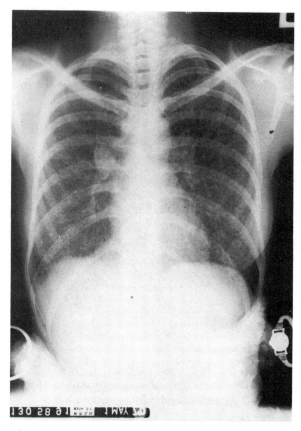

Figure 2–4. *Chest roentgenogram of a patient with class 2 sarcoidosis. Nodular parenchymal infiltrates are present along with bilateral hilar adenopathy.*

Table 2–11. *Differential Diagnosis of Infiltrates Seen in Sarcoidosis*

Wegener's granulomatosis
Eosinophilic pneumonia
Hypersensitivity pneumonitis
Idiopathic pulmonary fibrosis
Interstitial pneumonitis secondary to collagen-vascular disease
Miliary tuberculosis
Carcinomatosis
Pneumoconiosis

prognosis rarely requiring therapy. The most characteristic dermatologic lesion is a maculopapular eruption which may be found anywhere on the body, but it appears to have a special predilection for sites of previous trauma such as tattoos and scars.

Ocular manifestations occur in 25 percent of patients and include the following: anterior uveitis, posterior uveitis, conjunctival nodules, and keratoconjunctivitis sicca. When conjunctival lesions are seen, biopsies will yield a diagnosis 50 percent of the time, whereas blind biopsies have a very low yield. It is also important to remember that uveitis may lead to blindness, and its presence is a definite indication for corticosteroid treatment.

The lacrimal glands, parotid glands, and salivary glands also may be involved. Blind biopsies of salivary glands are positive 25 to 50 percent of the time. Peripheral lymphadenopathy is present 27 percent of the time. Musculoskeletal involvement includes myositis and polyarthritis.

Heart involvement may lead to cardiomyopathy and heart failure, conduction disturbances, and arrhythmias. Liver biopsies are positive in 75 percent of patients with type 2 disease and in 60 percent of patients with type 3 disease. The most common laboratory abnormality is an elevated alkaline phosphatase level. Hypercalcemia and hypercalciuria are present in 15 to 30 percent of patients. Alveolar macrophages produce increased amounts of 1,2-dihydroxyvitamin D. Nephrocalcinosis, nephrolithiasis, and chronic renal disease may occur. Hypercalcemia responds well to corticosteroids.

Central nervous system (CNS) and pituitary involvement result in diabetes insipidus and deficiencies of adrenocorticotropic hormone (ACTH) and thyroid-stimulating hormone (TSH). More common CNS manifestations include cranial neuropathies and aseptic meningitis. Hematologic abnormalities include anemia secondary to either autoimmune hemolysis or chronic disease and thrombocytopenia.

A diagnostic evaluation should include a careful history with special attention to respiratory symptoms, ocular symptoms, and such constitutional symptoms as fever, night sweats, and weight loss. It must be remembered that 40 percent of all sarcoidosis patients are asymptomatic and are discovered only after routine screening chest roentgenograms.

Once the diagnosis is suspected, special attention should be directed to peripheral lymph nodes, salivary glands, lungs, heart, skin, eyes, and neurologic examination. The patient should be sent to an ophthalmologist for slit-lamp examination to exclude uveitis.

Serial chest roentgenograms are essential. If lesions have been stable for 2 years, it is unlikely that they will progress. Routine blood work should include a complete blood count (CBC) and platelet count and determinations of serum calcium, serum proteins, liver enzymes, and renal function indices.

Pulmonary function tests, when abnormal, reveal a restrictive defect and a decreased single-breath diffusion capacity for carbon monoxide. Serial determinations of forced vital capacity and the diffusion capacity for carbon monoxide are most useful in selecting patients for treatment and monitoring therapeutic responses.

Special tests such as angiotensin-converting enzyme (ACE) levels, while not helpful in making a diagnosis, may be helpful in predicting progression of disease and response to therapy [21]. Angiotensin-converting enzyme levels which remain elevated portend a worse prognosis.

A definitive diagnosis of sarcoidosis is established when a compatible clinical picture is accompanied by tissue showing noncaseating granulomas [14]. The histologic differential diagnosis of noncaseating granulomas must be kept in mind and includes berylliosis, hypersensitivity pneumonitis, regional enteritis, fungal infection, drug reactions, and occasionally, tuberculosis.

Treatment

Sarcoidosis is treated with corticosteroids. The disease often spontaneously regresses. Because of this, the effectiveness of corticosteroid therapy is difficult to establish. There are, however, guidelines for therapy.

Absolute indications for corticosteroid therapy include severely symptomatic or progressive pulmonary involvement or involvement of other vital organs such as the eyes, heart, and CNS. General indications include unrelenting constitutional symptoms. Therapy usually consists of prednisone at 40 to 60 mg per day, and this is continued for 6 to 8 months.

The prognosis of sarcoidosis is in general quite good. The mortality rate is less than 5 percent. Fatal cases result from significant CNS or myocardial involvement.

Community-Acquired Pneumonia

The number of agents which are responsible for pneumonia is large. Defining an etiologic agent as the cause of pneumonia requires consideration of the clinical setting, the immunologic status of the patient, and any associated disease which increases susceptibility to infection [35].

The first issue is to decide whether the pneumonia was acquired in the community at large [25] or in a domiciliary setting. The more common causes of community-acquired pneumonia are listed in Table 2-12. The clinical presentation is often important in deciding which agent is the most likely etiology.

Diagnosis

Typical bacterial lobar pneumonias are characterized by an abrupt onset of fever, chills, pleuritic chest pain, and a cough productive of purulent sputum. Organisms commonly associated with this presentation include *S. pneumoniae, Klebsiella* species, oral anaerobes, *H. influenzae, S. aureus,* and *Legionella* species. In the geriatric age group, the symptoms are often modified, and thus older patients may present with more subtle findings.

Atypical pneumonias demonstrate either a segmental or subsegmental distribution on chest roentgenogram or diffuse infiltrates. The illness is less severe, and the cough is generally nonproductive. This presentation is associated with infections caused by *Mycoplasma pneumoniae,* respiratory viruses, and *Legionella* species.

The third category consists of chronic pneumonias in which infiltrates and symptoms have been present for at least 3 to 4 weeks. Etiologic agents in this category include *M. tuberculosis,* anaerobic organisms (often with abscess formation), and fungi (*Histoplasma* and *Coccidiodes*). Alveolar cell carcinoma, which can present as a lobar or diffuse alveolar infiltrate on chest roentgenogram, must be distinguished from a chronic infectious process. Also, an obstructed bronchus (foreign body or endobronchial carcinoma) must be considered in chronic, unresolving pulmonary infiltrates.

For the above-mentioned agents there are clinical circumstances which predispose certain individuals. These are outlined in Table 2-13.

The physical findings of acute lobar pneumonia include fever and tachypnea. Chest examination reveals signs of pulmonary consolidation. These include dullness to percussion, increased fremitus, inspiratory crackles, bronchial breath sounds, and egophony. If a parapneumonic effusion is present, a pleural rub may be heard. If the effusion is large, fremitus and breath sounds will be decreased. In atypical pneumonias, the physical

Table 2–12. *Common Causes of Community-Acquired Pneumonia*

Streptococcus pneumoniae
Staphylococcus aureus
Hemophilus influenzae
Mixed anaerobes
Other gram-negative bacteria
Mycoplasma pneumoniae
Viruses
Fungi: *Coccidiodes* and *Histoplasma*
Mycobacterium tuberculosis

Table 2–13. *Predisposing Conditions*

Alcoholism: *S. pneumoniae, Klebsiella,* oral anaerobes,
  M. tuberculosis

Chronic bronchitis: *S. pneumoniae,*
  H. influenzae

Advanced age: *S. pneumoniae,* gram-negative bacilli, *H.*
  influenzae

Poor oral hygiene: oral anaerobes

Endobronchial obstruction: *S. pneumoniae,* oral anaerobes

Southwestern United States: *Coccidiodes*

Central United States/Mississippi River Valley: *Histoplasma*

Depressed mental status: oral anaerobes

findings may be much more subtle and consist of only inspiratory crackles.

The chest roentgenogram confirms the diagnoses of pneumonia. Pneumonias produce alveolar infiltrates which are characterized by either being homogeneous consolidations (lobar or sublobar) or diffuse, patchy, ill-defined nodules. In either case, they are associated with air bronchograms, and they obscure normal structures (silhouette sign), such as cardiac borders, diaphragm, and pulmonary vessels. Silhouette signs may be used to localize alveolar infiltrates. For example, a right lower lung field consolidation may be located in either the right middle or the right lower lobe. If it obliterates the right heart border, it is in the middle lobe. If it obliterates the right hemidiaphragm, it is in the lower lobe.

Laboratory findings reveal elevated white blood cell counts with a shift toward immature forms in most acute bacterial pneumonias. Anemia of chronic disease is found in tuberculosis and long-standing anaerobic infections. A hemolytic anemia accompanied by increased cold agglutinins appears with *Mycoplasma* pneumonia.

Treatment

Patients suspected of having pneumonia should have a chest roentgenogram, complete blood count, sputum Gram's stain and culture, blood cultures, and cold agglutinins if *Mycoplasma* is a

serious consideration. Of paramount importance is the selection of initial antibiotic therapy. This decision is made after considering the factors discussed above, the results of the sputum Gram stain, and the patient's clinical status. Broader initial antibiotic coverage is required for septic patients.

The importance of obtaining an adequate sputum sample cannot be overemphasized. The sputum Gram stain should first be examined to assess the number of epithelial cells and neutrophils per low-power field. Adequate specimens contain less than 10 epithelial cells per field. Sputum cultures may support the finding of the sputum Gram stain, but in most cases they should not be used to dictate therapy, unless initial therapy is ineffective. A positive blood or pleural fluid culture more directly indicates the etiologic agent.

The following is a brief discussion of the management of the more common etiologic agents. For a more detailed discussion of specific organisms, see Chap. 7.

Streptococcus pneumoniae remains the most common cause of bacterial community-acquired pneumonia. The mortality rate, when bacteremia is present, is approximately 25 percent [41]. The clinical course may be complicated by the development of the adult respiratory distress syndrome (ARDS). The treatment of choice is procaine penicillin G, 600,000 to 1.2 million units per day in divided doses. In critically ill or septic patients higher doses are often recommended, because of the potential for strains that are resistant to the usual doses of penicillin. In penicillin-allergic patients, 1 to 2 gm erythromycin per day by mouth or intravenously is effective. Patients with chronic underlying disease, patients 60 years of age or older, and patients who are asplenic should receive a one-time dose polyvalent pneumococcal vaccine.

Staphylococcus aureus pneumonias often follow influenza infection. They also may result from bacteremic spread (i.e., right-sided endocarditis or septic thrombophlebitis). The treatment of choice is a semisynthetic penicillin (e.g., methicillin) given intravenously. Methicillin resistance is rare in community-acquired infections; when present, however, it usually occurs in intravenous drug abusers. Methicillin-resistant strains are treated with intravenous vancomycin.

Mycoplasma pneumoniae is the responsible agent in 20 percent of pneumonias in patients over the age of 40 years. Headache, nasopharyngeal symptoms, tender cervical adenopathy, and myalgias suggest the diagnosis. While most laboratories cannot culture this organism, serologic studies often suggest the diagnosis. A complement-fixing antibody titer greater than 1:128 or a fourfold rise in titer is suggestive. Cold agglutinin titers greater than 1:64 or which increase fourfold are seen in half the cases. The recommended treatment is erythromycin (1 to 2 gm per day).

Legionella are a recently recognized cause of community-acquired pneumonia. These organisms live for extended periods in water and moist soil. This helps explain why outbreaks have been associated with excavation of buildings. These organisms are commonly found in hospital shower heads, humidifiers, respiratory care devices, and tap water. *Legionella* can be cultured in special laboratories. In addition, an indirect fluorescent antibody test demonstrating a titer of 1:256 or greater is suggestive, although not specific. Moreover, direct fluorescent antibody tests are available to study sputum, bronchoalveolar lavage fluid, and lung tissue and may be positive in 50 percent of cases. The mortality rate is 20 percent in the general population and 80 percent in immunosuppressed patients. The treatment of choice is erythromycin, 1 gm given intravenously every 4 hours. Rifampin may be added if the patient does not respond to erythromycin.

Hemophilus influenzae commonly colonizes the airways of patients with chronic bronchitis. The diagnosis is suggested by a sputum Gram stain finding of gram-negative pleomorphic organisms. The Gram stain characteristics are essential for this diagnosis. *H. influenzae* is second only to *S. pneumoniae* in causing community-acquired pneumonia in older or chronically ill patients. In otherwise healthy young adults it follows *S. pneu-*

moniae, Mycoplasma pneumoniae, and viruses. The treatment of choice is ampicillin. Ampicillin resistance reaches 25 percent in certain geographic areas, and this is an important consideration when choosing initial therapy. Ampicillin-resistant strains may be treated with chloramphenicol or one of the newer cephalosporins.

The most common cause of community-acquired gram-negative pneumonias [33] is *Klebsiella*. Other responsible agents include *Escherichis coli, Pseudomonas, Acinetobacter,* and *Serratia*. While healthy individuals may develop *Klebsiella* pneumonia, it is usually found in elderly patients (especially nursing home residents) or in individuals with chronic underlying diseases, such as alcoholism and diabetes mellitus. Additionally, gram-negative pneumonias should be suspected in patients recently discharged from a hospital. Bacteremia may be present in 20 to 30 percent of patients and is associated with a mortality rate approaching 80 percent. Treatment includes the use of aminoglycosides combined with a cephalosporin.

Mixed anaerobic infections are found in patients with altered states of consciousness (seizures, following general anesthesia, and in alcoholics) which predispose to aspiration, in patients with gingivitis and pyorrhea, and in patients with an endobronchial obstruction (bronchogenic carcinoma). Penicillin (4 to 6 million units per day) is quite effective in treating anaerobic pulmonary infections despite the fact that not all anaerobic isolates demonstrate in vitro susceptibility. In patients who do not respond to intravenous penicillin, clindamycin is an excellent alternative agent.

Viral pneumonia results from many agents. Influenza A is a common cause of pneumonia during endemics. It is most often seen in older patients, particularly those with underlying disease such as chronic obstructive pulmonary disease and cardiovascular disease. While a primary viral pneumonia occurs less frequently in younger patients, a superimposed bacterial pneumonia is seen in this group.

Amantadine helps relieve symptoms and speeds the recovery in influenza A infections, but its primary role as a prophylactic agent in an endemic or susceptible population is questionable.

Respiratory syncytial virus may cause a pneumonia in adults which is similar to influenza A pneumonia. Adenovirus infections are rare, but when they do occur, they cause a severe necrotizing pneumonia which may progress to adult respiratory distress syndrome. These infections are seen in children and in young adults living in crowded living quarters (i.e., military recruits). Finally, chicken pox more commonly involves the lungs when acquired by adults. Approximately 16 percent of adults with chicken pox have pneumonia.

Chronic Pneumonias

Tuberculosis

Worldwide, tuberculosis remains a major health problem. It has been estimated that half the world's population is infected with tuberculosis, and it causes millions of deaths each year. The incidence in developed countries fell as socioeconomic conditions improved and effective public health measures were instituted. The development of effective chemotherapeutic agents accelerated the decline [15]. The recent increase in the yearly incidence of tuberculosis in the United States is thought to be due to the AIDS epidemic and/or increased immigration.

Tuberculosis is spread by aerosolization of respiratory secretions, with human beings as its only known reservoir. These aerosolized droplets deposit in the distal airways, where they are engulfed, but not necessarily killed, by macrophages. Infected macrophages move to regional lymph nodes and eventually enter the bloodstream. This hematogenous phase explains why tuberculosis is found not only in the lungs, but also in such multiple sites as bone, central nervous system, liver, kidneys, and adrenal glands. A T-cell-mediated immune response is noted in 4 to 12 weeks, and this is manifested by a positive skin test to purified protein derivative (PPD). In this initial stage, 95 percent of individuals do not develop a clinical disease. However, within 2 years, 5 to 6 percent will develop active disease. After 2 years, the risk of developing active disease falls to 0.25 to 0.5 percent per year.

Diagnosis

The most common presenting symptoms are productive cough, hemoptysis, chest pain (which is often pleuritic), and constitutional symptoms such as fever, night sweats, fatigue, malaise, and weight loss. Interestingly, 20 percent of patients may be asymptomatic on initial presentation. Routine laboratory tests may reveal an anemia of chronic disease. Hyponatremia is found in 10 percent of patients with active disease and is thought to be due to inappropriate antidiuretic hormone secretion.

Classic findings on chest roentgenogram are fibronodular infiltrates in the posterior and apical segments of the upper lobes, which contain patchy areas of confluent densities in addition to areas of cavitation. There is often hilar retraction. This classic presentation is becoming less common, with up to 30 percent of patients now presenting with "atypical" radiographic findings such as lower lobe infiltrates, single or multiple nodules, hilar adenopathy, and pleural effusions. Tuberculosis also may be present as a disseminated hematogenous disease with a miliary pattern on chest roentgenogram.

A definitive diagnosis is obtained by identifying the acid-fast organism in a clinical specimen, usually sputum. If the patient has a nonproductive cough, attempts should be made to induce sputum with inhaled hypertonic saline. Sputum smears using the Ziehl-Neelsen stain and the newer fluorescent stains are relatively rapid but insensitive, missing 25 to 40 percent of patients with moderate to far-advanced pulmonary tuberculosis. Culture methods, which are more specific and sensitive, classically take 3 to 6 weeks, although newer radiometric methods are becoming increasingly available and may shorten this to 7 to 10 days. In 15 percent of patients, tuberculosis organisms are not seen or cultured and the diagnosis is made on clinical grounds, relying on skin tests, radiographic findings, exposure history, and response to therapy.

TREATMENT

There are two basic principles in the treatment of tuberculosis. First, these organisms must be treated with multiple drugs to which they are susceptible. Second, treatment must be continued for an adequate length of time. There are two standard regimens for treating tuberculosis: a 9-month regimen and a 6-month regimen [1,30]. They are outlined in Table 2-14.

Isoniazid and rifampin are the principal chemotherapeutic agents used. Ethambutol or streptomycin are often added to the initial therapy until isoniazid resistance is excluded by susceptibility testing. Pregnant women receive identical therapy except that pyrazinamide and streptomycin are not included. Pyrazinamide is excluded because of potential teratogenicity, and streptomycin is not used because of known teratogenicity. Immunosuppressed patients are treated for 9 to 12 months with isoniazid and rifampin. Extrapulmonary tuberculosis is treated similar to pulmonary tuberculosis.

Before therapy is begun, baseline blood studies include determinations of liver enzymes, bilirubin, creatinine, and blood urea nitrogen (BUN), a

Table 2–14. *Standard Therapy for Tuberculosis*

1. Nine months of isoniazid and rifampin, usually accompanied in the initial phase by ethambutol. After the initial 1 to 2 months of daily therapy, these drugs may be given twice weekly for ease of monitoring compliance.
2. Two months of isoniazid, rifampin, and pyrazinamide, usually accompanied by ethambutol or streptomycin, followed by 4 months of isoniazid and rifampin.

complete blood count, a platelet count, and a uric acid determination. Patients should be monitored for symptoms monthly and blood studies should be checked only if symptoms suggest toxicity.

Properties, dosages, and side effects of the five most commonly used drugs in tuberculosis are outlined in Table 2-15. When drug resistance is found (usually isoniazid and sometimes streptomycin), the patient should be treated with two additional drugs to which the organism is susceptible.

Another group of patients who warrant treatment are some of those who are infected by tuberculosis but do not manifest active disease. Patients are considered infected if they have a significant reaction to the Mantoux skin test using 5 T.U. of intradermal purified protein derivative. A significant reaction is defined as 10 mm or more of induration, but this is modified in special circumstances (see below). Isoniazid preventative therapy is given to infected patients when the risks of developing active tuberculosis are greater than the risks of isoniazid hepatotoxicity. Isoniazid is indicated in the following conditions:

1. *Close contacts.* All close contacts of a patient diagnosed with active tuberculosis should be screened with skin tests. Contacts with significant skin reactions (>5 mm of induration) should be treated with isoniazid. Contacts with insignificant skin tests are divided into two groups. Patients at increased risk to develop disseminated disease (i.e., young children) are treated. Patients at low risk to develop disseminated disease (i.e., normal adults) are observed. Skin tests are repeated in 3 months. If the skin reaction becomes significant, isoniazid is begun, if not already started. If the skin reaction is insignificant, isoniazid, if begun, is stopped.
2. *Newly infected.* Patients who convert their skin test to significant within 2 years are at high risk to develop active tuberculosis.
3. Patients with a significant skin test and an *abnormal chest roentgenogram* showing typical fi-

Table 2–15. Properties, Dosages, and Side Effects of the Five Most Commonly Used Drugs in Tuberculosis

Chemotherapeutic agent	Effect on organism	Adult daily dose	Maximum daily dose	Twice-weekly dose	Major adverse reactions	Tests for side effects
Isoniazid	Bactericidal	5 mg/kg PO or IM	300 mg	15 mg/kg; 900 mg max.	Hepatitis, neuropathy, hypersensitivity	SGOT/SGPT (not as a routine)
Rifampin	Bactericidal	10 mg/kg PO	600 mg	10 mg/kg; 600 mg max.	GI upset, thrombocytopenia, fever, hepatitis	SGOT/SGPT (not as a routine)
Pyrazinamide	Bactericidal	15 to 30 mg/kg PO	2 gm	50 to 70 mg/kg	Hepatotoxicity, hyperuricemia, arthralgias, skin rash, GI upset	Uric acid, SGOT/SGPT
Streptomycin	Bactericidal	15 mg/kg IM	1 gm*	25 to 30 mg/kg IM	Ototoxicity, nephrotoxicity	Vestibular function, BUN/creatinine
Ethambutol	Bacteriostatic	15 to 25 mg/kg PO	2.5 gm	15 to 25 mg/kg	Optic neuritis	Red-green color discrimination, visual acuity

*Over age 60, limit streptomycin to 10 mg/kg; maximum daily dose 750 mg.

bronodular infiltrates (but not just calcified granulomas).

4. Patients in the following special clinical situations with significant skin reactions: (a) silicosis, (b) diabetes mellitus requiring insulin, (c) prolonged corticosteroid use (greater than 15 mg per day for more than 2 to 3 weeks), (d) immunosuppression, (e) hematologic malignancies, (f) AIDS, (g) renal failure requiring dialysis, and (h) chronic malnutrition.

5. Patients with a significant skin reaction under age 35 years. In none of the preceding four categories is age a criterion.

Histoplasmosis

Histoplasmosis [16] is a disease caused by the soil fungus *Histoplasma capsulatum*. These organisms are found in moist soil of temperate climate zones, especially in bird and bat habitats. The incidence is increased in the great river valleys of the central and southeastern United States.

Infection is caused by inhalation of aerosolized organisms, and this is facilitated by dry, windy, and dusty environmental conditions. The pathophysiology of infection is similar in many ways to tuberculosis. Yeast proliferate in small airways and alveoli and, after 1 to 2 weeks, spread to regional lymph nodes. This is followed by hematogenous spread. Almost 80 percent of primary infections are asymptomatic and appear to be quite common. Upwards of 50 percent of people living in endemic areas have splenic calcifications characteristic of histoplasmosis. At about 2 weeks, the skin test becomes positive and the granulomas formed contain walled-off organisms of *H. capsulatum*.

DIAGNOSIS

There are three clinical syndromes in histoplasmosis: (1) acute histoplasmosis, either primary or reinfection, (2) disseminated histoplasmosis, acute and chronic, and (3) chronic pulmonary histoplasmosis.

Acute histoplasmosis is associated with a flulike illness. Chest roentgenograms reveal a diffuse bronchopneumonia with predilection for the lower lobes, as well as hilar adenopathy. This form of the disease usually resolves spontaneously and may leave residual calcifications. A hypersensitivity reaction with arthralgia, arthritis, and erythema nodosum may occur. Hilar adenopathy is rare in reinfection acute histoplasmosis.

Disseminated histoplasmosis is the most severe form and implies that the host is immunocompromised. Corticosteroids and cytotoxic agents appear to increase the risk of developing dissemination. It is more common in men. Symptoms include fever, weight loss, and malaise. On physical examination, the most characteristic finding is an oropharyngeal ulcer, which is found in 75 percent of patients. Sputum cultures are usually negative. Pulmonary manifestations vary and may be absent. The diagnosis is made by performing a biopsy on other organs. Patients with normal immune systems may develop disseminated histoplasmosis which progresses slowly without an acute phase.

Chronic pulmonary histoplasmosis is most commonly found in men with chronic obstructive pulmonary disease. There is an early pneumonic form associated with a flulike illness and interstitial round cell infiltrates in the apical and posterior segments of the upper lobes, which may go on to develop fibrosis. There is also a late cavitary form which appears to be secondary to persistent infection of emphysematous cysts which periodically spill organisms into the surrounding parenchyma.

Late sequelae of histoplasmosis include erosion of calcified nodes into airways to form broncholiths. In addition, involvement of mediastinal lymph nodes may result in mediastinal fibrosis, which in turn causes entrapment of the superior vena cava, trachea, esophagus, or pulmonary arteries and veins.

TREATMENT

Acute histoplasmosis in normal hosts with mild symptoms does not require therapy. Severely ill patients require amphotericin B for a total dose of 500 mg. Patients with acute disseminated disease are treated with 2 to 3 gm of amphotericin B given over 6 weeks. Ketoconazole, which is less toxic and can be given orally, has been used in patients with slowly progressive disseminated disease and slowly progressive cavitary disease at doses of 400 mg or more per day.

Coccidioidomycosis

Coccidioidomycosis [11] is caused by the fungus *Coccidioides immitis,* which is found in desert soil in southern California, Nevada, Arizona, New Mexico, and Texas. The organisms proliferate in the rainy season and form arthrospores in the hot, dry seasons. Infection is by inhalation of arthrospores, which is facilitated by windy and dusty conditions along with excavation of infected soil. Humans and lower mammals are infected. In the distal airways the arthrospore develops into a spherule in which daughter cells, or endospores, form. Human-human transmission via the respiratory tract has not been reported. The cell-mediated immune response, as measured by skin testing, becomes positive in 2 to 3 weeks.

Diagnosis

Coccidioidomycosis can be separated into three clinical syndromes: (1) primary infection, (2) persistent or progressive pulmonary infection, and (3) disseminated infection.

Primary infection is asymptomatic in 40 to 60 percent of patients. Symptoms which do occur are nonspecific and are similar to a flulike illness with fever, chills, malaise, and arthralgias. Common findings on physical examination include pharyngitis and rash. Rashes are more common in women and are often an erythromatous maculopapular exanthem. Erythema nodosum is also seen. Pulmonary findings include signs of consolidation.

The chest roentgenogram is usually abnormal in acute infections. Infiltrates are quite variable as to location and character. Hilar adenopathy is present 20 percent of the time. Sputum smear and culture are positive in 40 to 70 percent of subjects with symptomatic primary disease. *Coccidioides immitis* is not part of normal flora. The diagnosis may be made by the appropriate interpretation of skin tests and serology. Complement-fixation (CF) titers correlate with disease activity in most cases. It must be remembered that not all patients with dissemination will have high complement-fixation titers and that a high titer alone is not diagnostic of dissemination.

Acute infections are most often self-limiting. Certain groups are at increased risk to develop disseminated disease. These include pregnant women, patients who are immunosuppressed (e.g., receiving corticosteroids or cytotoxic agents), blacks, Philippinos, and Native Americans. Patients at risk to develop persistent or disseminated disease often have complement-fixation titers that remain high, have pulmonary infiltrates and hilar adenopathy which do not resolve after 6 to 8 weeks, and demonstrate weight loss.

Persistent or progressive disease is manifested by (1) chronic pulmonary infiltration which may relentlessly destroy parenchyma, (2) pulmonary nodule(s), or (3) cavities which may hemorrhage, rupture into the pleural space, or spontaneously close. Isolated nodules must be differentiated from malignancy; these nodules rarely are the source of dissemination.

The most frequent sites of dissemination are skin, bones, soft tissue, and meninges. Meningitis is the most ominous form of disease. A lumbar puncture should be performed when dissemination is suspected. Complement-fixation titers should be performed on the cerebrospinal fluid in addition to other routine tests. Bone scans also may be quite useful in disseminated disease.

Treatment

Disseminated infections should be treated with amphotericin B, up to a 3-gm total dose. Meningitis requires intrathecal amphotericin B administration. Acute infections usually do not require treatment unless the patient falls into one of the high-risk groups. Indications for treatment in the persistent category include serologic evidence of active disease (complement-fixation titer remains increased or continues to rise) or progression on chest roentgenogram. Miconazole and ketaconazole also may be used to treat coccidioidomycosis except when meningitis is present. These two drugs are much less toxic than amphotericin B, but they may not be as effective.

Hospital-Acquired Pneumonias

The approach to a patient who develops pneumonia while in hospital is similar to that for a patient with community-acquired pneumonia with the exception that different therapies must be contemplated [20,27,35]. This often changes the choice of initial antibiotics.

Factors that predispose hospitalized patients to pneumonia include (1) previous antibiotic therapy, (2) aspiration of oral and gastric secretions, (3) hematogenous spread from an infected focus (gastrointestinal or urinary tracts), (4) endotracheal intubation, (5) the use of respiratory therapy equipment, and (6) intravenous catheters.

Organisms most often responsible for hospital-acquired pneumonias are listed in Table 2-16. Soon after entering the hospital, a patient's oropharynx becomes colonized with coliforms. This is particularly true for patients being treated with an antibiotic such as penicillin which is effective against organisms found in normal oral flora, and then there is proliferation of gram-negative bacteria. If this patient then aspirates (e.g., during anesthesia), a gram-negative pneumonia may occur. *Legionella, Pseudomonas,* and *Serratia* can be cultured from the water supply of hospitals and in respiratory therapy equipment.

Patients who require endotracheal intubation lose an important bacterial defense mechanism, a normally functioning larynx and the cough reflex. The trachea and bronchi of normal individuals are sterile. Within hours after endotracheal intubation, the airways become colonized with multiple organisms. One of the key clinical questions in an intubated patient is whether a positive sputum culture represents colonization or a true parenchymal infection. The patient's temperature, white blood count, chest roentgenogram, and sputum Gram stain dictate whether therapy is indicated.

Treatment

The most popular antibiotic regimens for empiric therapy in hospital-acquired pneumonias include coverage for gram-positive organisms including *S. aureus* (semisynthetic penicillin or first-generation cephalosporin) and an aminoglycoside to treat gram-negative bacilli. Hospitalized patients who have been on chronic broad-spectrum antibiotics are at an increased risk of superinfection with fungi, especially *Candida albicans.* Since *Candida* is often part of the normal flora, the decision to use amphotericin B when *Candida* is grown from sputum or urine is difficult. Criteria for initiating amphotericin B therapy include positive blood cultures, evidence of tissue invasion (positive lung biopsy, fundoscopic lesions), and the simultaneous culture of *Candida* from multiple sites (positive cultures from sputum, urine, and stool).

Table 2–16. *Organisms Commonly Responsible for Hospital-Acquired Pneumonias*

Streptococcus pneumoniae
Staphylococcus aureus
Pseudomonas spp.
Klebsiella spp.
Escherichia coli
Legionella spp.

Pneumonia in Immunocompromised Patients

Fever and pulmonary infiltrates are common occurrences in immunocompromised patients [12,36]. Since these infiltrates may represent infectious pneumonia and are often fatal, there is a sense of urgency concerning diagnosis and initiation of therapy. In fact, empiric therapy is initiated prior to a diagnosis in many cases. The decision regarding therapy is often complex, since the number and variety of potential agents are vast. In addition, there are noninfectious causes of fever and pulmonary infiltrates in these patients (Table 2-17). Congestive heart failure must be considered in the differential diagnosis of diffuse pulmonary infiltrates. These patients also may become fluid overloaded, and certain chemotherapeutic agents such as adriamycin cause myocarditis.

Diagnosis

It is not only important to start empiric therapy without delay, but it is also necessary to establish a diagnosis early. For example, the treatment for a drug-induced pneumonitis or radiation pneumonitis often dictates corticosteroids. However, the use of corticosteroids in the presence of an untreated infection may result in dissemination.

A careful history must include previous chemotherapy agents. If a patient has received radiation, the total dose and radiated parts should be documented. In the physical examination, signs of congestive heart failure should be sought. Nonpulmonary signs of infection such as retinal lesions consistent with fungemia also should be sought.

Immunocompromised patients with infectious pneumonias often do not produce sputum, particularly if they are neutropenic. Therefore, the sputum Gram stain, which is often so helpful in other patients with pneumonia, may not be available.

The two most helpful clinical clues for determining the etiology of pneumonia in an immunocompromised patient include (1) the type of immunosuppression (Table 2-18) and (2) the chest radiographic pattern.

Neutropenic patients are susceptible to gram-negative bacilli and *Aspergillus* species. Patients with B-cell dysfunction, as in hypogammaglobulinemia, multiple myeloma, and chronic lymphocytic leukemia, often become infected with encapsulated bacteria such as *S. pneumoniae* and *H. influenzae*. Patients with splenectomy also fall into this category. Defects in cell-mediated immunity (AIDS) predispose to infections with fungi (*Candida* and *Cryptococcus*), viruses (cytomegalovirus), and *Pneumocystis* and *Mycobacteria*. Long-term treatment with corticosteroids may cause multiple defects in the immune system. Patients on chronic glucocorticoid therapy are susceptible to *Pneumocystis*, cytomegalovirus, and *Nocardia*, along with the more common gram-negative bacilli and *S. aureus*.

The chest roentgenogram also aids in the diagnosis (Table 2-19). Localized pneumonias are more commonly seen with gram-negative bacilli, *S. aureus*, and *Aspergillus*, while diffuse infiltrates are more common with viruses (cytomegalovirus) and *Pneumocystis*.

As with other pneumonias, blood, pleural fluid, and at times sputum cultures may be helpful in establishing the diagnosis. Often, however, more invasive techniques must be used in the immunocompromised host. The two most commonly

Table 2–17. *Causes of Fever and Pulmonary Infiltrates in Immunocompromised Patients*

Infections
Drug reaction
Hemorrhage
Underlying malignancy
Leukostasis
Radiation pneumonitis
Pulmonary infarction

Table 2–18. *Types of Immunosuppression and Commonly Associated Pathogens*

Disorder	Pathogens

I. Granulocytopenia and altered inflammatory response:
  A. Myeloproliferative disorders (acute and chronic myelocytic leukemia)
  B. Drug therapy (corticosteroids, chemotherapy)
	Gram-negative bacilli (*Pseudomonas, E. coli, Klebsiella, Serratia*)
	S. aureus
	Aspergillus
	Candida
	Nocardia
	H. influenzae

II. Defective cell-mediated immunity:
  A. Lymphomas
  B. Diffuse carcinomas and sarcomas
  C. Renal failure
  D. Radiation
  E. Drugs (corticosteroids, alkylating agents, antimetabolites)
	Cryptococcus
	M. tuberculosis
	Viruses, (cytomegalovirus)
	Pneumocystis
	Nocardia
	Candida
	Legionella
	Listeria

III. Defective antibody production:
  A. Lymphocytic leukemia
  B. Multiple myeloma
  C. B-cell lymphoma
  D. Hypogammaglobulinemia
  E. Drugs (corticosteroids, alkylating agents, antimetabolites)
  F. Splenectomy
	S. pneumoniae
	H. influenzae
	Pseudomonas
	Other gram-negative bacilli
	Cytomegalovirus
	Pneumocystis

Table 2–19. *Types of Infiltrates in Immunocompromised Patients*

Localized:
  Pulmonary infarction
  Carcinoma
  Hemorrhage
  Infection:
    Aspiration pneumonia
    "Routine" bacteria
    Legionella
    Nocardia
    Fungal
    M. tuberculosis
  Radiation pneumonitis
Diffuse:
  Drug reaction
  Pneumocystis
  Cytomegalovirus and other viruses
  Congestive heart failure
  Leukostasis
  Invasive *Aspergillus* and *Candida*
  Lymphangitic carcinomatosis

used procedures are (1) bronchoscopy utilizing bronchoalveolar lavage and transbronchial lung biopsy and (2) open lung biopsy.

Bronchoscopy offers the advantages over open lung biopsy of being less invasive, not requiring general anesthesia, and taking less time. Transbronchial biopsies help establish the diagnosis of invasive fungal disease, recurrence of a malignancy, and drug-induced cytotoxicity. Transbronchial biopsies may be limited by a preexisting bleeding diathesis and or because of sampling error. Bronchoalveolar lavage, on the other hand, is relatively safe in the presence of bleeding diatheses and is ideal to diagnose *Pneumocystis, Legionella,* and *Mycobacterium* infection and occasionally malignancy (cytology). Bronchoalveolar lavage is not useful for the diagnosis of drug-induced interstitial pneumonitis.

Open lung biopsies, although invasive, offer the advantages of being more definitive, being relatively safe in patients with bleeding diatheses, and allowing larger samples of tissue to be obtained so that patchy diseases are not missed.

Treatment

The first decision regarding the approach to the immunocompromised patient with pulmonary infiltrates and fever is whether empiric therapy should be initiated and followed by a short period of observation or whether an invasive diagnostic procedure should be performed immediately. Certain agents such as *Pneumocystis* can be diagnosed in a matter of hours by bronchoscopy and special stains of clinical material. The decision concerning the timing of invasive procedures is often based on the clinical condition of the patient. If the patient appears to have deteriorated rapidly, invasive procedures are initiated early.

Empiric therapy is determined by the clinical situation. Patients with focal infiltrates on chest roentgenogram are usually begun on an aminoglycoside and cephalosporin, ticarcillin or carbenicillin. The patient is monitored carefully for 24 to 48 hours. If no response occurs, an invasive procedure is performed or the patient is given an empiric trial of amphotericin B and/or erythromycin.

When diffuse infiltrates are present, the patient is begun on the same initial antibiotic regimen as above except that trimethoprim-sulfamethoxazole is added. If there is no response, a diagnostic procedure is performed.

Pneumonia in Patients with AIDS

Patients with the acquired immune deficiency syndrome (AIDS) are at risk for developing multiple infections because of their immunocompromised state [17,29]. Because pneumonias in AIDS often present in an atypical fashion and are associated with a characteristic group of microorganisms, they will be discussed separately. Pneumonias account for 80 percent of all AIDS-related infections and are the most common cause of death.

Diagnosis

AIDS patients with pneumonia commonly present with cough (usually nonproductive) and dyspnea. Systemic symptoms such as fever, night sweats, and weight loss are less prominent. The onset of symptoms is often quite gradual, particularly with *Pneumocystis*.

The physical examination may not be helpful, except in the rare patient with a "routine" bacterial pneumonia. The most common abnormal findings are fever, tachypnea, and oral candidiasis.

The chest roentgenogram will reveal alveolar and interstitial infiltrates and should be the initial screening test. A normal chest roentgenogram,

however, does not exclude a pulmonary infection. Other tests which may be abnormal prior to radiographic changes include an arterial blood gas revealing hypoxia, hypocarbia, and a widened alveolar-arterial (A-a) oxygen gradient. An even more sensitive test is the serial measurement of diffusing capacity. Gallium lung scans often demonstrate increased uptake, indicating early inflammatory disease.

A list of organisms causing pulmonary infections in AIDS patients is found in Table 2-20. *Pneumocystis carinii* pneumonia is the most common. It accounts for 90 percent of all infections

Table 2–20. *Pulmonary Infections in AIDS Patients*

Common:
 Pneumocystis
 Cytomegalovirus
 M. avium complex
Uncommon;
 M. tuberculosis
 Cryptococcus
 Histoplasma
 Coccidioides
 Legionella
 Herpes simplex virus
 Pyogenic bacteria
 Taxoplasma

occurring in AIDS. Other pathogens may coexist. In addition, there is a subset of AIDS patients who appear to have a B-cell defect that renders them particularly susceptible to recurrent *S. pneumoniae* infections.

To determine the cause of pneumonia in AIDS, sputum should be examined with Gram, acid-fast, and methenamine-silver stains. The last two stains are specific for mycobacteria, fungi, and *Pneumocystis.* Figure 2-5 shows a lung biopsy specimen from a patient with *Pneumocystis.* It is often necessary to induce sputum (nebulized saline) because the majority of AIDS patients with pneumonia have a nonproductive cough. Bronchoscopy with transbronchial biopsies and bron-

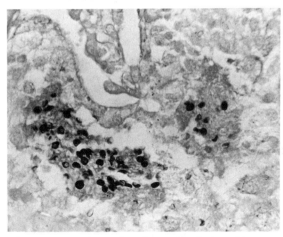

Figure 2–5. *Methenamine-silver stain of a lung biopsy revealing typical findings of* Pneumocystis carinii, *which stain black.*

choalveolar lavage is often necessary to establish a definitive diagnosis. In patients with bleeding diatheses, bronchoalveolar lavage alone is relied on.

Treatment

The agents of choice for *Pneumocystis* pneumonia are trimethoprim-sulfamethoxazole and pentamidine. These agents both cause significant untoward reactions. Reactions to trimethoprim-sulfamethoxazole include fever, rash, leukopenia, and thrombocytopenia. Reactions to pentamidine include leukopenia, hepatitis, and azotemia.

Mycobacterium tuberculosis is treated with standard antituberculosis chemotherapy. However, *M. avium* infection in AIDS is essentially untreatable. Similarly, no treatment is available for cytomegalovirus, which is cultured from bronchoscopy specimens approximately a third of the time. Coccidiomycosis, histoplasmosis, and systemic candiasis are treated with amphotericin B. *Cryptococcus* is treated with amphotericin B plus 5-flucytosine. Herpes virus infections are treated with IV acyclovir.

Supportive care includes supplemental oxygen in patients who are hypoxemic. The use of mechanical ventilation requires special consideration and should be addressed as early in the course of pneumonia as possible. The mortality rate for patients with their first episode of *Pneumocystis* pneumonia who require mechanical ventilation is 85 percent. The mortality rate increases to greater than 95 percent for subsequent episodes. Many patients decide not to be mechanically ventilated. Virtually all patients with AIDS die of opportunistic infections within 2 years of the diagnosis.

Pulmonary Thromboembolic Disease

Approximately 50,000 people die annually as a result of deep venous thrombosis and secondary pulmonary embolism. Most emboli arise in the deep veins of the leg, and the majority of patients who die do so suddenly from a massive embolus. Therefore, a major effort should be made to identify high-risk patients.

Pathophysiology

There are three factors which predispose to the formation of venous thrombi: (1) venous stasis, (2) activated blood coagulation, and (3) endothelial injury. Once a thrombus is formed, two outcomes are possible: either total resolution because of activation of the fibrinolytic system or organization and incorporation of the thrombus into the venous wall. With the latter there is potential for the thrombus to propagate and dislodge to become an embolus. Whichever sequence occurs, the event is complete in 7 to 10 days.

Several important cardiac and pulmonary consequences of pulmonary emboli should be remembered. If the embolus is large enough to sufficiently reduce the cross-sectional area of the pulmonary arterial system, acute cor pulmonale may result. Hypoxemia results from ventilation/perfusion mismatch. There is also loss of surfactant, which may result in atelectasis. A pulmonary infarction or necrosis secondary to embolic occlusion of a vessel occurs following 10 to 20 percent of pulmonary emboli. Infarction is more likely to occur in the setting of congestive heart failure.

Diagnosis

The clinical recognition of pulmonary embolism remains a problem [2]. It is estimated from postmortem data that 50 percent of clinically significant emboli are missed premortem. The risk factors for pulmonary embolism are outlined in Table 2-21. Dyspnea is the most common clinical

Table 2–21. Risk Factors for Pulmonary Emboli

Age over 40 years
History of previous deep venous thrombosis
Congestive heart failure
Prolonged inactivity
Obesity
Varicose veins
Special surgical procedure:
  Hip and knee surgery
  Extensive pelvic surgery
Estrogen-containing compounds
Dehydration

manifestation. Hemoptysis is more common with a pulmonary infarction. Pleuritic chest pain may occur. Severe substernal chest pain and syncope occur in the event of a massive pulmonary embolus. The differential diagnosis includes an acute myocardial infarction, aortic dissection, pneumonia, and pneumothorax.

Physical findings of a pulmonary embolism include temperature elevations, tachypnea, and tachycardia. A pleural friction rub and chest wall tenderness may be present after infarction, and localized crackles and wheezes also may be present. With massive pulmonary emboli, signs of pulmonary hypertension (loud P_2) and right ventricular overload (right ventricular heave and right-sided S_3) occur.

The most common electrocardiographic abnormality is sinus tachycardia. The so-called classic findings of right-axis shift, $S_1Q_3T_3$ pattern and a new complete right bundle-branch block are infrequent. Acute pulmonary embolism is one of the causes of the development of acute atrial fibrillation. The electrocardiogram is important to exclude an acute myocardial infarction. Similarly, the chest roentgenogram is helpful in excluding other diagnostic possibilities such as pneumothorax. The chest roentgenogram in acute pulmonary embolism may be normal. Nonspecific abnormalities include platelike basilar atelectasis with an elevated hemidiaphragm, pleural effusion, segmental oligemia, pleural-based wedge-shaped infiltrates (the Hampton's hump of infarction), and major vascular cutoffs.

Arterial blood gas determinations usually are not helpful in the diagnosis of pulmonary emboli, but they are indicated to assess the severity of the event and the need for supplemental oxygen. A normal P_{O_2} is seen in 10 to 15 percent of angiographically proven pulmonary emboli. Typically, hypoxemia, hyperventilation, and respiratory alkalosis occur, but these are findings which are also present in pneumonia, pneumothorax, left-sided ventricular failure, and an acute asthma attack.

The studies which are the most helpful in diagnosing thromboembolic disease are (1) ventilation/perfusion (V/Q) lung scans, (2) pulmonary angiograms, (3) venography, and (4) impedance plethysmography.

Pulmonary angiography is the definitive test. It is relatively safe when done in a selected fashion, distal to the main pulmonary artery, and in areas which are suspicious on the ventilation/perfusion scan. The risk is increased in patients with pulmonary hypertension and congestive heart failure. Less invasive methods have been sought to obviate the need for pulmonary angiography. Recent well-controlled randomized studies have helped define the role of lung scans, venography, and venous plethysmography [18,19]. A perfusion lung (Q) scan reveals defects in areas of a lung that have lost their pulmonary arterial blood supply. If a six-view perfusion lung scan is normal, pulmonary embolism is not the cause of a patient's symptoms. An abnormal perfusion scan, however, is nonspecific. Reduced perfusion is seen in emphysema, pneumonia, and cystic lung disease. In these latter situations, the ventilation (V) scan is abnormal; however, the ventilation scan usually remains normal with pulmonary thromboembolic disease.

Perfusion scan defects are often separated into three categories: (1) large or segmental defects, (2) subsegmental defects, and (3) indeterminate defects (those occurring in preexisting abnormalities on chest roentgenogram). A segmental mis-matched defect is diagnostic of a pulmonary embolus (no perfusion with maintenance of ventilation). This combination is highly predictive of a pulmonary embolism, and no further studies are indicated. In all other situations the lung scan is not diagnostic.

This does not mean, however, that a lung scan is not useful. It is the first test that should be done. If the perfusion scan is normal, pulmonary embolism is excluded. If a large defect is seen in an area of normal perfusion, the diagnosis of pulmonary embolism is made. If a pulmonary angiogram is necessary, the ventilation scan assists the angiographer in selecting which pulmonary arteries to inject.

When a nondiagnostic lung scan is obtained with a compatible clinical picture, deep venous thrombosis (DVT) may be sought by venography or venous plethysmography. The incidence of deep venous thrombosis in patients with nondiagnostic lung scans is 15 to 30 percent. Since the therapy for deep venous thrombosis and pulmonary thromboembolism does not differ in most situations, it is usually not necessary to pursue the diagnosis of pulmonary embolism with pulmonary angiography in the face of deep venous thrombosis. In situations where a deep venous thrombosis is not documented and the ventilation/perfusion scan is nondiagnostic, pulmonary angiography should be performed.

Treatment

Prevention is the mainstay of therapy for thromboembolic disease. Patients with an increased risk for deep venous thrombosis must be identified, and prophylactic measures which decrease the incidence of thrombosis must be undertaken.

The prophylactic regimens available to decrease the incidence of deep venous thrombosis and pulmonary emboli include low-dose heparin, oral coumarin, intravenous dextran, and antiplatelet agents such as aspirin. In addition, in patients in whom the risk of bleeding complications are increased, intermittent pneumatic compression of the lower extremities has been developed to de-

Table 2–22. *Prophylactic Treatment Measures*
for Various Categories of High-Risk Patients

Category	Incidence of clinically silent deep venous thrombosis	Prophylactic treatment of choice
Elective general surgery patients over 40 years of age	10–20 percent	Low-dose heparin*
Hip fractures	30–40 percent	Coumarin to prolong prothrombin time (PT) 1.5 × normal†
Elective hip surgery	30–40 percent	Coumarin or dextran
Major knee surgery	60 percent	Intermittent pneumatic compression
Prostate surgery	20–30 percent	Intermittent pneumatic compression
Neurosurgery	20–30 percent	Intermittent pneumatic compression
High-risk medical patient	Varies	Low-dose heparin

*Low-dose heparin is 5000 units subcutaneous every 8 or 12 hours.
†To decrease hemorrhage, coumarin should be started 24 hours after surgery. If surgery is delayed, coumarin is begun immediately and then stopped 48 hours before surgery.

crease venous stasis. By weighing the effectiveness of prophylactic measures against their complications, recommendations have been made for different groups of high-risk patients [10,19]. These recommendations are outlined in Table 2-22.

Once the diagnosis of pulmonary embolism is made, the standard treatment is continuous intravenous heparin at doses adjusted to maintain the partial thromboplastin time (PTT) twice normal. While heparin inhibits new thrombus formation, it does not reduce the risk of emboli from a previously formed thrombus and does not enhance the resolution of a thrombus. Heparin does, however, allow fibrinolysis to proceed unopposed. Additional embolic events in the first 48 hours after the initiation of therapy should not be considered a heparin failure. Heparin therapy is continued for 7 to 10 days followed by coumarin therapy for 3 to 6 months. Coumarin is given orally, and the dose should prolong the prothrombin time (PT) 1.5 times normal. Since patients are not considered adequately anticoagulated until the prothrombin time has been prolonged for 3 to 5 days, it should be initiated while the patient is receiving IV heparin to ensure that there has been a 3- to 5-day overlap of heparin and coumarin.

Complications from heparin therapy include bleeding and thrombocytopenia. Risks for bleeding include (1) age over 60 years, (2) local lesions in the gastrointestinal and urinary tracts, (3) uremia, and (4) thrombocytopenia. The main complication from coumarin is bleeding. Drugs given concomitantly which increase this risk include aspirin, cimetidine, phenylbutazone, anabolic steroids, amiodarone, and sulfonamides.

Thrombolytic therapy with either streptokinase or urokinase has also been used for pulmonary emboli and deep venous thrombosis. These agents offer the advantage of lysing existing thrombi with early restoration of the circulation. They do, however, have the disadvantage of increasing the risk of major bleeding complications. Thrombolytic therapy is indicated in the setting of a massive pulmonary embolus (obstructing greater than 50 percent of the pulmonary artery bed) which is hemodynamically compromising. Absolute contraindications to thrombolytic therapy are active internal bleeding and a recent (within 2 months) cerebrovascular accident or other acute intracranial process. Major relative contraindications are recent (within 10 days) surgery, obstetrical delivery during childbirth, organ biopsy, puncture of a nonaccessible vessel, and serious trauma. Severe hypertension (>200/100 mmHg) is also included in this category.

The final therapy to be considered is inferior vena caval interruption. The placement of intraluminal devices which prevent the passage of large clots but do not totally obstruct the vena cava are preferred over ligation procedures. Indications for this type of therapy are (1) acute venous thrombolic disease in patients with an absolute contraindication to anticoagulation, (2) massive pulmonary embolus in which recurrent pulmonary emboli may be fatal, and (3) the rare patient with recurrent pulmonary emboli while on adequate anticoagulation.

Adult Respiratory Distress Syndrome

The adult respiratory distress syndrome (ARDS) [3] is a clinical syndrome characterized by acute dyspnea, profound hypoxemia, decreased pulmonary compliance, and diffuse pulmonary infiltrates. It often occurs in previously healthy people without underlying lung disease. There are many causes for adult respiratory distress syndrome, but the final common pathway of injury to the lung is quite similar. Treatment in most instances is therefore usually the same regardless of etiology.

Pathophysiology

The major pathophysiologic alteration in adult respiratory distress syndrome is an increase in lung capillary permeability resulting in fluid accumulation within alveolar walls and spaces (noncardiogenic pulmonary edema) [38]. In normal individuals there is a net movement of fluid without proteins from the capillaries to the interstitial space. Intracapillary pressure, which tends to move fluid into the interstitial space (alveolar wall), is greater than the capillary colloid oncotic pressure, which tends to move fluid into the capillaries. The excess fluid is normally removed by lymphatics.

In adult respiratory distress syndrome there is damage to both the capillary endothelial cells and the alveolar epithelial cells. Endothelial cell injury leads to increased capillary permeability, which allows protein-rich fluid to leak into the interstitial space. As the protein concentration in the interstitial space increases, the colloid osmotic pressure difference between the capillaries and the interstitial space decreases. The result is increased movement of fluid into the interstitial space. This is in contrast to cardiogenic pulmonary edema, in which increased intracapillary pressure alone, without changes in permeability, increases the net flow of fluid out of the capillaries into the interstitial space.

As the protein-rich fluid leak continues, the interstitial space and lymphatics become engorged. The lungs become stiffer (decreased compliance), and the patient experiences dyspnea.

Epithelial cell damage also results in increased permeability and fluid shifts from the interstitial space into the alveoli. The fluid disrupts the surface-active factors (i.e., surfactant) which normally prevent alveolar collapse, especially at low lung volumes; this leads to atelectasis. Filling of the alveoli with fluid and the development of atelectasis both lead to decreased or absent ventilation in areas of the lung which are still perfused. The result is a right to left shunt, which explains why the hypoxemia of adult respiratory distress syndrome is characteristically poorly responsive to supplemental oxygen.

Factors which potentially enhance or cause the lung damage in this syndrome include complement activation, arachidonate metabolites, activation of the coagulation system, sequestration of activated polymorphonuclear cells (which release toxic oxygen metabolites and proteinases), and platelet activation.

Diagnosis

The clinical presentation of adult respiratory distress syndrome is preceded by a noxious event (Table 2-23) [13] which is followed by an interval (usually 12 to 24 hours) of relatively normal lung

Table 2–23. *Etiologies of Adult Respiratory Distress Syndrome*

Shock:
    Hemorrhage
    Cardiogenic
    Septic
    Anaphylactic
Massive aspiration of gastric contents
Multiple trauma
Fat emboli
Diffuse intravascular coagulation
Endotoxemia
Drug overdose:
    Opiates
    Aspirin
Overwhelming pneumonia
Severe pancreatitis
Burns
Amniotic fluid emboli
Air emboli

function. Then the rapid and progressive onset of dyspnea and hypoxemia occurs. Clinical signs include tachypnea, labored respirations, intercostal retractions, and cyanosis. Auscultation of the lung is often unremarkable. Breath sounds are usually harsh, with a short inspiratory phase and a normal expiratory phase. Crackles and wheezes are uncommon.

Chest roentgenograms initially show fine reticular infiltrates which progress to extensive bilateral alveolar infiltrates. Arterial blood gases show hypoxemia and, initially, hypocarbia. The hypoxemia is difficult to correct with supplemental oxygen. The static compliance of the lung decreases, but it is usually only measured after the patient is placed on a mechanical ventilator. The static compliance calculation is made by dividing the tidal volume (in milliliters) by the pressure (in centimeters of water) generated by the chest wall's and lung's tendencies to collapse while the expiratory valve of the ventilator is occluded after full inspiration.

The diagnosis of adult respiratory distress syndrome depends on a compatible clinical predisposing event, diffuse alveolar infiltrates on chest roentgenogram without evidence of left ventricular failure, profound hypoxemia which does not correct with supplemental oxygen, and a decreased static lung compliance (less than 50 ml/cmH$_2$O). The most important diagnosis to exclude is cardiogenic pulmonary edema. In contrast to adult respiratory distress syndrome, cardiogenic pulmonary edema is characterized by a large heart, Kerley B lines on chest roentgenogram, frequent occurrence of pleural effusions, and elevated left-sided filling pressure as estimated by the pulmonary artery wedge pressure.

Treatment

Management of adult respiratory distress syndrome includes treatment of the underlying disease (i.e., sepsis) and supportive care. Respiratory support of most patients involves intubation and mechanical ventilation.

The goal of respiratory support is to maximize oxygen delivery. Oxygen delivery is a function of cardiac output and oxygen content of the blood. Oxygen content is determined by the hemoglobin concentration and the percentage of hemoglobin which is saturated with oxygen. The P_{O_2} is the major factor which determines oxygen saturation. Therefore, to maximize oxygen transport, the P_{O_2} should be optimized while preserving the cardiac output. In addition, significant anemia should be corrected.

Volume-cycled mechanical ventilators are used to support patients with adult respiratory distress syndrome and may decrease the right-to-left shunt in two ways. High tidal volumes (10 to 15 ml/kg) help expand atelectatic areas of the lung. Positive end-expiratory pressure (PEEP) increases the functional residual capacity and therefore prevents atelectasis from occurring, especially at low lung volumes. High levels of PEEP may decrease cardiac output, and this effect must often be balanced against improvements in P_{O_2}.

Patients with this syndrome often require high inspired oxygen concentrations (up to 100 percent) to maintain the oxygen saturation at safe levels. Oxygen, however, is toxic to the lung. The oxygen concentration is titrated so that the lowest concentration (below 50 percent if possible) is used which will maintain a 90 percent oxygen saturation of hemoglobin. Decreasing the right-to-left shunt with PEEP is often an effective method for maintaining adequate oxygen saturation while at the same time allowing for a decrease in the inspired oxygen concentration.

Fluid management in this syndrome is complex. Hypovolemia will decrease the capillary leak and tend to improve adult respiratory distress syndrome. On the other hand, hypovolemia also may reduce cardiac output, especially in the presence of high levels of PEEP. The pulmonary artery wedge pressure is often measured to assess volume status. The optimal wedge pressure in this syndrome is the lowest pressure that will allow adequate cardiac output. The optimal pulmonary artery wedge pressure in this syndrome is approximately 10 cmH$_2$O.

Adult respiratory distress syndrome patients also should receive nutritional support, which must be considered when fluid requirements are assessed. Corticosteroids may have a role in adult respiratory distress syndrome associated with early gram-negative septic shock. The use of corticosteroids in other forms of this syndrome, however, remains controversial.

Antibiotics are very important, especially when sepsis is the etiology. In addition, a major complication of adult respiratory distress syndrome is superimposed infection. These patients are at significant risk to develop hospital-acquired pneumonias and should be approached as discussed earlier (see the section entitled Hospital-Acquired Pneumonias).

The mortality rate in adult respiratory distress syndrome is 50 percent. Patients with this syndrome may develop severe pulmonary fibrosis and become impossible to ventilate (i.e., maintain adequate P_{CO_2}) and oxygenate. Many patients die of infectious complications. Survivors usually regain their normal lung function, and a few will have persistent mild obstructive or restrictive defects.

Pleural Effusions

Pathophysiology

Pleural effusions [23] result both from primary pleural processes and disease remote from the pleura. Normal pleural space contains up to 10 ml fluid. Fluid moves into the pleural space via the parietal pleura, whose blood is supplied by the systemic circulation. Fluid leaves the pleural space through the visceral pleura, which is supplied by the pulmonary circulation. Cells and proteins are removed from the pleural space by the pulmonary lymphatics. Conditions which increase pulmonary vascular pressure (congestive heart failure), decrease oncotic pressure (nephrotic syndrome), obstruct lymphatics (malignancy), and increase capillary permeability (acute and chronic inflammation) all result in the formation of excess pleural fluid.

Diagnosis

Symptoms and signs of pleural effusions are often subtle until the effusions become large enough to compress lung tissue. Symptoms are often related to an underlying nonpleural process, such as an acute bacterial pneumonia causing a parapneumonic effusion. In some conditions associated with acute inflammation, pleuritic pain may be the presenting symptom. A large pleural effusion compressing adjacent lung often produces progressive dyspnea as the presenting complaint.

A pleural effusion must exceed 250 to 300 ml before it can be detected by physical examination. Dullness to percussion is the typical physical finding. In contrast to pulmonary consolidations, which also produce dullness to percussion, tactile fremitus and breath sounds will be decreased over the effusion. Owing to the compressive effect, signs of consolidation are present above the effusion. If the effusion is large enough (>1 liter), there also may be evidence of a contralateral mediastinal shift.

The chest radiograph is most important in detecting small pleural effusions. Effusions can be radiographically apparent if 250 to 300 ml fluid is present. Radiographic findings include a rounded meniscus at the costophrenic angle and a diffuse ground-glass density beneath the dome of the diaphragm, obscuring the pulmonary vessels (Fig. 2-6). A subpulmonic effusion (fluid trapped between a lower lobe and the diaphragm) should be suspected if the center of the hemidiaphragm appears flattened rather than its usual domed appearance and if there is obliteration of lower lobe vessels. On lateral chest radiograph pleural effusions often appear as a rounded density in the posterior costophrenic angle. If an effusion is sus-

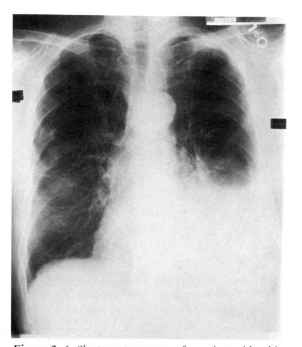

Figure 2–6. Chest roentgenogram of a patient with a history of ethanol abuse (note fractured ribs on the right) and pancreatitis. A large pleural effusion is present on the left side. The pleural fluid was an exudate with an elevated amylase level. The effusion was caused by pancreatitis.

pected, a lateral decubitus chest roentgenogram should be obtained.

The etiology of pleural effusions is sometimes determined by history and physical examination. In most cases, however, a thoracentesis is required for pleural fluid examination. A thoracentesis is not required in patients with obvious congestive heart failure whose effusion responds to diuresis and in diseases where the diagnosis is established by other means (i.e., pulmonary embolism, systemic lupus erythematosus). When an infectious etiology is considered, a thoracentesis should be performed without delay (see Treatment).

Following thoracentesis, color, turbidity, and odor of the fluid should be recorded. The fluid should be sent directly to the laboratory for the following determinations: white blood cell and differential counts, glucose, lactate dehydrogenase (LDH), protein, pH, and amylase if pancreatic disease or esophageal rupture is being considered. Gram and acid-fast stains should be performed, as well as appropriate cultures, which should include aerobic, anaerobic, and mycobacterial. Pleural fluid cytology also should be performed.

An important consideration in the differential diagnosis of pleural effusions is whether the fluid is a transudate or an exudate. Transudates are characterized by both low total protein and lactate dehydrogenase (LDH) levels. They usually result from alterations in hemodynamic factors such as elevated pulmonary vascular pressure or low oncotic pressure. Exudates result from inflammatory or malignant processes which either increase capillary permeability or interfere with lymphatic drainage. Exudates require one of the following: (1) pleural fluid protein/serum protein > 0.5, (2) LDH > two-thirds the upper limit of normal for serum LDH, and (3) pleural fluid LDH/ serum LDH > 0.6. Transudative effusions do not meet any of the preceding criteria. Table 2-24 lists the etiologies of transudates and exudates. Normally there are communications between the pleural and peritoneal spaces. This accounts for the transudative pleural effusions which occur

Table 2–24. Causes of Pleural Effusions

Transudates	Exudates
Congestive heart failure	Parapneumonic
Cirrhosis with ascites	Pulmonary embolism
Nephrotic syndrome	Neoplasm
Myxedema	Primary infections: bacteria, viruses, parasites
Peritoneal dialysis	Collagen-vascular disease (SLE, RA)
Acute atelectasis	Pancreatitis, pancreatic pseudocyst
	Esophageal rupture
	Drug reaction (nitrofurantoin, methysergide)
	Benign asbestos effusion
	Meig's syndrome
	Post-cardiac injury syndrome
	Yellow-nail syndrome (congenital lymphatic hypoplasia)
	Uremic pleurisy
	Chronic atelectasis
	Chylothorax
	Sarcoid

with ascites and peritoneal dialysis. Clear or straw-colored fluid is characteristic of transudates and is seen only occasionally with exudates. Cloudy fluids are due to increased numbers of white cells or increased levels of lipids. To distinguish between white blood cells and lipids, the fluid can be centrifuged and the supernatant examined. The supernatant is clear in fluids with increased white cells and will remain cloudy with lipid effusions. Lipid pleural effusions can be further separated into chylous effusions and pseudochylous effusions. Chylous effusions contain a high percentage of triglycerides. The most common etiology of chylous effusions is traumatic interruption or obstruction of the thoracic duct. Pseudochylous effusions contain large amounts of cholesterol or lecithin-globulin complexes and are often seen following chronic inflammatory

processes such as tuberculosis, rheumatoid arthritis, or malignancy.

It takes only 5000 to 10,000 red blood cells per milliliter for pleural fluids to appear serosanguineous. Grossly bloody effusions, on the other hand, are seen with tumors, trauma, pulmonary infarction (thromboembolism), after cardiac injury, and rarely, in tuberculosis.

A white blood cell count greater than 1000/ml usually indicates an exudative effusion. The total white cell count is not as useful as the differential counts. Neutrophilic predominance is found in acute inflammatory exudates (e.g., infections and collagen-vascular disease). Chronic inflammatory exudates often demonstrate lymphocyte predominance, which is most characteristic for tuberculosis and malignancy.

Important information is also gained from the pleural fluid glucose and pH. The presence of significant pleural inflammation interferes with the diffusion of glucose from serum to the pleural space. In addition, acids produced in the pleural space do not diffuse into the serum. This results in both pleural hypoglycemia and acidosis. This situation most often is the result of bacterial empyema, tuberculosis, rheumatoid arthritis, and diffuse malignant pleural involvement. Pleural fluid pH, but not the glucose, is also decreased in esophageal rupture with leakage of gastric contents into the pleural space.

When the diagnosis of exudative pleural effusion is not established by the aforementioned evaluation or if malignancy is suspected, a pleural biopsy should be performed. Biopsies are especially helpful in establishing the diagnosis of cancer and tuberculosis. Acid-fast stains and cultures of pleural fluid are positive in 50 to 70 percent. Pleural biopsy with histologic examination and tissue culture increases the yield to 80 percent. Similarly, pleural fluid cytology and pleural biopsy yield an 80 percent positivity rate for the diagnosis of malignancy. Pleural biopsy can be either an open or closed procedure (Abrams' needle).

Treatment

The treatment of pleural effusions depends not only on the etiology, but also on the degree to which the effusion is causing symptoms. Some effusions only require treatment of the underlying disease process (i.e., congestive heart failure). Others often require immediate and complete drainage (i.e., traumatic hemothorax).

Parapneumonic effusions are exudative acute inflammatory (neutrophils) effusions which accompany intraparenchymal infectious processes (i.e., pneumonia or lung abscess). An uncomplicated parapneumonic effusion will resolve as the underlying lung infection responds to treatment. These effusions have the potential for becoming empyemas (infected). Empyemas are quite viscous and form loculations within the pleural space that are difficult to drain, even with chest tubes. Besides being a cause of persistent fever, empyemas result in fibrous thickening of the pleura with entrapment of the underlying lung. This causes a restrictive ventilatory defect. Loculated empyemas (pleural abscesses) require surgical drainage.

There are also parapneumonic effusions which are not infected (i.e., empyema) but which cause residual pleural fibrosis. These effusions are called complicated parapneumonic effusions. As with an empyema, a complicated parapneumonic effusion may require open thoracectomy if drainage cannot be accomplished by a chest tube. This is why there is a certain urgency in the evaluation of parapneumonic effusions. If a complicated parapneumonic effusion or empyema is discovered early, treatment by chest-tube drainage may be adequate, thereby avoiding a thoracectomy and pleural stripping.

If the diagnostic thoracentesis reveals a turbid purulent fluid with many neutrophils (>20,000) or if the Gram stain or culture is positive, a chest tube should be inserted. Complicated parapneumonic effusions will have lower pH and glucose levels than uncomplicated ones. Since the pH falls before the glucose, it is a more sensitive indicator. If the pleural fluid pH is above 7.20, the parapneumonic effusion usually responds to antibiotic treatment alone and chest-tube drainage is not indicated. If the pH is less than 7.00, a chest tube should be inserted. For patients with fluid pH levels between 7.00 and 7.20, other factors must be considered, such as the size of the effusion (larger effusions more often requiring drainage than smaller effusions). The pH criteria listed above are only for parapneumonic effusions. Other types of effusions, such as those caused by rheumatoid arthritis, malignancy, and tuberculosis, may have a low pH and not require drainage.

The management of malignant pleural effusions depends on the degree to which the effusion causes symptoms (dyspnea). Large malignant effusions can usually be managed initially by complete drainage via thoracentesis. If the fluid reaccumulates rapidly, requiring frequent thoracenteses, the pleural space can be obliterated using sclerosing agents such as tetracycline.

Solitary Pulmonary Nodules

Pathophysiology

Solitary pulmonary nodules [24] are round or ovoid densities that are well-circumscribed, surrounded by aerated lung, and distinct from the pleura and mediastinum. They are less than 6 cm in size. Larger densities are usually referred to as masses (Fig. 2-7).

The three most common causes of solitary pulmonary nodules are (1) malignancies, (2) infectious granulomatous disease, and (3) hamartomas. Less common causes of solitary pulmonary nodules are lung abscess, healing pulmonary infarction, arteriovenous malformation, hematoma, and sequestration. The incidence and malignancy

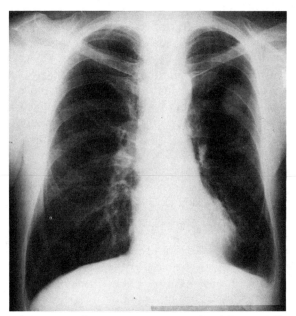

Figure 2–7. *Chest roentgenogram reveals a left upper lobe solitary pulmonary nodule. No old studies were available for comparison. At thoracotomy the lesion was found to be a primary lung adenocarcinoma.*

rate vary with geography; i.e., the incidence of benign disease is higher in areas endemic for coccidioidomycosis and histoplasmosis. Also, the older the patient with a new solitary nodule, the greater chance of it being malignant. At age 70 70 percent of solitary nodules are cancerous.

Diagnosis

The important clinical decision concerning a pulmonary nodule discovered by routine chest radiograph is whether to observe with follow-up chest roentgenograms or proceed with a diagnostic workup to exclude malignancy. Often the diagnostic evaluation process includes a thoracotomy. The early diagnosis of malignant nodules cannot be overemphasized, since there are good data to suggest that the smaller the malignant nodule, the greater the chance for surgical cure (i.e.,

nodules less than 4 cm have a 40 percent 5-year survival).

How does one decide whether a nodule is benign or malignant? The history and physical examination are usually not helpful. Patients are most often asymptomatic, with the nodule being discovered incidentally. Rarely, patients present with cough and hemoptysis. A history of smoking is important because it increases the chance of malignancy. Every effort should be made to obtain a previous chest roentgenogram. On physical examination, careful attention should be paid to cervical and supraclavicular nodes, since these are the primary areas of pulmonary lymphatic drainage outside the chest. Blood-borne metastases commonly go to the brain, bone, liver, adrenals, and other areas of the lung. A careful neurologic examination will help exclude brain metastases. A normal alkaline phosphatase level and lack of bone pain will help exclude bone metastases. Both the stool and urine should be evaluated for blood to help exclude an extrathoracic primary source with a single metastasis.

The two best indicators of benignity are characteristics of the nodule itself. The first is the presence of calcium, and the second is the rate of growth. Basically, four patterns of calcification are found in benign lesions. These are (1) a central area of calcification, (2) a ring of calcification, (3) diffuse speckles, and (4) a dense, irregular or "popcorn" calcification. An eccentric fleck of calcium can be seen in scar carcinomas and should not be used to judge a nodule benign.

The second factor is growth rate. Nodules that grow very rapidly or very slowly are less likely to be cancerous. This is why previous chest roentgenograms are so important. A lesion that has not changed in size in 2 years can be assumed to be benign. The doubling time for most carcinomas is estimated to be between 1 and 15 months. It is important to remember that when the volume of a sphere doubles, the diameter increases 1.26 times. Thus a nodule that is 3 cm in diameter will reach a diameter of 3.78 cm (3 × 1.26) when its volume doubles. To be conservative, many clinicians set limits at 10 days and 2 years and conclude that a lesion is most likely benign if it doubles in volume in less than 10 days or more than 2 years.

Treatment

When a patient presents with a solitary pulmonary nodule, a decision is then made whether to observe the nodule with follow-up chest roentgenograms every 6 months for 2 years or to pursue a diagnostic workup. Factors that indicate benignity and preclude further diagnostic studies are (1) an old chest roentgenogram that indicates no growth in 2 years, (2) a more recent chest roentgenogram demonstrating that the doubling time of the tumor is less than 10 days or greater than 2 years, and (3) typical benign calcification. Some clinicians also choose to watch lesions in patients less than 35 years of age without a smoking history.

If history and previous chest roentgenograms are not conclusive, further workup is indicated. The patient's pulmonary function should be measured to help predict whether a lobectomy can be tolerated. In addition, the patient's cardiac status and overall medical condition should be assessed to predict the overall risk of major surgery.

In patients at low risk for thoracotomy, one of two approaches is taken. Either the patient is sent for thoracotomy without less invasive diagnostic procedures or a biopsy is performed. Less invasive procedures include transthoracic needle biopsies and bronchoscopy with fluoroscopically guided transbronchial biopsy. A thoracotomy is avoided only if a benign lesion is definitively diagnosed by histology and/or special stains that indicate an infectious granuloma.

References

1. American Thoracic Society and Center for Disease Control. Treatment of tuberculosis and tuberculosis infection in adults and children. *Am. Rev. Respir. Dis.* 134: 355, 1986.
2. Bell, W. R., Simon, T. L., and De Mets, D. L. The clinical features of submassive and massive emboli. *Am. J. Med.* 62: 355, 1977.
3. Bone, R. C. (Ed.). Symposium on adult respiratory distress syndrome. *Clin. Chest Med.* 3: 1, 1982.
4. Burrow, B. (Ed.). Symposium on chronic respiratory disease. *Med. Clin. North Am.* 57: 545, 1973.
5. Christopher, K. L., Wood, R. P., II, Eckert, R. C., et al. Vocal-cord dysfunction presenting as asthma. *N. Engl. J. Med.* 308: 1566, 1983.
6. Crystal, R. G., Bitterman, P. B., Rennard, S. I., et al. Interstitial lung diseases of unknown causes: Disorders characterized by chronic inflammation of the lower respiratory tract. *N. Engl. J. Med.* 310: 154, 1984.
7. Crystal, R. G., Fulmer, J. D., Roberts, W. C., et al. Idiopathic pulmonary fibrosis: Clinical, histologic, radiographic, physiologic, scintigraphic, cytologic diagnosis and management of interstitial lung disease. *Ann. Intern. Med.* 85: 769, 1976.
8. Crystal, R. G., Roberts, W. C., Hunninghake, G. W., et al. Pulmonary sarcoidosis: The disease characterized and perpetuated by active lung T-lymphocytes. *Ann. Intern. Med.* 94: 73, 1981.
9. Crystal, R. G., Gadek, J. E., Forrans, V. J., Fulmer, J. D., Line, B. R., and Hunninghake, G. W. Interstitial lung disease: Current concepts of pathogenesis, staging, and therapy. *Am. J. Med.* 70: 542, 1981.
10. Dalen, J. E., and Hirsh, J. ACCP-NHLBI national conference on antithrombotic therapy. *Chest (Suppl.)* 89: 1, 1986.
11. Drutz, D., and Catanzaro, A. State of the art: Coccidioidomycosis. Part 1. *Am. Rev. Respir. Dis.* 117: 559, 1978; Part 2: 117: 727, 1978.
12. Fanta, C. H., and Pennington, J. E. Fever and new lung infiltrates in the immunocompromised host. *Clin. Chest Med.* 2: 19, 1981.
13. Fowler, A. A., Hamman, R. F., Good, J. T., et al. Adult respiratory distress syndrome: Risk with common predispositions. *Ann. Intern. Med.* 98: 593, 1983.
14. Gilman, M. J., and Wang, K. P. Transbronchial lung biopsy in sarcoidosis: An approach to deter-

mine the optimal number of biopsies. *Am. Rev. Respir. Dis.* 122: 721, 1980.

15. Glassroth, J., Robins, A. G., and Snider, D. E. Tuberculosis in the 1980s. *N. Engl. J. Med.* 302: 1441, 1980.

16. Goodwin, R. A., and Des Prez, R. M. Histoplasmosis: State of the art. *Am. Rev. Respir. Dis.* 117: 929, 1978.

17. Hopewell, P. C., and Luce, J. M. Pulmonary Manifestations of the Acquired Immunodeficiency Syndrome. In T. L. Petty and D. C. Flenley (Eds.), *Recent Advances in Respiratory Medicine,* 4th Ed. Edinburgh: Churchill-Livingstone, 1986.

18. Hull, R. D., High, J., Carter, C., et al. Pulmonary angiography, ventilation lung scanning and venography for clinically suspected pulmonary embolism with abnormal perfusion lung scan. *Ann. Intern. Med.* 98: 891, 1983.

19. Hull, R. D., Raglcob, G. E., and Hirsh, J. Pulmonary Thromboembolism. In T. L. Petty and D. C. Flenley (Eds.), *Recent Advances in Respiratory Medicine,* 4th Ed. Edinburgh: Churchill-Livingstone, 1986.

20. La Force, M. F. Hospital-acquired gram-negative rod pneumonias: An overview. *Am. J. Med.* 70: 664, 1981.

21. Lieberman, J., Schleissner, L. A., Nosal, A., et al. Clinical correlation of serum angiotensin-converting enzyme (ACE) in sarcoidosis. *Chest* 84: 522, 1985.

22. Liebow, A. A., and Carrington, C. B. Alveolar Diseases: The Interstitial Pneumonias. In M. Simon (Ed.), *Frontiers of Pulmonary Radiology.* New York: Grune & Stratton, 1969. P. 102.

23. Light, R. W. (Ed.). Pleural diseases. *Clin. Chest Med.* 6: 1, 1985.

24. Lillington, G. P. The solitary pulmonary nodule—1974. *Am. Rev. Respir. Dis.* 110: 699, 1974.

25. MacFarlane, J. T., Ward, M. J., Finch, R. G., and MacRal, A. D. Hospital study of adult community-acquired pneumonia. *Lancet* 2: 255, 1982.

26. McFadden, E. R., Jr., Kiser, J., and de Groot, W. Acute bronchial asthma: Relations between clinical and physiologic manifestations. *N. Engl. J. Med.* 288: 221, 1973.

27. Marlow, J. B. Hospital-acquired bacterial pneumonias. *Compr. Ther.* 8: 29, 1982.

28. Mitchell, D. N., and Scadding, J. G. Sarcoidosis: State of the art. *Am. Rev. Respir. Dis.* 110: 774, 1974.

29. Murray, J. F., Felton, C. P., Gary, S., et al. Pulmonary complications of the acquired immunodeficiency syndrome: Report of a National Heart, Lung and Blood Institute workshop. *N. Engl. J. Med.* 310: 1682, 1984.

30. National ACCP Consensus Conference on Tuberculosis. Consensus statement. *Chest (Suppl.)* 87: 1, 1985.

31. Nocturnal Oxygen Therapy Trial Group. Continuous or nocturnal oxygen therapy in hypoxemic chronic obstructive lung disease. *Ann. Intern. Med.* 93: 391, 1980.

32. Petty, T. L. (Ed.). *Chronic Obstructive Pulmonary Disease.* New York: Marcel Dekker, 1978.

33. Pierce, A. K., and Sanford, J. P. Aerobic gram-negative bacillary pneumonias. *Am. Rev. Respir. Dis.* 110: 647, 1974.

34. Powell, J. R., Voseh, S., Hopewell, P., Costello, J., Sheiner, L. B., and Regelman, S. Theophylline deposition in acutely ill hospitalized patients. The effect of smoking, heart failure, severe airway obstruction and pneumonia. *Am. Rev. Respir. Dis.* 118: 229, 1978.

35. Reynolds, H. Y. (Ed.). Respiratory infections. *Clin. Chest Med.* 2: 1, 1981.

36. Rosenow, E. C. Pulmonary disease in the immunocompromised host. Part 1. *Mayo Clin. Proc.* 60: 473, 1985; Part 2: 60: 610, 1985.

37. Scoggin, C. H. Acute Asthma and Status Asthmatics. In S. A. Sahn (Ed.), *Pulmonary Emergencies.* New York: Churchill-Livingstone, 1982. P. 127.

38. Staub, N. "State-of-the-art" review: Pathogenesis of pulmonary edema. *Am. Rev. Respir. Dis.* 109: 358, 1971.

39. Thurlbeck, W. M. *Chronic Airflow Obstruction in Lung Disease.* Philadelphia: Saunders, 1976.

40. Turner-Warwick, M. (Ed.). Interstitial lung disease. *Semin. Respir. Med.* 6: 1, 1984.

41. Van Metre, T. Pneumococcal pneumonia treated with antibiotics: The prognostic significance of certain clinical findings. *N. Engl. J. Med.* 251: 1048, 1954.

42. Watters, L. C., Schwarz, M. I., Cherniack, R. M., Waldron, J. A., Dunn, T. L., Stanford, R. E., and King, T. E. Idiopathic pulmonary fibrosis pretreatment bronchoalveolar lavage cellular constituents and their relationships with lung histopathology and clinical response to therapy. *Am. Rev. Respir. Dis.* 135: 696, 1987.

Renal Diseases, Fluid and Electrolyte Disorders, and Hypertension

3

Joseph I. Shapiro and
Robert W. Schrier

Disorders of Plasma Sodium Concentration

Disorders of the plasma sodium concentration are best considered as disorders of water metabolism [38,69]. It should be stressed that the plasma sodium concentration provides the physician with no information about the net quantity of sodium present in the body, but merely the relative quantities of water and sodium. As a general rule of thumb, the plasma sodium concentration is a reasonable index of the plasma osmolality. The following formula can be used to estimate the plasma osmolality:

Plasma osmolality
$$= 2 \times \text{plasma sodium concentration (mEq/liter)}$$
$$+ \frac{\text{plasma glucose (mg/dl)}}{18}$$
$$+ \frac{\text{blood urea nitrogen (mg/dl)}}{2.8}$$

As can be seen from this formula, the plasma sodium concentration is the major determinant of the plasma osmolailty under most circumstances.

Deviations from this rule occur in marked hyperglycemic states, chronic renal failure, and conditions where unmeasured osmols are present in substantive concentrations (e.g., ethanol, methanol, ethylene glycol, or mannitol intoxication).

Hypernatremia

Hypernatremia is generally seen in patients who either have impaired access to water or an impairment in thirst. Abnormalities in renal concentrating ability are usually not associated with hypernatremia in the absence of the aforementioned predisposing conditions; this is so because increased water intake compensates for most increases in urinary water losses. Although hypernatremia is most often associated with dehydration, it can be associated with normal or increased total-body sodium. A schema for the approach to the patient with hypernatremia is shown in Fig. 3-1.

131

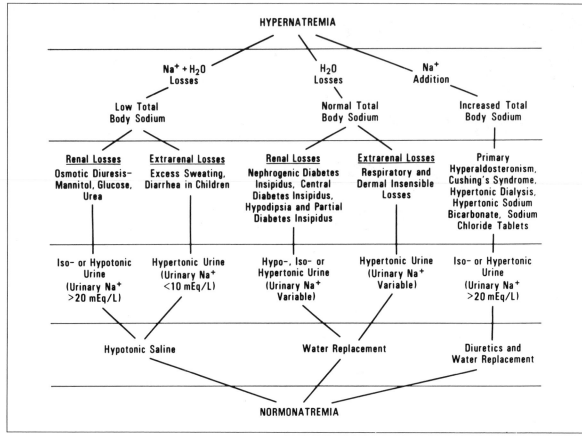

Figure 3—1. *Diagnostic and therapeutic classification of hypernatremia. (Adapted from T. Berl, R. J. Anderson, K. M. McDonald, and R. W. Schrier. Clinical disorders of water metabolism,* Kidney Int. *10: 123, 1976. Used by permission.)*

DIAGNOSIS

The symptoms of hypernatremia may range from virtually no symptoms to stupor, seizures, and coma. Whereas there are no predictable physical findings associated with hypernatremia, the state of total-body sodium may be apparent from the physical examination (e.g., edema or orthostatic hypotension). The laboratory findings associated with hypernatremia include increases in plasma osmolality, as well as changes in laboratory values associated with the underlying cause or condition associated with hypernatremia. The urinary sodium concentration should help in assessing the total-body sodium state of the patient [69] (see Fig. 3-1).

TREATMENT

Chronic therapy of the hypernatremic states involves ensured access to water and even prescribed daily water intakes in the patient with hypodipsia or adipsia. Correction of any underlying renal concentrating defects, if possible, should, of course, be undertaken.

The latter can be accomplished only if the cause of the renal concentrating defect is ascertained. These conditions can be roughly separated into those due to inadequate circulating antidiuretic

Table 3–1. Polyuric States: Response of Urinary Osmolality to Dehydration and Vasopressin (ADH)

Disorder	U_{OSM} (mOsmol/kg) NPO × 12 hours	After ADH
Complete central DI	<250	350–500
Partial DI	>350	25 percent or greater increase
Nephrogenic DI	<600	No change (± 10 percent)
Psychogenic polydipsia	500–800	No change (± 10 percent)
Normal	>800	No change (± 10 percent)

Note: NPO = nothing by mouth (nil per os); DI = diabetes insipidus; ADH = antidiuretic hormone.

hormone (i.e., arginine vasopression, AVP) and antidiuretic hormone-resistant states. This differential diagnosis can be determined on the basis of the following dehydration test. The patient is fluid-deprived to achieve a 3 to 5 percent loss of body weight while recording hourly urine volumes and urine and plasma osmolalities. Aqueous vasopression is administered immediately after completion of this fluid deprivation test.

Table 3-1 shows the results in patients with various polyuric disorders studied with this test. It should be stressed that dehydration studies are potentially dangerous, particularly in the patient with complete central diabetes insipidus, and should be done under careful physician observation and not overnight [69].

Patients with central diabetes insipidus are best treated with intranasal deamino dAVP (ddAVP), an antidiuretic hormone analogue with long-acting properties. Patients with chronic nephrogenic diabetes insipidus may be treated by thiazide diuretics, which decrease extracellular fluid volume and thus distal fluid delivery and urine flow. This treatment should be accompanied by moderate restriction of sodium intake [69].

Hyponatremia

Hyponatremia may be associated with a low, normal, or increased plasma osmolality [69]. Two types of hyponatremia are associated with normal or elevated plasma osmolality. In the first type, the plasma sodium concentration in the plasma water is normal, but the relative concentration of water in total plasma is depressed because of an increase in solids, i.e., so-called pseudohyponatremia. The classic examples of pseudohyponatremia are hyperproteinemic or hyperlipidemic states. The second variety is a true dilutional hyponatremia where plasma water content is increased by a shift of intracellular fluid into the extracellular fluid space. This occurs in uncontrolled hyperglycemia, as well as during mannitol infusions. An increase in the plasma glucose level of 100 mg/dl will lead to a dilutional decrease in plasma sodium concentration of about 1.6 mmol/liter. The majority of hyponatremic states are associated with hypo-osmolality. These hyponatremic hypo-osmolar states may be associated with either low, normal, or increased body sodium [69]. A diagnostic and treatment approach to hyponatremic states is shown in Fig. 3-2.

DIAGNOSIS
Severe hyponatremia may be associated with abnormalities in central nervous system function ranging from no symptoms or mild confusion to seizures and coma [4]. Physical examination findings in hyponatremia are generally related to the state of sodium balance (e.g., edema, orthostatic hypotension).

TREATMENT
Therapy of hyponatremia associated with a normal body sodium level is dependent on the severity of the hyponatremia. Severe hyponatremia associated with marked central nervous system symptoms of coma and/or seizures mandates emergency therapy. This therapy usually involves administration of hypertonic saline with a loop diuretic such as furosemide [5].

In less emergent states of asymptomatic hypo-

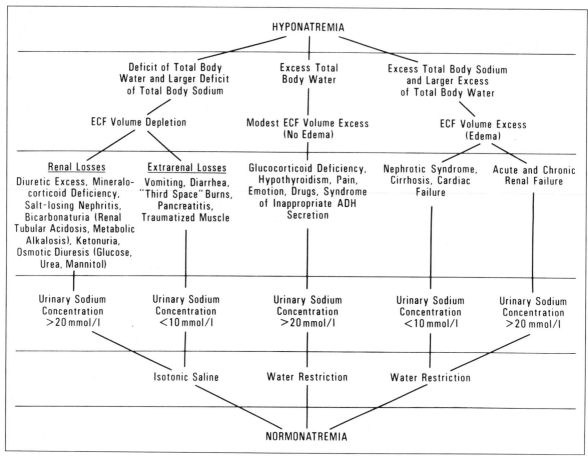

Figure 3–2. Diagnostic and therapeutic classification of hyponatremia. (Adapted from T. Berl, R. J. Anderson, K. M. McDonald, and R. W. Schrier. Clinical disorders of water metabolism, Kidney Int. 10: 123, 1976. Used by permission.)

natremia associated with a normal total-body sodium level, restricting fluids to 500 to 800 ml per day is generally adequate therapy. With the chronic syndrome of inappropriate antidiuretic hormone (SIADH), fluid restriction, either alone or with increases in dietary sodium, should be instituted. If this is inadequate therapy (e.g., noncompliance), adjunctive therapy with loop diuretics, demeclocycline (which decreases urinary concentrating ability), or oral urea (which provides an osmotic load) has been employed to increase renal water losses.

Therapy of hyponatremia associated with increases of total-body sodium level (e.g., cardiac and hepatic failure) involves fluid restriction and the judicious use of diuretics. Hyponatremia associated with decreases in total-body sodium level is best accomplished with infusions of isotonic saline.

As with the hypernatremic states, therapy of hyponatremia should not be overaggressive. Although controversial, it appears that overly rapid correction of severe hyponatremia may be associated with a syndrome of central pontine myelinolysis [43]. The formula for calculating the desired water losses to correct hyponatremia is as follows:

Solute-free water excess (liters)
$$= \left(1 - \frac{\text{measured plasma sodium}}{\text{desired plasma sodium}}\right) \times 0.6 \text{ (liter/kg)}$$
$$\times \text{ body weight (kg)}$$

With this approach, urinary electrolyte losses (i.e., Na, Cl, K) can be replaced with a small volume of hypertonic (3 percent) saline, and thus a net negative water balance is achieved without a decrease in total-body electrolytes. For example, if a furosemide-induced diuresis of 1 liter per hour is accompanied by electrolyte replacement with 150 ml 3 percent saline per hour, then, in essence, 850 ml electrolyte-free water is removed from the body. Potassium chloride (e.g., 20 mEq) also may be added to hypertonic saline solution to avoid potassium depletion.

Acid-Base Disorders

The body regulates systemic pH using essentially two systems. These are the respiratory system, which changes acid-base status by changing the partial pressure of carbon dioxide, and the renal (metabolic) system, which has the capacity to excrete excess amounts of either bicarbonate or acid, the latter in the forms of ammonium and titratable acid.

Acid-base problems are generally categorized as either respiratory, metabolic, or mixed disorders [39,40]. When an acid-base disorder of either a simple respiratory or metabolic nature is present, the noninvolved system will attempt to correct the disturbance in pH. This process is called compensation and reflects the integrity of the noninvolved system. As a general rule, compensation does not result in a normal pH. However, some degree of compensation is indeed normal, and the absence of appropriate compensation must suggest a separate disturbance. This will be covered in more detail in the following discussion.

Simple Metabolic Acidosis
Simple metabolic acidosis can best be defined as a decrease in systemic pH associated with a decrease in the plasma bicarbonate concentration. Acidemia is the term used to describe a fall in pH below 7.35 irrespective of the cause. The symptoms of metabolic acidosis generally vary according to the underlying cause. Metabolic acidosis is best approached by categorization using the anion gap [20,56]. The anion gap is described by the following equation:

Anion gap (mmol/liter)
= plasma sodium − (plasma chloride + plasma bicarbonate) (all in mmol/liter)

Metabolic acidoses can be divided into those associated with a normal anion gap, which is usually about 12 ± 2 mmol/liter in most laboratories, and those associated with an increased anion gap. There are two categories because metabolic acidosis can be due to accumulation of organic anions with an increase in the anion gap or loss of alkali without an increase in the anion gap. Tables 3-2 and 3-3 list the major causes of metabolic acidosis with an increased and normal anion gap, respectively.

During metabolic acidosis, the respiratory system will attempt to compensate for the change in systemic pH by increasing ventilation and lowering the P_{CO_2}. The decrease in P_{CO_2} that normally accompanies the disorder of metabolic acidosis is given by the following equation:

Decrease in P_{CO_2} (mmHg)
= 1 to 1.5 × decrease in plasma bicarbonate (mmol/liter)

Table 3–2. Metabolic Acidosis with Increased Anion Gap

Underlying Disorder	Mechanism
Diabetic ketoacidosis	Increased production of ketoacids: acetoacetic acid, beta-hydroxybutyric acid
Lactic acidosis	Increased production of lactic acid
Starvation	Mild overproduction of ketoacids
Nonketotic hyperosmolar coma	Increased production of organic acids other than ketoacids
Inborn errors of metabolism	Increased production of various organic acids
Ingestion of toxic substances:	
Salicylate overdose	Increased organic acid production plus dissociation of salicylic acid
Methyl alcohol ingestion	Formic acid accumulation plus organic acid overproduction
Ethylene glycol ingestion	Glycolic acid accumulation
Paraldehyde overdose	Unidentified organic acid production
Renal failure	Decreased excretion of the usual daily metabolic acid load

Table 3–3. Metabolic Acidosis with Normal Anion Gap (Hyperchloremic)

Underlying Disorder	Mechanism
Diarrhea	Loss of HCO_3^--rich (30–50 mmol/liter), K^+-rich bowel fluid
Small bowel or pancreatic drainage	Loss of HCO_3^--rich fluid
Ureterosigmoidostomy or malfunctioning ileal loop conduit, i.e., obstructed or loop too long	Exchange of HCO_3^- for Cl^- from urine in contact with bowel mucosa
Anion-exchange resins, cholestyramine	Exchange of Cl^- from resin for HCO_3^- across gut mucosa
Carbonic-anhydrase inhibitors, e.g., acetazolamide	Blocks renal HCO_3^- reclamation
Renal tubular acidosis: Distal (type I)	Inability to acidify urine maximally (e.g., hepatic cirrhosis, hyperglobulinemia, amphotericin B, hypercalcemic states)
Proximal (type II)	Decreased ability to reclaim normal quantities of filtered HCO_3^- (e.g., Fanconi's syndrome, cadmium poisoning, amyloid)
Hyperparathyroidism	Parathyroid hormone reduces proximal HCO_3^- reclamation
Hypoaldosteronism	Decreased H^+ secretion and NH_3 production
Dilutional acidosis	Rapid expansion of extracellular fluid dilutes HCO_3^- concentration slightly—no more than 10 percent
Parenteral alimentation	Some formulas contain excess organic cations (balanced by Cl^-), which yield H^+ on metabolism (e.g., Neoaminosol and FreAmine)
HCl, NH_4Cl, arginine HCl	All equivalent to adding strong acid to body fluids

Changes in P_{CO_2} of a lesser or greater degree than given by this relationship suggests a separate respiratory disorder [39].

DIAGNOSIS

Symptoms associated with metabolic acidosis are generally related to the underlying cause. Lowering of systemic pH due to metabolic acidosis may, because of respiratory compensation, be associated with dyspnea, as well as the physical findings of tachypnea. Also, acidosis can cause hypotension by decreasing myocardial contractility and diminishing vascular resistance.

TREATMENT

The therapy of metabolic acidosis is best directed toward the etiology of the disturbance. Exceptions to the etiology-oriented approach exist with life-threatening degrees of acidosis (i.e., an arterial pH of less than 7.0 to 7.1). Although controversial [7,30], administration of bicarbonate is still advocated in this setting of a very low arterial pH [54]. The usual approach to this problem involves calculating the rise in bicarbonate necessary to achieve an arterial pH of 7.15 to 7.20 using 50 to 80 percent of the body weight as the volume of distribution for bicarbonate. If respiratory compensation is not optimal, e.g., relative hypoventilation secondary to lung disease, increased ventilation with a ventilator may be required.

Chronic causes of metabolic acidosis are usually related to the failure of the kidney to excrete sufficient acid (e.g., the renal tubular acidoses [53] or the acidosis of chronic renal failure). In this setting, normalization of the serum bicarbonate to a level of about 20 is probably required to prevent skeletal demineralization [13]. The danger of hypertension and pulmonary edema, however, must be monitored. Alkali therapy is quite important for normal growth in children with proximal and distal renal tubular acidosis. Usually, with distal renal tubular acidosis, this goal can be achieved with 1 to 3 mEq/kg per day individual doses, but patients with proximal renal tubular acidosis may require much higher doses. This alkali is generally given as an oral formulation, either as sodium bicarbonate or as sodium citrate (which is converted by the body into bicarbonate). Since oral bicarbonate may cause bloating, the latter is generally better tolerated by patients.

Metabolic Alkalosis

Simple metabolic alkalosis can be described as an elevation of systemic pH associated with an increase in the plasma bicarbonate concentration. Alkalemia is a term used to describe a pH of 7.45 independent of the cause. Metabolic alkalosis is best categorized according to the extracellular fluid volume. There are two types of metabolic alkalosis, one associated with a decrease in total-body sodium level and extracellular fluid volume and another associated with a normal or increased total-body sodium level and extracellular fluid volume [39]. Synonyms more commonly used are sodium chloride-responsive metabolic

alkalosis and sodium chloride-resistant metabolic alkalosis, respectively. Since the urinary chloride concentration is generally low in sodium chloride-responsive metabolic alkalosis and is generally high in sodium chloride-resistant metabolic alkalosis, urinary chloride concentration is used to distinguish between these two varieties of metabolic alkalosis. Table 3-4 lists the causes of metabolic alkalosis. It should be stressed that although diuretics are classically considered to cause sodium chloride-responsive metabolic alkalosis, if the diuretic action is still present at the time the urine chloride is measured, it probably will be increased.

As in the case of metabolic acidosis, the respiratory system will, indeed, attempt to compensate for metabolic alkalosis. In general, the appropriate compensation involves hypoventilation and an increase in P_{CO_2} of about 0.25 to 1.0 mmHg for every 1 mmole/liter increase in the plasma bicarbonate level [39].

DIAGNOSIS

Severe metabolic alkalosis (pH > 7.6) may be associated with seizures, cardiac arrhythmias, and death. The muscle weakness associated with metabolic alkalosis is generally due to the concomitant decrease in plasma potassium concentration.

TREATMENT

The treatment of metabolic alkalosis is best directed at the underlying cause. As suggested by the name, sodium chloride-responsive metabolic alkalosis generally responds to replacement of sodium chloride. The sodium chloride is generally administered on isotonic saline infusions or, in milder cases, by increasing dietary sodium chloride intake. Sodium chloride-resistant metabolic alkalosis associated with an aldosterone adenoma or Cushing's syndrome generally requires a surgical approach. In cases of primary hyperaldosteronism secondary to hyperplasia (which does not respond well to surgery), aldosterone antagonism (i.e., administration of spironolactone) is recommended. Metabolic alkalosis caused by severe potassium depletion responds to potassium supple-

Table 3–4. Metabolic Alkalosis

Condition	Cause
NaCl-responsive (U_{Cl}^- < 20 mmol/liter):	
Diuretics	Generated by urinary Cl^- loss exceeding HCO_3^- loss; maintained by volume depletion, hyperaldosteronism, hypokalemia
Vomiting, gastric drainage	Generated by HCl loss; maintained by volume depletion, hyperaldosteronism, hypokalemia
Villous adenoma of colon	Secretes fluid rich in protein, K^+, and Cl^-
Congenital chloride diarrhea	Intestinal defect in Cl^- absorption
Cystic fibrosis	Excess skin Cl^- losses
Posthypercapnia	Not enough Cl^- to replace excess HCO_3^- generated as compensation for hypercapnia
NaCl-resistant (U_{Cl}^- > 20 mmol/liter):	
Excess mineralocorticoid activity:	Stimulates distal nephron Na^+ reabsorption and H^+ and K^+ secretion
Primary hyperaldosteronism (adenoma or hyperplasia)	
Ectopic ACTH production*	
Cushing's syndrome	
Bartter's syndrome	
Licorice ingestion	
Severe potassium depletion (<2.0 mmol/liter)	Impaired tubular chloride reabsorption
Unclassified:	
Excess alkali intake	Alkali intake exceeds excretory capacity
Milk-alkali syndrome	Alkali intake exceeds excretory capacity, particularly if nephrocalcinosis occurs
Hypercalcemia not due to PTH*	Release of bone alkali
Hypoparathyroidism	Increased proximal HCO_3^- reabsorption

*ACTH = adenocorticotropic hormone; PTH = parathyroid hormone.

mentation. Metabolic alkalosis is not generally treated as an emergency, except in extreme cases. If the systemic pH is greater than 7.60 and is associated with central nervous system abnormalities or cardiac arrhythmias, controlled hypoventilation using a ventilator, employing oxygen supplementation, and sedation is the preferred therapy. An infusion of hydrochloric acid or ammonium chloride is generally too slow to be emergently effective and also may have adverse effects.

Respiratory Acidosis

Respiratory acidosis occurs when ventilation fails and the carbon dioxide content in the blood increases. This results in a decrease in arterial pH. In acute respiratory acidosis, the systemic pH may fall to quite low levels, since the renal system has not had time to appropriately compensate. With chronic respiratory acidosis, renal compensation is actually quite efficient in modifying the decrease in pH. As a general rule of thumb, in chronic respiratory acidosis, for each 10-mmHg increase in the P_{CO_2}, plasma bicarbonate concentration will increase about 4 ± 4 mmol/liter [40].

The therapy of respiratory acidoses is directed at the underlying causes, which are discussed in detail in the section on pulmonary disorders.

Respiratory Alkalosis

Respiratory alkalosis is the most common acid-base disorder. This occurs when ventilation increases and the partial pressure of carbon dioxide falls. This fall in P_{CO_2} causes a rise in systemic pH. In acute respiratory alkalosis, again, there is very little time for the renal system to buffer the change in pH, and the systemic pH may reach very high levels. However, in chronic respiratory alkalosis, the systemic pH is generally maintained near normal, since the kidneys are quite efficient in excreting bicarbonate. As a rule of thumb with chronic respiratory alkalosis, for each 10-mmHg fall in P_{CO_2}, the plasma bicarbonate concentration decreases by about 2 to 5 mmol/liter. It is unusual for the serum bicarbonate concentration to fall to less than 15 mmol/liter in compensation for chronic respiratory alkalosis, and thus, if a lower serum bicarbonate concentration is present, a primary metabolic acidosis must be suspected [40].

Mixed Acid-Base Disorders

Mixed acid-base disorders involve a combination of the aforementioned disturbances. The most severe of the mixed disorders are combinations of respiratory and metabolic alkaloses or combinations of metabolic and respiratory acidoses. The danger of these combinations is the marked effect that these disorders have on altering the arterial pH. Combinations of metabolic acidosis and al-

kalosis are possible, and when combined with a respiratory disturbance, they create the so-called triple acid-base disorder.

The diagnosis of these triple acid-base disorders depends on the disproportionate increase in the anion gap compared with the disturbance of plasma bicarbonate concentration. An example would be a patient with severe vomiting superimposed on sepsis with associated hyperventilation and lactic acidosis [46]. The vomiting causing a loss of protons coincident with the lactic acidosis generating protons might result in a "normal serum bicarbonate concentration," and the patient would appear at first glance to have a simple respiratory alkalosis. However, examination of the anion gap (which would be quite increased) would show that three disturbances actually are present.

The treatment of mixed disturbances is best directed at the etiologies involved. Since life-threatening changes in pH require therapy directed at correcting the pH as quickly as possible, control of ventilation may be required to treat severe disturbances in pH.

Disorders of Potassium Metabolism

Hyperkalemia

Hyperkalemia is an electrolyte disorder that all physicians should be able to manage because it may cause sudden death. The causes of hyperkalemia can be considered under four general categories (Table 3-5): factitious, secondary to a cellular potassium shift, secondary to a potassium load, and as a result of failure to excrete potassium in the urine [26].

The body's first response to a potassium load is to shift potassium from the extracellular fluid to the intracellular fluid, where most of the total-body potassium resides [1]. This is accomplished through several systems, including the sympathetic nervous system and circulating catecholamines [63], the renin-angiotensin-aldosterone system [32], and insulin [14]. Patients at greatest

risk to develop hyperkalemia have disturbances either in insulin secretion or action (e.g., diabetes mellitus), in the renin-angiotensin-aldosterone system, and/or in the sympathetic nervous system and circulating catecholamines. Failure to excrete potassium in the urine, as seen commonly in

Table 3–5. *Causes of Hyperkalemia*

Mechanism	Example
Factitious	Thrombocytosis, hemolysis
Cellular shift	Digoxin, acidosis, diabetes
Potassium load	Dietary indiscretion (exogenous), rhabdomyolysis (endogenous)
Decreased excretion	Oliguric acute renal failure, type IV renal tubular acidosis

acute renal failure and type IV renal tubular acidosis, also predisposes to hyperkalemia [65]. The symptoms of hyperkalemia may include weakness or constipation, but frequently hyperkalemia may cause no symptoms at all. This does not mean that the disorder is not critical, since the first symptom of hyperkalemia may indeed be sudden death. The electrocardiogram is an extremely useful test in the setting of hyperkalemia. Early ECG changes are limited to peaking of the T waves. As hyperkalemia becomes more severe, there may be a decrease in the P-wave amplitude and a widening of the QRS complex, and eventually, the electrocardiogram may develop a "sine-wave" appearance.

Since hyperkalemia may result in sudden death through cardiac standstill at virtually any level above 6 mmol/liter, elevations of serum potassium above this concentration should be investigated with an electrocardiogram. Evidence of electrocardiographic abnormalities and a potassium concentration over 6 mmol/liter mandates immediate therapy. Levels above 6.5 to 7 mmol/liter, even without electrocardiographic abnormalities, also should receive immediate therapy. The most emergent and effective therapy of hyperkalemia is the administration of calcium (5 to 10 mmol as a slow IV bolus). Intravenous calcium, given either as a gluconate or a chloride salt, does not affect the serum potassium level, but it does antagonize the effect of potassium on the cellular electric membrane potential of cardiac tissue. Calcium increases the threshold potential for cardiac muscle excitation, whereas hyperkalemia raises the resting membrane potential (to a less negative number). The effect of intravenous calcium occurs almost instantly, and the effect persists as long as the elevation of serum calcium concentration persists. Insulin therapy enhances potassium movement into cells and also has a rapid onset of action. Insulin (15-unit bolus followed by an infusion of 1 to 10 units per hour) is quite effective and is extremely useful in a setting of insulin deficiency associated with hyperglycemia (diabetes mellitus), but it also may be used in normoglycemic individuals if administered with intravenous glucose (25 to 50 gm as a 50 percent dextrose bolus or a 10 percent dextrose infusion). Bicarbonate (50- to 100-mmol IV bolus) also shifts potassium into cells and acts immediately; bicarbonate should be used to treat hyperkalemia unless contraindicated by volume overload. Less immediate therapy of hyperkalemia involves the use of ion-exchange resins such as Kayexalate and, if there is sufficient renal function, the use of loop diuretics to increase urine flow and potassium excretion.

Hypokalemia

Hypokalemia, although potentially life-threatening through induction of ventricular arrhythmias, is usually less emergent than hyperkalemia. The therapy of hypokalemia must be more gradual, since the body cannot tolerate rapid infusions of potassium. The symptoms of hypokalemia include muscle weakness and central nervous system abnormalities. Cardiac arrhythmias may occur, especially with concomitant digitalis therapy. Hypokalemia is usually seen in the setting of diarrhea, vomiting or other gastrointestinal losses, or renal potassium wasting as observed with loop or thiazide diuretics, systemic magnesium deficiency, renal tubular acidosis type I and II, and Bartter's syndrome [26]. More recently, hypokalemia has been described to occur with therapeutic agents that rapidly shift potassium into cells (e.g., beta-adrenergic agents used as bronchodilators, the therapy of acute asthma or chronic obstructive pulmonary disease).

The electrocardiographic changes of hypokalemia include diminution of the T wave and increased prominence of the U wave. This may mimic the prolonged QT interval that occurs in the setting of hypocalcemia.

The therapy of hypokalemia depends on its severity. Severe hypokalemia associated with arrhythmias may require an intravenous potassium chloride infusion. Potassium is usually infused no faster than 20 mmol per hour, although in rare instances this rate may be exceeded. Infusion of high concentrations of potassium must be performed with a central venous catheter because of the irritant nature of such solutions. Less severe hypokalemia may be treated with oral supplementation with either potassium chloride or potassium citrate or by increasing the intake of high-potassium foods (e.g., bananas, citrus fruits, tomatoes, and potatoes).

Abnormalities of Calcium, Magnesium, and Phosphate Metabolism

Hypercalcemia

DIAGNOSIS

Hypercalcemia (calcium level greater than 10.5 mg/dl) demands a search for the disorders shown in Table 3-6. The most common cause of hypercalcemia is malignancy, whereas primary hyperparathyroidism is the second most common cause [59]. The symptoms of hypercalcemia per se may include changes in mentation, somnolence, and even coma. Bone pain, abdominal pain, and constipation are also frequently noted. The physical findings are dictated to some degree by the underlying disease. The laboratory values present with hypercalcemia are clues to the disorder. In primary hyperparathyroidism, urine phosphate wasting occurs and a mild renal tubular acidosis may be present. These disturbances in phosphate handling and acid-base homeostasis diminish

Table 3–6. *Causes of Hypercalcemia*

Increased calcium load:
  Largely from bone:
    Primary hyperparathyroidism
    Neoplasms: parathyroid hormone-like substances,
      prostaglandins, osteoclast activators, direct bone
      destruction
    Prolonged immobilization
  From gut and bone:
    Vitamin D overdose
    Sarcoidosis
    Adrenal insufficiency
    Vitamin A overdose
    Infantile hypercalcemia
  Largely from gut:
    Milk-alkali syndrome
    Calcium-exchange resins
Decreased calcium removal:
  Hypophosphatemia: decreased bone calcification
  Increased renal calcium reabsorption:
    Thiazides
    Adrenal insufficiency

serum phosphorus and increase plasma chloride concentrations. Thus, in cases of hypercalcemia due to hyperparathyroidism, the plasma chloride to plasma phosphorus ratio is usually high (greater than 33:1).

The improved radioimmunoassay for parathyroid hormone (PTH) has greatly aided in the differential diagnosis of hypercalcemia. Elevated *N*-terminal parathyroid hormone levels are not frequently observed in diseases other than primary hyperparathyroidism. Elevations in urinary cyclic AMP levels reflecting parathyroid hormone action also may be helpful in some cases. Measurements of 1,25-dihydroxyvitamin D_3 and 25-hydroxyvitamin D_3 levels also may be helpful in the differential diagnosis of hypercalcemia (e.g., increased level of 1,25-dihydroxyvitamin D_3 seen with sarcoidosis, increased 25-hydroxyvitamin D_3 seen with vitamin D intoxication).

TREATMENT

The treatment of hypercalcemia is, in nonemergent cases, dictated by the underlying disease. In emergent cases with severe elevations of the serum calcium level and abnormalities in mental status, several approaches are possible. The first approach is to increase urinary calcium excretion. This is accomplished by a solute diuresis induced by infusing isotonic sodium chloride and administering loop diuretics. It must be stressed that the loop diuretics are used to maintain the solute diuresis following volume expansion with 2 liters of isotonic saline. If diuretics induce volume depletion, urinary calcium excretions may actually decrease. In resistant cases, steroids may decrease vitamin D-responsive calcium absorption from the gut, as well as tumor-mediated bone reabsorption (e.g., multiple myeloma). Mithramycin

(12.5 to 25 µg/kg IV) is usually quite effective in acutely lowering the serum calcium concentration, apparently by inhibiting bone reabsorption. Calcitonin (100 MRC units IM) also may be effective in decreasing the serum calcium concentration by the same mechanism. Calcitonin is usually administered with steroids (60 mg per day) which blunt tachyphylaxis to calcitonin. Recent experimental work with diphosphonates indicates that these agents may be helpful in acutely lowering the serum calcium concentration. Intravenous phosphate infusions, which have previously been touted as useful in the setting of hypercalcemia, may be associated with visceral calcium-phosphorus precipitation as well as significant hypotension and therefore should be avoided [59].

Hypocalcemia

Hypocalcemia (plasma calcium concentration of less than 9 mg/dl) may be due to a variety of conditions. It is most commonly associated with lowering of the serum albumin level, which may be due to many underlying disorders. In this setting, the hypocalcemia is not physiologically important, since the ionized calcium is normal. Thus measurements of ionized calcium or mathematical correction of the calcium concentration for hypoalbuminemia is needed to confirm physiologically important hypocalcemia. As a rule of thumb, the serum calcium concentration should be 0.8 mg/dl lower for each 1 gm/dl decrease in albumin concentration.

The causes of hypocalcemia associated with a lowering in the ionized serum calcium level are listed in Table 3-7. These causes can be roughly divided into those associated with a lack of parathyroid hormone, parathyroid hormone resistance, decreases in vitamin D, or increases in calcium removal or sequestration [59]. The symptoms associated with hypocalcemia may range from virtually no symptoms to symptoms of neuromuscular irritability which may progress to frank tetany. The severity of the hypocalcemia may be assessed to a large degree on physical ex-

Table 3–7. *Causes of Hypocalcemia*

Decreased calcium delivery:
  Lack of parathyroid hormone:
    Surgical ablation, e.g., after thyroidectomy
    Idiopathic hypoparathyroidism
    Magnesium deficiency
  Parathyroid hormone resistance:
    Pseudohypoparathyroidism
    Magnesium deficiency
    Vitamin D deficiency
  Vitamin D deficiency:
    Malabsorption
    Advanced renal or liver disease
    Vitamin D-dependent rickets (enzyme defects)
    Anticonvulsants
Increased calcium removal:
  Hyperphosphatemia
  Osteoblastic metastases (e.g., carcinoma of prostate)
  Acute pancreatitis

amination by the presence of tetany and/or the presence of a positive Chvostek's sign. The emergent therapy of severe hypocalcemia is rapid infusion of calcium chloride or calcium gluconate over several minutes and repeated as needed. In the setting of hypocalcemia associated with severe magnesium deficiency, replenishment of magnesium stores must be accomplished in order to normalize the serum calcium. In cases of hypocalcemia associated with significant hyperphosphatemia, as seen in renal insufficiency, great caution must be used in infusing calcium, since calcium-phosphorus precipitation in viscera may be induced. Fortunately, the lowering of serum calcium concentration associated with hyperphosphatemia in renal failure is rarely significant enough to produce symptoms and therefore usually does not require emergent therapy. When it does, hemodialysis therapy is most appropriate, since this approach will both raise the serum calcium and lower the serum phosphorus concentrations.

Abnormalities of Magnesium Metabolism

Hypermagnesemia is most commonly seen in patients with renal failure who ingest magnesium-containing medications. The other common setting occurs in patients with preeclampsia who are being treated with magnesium. With concentrations greater than 10 mg/dl, tendon reflexes are usually absent and flaccid paralysis may develop; problems with cardiac conduction and hypotension due to peripheral vasodilatation also may occur. Therapy of life-threatening cardiac respiratory and neurologic complications consists of infusion of 2.5 to 5 mmol calcium, usually as a gluconate salt. Furosemide and saline administration will enhance renal magnesium excretion, but this will be too slow to provide emergent therapy. Hemodialysis may be necessary in cases of symptomatic hypermagnesemia in patients with chronic renal insufficiency [15].

Hypomagnesemia with levels less than 1.2 mg/dl may cause symptoms of tetany, seizures, and psychosis. The mediation of many of these symptoms may involve a secondary depression of the serum calcium concentration which is caused by both an inhibition of parathyroid hormone release and an impairment of tissue response to parathyroid hormone. The most common settings for hypomagnesemia include alcoholism, malabsorption, and ketoacidosis, although chronic treatment with loop diuretics as well as nephrotoxic antibiotics such as aminoglycosides may cause renal magnesium wasting. Treatment of severe hypomagnesemia requires infusing about 60 mmol magnesium over 12 hours, followed by oral doses and correction of the underlying disorders [15,51].

Abnormalities of the Plasma Phosphorus Concentration

Plasma inorganic phosphate is usually maintained in the 3 to 4.5 mg/dl range. Marked elevations in plasma phosphorus levels above 7 or 8 mg/dl usually occur only in patients with concomitant renal failure. Increases in plasma phosphorus concentration may cause reciprocal decreases in the serum calcium concentration. Moreover, elevations in plasma phosphorus con-

centration may cause precipitation of calcium phosphorus in blood vessels and other tissues. Elevations of plasma phosphorus concentration are not treated emergently unless the accompanying hypocalcemia is life-threatening. With hyperphosphatemia, the treatment of choice is hemodialysis, although infusions of glucose and insulin also may result in rapid decreases in the plasma phosphorus concentration. The therapy of chronic hyperphosphatemia is dietary restriction of high-phosphorus foods (e.g., milk and other dairy products) and the addition of phosphorus binders to the diet [72]. Most of these phosphorus binders have traditionally been aluminum-containing. More recently, the finding of aluminum toxicity in renal failure causing osteomalacia, encephalopathy, and severe anemia has stimulated efforts to use non-aluminum-containing binders, such as calcium carbonate.

Profound hypophosphatemia may accompany alcoholism with concomitant malnutrition, uncontrolled diabetes mellitus, administration of parenteral alimentation, refeeding after starvation, prolonged alkalotic states (especially respiratory alkalosis), the healing phase of severe burns, and ingestion of large amounts of phosphorus-binding agents for prolonged periods of time. Lowering of the plasma phosphorus concentration to less than 1 mg/dl may be associated with severe muscle weakness and even rhabdomyolysis, suppression of respiration, defective leukocyte function, hemolytic anemia, defects in platelet function, and encephalopathy of varying severity. Treatment of hypophosphatemia, if mild, consists of oral replacement with high-phosphorus foods (such as skim milk) or oral phosphorus solutions. Parenteral replacement of phosphorus must be done with great care. Recommendations generally limit infusions of phosphorus to 0.08 mmol/kg over 4 hours in asymptomatic patients and 0.16 mmol/kg over 4 hours in symptomatic patients. Frequent monitoring of the plasma phosphorus concentration during parenteral replacement is essential [44].

Edematous Disorders

Pathophysiology

Edema is the physical manifestation of an increase in the interstitial component of the extracellular fluid volume. Edema may be either localized or generalized. Edema occurs when Starling forces favor formation of interstitial fluid and this formation of interstitial fluid is in excess of what can be handled by the lymphatic system [68].

Localized edema usually occurs secondary to either venous obstruction, increased capillary permeability, or a lymphatic obstruction. Obstruction of the venous drainage of a capillary network (e.g., thrombophlebitis) leads to an increase in capillary hydrostatic pressure, which promotes the net exit of solute and water. Damage to the capillary epithelium occurring with burns or allergic reactions increases the permeability of the capillary membrane to protein. The resultant decrease in capillary oncotic pressure then favors further formation of edema. Finally, obstruction of lymphatic drainage also may result in edema formation (e.g., malignancy).

Generalized edema is most notable in areas where the venous pressure is higher (e.g., the lower extremities) and in the areas of decreased tissue turgor (e.g., the periorbital region). Generalized edema tends to be pitting in nature. It should be stressed that even patients with barely detectable edema usually have an increase of 2 to 3 liters of fluid in their interstitial space. Therefore, overt edema indicates a tremendous excess of interstitial fluid. Anasarca is a term that refers to massive generalized edema. Hydrothorax and ascites are special forms of local edema and may accompany generalized edematous disorders.

The causes of generalized edema include congestive heart failure, nephrotic syndrome, acute glomerulonephritis, chronic renal failure, cirrhosis of the liver, severe protein malnutrition, protein-losing enteropathy, and idiopathic cyclical edema [70]. It is noteworthy that all these causes of edema represent disturbances in the Starling forces. For example, with left ventricular heart failure there are increases in pulmonary venous pressure that cause increases in the pulmonary capillary pressure, which can result in pulmonary edema. In right-sided congestive heart failure there are increases in systemic venous pressure, which favor transudation of fluid from systemic capillaries. In the nephrotic syndrome a decrease in serum albumin concentration results in a decrease in the plasma oncotic pressure, which favors transudation of fluid into the interstitial space. It should be stressed that enhanced renal sodium conservation occurs and perpetuates edema in congestive heart failure, liver cirrhosis, and the nephrotic syndrome. This sodium retention appears to be stimulated by a decrease in effective arterial blood volume, which is related to the decrease in cardiac output characteristic of congestive heart failure, the peripheral vasodilation of cirrhosis, and the decrease in plasma oncotic pressure of nephrotic syndrome [68,70].

It is noteworthy that disorders that lead to increased renal sodium retention secondary to primary hyperaldosteronism and renal water retention, e.g., the syndrome of inappropriate antidiuretic hormone (SIADH), usually do not lead to generalized edema. With both primary hyperaldosteronism and the syndrome of inappropriate antidiuretic hormone, the initial increase in extracellular fluid volume increases renal sodium and water excretion, thus allowing "escape" from continued salt and water retention of aldosterone and antidiuretic hormone. The exact pathophysiologic mechanisms involved in this escape are at the present unclear, but it appears that increases in solute and water delivery to more distal nephron segments are important. Since decreased distal fluid delivery occurs with congestive heart failure, cirrhosis, and the nephrotic syndrome, the escape phenomenon does not occur and renal sodium and water retention persists.

Treatment

Therapy of the edematous disorders should initially be directed at the underlying cause. Local edema is treated by therapy of the local condition. For example, venous thrombosis is best treated with anticoagulant therapy. Generalized edema resulting from congestive heart failure is best treated by a combination of decreasing cardiac afterload with vasodilators, increasing contractility with digitalis, and decreasing preload with diuretics. It should be stressed that bed rest is an excellent means of decreasing edema in virtually all the generalized edematous disorders. This is so because bed rest diminishes hydrostatic pressure, favoring edema reabsorption in the lower extremities; this results in an increase in the circulating effective blood volume, which favors increased cardiac output, better renal perfusion, and increased renal excretion of salt and water. Even in congestive heart failure, bed rest, albeit in a sitting position, is beneficial, since it decreases cardiac output requirements.

Diuretics used to treat edema may be subdivided on the basis of their nephronal site of action. Mannitol and acetazolamide are proximal tubular diuretics. They inhibit proximal tubular reabsorption and cause a diuresis by increasing delivery of salt and water to more distal nephronal sites. Furosemide, ethacrynic acid, and bumetanide inhibit sodium chloride reabsorption in the ascending limb of Henle and are the most potent diuretics. Thiazide diuretics act in the distal convoluted tubule and cortical collecting duct to inhibit sodium reabsorption. Potassium-sparing diuretics act by inhibiting aldosterone action (e.g., spironolactone) or by inhibiting secretion of potassium and hydrogen ions at nonaldosterone sites in the distal nephrons (triamterene, amiloride) [64].

It should be stressed that diuretics may have significant side effects. Overaggressive diuresis may cause severe decreases in intravascular volume and arterial pressure. Proximal, loop, and thiazide diuretics may cause severe potassium depletion, hypokalemia, and metabolic alkalosis, whereas the potassium-sparing diuretics may cause hyperkalemia and metabolic acidosis [64,68].

Chronic Renal Failure

Chronic renal failure occurs when glomerular filtration is irreversibly impaired. Because of a surfeit of nephrons, the symptom complex of uremia due to retention of nitrogenous wastes in chronic renal failure does not usually occur until the glomerular filtration rate (GFR) is 10 percent or less of normal.

The normal glomerular filtration rate is approximately 100 ml per minute in an average-size 30-year-old male. This corresponds with a serum creatinine value of approximately 1.0 mg/dl. It must be stressed, however, that marked changes in glomerular filtration rate can occur with minimal elevations in the serum creatinine concentration. For example, if the serum creatinine concentration increases from 1 to 2.0 mg/dl, the glomerular filtration rate decreases by 50 percent from 100 to 50 ml per minute. Patients with a smaller muscle mass normally have lower serum creatinine concentrations, since creatinine production and excretion are proportional to muscle mass. In such patients, a serum creatinine level of 1.2 to 1.4 mg/dl could possibly represent a 50 percent decrease in function if the patient's normal serum creatinine level is 0.6 to 0.7 mg/dl. However, the laboratory will call this value "normal."

Creatinine clearance is the most commonly employed clinical estimate of glomerular filtration rate and is calculated by the following formula:

$$\text{Creatinine clearance (ml/min)} = \frac{\text{urine creatinine (mg/dl)}}{\text{serum creatinine (mg/dl)}} \times \text{urine flow rate (ml/min)}$$

Creatinine clearance actually overestimates glomerular filtration rate to some degree, since creatinine is not only filtered, but is also actively secreted by renal tubular cells. Some drugs actually decrease creatinine clearance without affecting glomerular filtration rate. These include trimethoprim and cimetidine, both of which inhibit creatinine secretion without affecting glomerular filtration rate. The most accurate estimate of glomerular filtration rate available is the clearance of inulin. However, this approach is not very convenient, because inulin must be infused intravenously to perform an inulin clearance determination.

Pathophysiology

As glomerular filtration rate decreases, certain adaptations occur. The remaining nephrons must excrete more sodium than before so as to maintain total-body sodium balance. This is true for other solutes, such as phosphate, for which renal adaptation has been well characterized. Parathyroid hormone concentration rises as glomerular filtration rate decreases, and serum calcium and phosphorus concentrations are maintained in the normal range (until creatinine clearance is decreased to less than 20 percent of normal). This occurs because parathyroid hormone decreases tubular phosphate reabsorption per nephron, thus allowing maintenance of phosphorus excretion despite a reduced number of nephrons. Systemic acid-base balance is usually maintained until creatinine clearance has decreased to below 25 to 30 percent of normal. Sodium and potassium homeostasis is usually maintained until there is far-advanced renal insufficiency (i.e., creatinine clearance less than 5 percent of normal), except when there are tubular abnormalities out of proportion to the decreases in glomerular filtration rate [2]. Most notable of these is the syndrome of hyperkalemic metabolic acidosis, which is seen most frequently in the setting of chronic renal insufficiency associated with diabetes mellitus. This syndrome is frequently associated with hyporeninemia and hypoaldosteronism, although in some cases there may be tubular resistance to aldosterone [47]. A rare syndrome of salt-losing nephropathy also has been described. In this setting, the tubules exhibit a marked impairment in sodium reabsorption and therefore are unable to maintain sodium homeostasis as large quantities of sodium are excreted in the urine. While the clinically apparent form of the syndrome is quite unusual, abnormalities in renal sodium conservation (to some degree) may be demonstrated in the majority of patients with chronic renal insufficiency. Specifically, in patients with chronic renal insufficiency (GFR < 25 ml per minute), the response to an increase or decrease in sodium and water intact is impaired and delayed. Thus these patients can more easily become salt and water depleted or salt and water overloaded than individuals with normal renal function.

The symptom complex of uremia that is associated with chronic renal failure has a variety of manifestations that involve virtually all organ systems. The central nervous system is probably earliest involved, with symptoms of sleep disturbances, loss of memory, increased irritability, and increased mood swings. The peripheral nervous system also may become involved with a sensory neuropathy that may be accompanied by an overt motor neuropathy. Restless-leg syndrome is characteristic of the neuropathy seen with uremia. The gastrointestinal system may be involved in uremia, with nausea, vomiting, and colitis. Pericarditis may occur with renal failure, and it may progress to pericardial tamponade. A syndrome of uremic cardiomyopathy has been suggested; however, most cases of heart failure in uremia are due to fluid overload and hypertension. Pleural effusions may occur, and a syndrome of uremic pneumonitis has been suggested [2].

The pathophysiology of uremia is unclear. Possible causes include (1) increases in the concentrations of small molecules such as urea and creatinine which contain nitrogen, (2) the so-called trade-off hypothesis, in which substances (e.g., parathyroid hormone) that increase in uremia to maintain solute balance are associated with toxic effects, and (3) a middle-molecule hypothesis that

Table 3–8. *Causes of Chronic Renal Failure*

Chronic glomerulonephritis:
  Primary
  Secondary (e.g., diabetes, amyloidosis)
Interstitial renal disease:
  Analgesic nephropathy
  Reflex nephropathy
  Chronic pyelonephritis
  Obstructive uropathy
Hereditary renal disease:
  Cystic disease
Hypertension

Table 3–9. *Potentially Reversible Causes of Progressive Azotemia in Patients with Chronic Renal Disease*

Decreased renal perfusion:
  Volume depletion
  Congestive heart failure
  Constrictive pericarditis or pericardial tamponade
  Drug-related hypotension
Uncontrolled hypertension
Urinary tract obstruction
Upper urinary tract infection
Nephrotoxic drug therapy
Hypersensitivity interstitial nephritis
Biochemical abnormalities:
  Hypercalcemia
  Hypokalemia
  Hypocalcemia: ? renal failure
  Hyperphosphatemia: ? renal failure

states that molecules with molecular weights of 5,000 to 10,000, such as vitamin B_{12}, accumulate and cause toxicity. At the present time, there is no definitive proof for a dominant role of these three hypotheses, and indeed, all of them may be involved in causing the uremic syndrome [2].

Diagnosis

The common causes of chronic renal failure are summarized in Table 3-8. These include glomerular as well as interstitial causes of renal disease. It should be stressed that any of the causes of acute renal failure may be superimposed on chronic renal failure. This can result in a patient with well-compensated chronic renal disease becoming uremic. For example, as already discussed, the renal homeostatic response to sodium depletion is impaired as functioning nephrons are lost and patients become more sensitive to minor degrees of volume depletion. Similarly, urinary tract obstruction or urinary tract infection may occur and impair creatinine clearance in these patients, thus leading to uremic symptoms. Potentially reversible causes of progressive azotemia in patients with chronic renal disease are listed in Table 3-9.

Treatment

The treatment of patients with chronic renal insufficiency which has not progressed to the state where dialysis or transplantation is necessary involves several considerations. First of all, if there is a treatable component of the underlying cause of the chronic renal insufficiency, it should be addressed. Regardless of the cause of the renal insufficiency, hypertension must be controlled. Recent data suggest that there may be potential advantages to drugs that interfere with the renin-angiotensin system (e.g., converting-enzyme inhibitors), but at this time, this still remains to be proven in humans. Serum phosphorus concentration should be normalized with the use of phosphorus binders [37]. Since aluminum toxicity has been traced in some patients to the aluminum in aluminum-containing antacids, calcium-containing antacids may be preferable [31]. Caloric intake should be maintained at optimal levels. Protein restriction, although shown to be theoretically beneficial in animal studies, has not yet been proven to be advantageous in adults, and thus at this point its clinical use is controversial [33,74]. Acidosis, when present, should be treated with bicarbonate or citrate supplementation to prevent acidosis-induced loss of calcium from bones [13].

Although potassium balance usually is maintained until the glomerular filtration rate falls to very low levels (less than 5 ml per minute), patients should be cautioned to avoid excess consumption of high-potassium foods. In some patients who have hyperkalemic distal renal tubular acidosis as part of their syndrome, the use of potassium binders such as Kayexalate may be required. Continuous attention must be given to dosage adjustment and potential toxicity of medications taken in the setting of a reduced glomerular filtration rate. It must be stressed that iatrogenic disease with drug therapy is quite common in advanced chronic renal insufficiency.

End-stage renal failure usually refers to the time when transplantation of a donor kidney or initiation of dialysis is required. Severe uremic symptoms (e.g., symptoms of seizures, coma, motor neuropathy, and pericarditis) are an absolute indication for initiation of dialysis. Lesser degrees of severity of uremic symptoms also require initiation of replacement of renal function, albeit on a less emergent level. Other indications for dialysis include electrolyte and fluid balance disturbances unresponsive to conservative means. It should be stressed that the degree of azotemia or level of glomerular filtration rate at which the patient will benefit from dialysis therapy will differ from patient to patient. Although somewhat controversial, most nephrologists would agree that diabetic patients require institution of dialysis at a higher glomerular filtration rate than nondiabetic patients. Even without symptoms, it is usual to begin dialysis therapy or initiate transplantation when the serum creatinine level exceeds 12 to 15 mg/dl, when the blood urea nitrogen (BUN) level exceeds 100 mg/dl, or when a calculated creatinine clearance rate is less than 3 to 5 ml per minute [49].

The prescription for dialysis therapy is quite controversial at this point. Maintenance of certain blood urea nitrogen and creatinine concentrations does not appear to be the most important guide to therapy. Control of anemia, while useful on a total dialysis population basis, is probably not of practical use in an individual patient. The usual dialysis prescription involves dialysis for 4 to 5 hours 3 days per week, but this will vary depending on the patient's condition, dialysis center policies, and the physician's bias [49]. Kinetic

modeling of dialysis therapy has been advocated by some, but at this point it is not routinely applied to the general population.

When possible, renal transplantation provides the most logical therapy for end-stage renal insufficiency. The major obstacle to transplantation continues to be the rejection process. The addition of cyclosporine to the transplant physicians' armamentarium has improved transplantation statistics in many centers and has lowered the dosage of steroids required by many patients. Cyclosporine nephrotoxicity, however, still remains a problem.

Dialysis therapy is most usually done by the blood (hemodialysis) route. Hemodialysis requires access to sufficient blood flow to ensure adequate removal of toxins and fluids during the conventional 4- to 5-hour dialysis which is performed approximately three times a week in most patients. The usual route of access is an arterial venous fistula that is constructed surgically. In patients who do not have an adequate venous system, a Gortex graft is interposed between artery and vein. In some patients, chronic indwelling venous catheters must be used on more than just a temporary basis.

Chronic peritoneal dialysis is another method of treating end-stage renal failure. This usually involves placement of a Tenckfoff or modified Tenckfoff catheter in the peritoneal cavity and then performing peritoneal dialysis on either a continuous schedule (CAPD) or on an intermittent cyclic basis (IPD). The continuous method has the advantage of excellent middle-molecule clearance, as well as a rather easy to learn methodology, which allows patients to perform their own dialysis in most cases. Cycling peritoneal dialysis also has been used employing an automatic cycling machine that performs the exchanges while the patient sleeps at night. These peritoneal techniques, however, are complicated by relatively frequent episodes of peritonitis (approximately one episode per patient-year). This peritonitis incidence is somewhat dependent on the rigidity with which patients adhere to sterile techniques [49].

Acute Renal Failure

Acute renal failure (ARF) may be defined as a sudden decrease in glomerular filtration rate which leads to progressive increases in plasma creatinine and blood urea nitrogen concentrations [66,67]. Acute renal failure may occur with or without oliguria. Oliguria is usually defined as a urine output less than 400 cc per day in an adult. The causes of acute renal failure are usually divided into three general categories. These categories are prerenal azotemia, postrenal azotemia, and intrarenal azotemia [66,67]. Prerenal azotemia is the most common cause of acute renal failure [35] and is due to abnormalities in renal hemodynamics, either secondary to decreased cardiac output, as seen with congestive heart failure, pericardial tamponade, or volume depletion (e.g., dehydration, hemorrhage), systemic vasodilatation, as seen in cirrhosis (where, although cardiac output is quite high, functional renal perfusion is decreased), or actual anatomic abnormalities of the renal vasculature, as seen in bilateral renal artery occlusion or stenosis. Postrenal azotemia is synonymous with urinary tract obstruction at any level. Obstruction is often due to intraluminal causes (e.g., stones or necrotic tumor obstructing a ureter), but it may be due to external compression of the ureters (e.g., lymphomas or fibrosis involving the retroperitoneal space). The most common cause of postrenal azotemia is obstruction of the urinary draining system at the level of the urethra, as occurs with prostatic hypertrophy or prostatic carcinoma. Intrarenal azotemia may be due to a variety of causes. These causes include acute tubular necrosis (ATN), which is the most common cause of intrarenal azotemia, and other renal lesions caused by glomerulonephritis, atheroembolic disease, and acute interstitial nephritis (AIN) [66,67].

Diagnosis

Prerenal azotemia must be suspected in all patients with azotemia, particularly in patients with a history of recent weight loss, recent surgery, diuretic use, or hospitalization. Signs of volume depletion, cirrhosis, or congestive heart failure should be detectable on physical examination. An elevation in blood urea nitrogen to plasma creatinine ratio greater than 10:1 suggests a prerenal cause of azotemia. The urine sediment is usually not remarkable in patients with prerenal azotemia; however, hyalin and nonpigmented casts may be present. Urine electrolytes and urine osmolality should reflect tubular responses to decreased renal perfusion and may be very helpful in the diagnosis of prerenal azotemia. The urinary osmolality is often elevated, frequently greater than 500 mOsmol/kg. Urinary sodium, on the other hand, is usually quite low, less than 10 to 20 mmol/liter. The urine to plasma creatinine ratio is frequently greater than 30. The renal failure index, defined as the urine sodium level divided by the urine creatinine level times the plasma creatinine level, and the fractional excretion of sodium, defined as the urinary sodium level over the urinary creatinine level times the plasma creatinine level over the plasma sodium level times 100, are also helpful. A renal failure index or fractional excretion of sodium less than 1 percent in the setting of oliguria is quite suggestive of prerenal azotemia [52]. These data are summarized in Table 3-10. Chronic renal failure or diuretics will make this ratio invalid, as may the presence of bicarbonaturia in the setting of metabolic alkalosis or glucosuria with diabetes mellitus. In most cases, invasive measurements of central venous pressure, pulmonary capillary wedge pressure, and cardiac output are not necessary, but in some critically ill patients these parameters must

Table 3–10. *Laboratory Markers of Prerenal Azotemia and Acute Tubular Necrosis**

Marker	Prerenal Acute Renal Failure	Oliguric or Nonoliguric Acute Tubular Necrosis
Urine sediment	Hyalin and nonpigmented casts	Muddy brown granular casts and epithelial cells
Plasma creatinine	Rarely > 5 mg/dl	Usually rises to 5 mg/dl or greater
U_{OSM} (mosmol/kg)	> 500	< 400
$U_{Na}{}^+$ (mmol/liter)	> 20	< 40
U/P creatinine	> 30	< 20
Renal failure index†	> 1	< 1

*Values that fall between prerenal azotemia and acute tubular necrosis may indicate early evolution to acute tubular necrosis. Chronic postrenal azotemia (obstruction) has values similar to acute tubular necrosis. Occasionally, nonoliguric acute tubular necrosis may have $U_{Na}{}^+$ values of 20 mmol/liter.
†Renal failure index $= U_{Na}{}^+/(U/P$ creatinine)

be directly measured to accurately assess volume and cardiac status. Regardless of the cause of acute renal failure, intravascular volume should be optimized [66,67].

The hepatorenal syndrome is a form of prerenal azotemia that affects patients with advanced liver disease. Intrarenal vasoconstriction appears to be the cause of the decreased glomerular filtration rate in this syndrome. Tubular function is intact; therefore, the fractional excretion of sodium and renal failure indices are quite low. The renal vasoconstriction in this setting is reversible, as proven by transplanting these kidneys in patients suffering from the hepatorenal syndrome into recipients with chronic renal failure but having normal liver function. At the present time there is no known therapy that successfully reverses the hepatorenal syndrome. It should be stressed that acute renal failure in the setting of liver disease may not be due to the hepatorenal syndrome, but rather may be due to acute tubular necrosis [66,67].

Postrenal azotemia, because of its response to therapy, must be excluded in all patients with acute renal failure. Clues to the presence of obstruction include a history of stone disease, recent pelvic surgery, analgesic abuse (associated with papillary necrosis), diabetes mellitus (associated with neurogenic bladder or papillary necrosis), migraines treated with methysergide (which may cause retroperitoneal fibrosis), urinary infections,

or symptoms suggesting an abnormal urinary collecting system (including hesitancy, difficulty in maintaining a stream, nocturia, and intermittent oliguria or anuria). On physical examination, the abdomen must be examined for evidence of a distended bladder. Careful rectal and pelvic examinations are essential. In patients with indwelling bladder catheters, the patency of the catheter must be verified. Ultrasonography is a very sensitive screening test for the presence of urinary tract obstruction, although false-positive results do occur with a 10 to 15 percent frequency [19]. False-negative results also may occur with staghorn calculi and chronic renal failure with small, shrunken kidneys in which the intrarenal collection system has limited ability to dilate. The ultrasound examination is, however, the preferred study to exclude the diagnosis of urinary tract obstruction. A positive ultrasound examination may require a more definitive study (i.e., retrograde or antegrade pyelography) to document obstruction of the urinary collecting system. Excretory urography may exacerbate or cause acute renal failure in patients with significant risk factors (including diabetic nephropathy, multiple myeloma, and prerenal azotemia) and therefore should be avoided if possible.

Intrarenal azotemia may be due to a variety of causes. The most common cause is acute tubular necrosis, which may be oliguric or nonoliguric. The vast majority of cases of oliguric acute tubular

Table 3–11. Causes of Acute Renal Tubular Necrosis

Ischemic disorders:
  Shock: cardiogenic, septic, hemorrhagic
  Major trauma: accidental or surgical
  Pigment release: myoglobin, hemoglobin
  Prolonged major volume depletion
  Obstetrical emergencies
  Gastrointestinal disease, especially pancreatitis
Exogenous toxins:
  Antibiotics (e.g., aminoglycosides, amphotericin B)
  Heavy metals: mercury, lead
  Ethylene glycol
  Carbon tetrachloride
  Radiocontrast material

necrosis are associated with relatively high fractional excretions of sodium and renal failure indices less than 1 percent [52]. As many as 20 to 30 percent of patients with nonoliguric acute renal failure due to acute tubular necrosis may have fractional excretions of sodium that are less than 1 percent [3,52]. The causes of acute tubular necrosis are summarized in Table 3-11. Ischemia is a major underlying cause of acute tubular necrosis, as it is in dye-induced and nephrotoxic drug-induced acute tubular necrosis. Many cases of acute tubular necrosis are multifactorial, with more than one risk factor present [61].

The clinical course of acute tubular necrosis is variable. Oliguria is classically described as lasting from 10 to 14 days, but it may persist longer, particularly in older patients or in patients with severe complicating illnesses. A rise in urine volume usually heralds the recovery of renal function in the oliguric patient; however, the blood urea nitrogen and plasma creatinine levels may continue to rise as the onset of the diuresis occurs. The diuretic phase of acute tubular necrosis also lasts from 10 to 14 days. However, again, this duration may be variable [73]. After 3 to 4 weeks of azotemia in young and middle-aged patients, the diagnosis of acute tubular necrosis must be questioned and a renal biopsy should be considered to determine the presence of another type of intrarenal disorder such as cortical necrosis, acute glomerulonephritis, or acute interstitial nephritis

(see below). The patients who survive acute tubular necrosis usually regain near normal renal function. Renal concentrating and acidifying functions, however, may not be completely normal until 3 to 12 months following recovery.

Radiocontrast-medicated acute tubular necrosis is notable for several reasons. First of all, it is frequently associated with a low fractional excretion of sodium, even when associated with oliguria. Second, it typically has a mild course, with relatively short oliguric and diuretic phases as compared to the usual course of acute tubular necrosis [21].

Other causes of intrarenal acute renal failure include acute interstitial nephritis, acute glomerulonephritis, cholesterol emboli syndrome, and systemic vasculitis. Acute interstitial nephritis is usually due to drug reactions or infections, but 20 percent of cases are idiopathic [48]. Drugs commonly associated with this condition include antibiotics (e.g., penicillins, cephalosporins, sulfa), antiseizure medications (e.g., Dilantin), diuretics agents (e.g., thiazide and loop diuretics), and nonsteroidal anti-inflammatory agents, which recently have been reported to cause a syndrome of acute interstitial nephritis with high-grade proteinuria [8,48]. Acute glomerulonephritis must be suspected in cases of acute renal failure. It should be stressed that acute glomerulonephritis may not have the typical urinalysis findings of hematuria, proteinuria, and red blood cell casts in a setting with very low urine flows. The cholesterol emboli syndrome usually occurs in patients with severe atherosclerosis of the aorta who have recently had aortic manipulation, such as aneurysectomy or a recent radiographic study involving arterial catheterization. A certain portion of these patients, however, do not have this antecedent aortic manipulation and present spontaneously with cholesterol emboli syndrome. Clues to the diagnosis include evidence of arterial occlusion in the distal lower extremities, high-grade leukocytosis, eosinophilia, and the absence of other etiologic causes for the diagnosis of acute renal failure [66,67]. Renal failure associated with multiple myeloma may be due to a variety of causes, including radiocontrast nephropathy, renal calculi, infection, and amyloid. The most common cause of acute renal failure (besides prerenal azotemia) in the setting of multiple myeloma is a tubular precipitation syndrome (myeloma kidney). This is an important cause of acute renal failure in patients who develop this syndrome without exposure to ischemic injury or nephrotoxic agents [11].

The major causes of mortality in acute renal failure are infection and gastrointestinal hemorrhage. Invasive procedures including intravenous lines, central venous catheters and Swan-Ganz catheters, therefore, should be done with the utmost care. Indwelling urinary bladder catheters are not necessary unless bladder outlet obstruction is present. Despite modern management, the mortality rate in patients with acute renal failure due to acute tubular necrosis following surgical procedures and trauma is over 60 percent; acute tubular necrosis in a medical setting, about 30 percent; and during obstetrical acute tubular necrosis, about 15 percent [66,67].

Treatment

The therapy of acute renal failure also must be separated into individual entities of prerenal, postrenal and intrarenal azotemia. Prerenal azotemia must be treated by improving renal perfusion. If the renal failure is due to congestive heart failure, the approach must be to maximize cardiac output and thereby improve renal perfusion. If the renal failure is due to dehydration, the patient must be treated by fluid replacement. Obstructive uropathy is, of course, best treated by relief of the obstruction. If acute renal failure is intrarenal, the physician must distinguish between acute tubular necrosis and other intrarenal causes of acute renal failure. If glomerulonephritis is a strong possibility, it should be diagnosed promptly with a renal biopsy and treated as appropriate (e.g., high-dose steroids for lupus nephritis and rapidly progressive glomerulonephritis, perhaps with plasmapheresis). Similarly, the diagnosis of vasculitis

must be considered and made by abdominal angiography or the appropriate organ biopsy. Acute interstitial nephritis is best treated by removing the offending drug, although, in some cases, a short course of steroids may be beneficial (10 to 14 days of 60 to 80 mg prednisone per day).

If acute tubular necrosis is the cause of acute renal failure, correction of abnormalities in the extracellular fluid volume is still important. If adequate extracellular fluid volume is present, there may be benefit in administering large doses of loop diuretics such as furosemide (1 to 5 mg/kg IV over 30 minutes), with or without dopamine in renal vasodilator doses (1 to 3 mg/kg per minute) to initiate a diuresis [28]. The reasoning behind this approach is that this pharmacologic treatment often succeeds in initiating a diuresis (i.e., converts oliguric to nonoliguric renal failure). This makes fluid management more simple in these patients; moreover, nonoliguric acute renal failure statistically has a lower mortality rate than oliguric acute renal failure [3]. However, whether increasing urine flow with diuretics and/or renal vasodilators actually does improve mortality for a given patient is not clear at the present time.

Dialysis therapy may be necessary in treating acute renal failure. Absolute indications for dialysis include severe uremic symptoms (e.g., pericarditis, seizures, coma), severe electrolyte disturbances unresponsive to conservative management (e.g., hyperkalemia, acidosis, hyperphosphatemia with hypocalcemia), and volume overload unresponsive to diuretic therapy. It has become common practice to initiate dialysis in the setting of oliguria without any of these absolute indications when the blood urea nitrogen level reaches 100 mg/dl or the creatinine value reaches 10 mg/dl [66,67]. Dialysis is usually initiated via the blood route, i.e., hemodialysis, but it may be accomplished via the peritoneal route in some cases. Peritoneal dialysis has the advantage and disadvantage of being slower and more gradual. In patients with unstable hemodynamics, it may be preferable for this reason, but it should be stressed that it is also much slower in correcting electrolyte and fluid abnormalities as well as uremic symptoms. The dialysis prescription in the setting of acute renal failure is generally to maintain the blood urea nitrogen level under 100 mg/dl and the serum creatinine level under 10 mg/dl. Most important are the prevention of electrolyte and fluid disturbances and the avoidance of the uremic syndrome. Many pharmacologic agents must have their dosages adjusted appropriately depending on their dialysis clearance and the degree of underlying renal function.

In the last 10 years, a new technique, continuous arteriovenous hemofiltration (CAVH), has become more widely used for the treatment of acute renal failure. Experience with the technique has largely been restricted to Europe, although several series have been accumulated in the United States. Basically, this technique involves hemofiltering blood using the patient's own blood pressure. If used properly, this technique can result in acceptable control of azotemia, blood electrolyte concentrations, and acid-base balance. Moreover, impressive fluid removal is possible with this technique as well. The major disadvantages to this technique are the requirements for arterial access and the slowness of correction of severe electrolyte disturbances [41].

Nephrotic Syndrome, Nephritic Syndrome, Asymptomatic Proteinuria and Hematuria, and Rapidly Progressive Glomerulonephritis

Nephrotic Syndrome

The nephrotic syndrome is a symptom complex consisting of proteinuria, hypoproteinemia, edema, lipiduria, and hyperlipidemia [36]. The nephrotic syndrome is caused by a glomerular leakiness to plasma proteins, primarily albumin, which leads to severe protein losses in the urine, decreases in protein concentration in the serum, increases in urine and blood lipids, and marked salt and water retention. Other accompanying features of the nephrotic syndrome include a hypercoagulable state, which may lead to renal vein thrombosis, lower extremity thrombophlebitis, and pulmonary emboli, and the consequences of the increase in blood lipid concentration, which may lead to accelerated atherosclerosis. Other complications of the nephrotic syndrome are related to severe salt and water overload and include pleural and peritoneal fluid accumulations [36].

The nephrotic syndrome may be caused by primary glomerular diseases or the so-called idiopathic nephrotic syndrome, or secondary nephrotic syndrome, which is secondary to a variety of systemic diseases [27,36]. The major causes of the nephrotic syndrome and their frequency in adults are summarized in Table 3-12.

DIAGNOSIS

The approach to the nephrotic syndrome must be based on a systematic evaluation of potential causes. This involves a detailed history and physical examination with attention to signs and symptoms of systemic disorders and a laboratory evaluation in search of abnormalities suggestive of malignancy, vasculitis, other collagen-vascular

Table 3–12. Causes of Nephrotic Syndrome and Frequency in Adults

Idiopathic nephrotic syndrome (75 percent):
  Lipid nephrosis (15 percent)
  Membranous glomerulopathy (22.5 percent)
  Membranoproliferative glomerulonephritis (7.5 percent)
  Focal sclerosis (7.5 percent)
  Proliferative glomerulonephritis (22.5 percent)
Secondary nephrotic syndrome (25 percent)
  Diabetes mellitus (5 to 10 percent)
  Systemic lupus erythematosus (5 percent)
  Neoplasms: lymphomas, solid tumors (5 to 10 percent)
  Amyloidosis
  Infections: syphilis, *Plasmodium* malaria, shunt nephritis
  Toxic nephropathy: gold, mercury, penicillamine,
    "street" heroin, probenecid
  Transplant rejection
  Toxemia of pregnancy

disorders, glucose intolerance, or drug-induced and non-drug-induced allergic phenomena.

The urinalysis in cases of nephrotic syndrome will reveal the presence of proteinuria on dipstick and usually is remarkable for the presence of fatty casts and fat bodies in the urine. Fat bodies consist of renal tubular cells packed with cholesterol esters which appear as so-called Maltese crosses in polarized light. Twenty-four-hour urine collections have traditionally been obtained for measurement of creatinine and protein to grade the severity of the proteinuria. Nephrotic-range proteinuria has been somewhat arbitrarily defined as greater than 3.5 gm urinary protein execution in 24 hours normalized per 1.73 m² of body surface area. Recently, data have accumulated suggesting that the ratio between the protein and creatinine on a spot urine test (obtained at any time other than during the first morning void) correlates quite well with 24-hour ratios. Using this approach, a urine protein to creatinine ratio of 2.0 or greater can be considered diagnostic of nephrotic-range proteinuria.

Definitive diagnosis of the etiology of the nephrotic syndrome requires a renal biopsy. As a rule, the renal biopsy should be performed in all adults with the nephrotic syndrome unless significant contraindications to the biopsy technique exist (e.g., systemic bleeding disorder, presence of a single functioning kidney, patient refusal) or unless absolute contraindications to steroid or immunosuppressive therapy are present. Before renal biopsy is undertaken, a careful history concerning bleeding problems, laboratory tests of coagulation and bleeding time, and assessment of the presence of two kidneys with ultrasound and/or x-ray therefore should be performed. Localization of the kidney for renal biopsy is currently performed with either renal ultrasound or fluoroscopy [36].

Histologically, the idiopathic nephrotic syndrome usually presents as one of five typical patterns. These include lipoid nephrosis or nil disease, membranous glomerulopathy, membranoproliferative glomerulonephritis, focal glomerulosclerosis, and proliferative glomerulonephritis [27].

Lipoid nephrosis, or nil disease, is a clinicopathologic entity characterized by nephrotic syndrome associated with virtually no abnormal findings on light microscopy and fusion of foot processes demonstrable by electron microscopy. Immunofluorescence studies are usually negative in nil disease. Lipoid nephrosis is the most common cause of nephrotic syndrome in children (65 to 75 percent) and is a frequent cause of nephrotic syndrome in adults (15 percent). It is clinically characterized by the relatively abrupt onset of nephrotic syndrome with a relatively normal glomerular filtration rate and the absence of hematuria. In children, but not adults, the proteinuria is highly selective; i.e., only small molecular proteins leak in the urine. Pathogenesis of this disorder is not clear; however, abnormalities in T-cell function are suspected.

TREATMENT
The clinical course of lipoid nephrosis is usually one of spontaneous or therapeutically induced remissions in proteinuria and edema followed, in many cases, by relapses. The therapeutic approach usually consists of high doses of prednisone (60 to 80 mg per day) given for short courses (6 to 12 weeks). Frequent relapses on this regimen may benefit from a therapeutic course with an immunosuppressive agent such as chlorambucil or cyclophosphamide. The prognosis for long-term preservation of renal function is quite good [27,36].

Focal glomerulosclerosis is an idiopathic glomerulopathy characterized by nephrotic-range proteinuria, variable hematuria, mild hypertension, and a characteristic focal and segmental obliteration of the glomerulus. Immunofluorescence studies reveal deposition of C3, IgG, and IgM in the sclerotic areas. Electron microscopy confirms focal sclerosis and also shows diffuse foot-process fusion. The disease is difficult at times to distinguish from nil disease, since the first glomeruli involved by the sclerotic process are juxtamedullary and may not be sampled on the renal biopsy. In contrast to nil disease, focal glomerulosclerosis tends to be progressive in terms of loss of renal function and is usually unresponsive to therapy [27,36].

Membranous glomerulopathy is the most common cause of nephrotic syndrome in adults. Membranous glomerulopathy appears to be caused by in situ formation of immune complexes, with the secondary fixation of complement. On light microscopy, thickening of the glomerular basement membrane is present, as is evidence of immune deposits with special stains. On electron microscopy, electron-dense deposits are present in a subepithelial pattern with various degrees of basement membrane reaction to these deposits. Immunofluorescence shows a so-called lumpy-bumpy pattern of IgG and C3 along the capillary basement membrane. Clinically, one sees the nephrotic syndrome as the major feature of membranous nephropathy, with hypertension present in a variable proportion of patients. Hematuria on a microscopic level is common, although gross hematuria is uncommon. The clinical course of this disorder is usually slowly progressive; however, spontaneous remissions may occur in 25 to 35 percent of patients [27,36]. The value of therapy for this disorder is not yet certain, although it appears that high doses of alternate-day prednisone (100 to 120 mg) given for 2 months or 6 alternating months of steroids and cytotoxic agents may be beneficial in preserving renal function [10,58].

Membranoproliferative glomerulonephritis is also known as mesangiocapillary or lobular glomerulonephritis. It is an idiopathic glomerular disease that has the distinctive histologic findings of prominent mesangial proliferation with extension of mesangial material into the subendothelial region. The peak incidence ranges from ages 5 to 29 years and accounts for about 10 percent of the idiopathic nephrotic syndrome in adults.

About 50 percent of patients with membranoproliferative glomerulonephritis present with nephrotic syndrome, 30 percent present with proteinuria and hematuria, and the remainder present with predominantly nephritic complaints of hematuria or red cell casts and even gross hematuria. Hypertension and azotemia are common in almost half the patients on initial investigation. The C3 levels are depressed in almost all patients at some stage in the illness. On electron microscopy, this lesion may be separated into two major categories. Type 1 membranoproliferative glomerulonephritis appears to be an immune-complex disease associated with electron-dense deposits in subendothelial and mesangial locations. Type 2 membranoproliferative glomerulonephritis (dense-deposit disease) appears to be characterized by the presence of extremely electron-dense deposits within the tubular and glomerular basement membranes. Type 1 membranoproliferative glomerulonephritis appears to be associated with fixation of complement via the classical pathway, whereas the type 2 lesion appears to be associated with the so-called C3 nephritic factor [27,36].

Therapy for either of these disorders is at present controversial. It appears that steroid or other immunosuppressive therapy is not of value in adults with this disorder. However, some evidence has recently surfaced suggesting that anticoagulant or antiplatelet agents may be beneficial in preventing the progression of this disorder [17].

Secondary Nephrotic Syndrome

The nephrotic syndrome is frequently (25 percent) due to systemic disorders in adults. The causes may range from vasculitis or collagen-vascular disorders, which are discussed in another section, to diabetes mellitus, which is the most common cause of secondary nephrotic syndrome in adults [36]. Other causes are listed in Table 4-12.

Diabetic nephropathy accounts for a considerable proportion of nephrotic syndrome in adults. The onset is heralded by proteinuria, which often progresses to overt nephrotic syndrome. Proteinuria usually appears in patients with the juvenile form of diabetes mellitus between 14 and 20 years after the onset. Renal failure develops after 6 to 30 months in many of these patients. Hypertension commonly develops as the renal disease progresses. Control of hyperglycemia with insulin therapy does not appear to affect the course of the chronic renal disease once proteinuria is established. Investigations concerning the use of angiotensin-converting enzyme inhibitors in the progression of diabetic glomerulopathy are underway [34].

Other important disorders of renal function may occur in patients with diabetes mellitus. Papillary necrosis may occur, especially when diabetes is complicated by obstruction and upper urinary tract infection. Upper and lower urinary tract infections are more likely to occur in patients with diabetes mellitus than in normal subjects. Urinary tract obstruction secondary to neurogenic bladder may occur. Administration of radiocontrast material appears to cause acute renal failure in patients with diabetes with significantly higher incidence than in nondiabetic patients. Hyporeninemic hypoaldosteronism with hyperkalemia and renal tubular acidosis is also often seen in patients with long-standing diabetes mellitus [34].

Amyloidosis is another cause of secondary nephrotic syndrome which must be suspected in any patients with a chronic inflammatory disease, as well as in patients who have multiple myeloma. Rectal biopsy may be a useful diagnostic tool. The clinical course of amyloidosis is usually that of proteinuria with inexorably progressive renal failure without severe hypertension. Hepatitis B antigenemia may be associated with the nephrotic syndrome [45]. Similarly, systemic lupus erythematosus may be associated with the nephrotic syndrome [71].

Certain infections are associated with the nephrotic syndrome. These include syphilis, schistosomiasis, hepatitis B, and malaria. Other causes of secondary nephrotic syndrome are toxic or allergic reactions to drugs (most commonly seen with nonsteroidal anti-inflammatory agents), transplant rejection, and toxemia of pregnancy [36].

Acute Nephritic Syndrome

The acute nephritic syndrome is a syndrome characterized by hypertension, hematuria, and red blood cell casts in the urine. The acute nephritic syndrome can be seen in a variety of renal lesions, including a number of secondary lesions associated with collagen-vascular diseases and vasculitides, as well as in several primary renal lesions [22]. The most well-characterized form of acute nephritic syndrome is postinfectious acute glomerulonephritis. The classic form of this is poststreptococcal glomerulonephritis. Poststreptococcal glomerulonephritis follows infections of the pharynx or skin with nephritogenic streptococci after a latent period averaging about 10 days. The clinical features of this disorder include mild to moderate hypertension, mild fever, nausea, abdominal pain, edema, hematuria, and red blood cell casts. On occasion, volume overload with signs of left ventricular failure or encephalopathy may occur.

Diagnosis

The diagnosis of acute poststreptococcal glomerulonephritis is based on a typical clinical course as well as the isolation of group A streptococci from the pharynx or skin and/or the presence of typical rises in the ASOT, antistreptokinase, antihyaluronidase, or anti-DNAse at 1 to 3 weeks after infection. Rises in ASOT do not usually occur with skin infections, and the other markers are essential to make the diagnosis in this setting. Serum complement levels are decreased early in acute poststreptococcal glomerulonephritis, although they usually return to normal within 6 weeks. Histologic examination of poststreptococcal glomerulonephritis reveals a diffuse, exudative, and proliferative glomerulonephritis on light microscopy with evidence of electron-dense subepithelial humps on electron microscopy and a granular "lumpy-bumpy" pattern of complement component 3 (C3) and IgG on immunofluorescence study. None of these findings, though, is entirely specific for acute poststreptococcal glomerulonephritis [27].

TREATMENT

The prognosis for acute poststreptococcal glomerulonephritis appears quite good in children. The prognosis in adults is controversial, but it may be somewhat worse. Treatment of this disorder is entirely symptomatic, since there is no evidence that any therapy affects the clinical course.

Other lesions that may mimic acute poststreptococcal glomerulonephritis are a postinfectious syndrome following other infections, including pneumococcal pneumonia, various staphylococcal infections, various viral infections, and infective endocarditis or infected shunts [18,29,60].

Asymptomatic Proteinuria and Hematuria

Asymptomatic proteinuria and hematuria may occur in a variety of renal lesions. These signs, of course, may occur in virtually all renal lesions discussed earlier. In addition to these, other disorders are noteworthy. Focal glomerulonephritis associated with IgA deposits in the mesangium (Berger's disease) usually is associated with the syndrome of intermittent hematuria and/or persistent microscopic hematuria with mild proteinuria. This disorder tends to occur more often in men, is usually not, but occasionally is, progressive, and does not respond to any known therapy. This disorder appears to be part of a spectrum that includes Henoch-Schönlein purpura. Other focal proliferative glomerulonephritides not associated with IgA nephropathy also may be associated with asymptomatic proteinuria and hematuria. At the present time, no treatment is advocated for such disorders [36].

It should be stressed that microscopic hematuria and/or gross intermittent hematuria may be caused not by a glomerular lesion, but by a structural lesion in the urinary collecting system or renal parenchyma. Since this type of lesion may be malignant, it must be ruled out. Other causes of microscopic hematuria and/or gross hematuria include urinary calculi and the idiopathic loin-pain hematuria syndrome or benign familial hematuria.

Rapidly Progressive Glomerulonephritis

Rapidly progressive glomerulonephritis is a syndrome of glomerulonephritis which is associated with the rapid and often irreversible loss of renal function. Rapidly progressive glomerulonephritis (RPGN) is histologically characterized by extensive extracapillary proliferation, i.e., crescents, which are usually present in greater than 50 percent of the glomeruli sampled in the biopsy specimen. The combination of the clinical features (progressive deterioration of renal function, microscopic hematuria with red cell casts, and proteinuria) and the characteristic biopsy appearance allows for the diagnosis. Table 3-13 lists the most important causes of rapidly progressive glomerulonephritis [27].

Goodpasture's syndrome is the clinical syndrome of glomerulonephritis (usually of the rapidly progressive type) and lung hemorrhage associated with anti-glomerular basement-membrane (anti-GBM) antibody. Documentation of this last feature requires either the demonstration of anti-glomerular basement-membrane antibody in the serum or the finding of linear deposition of IgG along the glomerular capillary basement membrane on immunofluorescence staining of a biopsy specimen.

Goodpasture's syndrome is classically a disease of young males. Pulmonary symptoms may occur prior to the renal disease in up to 70 percent of

Table 3-13. *Causes of Rapidly Progressive Glomerulonephritis (RPGN)*

Antiglomerular basement-membrane disease:
  Goodpasture's syndrome
  Anti-glomerular basement-membrane nephritis without lung hemorrhage
Idiopathic rapidly progressive glomerulonephritis
Systemic disease:
  Systemic lupus erythematosus
  Bacterial endocarditis
  Henoch-Schönlein purpura
  Polyarteritis nodosa
  Wegener's granulomatosis
  Poststreptococcal glomerulonephritis
  Mixed cryoglobulinemia
  Occult visceral sepsis

patients. Lung hemorrhage usually leads to symptoms of hemoptysis and dyspnea, as well as an abnormal chest radiograph. Iron-deficiency anemia due to this bleeding is common in this disorder.

The clinical course of Goodpasture's syndrome is usually one of progressive renal failure necessitating dialysis or transplantation. Therapy of the syndrome is currently approached with a combination of plasmapheresis and immunosuppression using steroids and either azathioprine or cyclophosphamide [27].

The association of rapidly progressive glomerulonephritis and lung hemorrhage is not specific for Goodpasture's syndrome, and it may occur in other diseases, such as systemic lupus erythematosus, bacterial endocarditis, Henoch-Schönlein purpura, and polyarteritis nodosa. It should be stressed that these diseases must be distinguished from Goodpasture's syndrome for optional therapy. For vasculitides leading to the syndrome of rapidly progressive glomerulonephritis, an approach of immunosuppressive agents without plasmapheresis appears to be as effective as using immunosuppressive agents with plasmapheresis if pulses of high-dose parenteral steroids are included in the regimen.

An idiopathic rapidly progressive glomerulonephritis syndrome associated with anti-glomerular basement-membrane antibodies without lung hemorrhage may be a clinically distinct entity from Goodpasture's syndrome. However, clinically, the approach to this disorder is the same (i.e., plasmapheresis and immunosuppression).

With rapidly progressive glomerulonephritis associated with anti-glomerular basement-membrane antibody in the circulation, dialysis is usually the treatment of choice for end-stage renal disease. Transplantation may be accomplished successfully only after the anti-glomerular basement membrane antibody titer drops to an undetectable level [27].

Lupus Nephritis and other Connective-Tissue Diseases Affecting the Kidney

Systemic lupus erythematosus (SLE) and other connective-tissue diseases may involve the kidney. In the case of systemic lupus erythematosus, on pathologic criteria of involvement, virtually 100 percent of patients show renal lesions. Clinical renal disease, however, occurs only in about two-thirds of patients [71]. Clinical manifestations include isolated urinary sediment abnormalities, acute glomerulonephritis, nephrotic syndrome, and rapidly progressive glomerulonephritis. Clinical activity of the renal disease correlates reasonably well with the presence of urinary sediment abnormalities, decreases in serum complement and titers of antibody to double-stranded DNA. The pathologic findings of systemic lupus erythematosus in the kidney are as varied as the clinical manifestations and include glomerular lesions (e.g., minimal mesangial changes, focal proliferative lesions, diffuse proliferative lesions, membranous lesions) and tubulointerstitial disease. The prognosis is quite variable, but it appears to be better for the less severe histologic lesions and more guarded for cases associated with severe histologic changes. Therapy of systemic lupus erythematosus includes prednisone as well as immunosuppressive agents. Although controversial, it appears that immunosuppressive agents such as cyclophosphamide and azathioprine may improve the prognosis of severe lupus nephritis. The optimal type of immunosuppression, however, is not known at this time and remains a topic of intense investigation [16,71].

The kidney is often involved in various vasculitides [22]. Henoch-Schönlein purpura is a special syndrome linking a leukocytoclastic vasculitis with clinical manifestations of palpable purpura, abdominal pain, vomiting, lower intestinal bleeding, arthralgias, epistaxis and hemoptysis with renal manifestations of hematuria (with or without red blood cell casts in the urine), and variable decreases in the glomerular filtration rate. Clinically important renal disease occurs in about a third of patients with this disorder. IgA nephropathy (Berger's disease) appears to be part of the same spectrum as Henoch-Schönlein disease. The renal disease of Henoch-Schönlein disease tends to be more severe in adults than in children. There are no specific laboratory tests, although the serum IgA levels may be elevated, as may be the levels of serum IgA immune complexes in afflicted patients. On renal biopsy, mesangial IgA deposits may be found in patients with Henoch-Schönlein disease. It appears that the renal vasculitis is not responsive to therapy, although some trials are currently underway to study the effect of immunosuppression and/or plasmapheresis in this entity.

Polyarteritis nodosa may exist in a macroscopic as well as microscopic form. The macroscopic form classically involves large vessels, occurs most commonly in males above the age of 50, and presents with systemic findings including arthralgias, peripheral neuropathy, fever, and hemolytic anemia. Hypertension is common and may progress to a malignant stage. Renal disease occurs in about 80 to 90 percent of such patients and is manifested typically by hematuria and variable changes in the glomerular filtration rate. The nephrotic syndrome is uncommon. Progressive renal disease may occur in this setting and is often exacerbated in association with hypertension. The diagnosis can be made by the combination of the clinical picture, pathologic identification of the vascular lesions usually in tissues other than the kidney, and the characteristic angiographic appearance, which includes typical microaneurysms in the renal arterial vessels and the medium-sized muscular arteries of other abdominal viscera. Abusers of intravenous amphetamines may develop a clinical pathologic disorder that mimics polyarteritis nodosa. Hepatitis B antigen is present in the sera of as many as 50 percent of patients with the macroscopic form of polyarteritis nodosa [18,22].

The microscopic form of polyarteritis nodosa, also called hypersensitivity angiitis, has similar systemic manifestations as those described for the macroscopic form. Differences that are noteworthy are that hypertension is unusual in the microscopic form and that bronchial asthma and eosinophilia (which are unusual in the macroscopic form) are common in the microscopic form. The renal disease associated with hypersensitivity angiitis may be rapidly progressive. Renal biopsy examination often demonstrates fibroid necrosis in glomerular tufts and crescentic epithelial-cell proliferation. Treatment with prednisone and immunosuppression appears effective in both the macroscopic and microscopic forms of polyarteritis nodosa [22,23].

Wegener's granulomatosis is an unusual, but important, form of vasculitis which may involve the kidney. This systemic disorder typically involves granulomatous arteritis of the upper respiratory tract (including sinuses, middle ear, and nasopharynx), necrotizing pneumonitis of the lower respiratory tract, and a renal lesion of necrotizing glomerulonephritis. The extrarenal lesions are quite responsive to steroid therapy, but the renal lesion may respond only to cyclophosphamide therapy. Cyclophosphamide is therefore excellent therapy for all manifestations of this disease and is the treatment of choice [23].

Infective endocarditis may present with a renal lesion that is similar to that seen with shunt infections or visceral abscesses. These patients develop immune-complex glomerulonephritis with hematuria and proteinuria. In this condition, plasma C3 levels frequently are reduced. Nephrotic syndrome appears to be more common in shunt nephritis than in endocarditis associated nephritis. Treatment of the underlying infection is the appropriate therapy for these disorders [29].

Essential mixed cryoglobulinemia may be associated with a glomerular lesion that manifests itself as chronic progressive renal disease, acute renal failure, nephrotic syndrome, asymptomatic proteinuria, and/or hematuria. Systemic manifestations of cryoglobulinemia include palpable purpura, cold-induced necrosis of the digits, and hepatosplenomegaly. Although no therapy is of definitive benefit, treatment with plasmapheresis and cytotoxic medications appears to be effective in some patients [22].

Hepatitis B antigenemia appears to be associated with a variety of renal lesions. As mentioned before, the macroscopic form of polyarteritis nodosa is frequently associated with hepatitis B antigenemia. Hepatitis B antigenemia also is associated with other histologic renal lesions, including membranoproliferative glomerulonephritis, membranous glomerulopathy, and focal and diffuse proliferative glomerulonephritis. The pathogenesis of these lesions is unknown, although they are believed to involve immune-complex deposition [45].

The kidney may be involved in other forms of connective-tissue diseases. Renal involvement in progressive systemic sclerosis (scleroderma) has been noted with variable frequency. The histologic appearance is indistinguishable from that of malignant hypertension. Patients with Sjögren's syndrome also may have an associated glomerulonephritis, but more commonly the renal involvement consists of interstitial nephritis and distal renal tubular acidosis. Mixed connective-tissue disease (MCTD) is occasionally associated with renal manifestations similar to those seen with systemic lupus erythematosus, but in general, this entity spares the renal and central nervous systems.

Cystic Diseases of the Kidney

Cystic diseases of the kidney may range from simple cysts that cause virtually no symptoms to polycystic diseases in which the kidney parenchyma is replaced by nonfunctioning cysts with ultimate progression to renal insufficiency.

Polycystic kidney disease is an autosomal-dominant genetic disorder that produces gradual loss of the renal parenchyma with replacement by multiple renal cysts. Polycystic kidney disease is associated with cysts of the pancreas, liver, and spleen, as well as intracranial aneurysms. The disorder usually becomes clinically apparent between the ages of 20 and 40 years, presenting with hypertension, gross or microscopic hematuria, and abdominal pain. Palpably enlarged kidneys are found in the majority of patients. Diagnosis is based on family history and the presence of bilateral enlarged kidneys with multiple cysts. These cysts may be diagnosed on intravenous pyelography or ultrasonography, the latter noninvasive approach constituting the screening study of choice [25]. The clinical course of adult polycystic kidney disease is variable; however, most patients do reach end-stage renal failure in their fifth or sixth decade. Rarely, polycystic kidney disease may become manifest in childhood. Treatment is directed at protecting the kidney from factors that could hasten deterioration of renal function, including hypertension and urinary tract infection. Genetic counseling is certainly indicated for patients with polycystic kidneys detected before or during their reproductive years [77].

Medullary cystic disease, or nephronophthisis, is a familial disorder that causes the characteristic pathologic lesion of microscopic cysts in the medulla with associated interstitial fibrosis. This disorder is morphologically indistinguishable from juvenile nephronophthisis (see below). The juvenile form is inherited as an autosomal-recessive trait, whereas the adult form appears to be primarily an autosomal-dominant disorder. The clinical manifestations include polyuria, anemia, renal salt wasting with prominent renal osteodystrophy, and progressive renal failure [77].

Infantile polycystic kidney disease differs from adult polycystic kidney disease in several respects. Generally, it is inherited in an autosomal-recessive manner, whereas the adult form is usually autosomal-dominant. As already mentioned, there are occasional reports of an autosomal-dominant inheritance pattern in children. The renal lesion in infantile polycystic kidney disease tends to be overshadowed by an extremely severe hepatic fibrosis that is usually present and is often the cause of death [77].

One or more simple renal cysts are commonly encountered as an incidental finding at autopsy in the elderly. In patients undergoing pyelography or ultrasound for other reasons, cysts must be distinguished from carcinomas undergoing cystic transformation. In many cases this can be done by the ultrasonographic appearance alone, but in other cases cyst aspiration, computed tomographic (CT) scanning, and even exploratory surgery may be required.

Recently, it has been noted that some patients with chronic renal failure may develop renal cystic disease and renal tumors while undergoing maintenance hemodialysis. This has been noted in chronic renal failure of diverse causes. Hemorrhage into the cysts may cause pain and sometimes gross hematuria. Malignant transformation may occur and must be excluded in a similar manner as single renal cysts [62].

Medullary sponge kidney, a nondestructive hereditary cystic disorder of the renal medulla, may be asymptomatic or cause renal calculi with pain, obstruction, or hematuria. This disorder is frequently associated with a distal renal tubular acidosis. Abdominal radiography may demonstrate nephrocalcinosis due to calcium deposition within cysts. Excretory urography usually reveals stasis of contrast material within dilated cystic collecting ducts, yielding a spongelike appearance of the renal papilla from which this disorder is named. This disorder usually does not cause progressive renal failure [77].

Interstitial Renal Disease

The term *interstitial renal disease* describes a variety of renal lesions that share the common pathologic finding of a primarily interstitial inflammatory process. Patients with interstitial renal disease tend to have mild to moderate proteinuria (generally less than 2 gm per day) and variable pyuria and hematuria, and they usually lack red blood cell casts. With chronicity, hypertension and slowly progressive azotemia become apparent with interstitial renal disease [12].

The different major causes of interstitial renal disease are shown in Table 3-14. The most important cause of interstitial renal disease is reflux nephropathy or vesicoureteral reflux (VUR). This lesion is frequently associated with recurring episodes of bacterial pyelonephritis and is a common cause of end-stage renal disease in adults. Early repair of vesicoureteral reflux may be beneficial in the prevention of subsequent renal failure, but once proteinuria is established, surgical repair is indicated only to treat uncontrolled recurrence of infection. The mechanism of the progression of renal failure in this disease is controversial, but it may be related to hyperfiltration of remaining nephrons.

Mechanical obstructive effects of calcium or non-calcium-containing stones in the collecting system may cause interstitial renal disease. Hypokalemia and hypercalcemia also have been shown to be associated with interstitial nephritis in the absence of stones. It is unclear whether hyperuricemia by itself causes progressive renal dysfunction. Several toxins can cause acute as well as

Table 3–14. *Causes of Interstitial Renal Disease*

Vesicoureteral reflux (VUR) (usually complicated by infection)

Granulomatous disease (e.g., tuberculosis)

Drug- or toxin-related (e.g., analgesic nephropathy, allergic interstitial nephritis)

Obstruction

Calculi

Electrolyte disturbances (e.g., hypercalcemia, hypokalemia)

Collagen-vascular disease (e.g., Sjögren's syndrome)

Myeloma kidney

chronic interstitial renal disease. Analgesics are an important cause of chronic interstitial nephritis. It appears that a combination of phenacitin and aspirin is most often associated with progressive renal insufficiency. Papillary necrosis occurs early in this disease and is followed by chronic interstitial changes. Sickle-cell disease also may cause progressive renal insufficiency. Papillary necrosis can occur both with the fully expressed homozygous disease and with the sickle-cell trait [12].

Acute interstitial nephritis is most commonly an allergic reaction to different medications. This has been best described for ampicillin and other penicillin drugs, but it has been reported for a host of drugs, including other antibiotics (sulfa, cephalosporins), diuretics (thiazide, furosemide), antiseizure medications (phenytoin), and allopurinol [48]. Recently, a large number of cases of interstitial nephritis associated with nonsteroidal anti-inflammatory drugs have been reported. As already mentioned, the interesting feature about this disorder appears to be the frequent concomitant occurrence of high-grade proteinuria with these drugs [8].

Bacterial pyelonephritis is a common cause of interstitial renal disease. It appears that bacterial pyelonephritis most often occurs from ascending lower urinary tract infection with gram-negative bacteria. In general, patients who have lower urinary tract infections will not develop pyelonephritis if their urinary tracts are anatomically and functionally intact. Pyelonephritis and urinary tract infections in general are discussed more thoroughly in Chapter 6.

Obstructive Nephropathy

Acute urinary tract obstruction leads to an acute rise in renal tubular pressure and a decreased glomerular filtration rate. Chronic obstruction is also associated with marked decreases in the glomerular filtration rate, although the tubular fluid pressure tends to normalize. Permanent loss of the renal mass may occur along with dilatation of the pelvicaliceal system and pressure atrophy. Superimposed infection and ischemia may contribute to the loss of renal parenchyma.

Causes of obstruction are listed in Table 3-15. Bilateral obstruction obviously is the most dangerous, since it compromises the functions of both kidneys and may lead to renal failure if not relieved [76].

Diagnosis

Symptoms of obstruction may range from no symptoms to severe flank, abdominal, or suprapubic pain. Symptoms of bladder outlet obstruction include hesitancy, dribbling, and intermittent cessation of the urine stream during voiding. Important clues to the presence of obstruction include pyelonephritis or recurrent lower urinary tract infections in females or any urinary tract infection in males. Marked fluctuation in urine volumes in azotemic patients does suggest partial intermittent urinary tract obstruction. Functional abnormalities secondary to partial urinary tract

Table 3–15. Causes of Urinary Tract Obstruction

Bilateral:
  Meatal or urethral stricture or valve
  Prostatic hypertrophy, cancer, or inflammation
  Neurologic or drug-induced bladder dysfunction

Often or usually bilateral:
  Bladder carcinoma
  Radiation injury of the uterus
  Pelvic tumors
  Retroperitoneal tumors
  Retroperitoneal fibrosis
  Pelvic inflammatory disease
  Carcinoma of ureter or renal pelvis

Usually unilateral:
  Stones or stone-induced stricture
  Papillary necrosis
  Ureteropelvic junction stricture or valve
  Inadvertent ligature
  Ureteral blood clots
  Aortic aneurysm

obstruction include decreases in glomerular filtration rate, a concentrating defect producing polyuria and nocturia, and a distal renal tubular acidifying defect that may be associated with hyperkalemia [6]. Superimposed infection may cause marked loss of the renal parenchyma, including papillary necrosis or even pyelonephrosis (replacement of renal parenchyma with pus). Instrumentation must be undertaken with great care in these patients to avoid introducing infection into the blood system.

Treatment

Treatment of obstruction involves the relief of the obstructing lesion. Bladder outlet obstruction is best relieved with placement of a Foley catheter or, if necessary, a suprapubic catheter. Relief of obstruction of the ureteral drainage system may be accomplished by placement of stents via a transbladder approach or via nephrostomy tubes placed percutaneously.

Following relief of bilateral obstruction, a postobstructive diuresis frequently occurs. The pathophysiologic mechanisms for this diuresis include increases in total-body solutes, osmotic diuresis secondary to increases in the blood urea nitrogen level, and a concentrating defect that has features of both medullary gradient washout and tubular insensitivity to antidiuretic hormone. It should be stressed, though, that iatrogenic overhydration frequently contributes to the maintenance of a postobstructive diuresis [76].

Renal Stone Disease

Renal stone disease is a common form of renal lesion. Series demonstrate renal calculi in anywhere from 1 to 10 percent of autopsies. Approximately 1 patient per 1000 individuals is hospitalized in this country for stone disease annually [75].

Diagnosis

The symptoms of renal stones may range from virtually no symptoms to excruciating pain. The pain is typically localized to the flank, with radiation into the groin. It is usually unilateral. This pain may be associated with marked costovertebral angle tenderness. The urinalysis often demonstrates microscopic hematuria when the patient has symptoms. The urinalysis may reveal crystals, but this is not a specific finding for stone disease.

Approximately 90 percent of renal calculi are radiopaque and may be seen on a flat plain radiograph of the abdomen. Intravenous pyelography is used for confirmation of the intraureteral nature of a stone [75].

Treatment

The therapeutic approach to renal stone disease is dictated by the type of disorder present. These disorders are summarized in Table 3-16. Renal stones are most commonly calcium oxalate in nature. Calcium oxalate stones are often associated with hypercalciuric states, but they also may be due to hyperoxaluric or hyperuricemic states as well. Often no abnormality in calcium oxalate excretion may be found [9]. A smaller percentage of stones are due to calcium phosphate. These are frequently associated with renal tubular acidosis or hyperparathyroidism. Cystine stones are usually associated with a disease known as cystinuria. Cystinuria is an autosomal-recessive genetic defect in amino acid transport. Hyperuricosuria may result in uric acid stones, which are the only common radiolucent calculi. Struvite stones, or triple-phosphate stones, as they are also known, are usually associated with infection due to urea-splitting organisms. This is the most common cause of staghorn calculi [75].

The evaluation for a first renal stone in a child or adult with recurrent stones includes 24-hour

Table 3–16. *Causes of Renal Calculi*

Cause	Percent of Cases
Specific disorders (30 percent):	
Hypercalciuria:	
Primary hyperparathyroidism	4
Renal tubular acidosis (distal)	4
Sarcoidosis, vitamin D excess, hyperthyroidism	3
Uric acid stones:	
Gout	4
Chronic diarrhea	2
Hyperoxaluria:	
Disease of the ileum or jejunoileal bypass	4
Primary	—
Cystinuria	1
Struvite stones (infection)	3
Medullary sponge kidney	4
Acetazolamide, alkali ingestion	1
Idiopathic disorders (70 percent):	
Idiopathic hypercalciuria	40
Hyperuricosuric, normocalciuric calcium stones	14
Idiopathic calcium stones	16

urine collections for creatinine, calcium, uric acid, oxalate, and cysteine, as well as determination of the serum calcium, phosphorus, uric acid, electrolyte, creatinine, and parathyroid hormone (if the serum calcium level is high or the serum phosphorus level is low) [57]. All stones should be treated by increasing oral intake of fluids 2½ to 3 liters per day, regardless of the underlying abnormality in mineral excretion. Cystinuria may be managed by increasing urine volume and maintaining the urine pH at an alkaline level with oral alkali. If necessary, d-penicillamine may be used. Hyperoxaluria is usually treated by avoidance of oxalate-rich foods and/or cholestyramine therapy. Idiopathic hypercalciuria may be approached in several ways. Some investigators feel that the nature of the defect in calcium metabolism must be defined, and they prescribe specific therapy for that defect. Other investigators have shown that oral thiazides are as effective as any other therapy, regardless of the underlying nature of the defect. Hyperuricosuria is best treated with allopurinol therapy. Infected struvite stones represent a very difficult problem that often requires surgical treatment of the calculi as well as aggressive treatment of the underlying infection [75].

Hypertension

Hypertension may be defined in a variety of ways. It is known that the risk of stroke, heart attack, and renal failure increases with increases in blood pressure. Although there is no sharp demarcation point in assessing cardiovascular risk, the increase in this risk does become greatest as blood pressures exceed 140 mmHg systolic and 90 mmHg diastolic. Some authors therefore use these systolic and diastolic numbers as a cutoff for normal blood pressure in adults. An alternate definition of hypertension is that it is the level of blood pressure at which the benefits of treatment outweigh the deleterious effects of such treatment [42]. Clearly, this latter operational approach will differ depending on treatment and the individual being treated. Although more difficult to apply to large groups of patients, the latter approach is what physicians must use with individual patients.

The major adverse effects of hypertension are on the body's vasculature. Examination of the ocular fundi permits visualization of the effects of hypertension on small vessels. Assessment of heart size by both clinical and visualization techniques allows the assessment of the effects of hypertension on this organ. Renal functional assessment by the serum creatinine and creatinine clearance values permits evaluation of the effects of hypertension on the kidneys. A careful history for evidence of cerebrovascular injury and a careful neurologic examination are essential in the evaluation of hypertension.

Diagnosis

The causes of hypertension are summarized in Table 3-17. It should be immediately evident that essential hypertension is the most common cause of hypertension, accounting for 90 percent of cases. However, as a result of the therapeutic implications of recognizing secondary causes, they must be sought for diligently in the appropriate setting. Coarctation of the aorta may be essentially excluded on physical examination of proximal and distal pulses. As we will see in the following discussion, history and physical examination will suggest the possibility of pheochromocytoma or renal artery stenosis in many cases. Urinalysis will be a clue toward the presence of renal parenchymal disease. The possibility of primary hyperaldosteronism or Cushing's syndrome should be suggested by the finding of a low serum potassium value. In the majority of patients with hypertension, the workup for secondary causes goes no further than the physician performing a careful history, physical examination, and urinalysis and obtaining routine laboratory data [50].

Essential hypertension affects a large portion of people in this country. The highest prevalence is found in black males, but virtually all ethnic

Table 3–17. *Major Causes of Hypertension*

Cause	Percent of Cases
Essential hypertension	90
Secondary hypertension:	10
Renal artery stenosis*	
Renal parenchymal disease*	
Primary hyperaldosteronism	
Pheochromocytoma	
Aortic coarctation	
Cushing's syndrome	
Renin-producing tumors	

*The more common causes of secondary hypertension.

groups are involved. Since hypertension, hyperlipidemia, smoking, family history, and diabetes are the major risk factors for symptomatic cardiovascular disease, evaluation of hypertension must include evaluation of these other risk factors. Essential hypertension generally involves patients 30 to 50 years of age at onset, is usually asymptomatic (a point that must be stressed in conversations with patients), is usually mild in nature (although it may, in fact, be the most common predisposing cause for malignant hypertension), is usually easily controlled, and has a familial predisposition. Patients may be assigned a working diagnosis of essential hypertension when major secondary causes of hypertension have been easily eliminated. It must be stressed, however, that a departure from the usual symptomatology of essential hypertension discussed earlier should provoke a more thorough search for secondary causes of hypertension.

Parenchymal renal disease is a major cause of secondary hypertension. It is usually related to salt and water overload occurring with parenchymal renal disease, but it may be due to increased renin secretion and other factors in a subset of this population. The presence of parenchymal renal disease can be detected on urinalysis and assessment of serum creatinine levels in the majority of patients. Hypertension in this setting must be treated aggressively, since hypertension may accelerate the progression of renal disease.

The major treatable form of secondary hypertension is renovascular hypertension. This must be suspected in all patients who have either severe hypertension or hypertension that comes at an early age, develops at a very late age, or is refractory to therapy. Renal artery atherosclerosis accounts for about 55 percent of renovascular hypertension, and arterial fibromuscular dysplasia is responsible for the remaining 45 percent. In this latter group, most patients are younger than 45 years of age, 90 percent are female, and response to therapy is excellent. Abdominal bruits, elevated plasma renin activities for the rate of urinary sodium excretion, and departure from the usual clinical features of essential hypertension suggest the diagnosis. It must be stressed that in patients who may have this entity it is not excluded with certainty until an arteriographic examination of the renal vessels is performed. Intravenous pyelography (rapid sequence) has been advocated by some in the diagnostic approach for this disorder. However, even though it is 75 percent sensitive, a negative test does not exclude a renal artery stenosis. Renal vein renin determinations, if positive (i.e., showing lateralization), are highly suggestive of surgical cure, but they are not usually routinely employed in the assessment of renovascular hypertension. The reason for this is that a negative study does not exclude a successful response to angioplasty or surgery.

Treatment

The treatment of choice for renal artery stenosis causing renovascular hypertension is surgical correction of the narrowing. This is currently best accomplished through balloon angioplasty, although in some cases a surgical approach must be employed. In certain high-risk patients, however, pharmacologic treatment with angiotensin-converting enzyme inhibitors and other antihypertensive agents may be preferable.

Pheochromocytoma is an unusual cause of hypertension. However, since it is usually accompanied by extremely severe hypertension and is amenable to surgical therapy, it must be considered. Paroxysmal or markedly labile hypertension, episodes of tachycardia, sweating, tremor, and headache, glucose intolerance and weight loss, and orthostatic hypotension should suggest this diagnosis. The appropriate screening test for pheochromocytoma is a urine collection for a combination of vanillylmandelic acid (VMA), metanephrines, and catecholamines. CT scanning is appropriate if a positive urine test is discovered.

Coarctation of the aorta should be considered in all young patients and even adults with hypertension. The appropriate screening test is physical examination where the leg blood pressure is lower than the arm blood pressure. Femoral artery pulses may be decreased or not palpable with this lesion. Chest radiography may reveal rib notching.

Primary aldosteronism and Cushing's disease are causes of secondary hypertension. These lesions cause hypertension via salt and water overload as a consequence of excess mineralocorticoid activity. Peripheral renin levels are usually suppressed in this disease. The diagnosis must be suspected in patients who have low serum potassium levels in the absence of diuretics or extremely low plasma potassium concentrations on diuretics (2.5 mEq/liter). The more thorough approach to the diagnosis of this disease involves determining nonsuppressible aldosterone levels with volume-expansion maneuvers and the presence of suppressed renin activity with volume-depletion maneuvers. CT scanning, again, is used to demonstrate the presence of tumors responsible for these endocrinopathies. These disorders are discussed in greater detail in Chapter 7.

In some patients with hypertension, the clinical presentation may be extremely severe. A syndrome of markedly high blood pressures with evidence of acute vascular injury has been termed *malignant hypertension*. This diagnosis is established by the presence of retinal hemorrhages and exudates in the presence of extremely high blood pressures, usually diastolic blood pressure greater than 140 mmHg. Some investigators require the presence of papilledema to make this diagnosis. The syndrome is often associated with evidence of ventricular decompensation, renal insufficiency, and severe neurologic symptoms. Malignant hypertension must be treated aggressively by decreasing blood pressure to safe levels with intravenous administration of antihypertensives. The preferred drug for this syndrome is nitroprusside, which can be infused by vein and can be titrated to maintain the diastolic blood pressure at about 100 mmHg. Rapid lowering of the blood pressure to normal levels in this syndrome may be accompanied by evidence of cerebrovascular insufficiency. Azotemia accompanying malignant hypertension will often worsen during initial treatment, but in the majority of patients it will improve later with such therapy. Malignant hypertension constitutes a true medical emergency and must therefore be managed aggressively.

Hypertension is best treated on an individual basis. Recent data have accumulated suggesting that normalization of blood pressure is beneficial even in patients with mild hypertension (diastolic blood pressures ranging from 90 to 95 mmHg) [24]. In such patients, however, nonpharmacologic therapy including salt restriction, weight loss, and increases in aerobic exercise may be sufficient to normalize blood pressure [42]. Pharmacologic therapy of hypertension is usually administered in a so-called step-care pattern. This involves initiating therapy with either a diuretic, usually of the thiazide class, or a beta blocker as the first approach. If a diuretic is chosen as step 1 but is insufficient to normalize blood pressure, either a beta blocker or a centrally acting drug is administered (step 2). In more severe cases, a third drug (step 3), usually a vasodilator, is added. It should be stressed that all medications used in the treatment of hypertension have their own complications. Table 3-18 lists the most commonly employed antihypertensives and common complications associated with such drugs [55].

Table 3–18. *Complications of Antihypertensive Medications*

Agent	Common Complications
Diuretics:	
Thiazide diuretics	Hypokalemia, metabolic alkalosis, glucose intolerance, hyperuricemia, volume depletion
Loop diuretics (e.g., furosemide)	Hypokalemia, metabolic alkalosis, hyperuricemia, volume depletion
Potassium-sparing diuretics (e.g., spironolactone, amioride, triamterene)	Hyperkalemia, renal tubular acidosis
Centrally acting drugs:	
Alpha-methyldopa	Impotence, orthostasis, hemolytic anemia
Clonidine	Somnolence, withdrawal syndrome
Vasodilators:	
Hydralazine	Drug-induced lupus, tachycardia
Minoxidil	Tachycardia, pericardial effusion
Converting-enzyme inhibitors:	
Captopril	Hyperkalemia, leukopenia, proteinuria
Beta-blocking agents	Cardiac failure, hyperkalemia, precipitate sick-sinus syndrome

References

1. Alexander, E. A., and Levinsky, N. G. An extrarenal mechanism: potassium adaptation. *J. Clin. Invest.* 47: 740, 1968.
2. Alfrey, A. C. Chronic Renal Failure: Manifestations and Pathogenesis. In R. W. Schrier (Ed.), *Renal and Electrolyte Disorders.* Boston: Little, Brown, 1986. Pp. 461–494.
3. Anderson, R. J., Linas, S. L., Berns, A. J., et al. Nonoliguric acute renal failure. *N. Engl. J. Med.* 296: 1134, 1977.
4. Arieff, A. I., and Guisandi, R. Effects on the central nervous system of hypernatremic and hyponatremic states. *Kidney Int.* 10: 104, 1976.
5. Ayus, J. C., Krothapelli, R. K., and Anett, A.

I. Changing concepts in treatment of severe symptomatic hyponatremia: Rapid correction and possible relation to central pontine myelinolysis. *Am. J. Med.* 78: 897, 1984.
6. Batlle, D. C., Arruda, J. A. L., and Kurtzman, N. A. Hyperkalemia distal renal tubular acidosis associated with obstructive uropathy. *N. Engl. J. Med.* 304: 373, 1981.
7. Bishop, R. L., and Weisfeldt, M. L. Sodium bicarbonate administration during cardiac arrest. *J.A.M.A.* 235: 506, 1976.
8. Brezin, J. H., Katz, S. M., Schwartz, A. B., and Chinitz, J. L. Reversible renal failure and nephrotic syndrome associated with nonsteroidal

anti-inflammatory drugs. *N. Engl. J. Med.* 301: 1271, 1979.

9. Coe, F. L., Kerk, J., and Norton, E. R.   The natural history of calcium urolithiasis. *J.A.M.A.* 238: 1519, 1977.

10. Coggins, C., and The Collaborative Nephrotic Syndrome Study Group.   A controlled study of short-term prednisone in adults with membranous nephropathy: Collaborative study of the adult nephrotic syndrome. *N. Engl. J. Med.* 301: 1301, 1979.

11. Cohen, D. J., Sherman, W. H., Osserman, E. F., and Appel, G. B.   Acute renal failure in patients with multiple myeloma. *Am. J. Med.* 76: 247, 1984.

12. Cotran, R. S., Tolkoff-Rubin, R. H., and Tolkoff-Rubin, W. E.   Tubulointerstitial Diseases. In B. M. Brenner and F. C. Rector (Eds.), *The Kidney.* Philadelphia: Saunders, 1986. Pp. 1143–1174.

13. Cunningham, J., Fraber, L. S., Clemens, T. L., et al.   Chronic acidosis with metabolic base disease: Effect of alkalosis on base morphology and vitamin D metabolism. *Am. J. Med.* 73: 199, 1982.

14. Defronzo, R. A., Sherwin, R. J., Dillingham, M., Hendle, R., Tarmborlane, W. V., and Felig, P.   Influence of basal insulin and glucagon secretion on potassium and sodium metabolism: Studies with somatostatin in normal dogs and normal and diabetic human beings. *J. Clin. Invest.* 61: 472, 1978.

15. Dirks, J. H., and Alfrey, A. C.   Normal and Abnormal Magnesium Metabolism. In R. W. Schrier (Ed.), *Renal and Electrolyte Disorders.* Boston: Little, Brown, 1986. Pp. 331–360.

16. Donadio, J. V., Holley, K. E., Ferguson, R. H., and Ilstrup, D. M.   Treatment of diffuse proliferative lupus nephritis with prednisone and combined prednisone and cyclophosphamide. *N. Engl. J. Med.* 299: 1151, 1978.

17. Donadio, J. V., Anderson, C. F., Mitchell, J. C., et al.   Membranoproliferative glomerulonephritis: A prospective clinical trial of platelet inhibitor therapy. *N. Engl. J. Med.* 310: 1421, 1984.

18. Duffy, J., Lidsky, M. D., Sharp, J. T., et al.   Polyarteritis and hepatitis B. *Medicine* 55: 19, 1976.

19. Ellenbogen, P. H., Scheible, F. W., Talmer, L. B., and Leopold, G. R.   Sensitivity of gray scale ultrasound in detecting urinary tract obstruction. *Am. J. Roentgenol.* 130: 731, 1978.

20. Emmett, M., and Narins, R. G.   Clinical use of the anion gap. *Medicine* 56: 38, 1977.

21. Fang, L. S. T., Sirota, R. A., Ebert, T. H., and Lichtenstein, W. S.   Low fractional excretion of sodium with contrast medium induced acute renal failure. *Ann. Intern. Med.* 140: 531, 1980.

22. Fauci, A. S., Haynes, B. F., and Katz, P.   The spectrum of vasculitis: Clinical, pathologic, immunologic and therapeutic considerations. *Ann. Intern. Med.* 89: 660, 1978.

23. Fauci, A. S., Katz, P., Haynes, B. F., and Wolfe, S. M.   Cyclophosphamide therapy of severe necrotizing vasculitis. *N. Engl. J. Med.* 301: 235, 1979.

24. Frohlich, E. D.   Treatment of Hypertension: The Case for Pharmacologic Treatment. In R. G. Norris (Ed.), *Controversies in Nephrology and Hypertension.* New York: Churchill-Livingstone, 1984. Pp. 93–108.

25. Gabow, P. A., Ikle, D. W., and Holmes, J. H.   Polycystic kidney disease: Premortem analysis of nonazotemic patients and family members. *Ann. Intern. Med.* 101: 238, 1986.

26. Gabow, P. A., and Peterson, L. S.   Disorder of Potassium Metabolism. In R. W. Schrier (Ed.), *Renal and Electrolyte Disorders.* Boston: Little, Brown, 1986. Pp. 207–250.

27. Glassock, R. J., Cohen, A. H., Adler, S., and Ward, H.   Primary Glomerular Diseases. In B. M. Brenner and F. C. Rector (Eds.), *The Kidney.* Philadelphia: Saunders, 1986. Pp. 1014–1084.

28. Graziani, G., Cantaluppi, A., Casati, S., et al.   Dopamine and furosemide in oliguric acute renal failure. *Nephron* 37: 39, 1984.

29. Gutman, R. A., Striker, G. E., Gilliland, B. C., et al.   The immune complex glomerulonephritis of bacterial endocarditis. *Medicine* 51: 1, 1972.

30. Hazard, P. B., and Griffin, J. P.   Sodium bicarbonate in the management of systemic acidosis. *South. Med. J.* 73: 1339, 1980.

31. Heat, J. G., and Nielsen, C. P.   Serum aluminum in hemodialysis patients: Relation to osteodystrophy, encephalopathy and aluminum hydroxide consumption. *Miner Electrolyte Metab.* 10: 345, 1984.

32. Himathongham, T., Dluhy, R. G., and Williams, G. H.   Potassium-aldosterone-renin interrelationships. *J. Clin. Endocrinol. Metab.* 41: 153, 1975.

33. Hostetter, H. T., Rennke, H. G., and Brenner, B. M.   The case for intrarenal hypertension in the initiation and progression of diabetes and other glomerulopathies. *Am. J. Med.* 72: 375, 1982.

34. Hostetter, T. H. Diabetic Nephropathy. In B. M. Brenner and F. C. Rector (Eds.), *The Kidney.* Philadelphia: Saunders, 1986. Pp. 1377–1402.

35. Hou, S. H., Bushinksky, D. A., Wish, J. B., Cohen, J. J., and Harrington, J. T. Hospital-acquired renal insufficiency. *Am. J. Med.* 74: 243, 1983.

36. Hutt, M. P., and Kelleher, S. P. Proteinuria and the Nephrotic Syndrome. In R. W. Schrier (Ed.), *Renal and Electrolyte Disorders.* Boston: Little, Brown, 1986. Pp. 565–590.

37. Ibels, L. J., Alfrey, A. C., Haut, L., et al. Preservation of function in experimental renal disease by dietary restriction of phosphate. *N. Engl. J. Med.* 298: 122, 1978.

38. Jamison, R. L., and Oliver, R. E. Disorders of urinary concentration and dilution. *Am. J. Med.* 72: 308, 1982.

39. Kaehny, W. D., and Gabow, P. A. Pathogenesis and Management of Metabolic Acidosis and Alkalosis in Renal and Electrolyte Disorders. In R. W. Schrier (Ed.), *Renal and Electrolyte Disorders.* Boston: Little, Brown, 1986. Pp. 141–186.

40. Kaehny, W. D., and Gabow, P. A. Pathogenesis and Management of Respiratory Acidosis and Alkalosis in Renal and Electrolyte Disorders. In R. W. Schrier (Ed.), *Renal and Electrolyte Disorders.* Boston: Little, Brown, 1986. Pp. 187–206.

41. Kaplan, A. A., Longnecker, R. E., and Folkert, V. W. Continuous arteriovenous hemofiltration. *Ann. Intern. Med.* 100: 358, 1984.

42. Kaplan, N. M. Treatment of Hypertension: The Case for Non-drug Treatment. In R. G. Norris (Ed.), *Controversies in Nephrology and Hypertension.* New York: Churchill-Livingstone, 1984. Pp. 73–92.

43. Kleinschmidt-deMasters, B. K., and Nurenberg, M. D. Rapid correction of hyponatremia causes demyelination: Relation to central pontine myelinolysis. *Science* 211: 1068, 1981.

44. Knochel, J. P. The pathophysiology and clinical characteristics of severe hypophosphatemia. *Arch. Intern. Med.* 85: 23, 1976.

45. Kohler, P. F., Cronin, R. E., Hammond, W. S., et al. Chronic membranous glomerulonephritis caused by hepatitis B antigen-antibody immune complexes. *Ann. Intern. Med.* 81: 448, 1974.

46. Kreisberg, R. A. Lactate homeostasis and lactic acidosis. *Ann. Intern. Med.* 92: 227, 1980.

47. Kurtzman, N. A. Acquired distal renal tubular acidosis. *Kidney Int.* 24: 807, 1983.

48. Linton, A. L., Clark, W. F., Driedser, A. A., Turnbull, D. I., and Lindsay, R. M. Allergic interstitial nephritis due to drugs. *Ann. Intern. Med.* 93: 735, 1980.

49. Manis, T., and Friedman, E. A. Dialysis therapy for irreversible uremia. *N. Engl. J. Med.* 301: 1260, 1979.

50. Maronde, R. F. The hypertensive patient: An algorithm for diagnostic workup. *J.A.M.A.* 233: 992, 1975.

51. Massry, S. G., and Seelig, M. S. Hypomagnesemia and hypermagnesemia. *Clin. Nephrol.* 7: 147, 1977.

52. Miller, T. R., Anderson, R. J., Linas, S. L., et al. Urinary diagnostic indices in acute renal failure: A prospective study. *Ann. Intern. Med.* 89: 47, 1978.

53. Morris, R. C. Renal tubular acidosis. *N. Engl. J. Med.* 304: 418, 1981.

54. Narins, R. G., and Cohen, J. J. Bicarbonate therapy for organic acidosis: The case for its continued use. *Ann. Intern. Med.* 106: 615, 1987.

55. Nies, A. J. Clinical pharmacology of antihypertensive drugs. *Med. Clin. North Am.* 61: 675, 1977.

56. Oh., M. S., and Carroll, H. J. The anion gap. *N. Engl. J. Med.* 297: 814, 1977.

57. Pak, C. Y. C., Britton, F., Pederson, R., et al. Ambulatory evaluation of nephrolithiasis: Clinical presentation and diagnostic criteria. *Am. J. Med.* 69: 19, 1980.

58. Ponticelli, C., Zucchelli, P., Imbasciati, E., et al. Controlled trial of methylprednisolone and chlorambucil in idiopathic membranous nephropathy. *N. Engl. J. Med.* 310: 946, 1984.

59. Popovtzer, M. M., and Knochel, J. P. Disorders of Calcium, Phosphorus, Vitamin D and Parathyroid Hormone Activity. In R. W. Schrier (Ed.), *Renal and Electrolyte Disorders.* Boston: Little, Brown, 1986. Pp. 223–298.

60. Ramen, L., Wise, B., Goodman, J. R., et al. Renal disease with *Staphylococcus albus* bacteremia: A complication associated with infected ventriculoatrial shunt. *J.A.M.A.* 212: 1671, 1970.

61. Rasmussen, H. H., and Ibels, L. S. Acute renal failure: Multifactorial analysis of causes and risk factors. *Am. J. Med.* 73: 211, 1981.

62. Ratcliffe, P. J., Dunnill, M. S., and Oliver, D. O. Clinical importance of acquired cystic diseases of the kidney in patients undergoing dialysis. *Br. Med. J.* 287: 1855, 1983.

63. Rosa, R. M., Silva, P., Young, J. B., et al. Adrenergic modulation of extrarenal potassium disposal. *N. Engl. J. Med.* 302: 431, 1980.

64. Rose, B. D. Clinical Use of Diuretics. In B. M. Brenner and J. H. Stein (Eds.), *Body Fluid Homeostasis*. New York: Churchill-Livingstone, 1987. Pp. 409–438.

65. Schambelan, M., Sebastian, A., and Biglieri, E. G. Prevalence, pathogenesis and functional significance of aldosterone deficiency and hyperkalemic patients with chronic renal insufficiency. *Kidney Int.* 17: 89, 1980.

66. Schrier, R. W. Acute renal failure. *Kidney Int.* 15: 205, 1979.

67. Schrier, R. W. Acute renal failure. *Hosp. Pract.* 3: 93, 1981.

68. Schrier, R. W., and Anderson, R. J. Renal Sodium Excretion, Edematous Disorders and Diuretic Use. In R. W. Schrier (Ed.), *Renal and Electrolyte Disorders*. Boston: Little, Brown, 1986. Pp. 79–140.

69. Schrier, R. W., and Berl, T. Disorders of Water Metabolism. In R. W. Schrier (Ed.), *Renal and Electrolyte Disorders*. Boston: Little, Brown, 1986. Pp. 1–78.

70. Skorecki, K. L., and Brenner, B. M. Body fluid homeostasis in man: A contemporary overview. *Am. J. Med.* 70: 77, 1981.

71. Siegel, N. G., and Hayslett, J. P. Renal Involvement in Systemic Lupus Erythematosus. W. W. Suki and G. Eknoyan (Ed.), *The Kidney in Systemic Disease*. New York: John Wiley & Sons, 1981. Pp. 55–76.

72. Slatopulsky, E., Rutherford, W. E., Rosenbaum, R., Martin, K., and Hruska, K. Hyperphosphatemia. *Clin. Nephrol.* 17: 138, 1977.

73. Swann, R. L., and Merrill, J. P. The clinical course of acute renal failure. *Medicine* 32: 215, 1953.

74. Walser, M., Mitch, W. E., and Collier, V. U. The effect of nutritional therapy on the course of chronic renal failure. *Clin. Nephrol.* 11: 66, 1979.

75. Williams, H. E. Nephrolithiasis. *N. Engl. J. Med.* 290: 33, 1974.

76. Wilson, D. R., and Schrier, R. W. Obstructive Nephropathy: Pathophysiology and Management. In R. W. Schrier (Ed.), *Renal and Electrolyte Disorders*. Boston: Little, Brown, 1986. Pp. 495–526.

77. Zeisler, T. W., Talner, C. B., and Blantz, R. C. Cystic Diseases of the Kidney. In B. M. Brenner and F. C. Rector (Eds.), *The Kidney*. Philadelphia: Saunders, 1986. Pp. 1872–1905.

Gastro-intestinal Disease

4

John Schaefer and Andrew Mallory

New medical information is accumulating at an almost overwhelming pace. Nowhere are these important changes occurring faster than in the field of gastroenterology. In this section we attempt to present a concise assessment of current concepts in basic pathophysiology, diagnosis, and treatment. Since gastroenterology is the broadest subspecialty in internal medicine, we have limited coverage to the areas of greatest clinical importance.

Acute Gastrointestinal Tract Hemorrhage

Acute gastrointestinal tract hemorrhage may be life-threatening. Fortunately, bleeding stops spontaneously in most patients during the course of general resuscitative procedures. Specific interventive measures, including surgery, are required only for a small minority of patients with persistent bleeding. Since patients continuing to bleed cannot be identified initially with certainty, all patients should be managed with combined medical and surgical consultation. Although modern diagnostic and therapeutic procedures are ever-improving, the overall mortality rate with acute gastrointestinal tract hemorrhage has remained near 10 percent over the past three decades. This unimproved mortality rate is deceptive because the more recent series of patients include a greater number of high-risk patients over age 60 and many with severe associated medical conditions [15,34].

Initial Assessment
The first priority in a hemorrhaging patient is to estimate the magnitude of blood loss. This is best assessed by carefully checking the vital signs and postural changes. All physical signs may remain normal with acute blood loss up to 500 ml. If acute bleeding continues to the range of 1000 ml, signs of hypovolemia develop, as indicated by a postural fall in systolic blood pressure of greater than 10 mmHg and a rise in pulse rate. In addition, patients are often anxious and show a delayed capillary refill of greater than 2 seconds. Acute blood loss of 2000 ml or more usually causes clinical shock. The systolic blood pressure is below 90 mmHg, and patients are pale, clammy, restless, and often mentally confused.

Acute Management
As soon as possible, one or two large-bore intravenous access lines are placed and blood is dispatched for type and crossmatch. Intravenous crystalloid therapy, usually with normal saline, is started immediately. Whole blood transfusions are started in patients in shock and in those with persistent postural changes and oliguria. Patients with coagulopathy may benefit from intravenous fresh-frozen plasma, platelet packs, and packed red blood cells. Intravenous therapy is continued

with variable vigor until blood volume is restored and hemorrhage ceases. Most clinicians prefer that the posthemorrhage hematocrit stabilize at no lower than 30 percent.

After a plan for resuscitative fluids has been instituted, a pertinent history and physical examination will reveal the status of the patient's general health and provide clues as to the source of hemorrhage. Hematemesis indicates that the site of bleeding is proximal to the ligament of Treitz. Melena also means an upper gastrointestinal source of hemorrhage with only rare exception. Massive upper intestinal hemorrhage may present with red blood per rectum, usually without clots. These patients often show signs of hypovolemia and usually have fresh blood in the nasogastric aspirate. Patients with bright red blood clots per rectum and stable vital signs probably have a lower intestinal bleeding site.

Prediction of the specific bleeding lesion from the history and physical examination is imprecise but still a worthy effort. Peptic ulcers are suspected in patients with true peptic symptoms or "indigestion" for which they take frequent antacids. Patients who abuse alcohol or who take nonsteroidal anti-inflammatory agents are candidates for erosive gastritis or gastric ulcers. Repetitive emesis or dry heaves often signal the presence of Mallory-Weiss esophageal tears. Findings of chronic liver disease always raise the possibility of variceal hemorrhage. Lower intestinal hemorrhage in an otherwise asymptomatic older patient suggests bleeding from either a colonic diverticulum or a right-sided colonic angiodysplasia. When all findings seem unrevealing, consider unusual causes of intestinal bleeding such as familial hemorrhagic telangiectasia, pseudoxanthoma elastica, and Meckel's diverticulum.

Ongoing Monitoring

A large nasogastric or orogastric tube, size 24F or larger, should be placed in all patients with upper gastrointestinal tract hemorrhage. The large caliber is necessary to remove clotted blood from the stomach; smaller tubes cannot adequately evac-

uate gastric contents and may provide misleading information. Initial irrigation is continued until all accumulated clots have been removed. Frequent irrigations thereafter, about every 15 minutes, provide an excellent on-line monitor for continuing hemorrhage and keep the stomach clear for an early diagnostic study or surgery. Saline or tap water may be used, and the fluid need not be chilled. Lavage is primarily for monitoring, and no therapeutic benefit is anticipated. Vital signs, urine output, and appearance of lavage fluid are recorded at frequent intervals.

Although a hematocrit is often one of the first tests obtained in patients with intestinal hemorrhage, it does not accurately assess the magnitude of acute blood loss. From a single episode of bleeding it takes approximately 8 hours for the hematocrit level to fall one-half its ultimate drop; this time is substantially shortened by intravenous fluid administration. For the same reason, a falling hematocrit by itself does not necessarily indicate ongoing hemorrhage. This delay in equilibration must be kept in mind for any useful interpretation of the hematocrit values.

These events should be recorded on a flowsheet or by frequent progress notes so that all the personnel caring for the patient have ready access to the same complete and accurate information. Virtually all the acute-care decisions in patients with upper gastrointestinal tract hemorrhage are made within 24 to 48 hours of admission.

Diagnosis

When the patient has stabilized and overt hemorrhage has ceased, an early diagnostic procedure is often advised. Fiberoptic panendoscopy, the diagnostically most accurate procedure for upper tract hemorrhage, is particularly valuable in selected high-risk patients. This includes most patients over age 60 and those with suspected hemorrhage from esophageal varices, gastric erosions, or a gastroesophageal mucosal tear. Younger patients and those with peptic symptoms are well assessed with an initial barium x-ray study. The early diagnosis of the source of bleeding allows for an appropriate choice of therapy if bleeding resumes. For instance, intravenous vasopressin or placement of a Sengstaken-Blakemore tube would be of no value and even of potential harm for a patient with a bleeding peptic ulcer.

Special problems are created by the small number of patients with unremitting massive hemorrhage. It is not possible to outline a standard approach for such patients. Decisions about attempting diagnostic procedures and performing emergency surgery must be individualized. Important considerations include the patient's age, associated medical conditions, ability to cooperate, probable source of hemorrhage, and hemodynamic stability. Opinions on approach among the attending physicians are seldom unanimous. It is occasionally useful to endoscope an uncooperative patient with persistent hemorrhage after induction of anesthesia with the airway protected by endotracheal intubation. Some general guidelines for emergency surgery to control ongoing hemorrhage include (1) need for transfusion of more than 5 units of blood in the first 24 hours of hospitalization, (2) need for more than 3 units of blood in the second 24 hours, and (3) clinically important rebleeding after bleeding has ceased for at least 24 hours. Early surgery is favored for patients over age 60 and for those with point-source hemorrhage from a peptic ulcer or Mallory-Weiss tear. Emergency surgery for erosive gastritis and variceal hemorrhage is undertaken with less enthusiasm.

The frequency of upper tract bleeding lesions varies between institutions depending on the population served. In all hospitals, hemorrhage from peptic ulcers is most common. Hospitals serving a population with a high prevalence of alcoholism see many patients with erosive gastritis, esophageal varices, and Mallory-Weiss lesions with a combined frequency exceeding hemorrhage from peptic ulcers. Unusual causes of hemorrhage such as heritable and acquired vascular lesions, hematologic, and vasculitic syndromes are more likely referred to tertiary care centers.

Acute colonic bleeding is usually manifest by red blood with clots per rectum. Postural signs are often absent, and nasogastric aspirate is free of blood. Early proctoscopic examination is valuable to exclude bleeding from hemorrhoids, inflammatory bowel disease, and rectosigmoid ischemia. Normal rectal mucosa and blood streaming from above indicates a more proximal lesion. As with upper intestinal tract lesions, bleeding usually stops spontaneously. Patients may then be prepared by catharsis for a barium enema or colonoscopy. If hemorrhage does not stop, a diagnostic angiogram or one of several radioisotope scanning procedures may localize the bleeding site. The diagnostic procedure of choice is best determined by local expertise and experience. Identification of the site is particularly beneficial should the patient require surgery for uncontrolled hemorrhage. This localization permits a hemicolectomy and spares the patient the increased morbidity of a total colectomy. Inflammatory bowel disease, angiodysplasia, and diverticular disease, often of the right side of the colon, are the most common sources of large-volume hemorrhage. Infrequently, a large polyp or an ulcerated colonic cancer presents with overt hemorrhage. In young adults, a Meckel's diverticulum must be kept in mind.

Diarrheal States

Diarrhea is defined as an abnormal increase in stool liquidity usually accompanied by an increase in daily stool weight (>200 gm) and frequency. Acute diarrhea has been present for less than 3 weeks; chronic diarrhea has been present for 3 or more weeks [33].

Most diarrhea can be classified as due to one or a combination of four mechanisms. In *osmotic diarrhea* (e.g., lactase deficiency, antacid therapy), the presence of poorly absorbed osmotically active solutes in the gut lumen results in a net influx of fluid into the bowel lumen. Stool fluid analysis reveals an osmotic gap; that is, [Na] + [K] × 2 is less than the osmolality of the stool as measured by freezing-point depression. Osmotic diarrhea characteristically ceases when the patient fasts. In *secretory diarrhea* (e.g., bile salt-induced, enterotoxins), net intestinal ion absorption is inhibited or intestinal ion secretion is stimulated. Diarrhea will continue even when the patient fasts. In *exudative diarrhea* (e.g., ulcerative colitis, shigellosis), there is an outpouring of mucus, blood, and protein from the inflamed intestinal mucosal surface. In diarrhea due to *deranged intestinal motility* (e.g., irritable bowel syndrome, postvagotomy syndrome), fluid stools may result from intestinal "hurry."

Acute Diarrhea

DIAGNOSIS

A listing of the more common causes of acute diarrhea appears in Table 4-1. Acute diarrhea of several days' duration, especially in an epidemic setting without high fever, rectal bleeding, or a history of travel, suggests a viral etiology. A bacterial cause (e.g., *Salmonella, Shigella, Campylobacter*) is suggested by high fever and bloody stools [3]. When the history suggests food poisoning, *Staphylococcus aureus* or *Clostridium perfringens* are most likely. Diarrhea caused by parasites (primar-

Table 4–1. *Common Causes of Acute Diarrhea*

Viral (e.g., Norwalk, Rotavirus)
Bacterial:
  Food poisoning (especially *Staphylococcus aureus,*
    Clostridium perfringens)
  Other:
    Salmonella
    Shigella
    Campylobacter
    E. coli
    Yersinia
    Vibrio parahemolyticus
Parasitic (e.g., *Entamoeba histolytica, Giardia lamblia*)
Drugs:
  Antacids
  Antibiotics
  Lactulose
  Chemotherapeutic agents

ily *Giardia lamblia* and *Entamoeba histolytica*) may present acutely, but it is more commonly chronic and will be discussed below. Drugs may cause acute or chronic diarrhea and will be discussed below.

A history of recent travel outside the United States, especially to tropical countries, suggests "traveler's diarrhea." Most commonly, toxigenic *E. coli* are responsible, but other organisms, including viruses, *Salmonella, Shigella, Campylobacter, Giardia,* and *Entamoeba,* are also seen. In the homosexual patient, rectal involvement with herpes, syphilis, gonorrhea, and chlamydia also must be considered.

In the patient with acute diarrhea, the physical examination is most useful in determining the state of hydration. The presence of gross or occult blood in the stool on rectal examination will suggest a bacterial (or amebic) etiology. Proctosigmoidoscopic examination may reveal specific (e.g., pseudomembranes of antibiotic-induced diarrhea) or nonspecific, but helpful findings (e.g., ulcers with normal intervening mucosa in amebiasis).

In the acute setting, a liquid stool for culture and examination for white blood cells and ova/parasites is most helpful. "Routine" stool cultures are usually adequate for most bacterial pathogens, but special cultures will be necessary if *Yersinia* and herpes are suspected. The presence of white blood cells in large numbers suggests mucosal inflammation (*Salmonella, Shigella, Campylobacter, Entamoeba,* pseudomembranous enterocolitis). Ova and parasite examinations are helpful if positive, but they are frequently negative, especially in the presence of *Giardia* infection. A fresh stool specimen (examined within 1 hour) is important when amebiasis is suspected. Stool assays for *Clostridium difficile* toxin may be useful. Serologic tests for *Entamoeba histolytica* and lymphogranuloma venereum may be necessary.

TREATMENT AND PROGNOSIS

General supportive measures include maintenance of hydration (oral fluids, especially carbohydrate-electrolyte mixtures), a low-lactose diet, and antidiarrheal agents (kaolin, pectin). Antidiarrheal agents that slow motility (e.g., loperamide, diphenoxylate) are relatively contraindicated in the presence of fever or rectal bleeding in view of evidence that certain bacterial diarrheal illnesses may be prolonged by these drugs.

Specific treatment will obviously depend on the underlying diagnosis. Salmonellosis requires only supportive treatment; antibiotics may prolong symptoms and intestinal carriage of organisms. However, with severe symptoms or if bacteremia or enteric fever is present, antibiotics are indicated (ampicillin, 1 to 2 gm per day; trimethoprim, 160 mg, and sulfamethoxazole, 800 mg, every 12 hours). Shigellosis is also usually self-limited, but with severe symptoms, the same antibiotics are indicated. In *Campylobacter* infections, erythromycin, 2 gm per day, appears to be useful in severe or prolonged infections. In giardiasis, quinacrine, 300 mg per day, and metronidazole, 750 mg per day, appear to be equally effective. In intestinal amebiasis, metronidazole, 750 mg tid, plus iodoquinol, 650 mg tid, should be used. Simply withdrawing the antibiotic may suffice in patients with mild symptoms of pseudomembranous enterocolitis caused by *Clostridium difficile.* If symptoms persist or are severe, metronidazole, 500 mg orally tid, or vancomycin, 125 mg orally qid, are usually effective.

Traveler's diarrhea is usually a mild, self-limited infection that requires no specific treatment. Bismuth subsalicylate (Pepto-Bismol) in large doses, 60 ml PO qid, may provide symptomatic improvement.

Chronic Diarrhea

Table 4-2 lists the more common causes of chronic diarrhea.

DIAGNOSIS

A detailed clinical history is often the single most important task of the physician in arriving at a diagnosis of the cause of chronic diarrhea. Frequent, small-volume diarrhea suggests a colonic

Table 4–2. Common Causes of Chronic Diarrhea

Infections:
  Immunocompetent patient:
    Bacterial: *Clostridium difficile*
    Parasitic: *Giardia lamblia, Entamoeba histolytica*
  Immunocompromised patient (e.g., acquired immune deficiency syndrome):
    Cryptosporidiosis, *Mycobacterium avium intracellulare,* cytomegalovirus
Drugs: especially antibiotics, antacids, lactulose, chemotherapeutic agents
Malabsorption: e.g., nontropical sprue, pancreatic insufficiency, lactase deficiency, bacterial overgrowth, Whipple's disease
Endocrine disorders: diabetes, hyperthyroidism
Irritable (functional) bowel disease
Inflammatory bowel disease: Crohn's disease, chronic ulcerative colitis
Other:
  Hormone-secreting tumors: gastrinoma, carcinoid, pancreatic cholera syndrome
  Colon carcinoma or other obstruction
  Colonic villous adenoma
  Laxative abuse
  Postoperative: after vagotomy, short bowel

source; less frequent, large-volume stools indicate a small bowel source. Alternating constipation and diarrhea suggest the irritable bowel syndrome.

Evidence of gastrointestinal bleeding suggests pseudomembranous enterocolitis, amebiasis, inflammatory bowel disease, or colon carcinoma. Marked weight loss and an "oil slick" in the toilet water, evidence of vitamin or mineral deficiencies, suggest malabsorption. Symptoms of arthritis are seen when diarrhea is due to inflammatory bowel disease, Whipple's disease, or *Yersinia* infection. Fever may suggest inflammatory bowel disease, lymphoma, infection, or Whipple's disease.

The findings on physical examination of fever, arthritis, and evidence of marked weight loss or occult blood in the stools suggest those conditions described above. Postural hypotension is seen with diabetes, amyloidosis, and Addison's disease causing diarrhea, but diarrheal fluid losses from any cause can be associated with volume depletion and orthostatic hypotension. Erythema nodosum or pyoderma gangrenosum suggests an inflammatory bowel disease. Other associations include hyperpigmentation with Whipple's disease, celiac sprue with Addison's disease, evidence of atherosclerosis (congestive heart failure, absent arterial pulses) with ischemic bowel, hepatomegaly with inflammatory bowel disease and lymphoma, and evidence of neuropathy with diabetes and amyloidosis.

With respect to laboratory findings, the presence of white blood cells on a fecal smear suggests *Clostridium difficile*-induced diarrhea or inflammatory bowel disease. A microscopic examination of liquid stool is needed to diagnose a chronic parasitic infection (see above). In the immunocompromised patient, special tests may be required to diagnose crytosporidiosis (stool examination by concentration or modified acid-fast techniques or small bowel biopsy), *Mycobacterium avium intracellulare* (stool culture, acid-fast staining of stool, small bowel biopsy), and cytomegalovirus (histologic demonstration of intranuclear inclusions or viral culture). The laboratory demonstration of malabsorptive disorders is described in detail below.

Alkalinization of the stool may demonstrate the presence of phenolphthalein (a common ingredient of laxatives) and suggest laxative abuse. Specific tests for diabetes and hyperthyroidism are discussed in Chapter 7. Hormone assays are used to diagnose gastrinoma (serum gastrin), carcinoid (urine 5-hydroxyindoleacetic acid), and pancreatic cholera syndrome (vasoactive intestinal polypeptide).

Plain films of the abdomen may detect pancreatic calcifications, which suggest pancreatic insufficiency. The upper gastrointestinal series may be useful in suggesting the short bowel syndrome, malabsorptive states (thickened folds, precipitated barium), or Crohn's disease (narrowed lumen, ulcers). The barium enema may suggest inflammatory bowel disease (see below), colon carcinoma, or laxative abuse (absent haustrations).

TREATMENT AND PROGNOSIS
General supportive measures are discussed above (see Acute Diarrhea). Specific therapy and prognosis obviously will depend on the etiology of the diarrhea and, in general, are described elsewhere in this chapter (Acute Diarrhea, Malabsorption, Irritable Bowel Disease, Inflammatory Bowel Disease) or in Chapters 6 and 7.

Disease of the Esophagus

Gastroesophageal Reflux and Esophagitis
Symptomatic gastroesophageal reflux is common [49]. Heartburn, a burning substernal discomfort, is the most frequent esophageal symptom in patients with reflux of gastroduodenal contents. Many people experience reflux and transient heartburn without demonstrable injury to the distal esophageal mucosa. For some, presumably with more frequent and prolonged reflux, distal esophageal inflammation, friability, erosions, and even deep ulceration may occur. This has recently been called gastroesophageal reflux disease (GERD). Most patients with this disease have reduced pressure in the lower esophageal sphincter. This is often associated with a sliding hiatus hernia, but most patients with hiatus hernia do not have clinically important esophageal reflux. Likewise, not all patients with reduced lower esophageal sphincteric pressure have injurious reflux. Patients with gastroesophageal reflux disease also have delayed esophageal clearance of refluxed material.

CONFIRMING TESTS
Heartburn is a reliable signal for reflux, and there are a variety of confirming tests. The barium esophagogram is a simple but insensitive test. Its main value lies in excluding other causes of esophageal symptoms and demonstrating esophageal strictures and mass lesions. A pH probe in

the distal esophagus reliably detects reflux of acid. This procedure is often performed at the time of esophageal motility testing. More recently, 12- to 24-hour monitoring of esophageal pH in ambulatory patients has quantitated the frequency and duration of spontaneous reflux during normal daily activity. Radioactive scintigraphic techniques for reflux of gastric contents are also available and may be of particular value in assessing small-volume pulmonary aspiration. If intermittent substernal pain is of esophageal origin, perfusion of the distal esophagus with acid (Bernstein's test) may provoke similar discomfort. Finally, fiberoptic esophagoscopy permits excellent visualization of the esophagus for evidence of overt mucosal injury, and mucosal biopsies for histologic examination can be obtained at the same time.

COMPLICATIONS

A small number of patients with gastroesophageal reflux disease develop complications. These complications most often occur in patients with long-standing, neglected esophagitis or in those with injury refractory to treatment. In response to prolonged, deep inflammation, submucosal fibrosis may lead to a distal esophageal stricture. Dysphagia for solids often heralds this stenosis. Another closely allied complication is a penetrating ulcer located at a variable distance from the esophagogastric junction. The ulceration, with or without an associated stricture, occurs in metaplastic columnar epithelium that has replaced the injured esophageal squamous epithelium. This lesion, Barrett's epithelium, carries an increased risk for development of adenocarcinoma. Additional complications of chronic reflux esophagitis include aspiration pneumonia and bleeding (most often low grade and chronic, but overt on occasion).

TREATMENT

Various treatment regimens are used depending on the severity and persistence of findings [6,41]. For patients with infrequent heartburn of recent onset, empiric conservative therapy can first be tried. Basic measures include use of antacids, elevation of the head of the bed on 6-inch blocks, weight loss if the patient is overweight, avoidance of bedtime snacks, and elimination of foods that lower the distal esophageal sphincter pressure, such as chocolate and alcohol. If reflux symptoms do not subside within several weeks on this basic treatment, upper gastrointestinal tract panendoscopy should be done to document the extent of esophageal inflammation, if any, and to exclude other pathology in the stomach and duodenum. An H_2-receptor blocker, e.g., ranitidine, 150 mg bid or 300 mg hs, is then added to the treatment regimen. Sucralfate, 1 gm qid, stimulating prostaglandin-induced cytoprotection, also may be added or substituted for antacids. Most patients will respond, but some do not. Noncompliance is a frequent cause of treatment failure. For patients with refractory symptoms and proven esophagitis, a cholinergic agent (Bethanecol, 10 to 25 mg qid) or, more recently, metoclopramide, 10 mg qid, may be added to augment the lower esophageal sphincter tone and improve gastric emptying. The full program is continued for 3 to 6 months. If symptoms persist and esophagitis is unchanged on endoscopic examination, an antireflux operation is advised. The antireflux procedures are approximately 75 percent successful. Less than 10 percent of compliant patients should require surgery. Other indications for surgery include persistent esophageal stricture, esophageal ulcer (Barrett's esophagus), and rarely, recurrent hemorrhage of esophageal origin. Intermittent esophageal dilatation may be useful for many patients with benign strictures and is essential for those who refuse or have contraindications for surgery.

Esophageal Cancer

Cancer of the esophagus is a particularly distressing disease [13]. Treatment remains controversial, and cure is infrequent. Fortunately, it is not a common cancer. In this country it occurs most often in black men. Etiology is unknown, but incriminated risk factors include abuse of tobacco and alcohol and conditions with chronic esophageal mucosal inflammation, e.g., caustic strictures, Barrett's esophagitis, and the stasis effects of achalasia.

Diagnosis of esophageal cancer is often delayed until late in the course of the disease. The esophagus is a pliable organ, and the cardinal symptom of dysphagia for solids ordinarily occurs only after the tumor has encircled the esophageal lumen. Even then the initial symptoms may be mild and ignored. Constant substernal pain usually reflects mediastinal spread of the tumor. A CT scan of the mediastinum is useful in the preoperative assessment. More than half of all patients are found preoperatively or at time of surgery to have tumor spread beyond the chance for surgical cure.

DIAGNOSIS

Persistent dysphagia must always be investigated. A barium esophagogram readily identifies the level and constricting nature of the lesion. Esophagoscopy with cytology and biopsy provides histologic confirmation of cancer in almost all cases. More than 95 percent of esophageal tumors are squamous cell cancers. Uncommonly, adenocarcinoma may arise from the columnar epithelium of Barrett's esophagus or rarely from the submucosal esophageal glands. Most often adenocarcinoma of the distal esophagus represents extension from gastric cancer.

TREATMENT

Therapy of esophageal cancer is not standardized, and palliation is often the main goal. Cancers of the upper third of the esophagus and most cancers of the middle third are not considered resectable. These patients are palliated with radiation therapy. The distal lesions are treated by surgical resection for palliation of obstructive symptoms and less often for "cure." For patients who are not surgical candidates or who have recurrent disease, esophageal patency may be maintained by mechanical dilation or placement of a hollow prosthesis through the tumorous area. Recently,

palliation by endoscopic laser ablation of the intraluminal tumor has proved useful. Investigational protocols for chemotherapy also may be tried. The 5-year survival rate for esophageal cancer is approximately 5 percent.

Other Esophageal Conditions

ACHALASIA

Achalasia is characterized by a dilated aperistaltic body of the esophagus associated with an idiopathic inflammatory destruction of the intramural autonomic ganglion cells. Manometric studies show increased tone of the lower esophageal sphincter (LES) and failure of relaxation with swallowing. Patients experience dysphagia for both solids and liquids. Esophageal emptying is markedly delayed, and retention may lead to aspiration. Weight loss is common. Brusk balloon dilatation of the lower esophageal sphincter usually relieves the obstructive symptoms. If this procedure fails, a surgical myotomy of the circular musculature of the lower esophageal sphincter is effective.

DIFFUSE ESOPHAGEAL SPASM

Diffuse esophageal spasm (DES) causes severe substernal pain easily confused with that of myocardial ischemia. The pain is caused by prolonged high-pressure nonperistaltic contractions of the body of the esophagus of uncertain cause. The substernal discomfort varies in duration and intensity, and the short-term response to therapeutic maneuvers is often difficult to assess. Some patients seem to benefit from administration of nitroglycerine or calcium-channel blocking agents. In extreme circumstances, a long myotomy (extended Heller procedure) of the middle and distal esophagus may give symptomatic relief.

SCLERODERMA

Esophageal involvement occurs in virtually every patient with scleroderma. The disease process destroys the smooth muscle of the distal esophagus, including the lower esophageal sphincter. Aperistalsis is also present. There is free esophageal reflux, and the patient is subject to all the symptoms and complications of severe gastroesophageal reflux disease. There is no therapy for the underlying process. Vigorous treatment of reflux affords symptomatic relief.

Gastric Carcinoma

Adenocarcinoma is by far the most common malignancy of the stomach [11,36]. Lymphoma, sarcoma, and other rare tumors constitute less than 10 percent of gastric malignancies. Worldwide there is marked geographic variation in the frequency of gastric carcinoma. For instance, the incidence in Japan is more than fivefold greater than the incidence in the United States. No single etiologic agent can be identified for these regional differences, but environmental factors, particularly dietary habits, are most often cited. Second-generation Japanese immigrants to the United States, for example, lose their enhanced propensity for gastric cancer. Fortunately, for unknown reasons, the incidence of gastric cancer in the United States and elsewhere has shown a steady decrease over the past 50 years. The current rate, below 10 per 100,000 population, is less than a third of the rate in 1930. Known risk factors include male sex over age 50, chronic atrophic gastritis (as with pernicious anemia and perhaps years after subtotal gastrectomy), adenomatous gastric polyps greater than 2 cm in size, and possibly blood group type A.

Diagnosis
Early in its course, gastric carcinoma does not produce any symptoms or physical findings. Gastric cancer is generally far-advanced before nonspecific dyspepsia, early satiety, weight loss, or a palpable mass lead to investigation. The diagnosis is usually suggested by radiologic findings and confirmed by gastroscopy with biopsy.

Japanese investigators report the successful diagnosis of gastric cancer in asymptomatic subjects found by endoscopic biopsy surveillance testing. Approximately 40 percent of gastric carcinomas in Japan are slow-growing and limited to the mucosa and submucosa. These tumors are called early gastric cancers, and the cure rate for these superficial lesions is excellent [20]. When these tumors are found by surveillance testing in an asymptomatic population, the surgical cure rate ranges between 70 and 90 percent at 5 years. Unfortunately, less than 10 percent of gastric carcinomas in the United States are of this type. The infrequency of early gastric cancer and the overall low incidence of gastric cancer in this country make surveillance testing impractical.

Treatment
The only effective treatment for gastric cancer is surgical resection for potential cure or for palliation in the presence of obvious distant spread. More than two-thirds of symptomatic patients operated on with hope of cure are found to have overt evidence of widespread disease at the time of surgery. Of interest, patients with long-standing symptoms and polypoid lesions tend to do better than patients with symptoms of short duration and ulcerative or infiltrative lesions. The overall surgical cure rate in the United States is 10 to 15 percent. Some patients transiently respond to multiagent chemotherapy, but improved survival has not been documented.

Benign Gastric Ulcer

Benign gastric ulcers occur equally in both sexes most often in the sixth and seventh decades of life. Unlike duodenal ulcers, the incidence of gastric ulcers does not seem to be decreasing.

The pathogenesis of gastric ulcers is unknown and probably multifactorial. Gastric reflux of duodenal contents, antral gastritis, and delayed gastric emptying are often found, but they are of uncertain etiologic importance. Since most patients with gastric ulcers are not hypersecretors of acid, the ulcerogenic diathesis seems more related to impaired mucosal defense. Thus a defect may occur in one or more of the following mucosal protective mechanisms. Gastric epithelial cells produce mucus, a portion of which forms a thin, adherent layer over the surface cells. Small quantities of bicarbonate are secreted into this adherent mucus gel. This neutralizes back-diffusing hydrogen ions and protects the surface cells from acid injury. The mucosal vitality and integrity are maintained by the orderly generation of new cells to replace the old. A generous microcirculation supports the entire process. All these factors seem to be stimulated in part by locally produced prostaglandins. At least in some instances agents that inhibit prostaglandin synthesis lead to gastric mucosal ulceration.

Diagnosis

The symptoms of a gastric ulcer are suggestive of, but generally not sufficiently specific for, accurate diagnosis. Patients may have diffuse epigastric or left upper quadrant discomfort relieved by antacids. Some have prominent nausea, vomiting, anorexia, and weight loss. The physical findings are not helpful aside from epigastric tenderness. In most instances, the initial diagnosis is made by radiographic examination of the upper gastrointestinal tract. The radiologist can detect over 80 percent of gastric ulcers and is quite accurate in assessing their benign nature. Most clinicians, however, believe patients with gastric ulcers should have endoscopy with multiple biopsies to exclude ulcerating cancer.

Treatment

Even though acid hypersecretion is not a prime cause of gastric ulcer, most gastric ulcers respond to an antiacid regimen [38]. With H_2-receptor antagonist therapy, gastric ulcers usually heal within 8 to 12 weeks [26]. Gastric ulcers tend to recur, and most respond to retreatment. The recurrence rate may be reduced by maintenance of H_2 blocker therapy (e.g., cimetidine, 400 mg hs, or ranitidine, 150 mg hs).

Prostaglandin therapy, not yet available for general use in this country, has a theoretically attractive appeal for treatment of gastric ulcers. In acceptable therapeutic dosages, prostaglandin analogues suppress secretion of gastric acid and perhaps also pepsin and gastrin. In addition, prostaglandins enhance the gastric mucosal defense mechanisms. In controlled trials, prostaglandin therapy has shown a healing rate comparable with that of H_2-receptor blockade. The beneficial results of sucralfate therapy have been largely ascribed to its local prostaglandin-stimulating effect. Side effects of prostaglandin therapy include only moderate diarrhea in a small percentage of patients, but an abortifacient potential may preclude use in women of childbearing potential.

All gastric ulcers should be followed to complete healing, and they should be checked for early recurrence within 3 to 6 months. Healing can be most practically assessed by radiographic follow-up, but some argue that endoscopic evaluation is necessary.

Surgical resection of gastric ulcers offers a very satisfactory permanent cure rate. Surgery is advised for those with major complications and for recurrences despite a maintenance H_2 blocker therapy. Gastric ulcers that fail to heal on adequate therapy and those where malignancy cannot be excluded also require surgical resection.

Gastritis

Gastritis is a term implying inflammation of the stomach wall, especially of the mucosal lining. The term is generic and often connotes a variable meaning to the clinician, endoscopist, pathologist, and radiologist. There is no unifying classification fulfilling the needs of all. The various forms of gastritis are usually modified by one or more of such terms as acute, chronic, erosive, superficial, focal, nonspecific, hypertrophic, or atrophic. Recently, the bacterium *Campylobacter pylori* has been found in association with antral gastritis and peptic ulceration. The clinical importance and possible pathogenetic significance of this finding are not yet established [4]. Two of the most frequent and important forms of gastritis are acute erosive gastritis and chronic atrophic gastritis.

Acute Erosive Gastritis

Acute erosive gastritis is one of the most serious forms of gastritis. It occurs in several common clinical settings. Erosive gastritis is most often seen in patients who ingest drugs that disrupt the gastric mucosal barrier. Nonsteroidal anti-inflammatory drugs and alcohol are frequent offenders. Erosive gastritis is also seen in patients under severe stress, such as occurs with multiple organ failure or uncontrolled sepsis. Both situations are characterized by multiple discrete or confluent superficial gastric mucosal erosions causing massive hemorrhage. The diagnosis is best confirmed by endoscopy. Treatment is supportive, with withdrawal of any suspected causative agent. Fortunately, the hemorrhage is often self-limited, particularly if there is a removable precipitating agent. The prognosis for drug-induced erosive gastritis is generally quite good. The prognosis for stress-induced erosive gastritis is much more ominous. Resectional surgery for control of hemorrhage is often necessary, and the mortality rate is high. Thus it is gratifying to know that there has been a decreased incidence of stress-related erosive gastritis in response to prophylactic measures. Gastric acid neutralization with hourly antacids or H_2-receptor blockade has been highly successful in preventing serious hemorrhage in chronically stressed patients [58].

Chronic Atrophic Gastritis

Patients with chronic atrophic gastritis usually have no gastric symptoms. The diagnosis may be first suspected by the absence of gastric rugal folds on radiographic examination or by a pale mucosa with visible vessels showing through an endoscopy. The histology shows a variable loss of gastric glands with or without a round-cell inflammatory infiltrate. The atrophic changes may be diffuse or focal in distribution. A small proportion of patients with diffuse involvement of the fundus of the stomach will develop achlorhydria and pernicious anemia. The etiology of atrophic gastritis is not known, but an immunologic injury has been implicated in some patients [28]. Many patients with atrophic gastritis and almost all with pernicious anemia have circulating antibodies to parietal cells. The etiologic importance of these antibodies is still debated, but some patients with pernicious anemia may have a beneficial response to corticosteroid therapy. There is also an increased incidence of concurrent autoimmune disorders in patients with pernicious anemia. Patients with long-standing atrophic gastritis seem to be at increased risk of development of gastric cancer. There is no treatment for atrophic gastritis. If malabsorption of vitamin B_{12} is impaired, monthly parenteral replacement suffices.

Duodenal Ulcer Disease

Duodenal ulcer occurs sometime during the lifetime of approximately 10 percent of the U.S. population, predominantly in men. The incidence peaks between the third and fifth decades of life. For reasons that are unknown, the incidence of duodenal ulcer disease has been decreasing in the past few decades.

The etiology of peptic ulcer disease is unknown. Evidence suggests the cause to be multifactorial with a variable combination and importance of factors in any given patient. Normal gastroduodenal physiology assumes an equilibrium between the potential ulcerogenic agents, i.e., acid and pepsin, and mucosal cytoprotective factors. Some patients with duodenal ulcer disease have abnormally high acid secretory rates, and the balance may be considered tipped in favor of the ulcerogenic forces. Indeed, the mean level of gastric acid secretion for patients with duodenal ulcer is higher compared to controls. There is, however, considerable overlap, and the majority of duodenal ulcer patients have acid secretory rates within the range of controls. For this group, a decrease in inherent mucosal defense is postulated. It is also reasonable to assume that many ulcer patients have a combination of enhanced ulcerogenic and decreased protective factors.

Diagnosis

The most characteristic symptom of duodenal ulcer disease is epigastric discomfort relieved by food or antacid. Nocturnal pain is common, but patients with uncomplicated duodenal ulcers seldom vomit or lose weight. All symptoms, however, are nonspecific and highly variable. Other conditions often mimic the traditional symptoms ascribed to peptic ulcer disease. Perhaps the most difficult to distinguish are patients with functional dyspepsia, particularly if an empiric diagnosis of ulcer disease has been offered in the past.

Complications of duodenal ulcer disease present with more characteristic findings. Pain that radiates to the back and is unrelieved by antacids suggests posterior penetration of the ulcer into retroperitoneal structures. An anterior penetrating duodenal ulcer may present as a free abdominal cavity perforation. Such patients have severe abdominal pain, generalized peritoneal signs of inflammation, rigid anterior abdominal musculature, and absent bowel signs. Abdominal radiographs show free peritoneal air in most, but not all, patients. Emesis of recognizable food particles ingested many hours or even days earlier and an abdominal succussion splash with shaking are indicative of chronic gastric outlet obstruction. Melena is the most common sign of duodenal ulcer hemorrhage; hematemesis and postural signs of acute hypovolemia are also often seen.

The physical examination in patients with an uncomplicated duodenal ulcer seldom contributes, but nonspecific epigastric tenderness is often present. A barium upper gastrointestinal series is quite accurate in detecting the initial episode of duodenal ulcer, but it has significantly less value in demonstrating a recurrent ulcer in the bulb deformed by previous ulceration. The diagnosis of duodenal ulcer is most confidently made by fiberoptic panendoscopy. Gastric analysis is of little diagnostic value in routine peptic ulcer disease because of the overlap in the gastric secretory pattern of patients with peptic ulcer and normal controls. Patients with an ulcer diathesis difficult to control or with refractory ulcers in atypical locations should have a serum gastrin level determination to screen for pancreatic gastrinoma (Zollinger-Ellison syndrome). In patients with the Zollinger-Ellison syndrome, the fasting serum gastrin level is almost always elevated over 150 pg/ml, and a value over 1000 pg/ml is diagnostic.

Treatment

Today, H_2-receptor antagonists are most commonly used for treatment of duodenal ulcers. With these agents, more than 90 percent of duodenal ulcers heal within 6 to 8 weeks. Antacid neutralization of luminal acid is comparably effective, but poor compliance limits its long-term usefulness. Recent clinical studies have shown that synthetic prostaglandin analogues can inhibit acid secretion and provide effective therapy for peptic disorders [25]. These agents also stimulate enhancement of mucosal integrity (cytoprotection). In the near future, oral prostaglandin agents may be released with both acid antisecretory and cytoprotective effects. The effectiveness of sucralfate as an antiulcer agent probably depends both on its ulcer-coating and barrier property and on its stability to stimulate gastric mucosal prostaglandin production. Other acid antisecretory agents under investigation include selective antimuscarinic compounds with fewer undesirable side effects and a long-acting inhibitor of the ATPase-dependent pump that releases hydrogen ions into the gastric contents [35,56].

On adequate therapy, patients with uncomplicated ulcers should become symptom-free within the first week of treatment. If symptoms persist, one must review the accuracy of diagnosis and check the patient's compliance. Unfortunately, once the duodenal ulcer is healed, most patients have frequent recurrences. Studies show recurrence rates ranging from 35 to 80 percent within 1 year. Symptoms are often unreliable. Many patients with recurrent symptoms have no evidence of ulcer, and ulcers often recur without symptoms. Endoscopy may be necessary for accurate diagnosis. Recurrent ulcers respond promptly to empiric therapy. For patients with a major complication or frequent recurrences impairing lifestyle, maintenance therapy with H_2-receptor blockers has proved valuable [47]. The rate of recurrence is reduced by one-half or more. Smoking delays ulcer healing, hastens recurrence, and largely negates the beneficial effect of prophylactic H_2-receptor blockade. Patients with major complications and those with troublesome recurrences despite maintenance H_2-receptor therapy require surgical therapy.

Pancreatic Diseases

Acute Pancreatitis

Acute pancreatitis is an inflammatory disorder of the pancreas classified pathologically as edematous or hemorrhagic (necrotic). Alcohol abuse and biliary tract disease are etiologically implicated in more than 80 percent of patients; an idiopathic category accounts for most of the remainder. Less common causes include hypercalcemia, hypertriglyceridemia, drugs (e.g., azathioprine, tetracycline, valproic acid, sulindac, methyldopa, furosemide, estrogens, thiazides, and sulfonamides), and trauma.

DIAGNOSIS

Patients usually present with severe epigastric pain often radiating directly to the back. Nausea and vomiting are commonly present. Fever, gastrointestinal bleeding, and jaundice are less common. In patients with hemorrhagic pancreatitis, shock and unresponsiveness may be present. Evidence of dehydration, abdominal tenderness with guarding, and absent or hypoactive bowel sounds is commonly seen. With severe disease (especially hemorrhagic pancreatitis), shock, mental confusion, or coma and evidence of retroperitoneal hemorrhage, e.g., periumbilical (Cullen's sign) or flank ecchymoses (Grey Turner's sign), may be apparent.

Laboratory values commonly include leukocytosis, increased (with dehydration) or decreased (with hemorrhage), hematocrit, azotemia, hyperglycemia, and mildly abnormal liver tests. The key to the diagnosis is the finding of hyperamylasemia or hyperamylasuria [50]. The serum amylase level is elevated in 75 percent of patients with acute pancreatitis; it may be normal, however, in alcohol-induced disease. The serum amylase level rises within 24 to 48 hours of onset of pain and usually returns to normal within 3 to 5 days. Urine amylase excretion is a more sensitive

Table 4–3. Causes of Hyperamylasemia
or Hyperamylasuria or Both

Pancreatic Disease	Nonpancreatic Disease
Pancreatitis	Renal insufficiency
Pancreatic carcinoma	Tumor hyperamylasemia
Pancreatic trauma	Salivary gland disease
	Macroamylasemia
	Biliary tract disease
	Penetrated peptic ulcer
	Perforated peptic ulcer
	Intestinal infarction
	Intestinal obstruction
	Burns
	Diabetic ketoacidosis

Source: Adapted from Salt, W. B., II, and Schenker, S. Amylase: Its clinical significance: A review of the literature. *Medicine*, 55: 273, 1976. Used with permission.

index because it rises earlier to a higher concentration and persists longer. Because amylase is present in other organs as well as the pancreas, an increase in serum or urine amylase is not specific for pancreatic disease. In general, however, nonpancreatic causes produce milder elevations (e.g., 200 to 500 Somogyi units/100 ml). Table 4-3 lists the more common causes of hyperamylasemia and hyperamylasuria.

Two principal isoamylases exist: (1) P-type derived from the pancreas, and (2) S-type derived from the salivary glands and other organs. S-type isoamylase predominates in normal serum. Although the isoamylases offer promise of increased specificity for the diagnosis of pancreatitis, they are not yet in general use. The serum lipase level is also usually elevated in acute pancreatitis and may add specificity to the diagnosis, since the pancreas is the main source of this enzyme.

Plain abdominal films may reveal a generalized or localized ("sentinel loop") ileus. Abdominal ultrasound and CT scans often reveal an enlarged pancreas in uncomplicated disease. These latter two tests are extremely useful in detecting complications of acute pancreatitis, such as abscess, pseudocyst, and bile duct obstruction (from the enlarged pancreas or associated gallstones) [43].

TREATMENT AND PROGNOSIS

Treatment of pancreatitis consists of vigorous intravenous fluid administration because many of these patients sequester large amounts of fluid in the retroperitoneum. Analgesia is usually required, and meperidine appears to be the most commonly used agent. Nasogastric suction is probably not necessary for patients with mild to moderate pancreatitis, but it should be used in severe cases. Antibiotics and anticholinergics are not helpful in most patients. The value of prophylactic antibiotics in hemorrhagic pancreatitis is controversial.

Complications are common. Pancreatic pseudocysts may result in continued pain and serum amylase elevation. Diagnosis is suggested by a palpable mass and is confirmed by an ultrasound or CT study. Treatment is surgical if the cyst is large or persistent. Development of a pancreatic abscess is suggested by fever, hypotension, and pain. Treatment requires antibiotics and surgical drainage. Other complications include pleural effusions, pulmonary atelectasis, gastrointestinal bleeding, hypocalcemia, and hyperglycemia. An unknown percentage of patients will progress to chronic pancreatitis, especially if alcohol is the etiology. The overall mortality rate for acute pancreatitis is approximately 5 percent.

Chronic Pancreatitis

Chronic pancreatitis is an inflammatory disease of the pancreas that has resulted in permanent damage to the gland. Alcoholism is the most common cause of the disease; less frequently, biliary tract disease, trauma, cystic fibrosis, hyperparathyroidism, hyperlipemia, and hereditary factors are responsible.

DIAGNOSIS

Patients may present with (1) intermittent attacks of acute abdominal pain resembling acute pancreatitis (i.e., chronic relapsing pancreatitis), (2) continuous epigastric pain, or (3) symptoms of malabsorption.

During episodes of pain, physical findings will resemble those described for acute pancreatitis. If malabsorption is present, there may be evidence of weight loss or fat-soluble vitamin deficiency.

Laboratory tests supporting the diagnosis include indices of pancreatic malabsorption (elevated 72-hour stool fat with normal D-xylose absorption and small bowel biopsy; see Maldigestion and Malabsorption) and a low bicarbonate concentration in pancreatic fluid after secretin stimulation. An abnormal result of a triolein breath test with correction by administration of pancreatic enzymes (see Maldigestion and Malabsorption) supports the diagnosis.

Abdominal plain films may reveal pancreatic calcifications. Pancreatography (e.g., performed through the endoscope) often shows a dilated, irregular duct.

TREATMENT AND PROGNOSIS

Analgesics are frequently necessary for pain. If malabsorption is present, oral pancreatic enzymes (2 to 4 pancreatic enzyme capsules with meals) may be given to facilitate digestion. A poor response may result from inactivation of enzyme by gastric acid and may improve with coadministration of sodium bicarbonate (1 to 3 gm). Insulin is required if diabetes mellitus develops. Recent evidence suggests that large oral doses of pancreatic enzymes may help prevent recurrent attacks of pain. Surgical procedures may be necessary for complications such as pseudocysts; the role of surgery in preventing recurrent attacks or in relieving chronic pain is, however, problematic and unproven.

Because of the chronic nature of the disease, drug addiction is common. Other complications include pseudocysts, diabetes, ascites, and common bile duct obstruction.

Pancreatic Carcinoma

Pancreatic carcinoma is the third most common gastrointestinal cancer in the United States. The incidence is higher in males. Associated risk factors are smoking, heavy alcohol intake, and perhaps chronic pancreatitis and diabetes mellitus. In most patients no obvious risk factors exist. Solid adenocarcinoma of duct-cell origin is the most common pancreatic neoplasm. The tumor occurs in the head of the pancreas in 70 percent, in the body in 20 percent, and in the tail in 10 percent.

DIAGNOSIS

Presenting symptoms are vague and nonspecific. The classic triad of abdominal pain, weight loss, and jaundice appear late in about two-thirds of patients with pancreatic cancer. The pain is usually steady and often radiates through to the back. Profound anorexia usually accompanies the weight loss. Jaundice most commonly indicates a large mass of tumor encasing the distal common bile duct. On rare occasions, however, a relatively small tumor in the ampullary region may obstruct the bile duct early in the course. If the tumor is located in the body or the tail of the gland, jaundice occurs even later and is usually a manifestation of liver metastases. Mental symptoms of depression and anxiety are common with a pancreatic carcinoma; acute pancreatitis and brisk gastrointestinal bleeding are uncommon. A migratory thrombophlebitis is most commonly seen with tumors of the body and tail.

Physical findings with pancreatic carcinoma are variable. An enlarged gallbladder in half the jaundiced patients suggests a pliable, nondiseased gallbladder distended by bile duct obstruction (Courvoisier's sign). A palpable tumor is present in about 20 percent of patients.

Routine laboratory tests (serum and urine amylase, glucose tolerance test, secretin-pancreozymin test) are neither sensitive nor specific. The carcinoembryonic antigen (CEA), which is elevated in 90 percent of advanced cases, lacks specificity, being elevated frequently in patients with other neoplasms (e.g., colon, stomach, breast) and with some benign conditions (e.g., cigarette smoking, cirrhosis, chronic obstructive pulmonary disease).

The standard upper gastrointestinal radiographic series is insensitive, but occasionally it provides useful information, especially for lesions in the head of the gland. The diagnostic accuracy of an ultrasound or CT scan is 80 to 90 percent for lesions greater than 3 cm in diameter. Cholangiography by a transhepatic percutaneous route with a Chiba needle or endoscopic retrograde cholangiopancreatography (ERCP) will confirm an extrahepatic block of the common bile duct in jaundiced patients. Endoscopic retrograde cholangiopancreatography can also be used to demonstrate pancreatic duct changes and is abnormal in perhaps 90 percent of patients. The accuracy of selective angiography is about 85 percent; its limited availability and high cost, however, are disadvantages. Fine-needle percutaneous biopsy of the pancreatic mass is the newest diagnostic approach and appears to offer reasonable sensitivity (80 percent) and excellent specificity (100 percent).

Most of the tests just described are positive only when the lesion is large and clinical suspicion is high. A test to detect early pancreatic carcinoma at a curable stage, therefore, is clearly needed. At present, a preliminary evaluation should consist of an ultrasound or CT scan of the liver and pancreas. If the study is abnormal, then the more invasive diagnostic procedures can be performed.

TREATMENT AND PROGNOSIS
Treatment of pancreatic carcinoma remains unsatisfactory. The overall resectability rate is less than 25 percent, and the overall 5-year survival is less than 1 percent. Surgical palliation to relieve or prevent common bile duct or duodenal obstruction or both is generally done. Chemotherapy offers little benefit. Radiation may occasionally relieve intractable pain.

Maldigestion and Malabsorption

Maldigestion and malabsorption may occur in a wide variety of pancreatic, biliary, and bowel diseases [19]. Some of the more common causes are listed in Table 4-4.

Diagnosis
Symptoms and signs of malabsorption will vary depending on such factors as nutrients malabsorbed, severity of malabsorption, and the underlying disease responsible for the malabsorption. Diarrhea is particularly common. Stools are large, frequent, foul, loose, and frothy in patients with generalized malabsorption related to small bowel disease. With pancreatic insufficiency, stools tend to be bulky but less frequent; gross fat or oil often is present and suggests steatorrhea. Weight loss is common with malabsorption and results from caloric deprivation. Other symptoms and signs include pallor and weakness (anemia of folate, iron, and vitamin B_{12} deficiency), hemorrhage (vitamin K malabsorption), anasarca (decreased albumin synthesis related to amino acid and peptide mal-

absorption), and tetany (vitamin D and calcium malabsorption).

When a maldigestion/malabsorption disorder is suspected, laboratory tests are usually required for determining the etiologic diagnosis. Some of the more commonly used are described below.

The *fecal fat excretion test* requires a 72-hour stool collection while the patient is ingesting 70 to 100 gm fat per day. Excretion of greater than 7 gm fat indicates fat malabsorption. This test is probably the best screening test for generalized malabsorption, but it is cumbersome and nonspecific.

The *serum carotene test* measures the blood level of this fat-soluble compound and is a crude indicator of the adequacy of fat absorption. Although low levels (<50 μg%) suggest fat malabsorption, ingestion of inadequate amounts of carotene-containing foods (liver, lettuce, carrots, and spinach) will result in low serum levels within 1 week. Elevated levels occur commonly with hypothyroidism, diabetes, hyperlipidemia, and anorexia nervosa and may result in false-negative tests.

Table 4–4. Maldigestion and Malabsorption Syndromes in the Adult

General:
  Biliary:
    Biliary tract obstruction
    Malabsorption of bile acids
  Pancreatic disease:
    Chronic pancreatitis
    Pancreatic carcinoma
  Small bowel disease:
    Sprue (nontropical and tropical)
    Small bowel resection
    Whipple's disease
    Crohn's disease
    Radiation enteritis
    Lymphangiectasia
    Ischemic bowel disease
    Lymphoma
    Amyloidosis
    Bacterial overgrowth
  Other:
    Inadequate mixing of chyme with digestive secretions, as with a Billroth II anastomosis
    Drug-induced, e.g., neomycin
    Hypogammaglobulinemia
    Parasitic infections, e.g., giardiasis
Selective:
  Lactase deficiency
  Ileal resection or disease: vitamin B_{12} and bile acid deficiency
  Abetalipoproteinemia
  Drugs, e.g., cholestyramine
  Rare congenital deficiencies, such as enterokinase, dipeptidase, and pancreatic lipase deficiencies

In the D-*xylose absorption test* [24], a dose of the sugar is given orally, serum is collected at 1 or 2 hours, and urine is collected for 5 hours. Low serum or urine values usually indicate a small bowel mucosal abnormality, since bile salts and pancreatic enzymes are not required for absorption. Delayed gastric emptying and intestinal bacterial overgrowth may cause low serum and urine D-xylose values; impaired renal function may cause low urine values.

Vitamin B_{12} absorption depends on an intact terminal ileum and the presence of intrinsic factor. In the *Schilling test,* a small dose of ^{60}Co-labeled vitamin B_{12} is given orally together with a large dose of unlabeled vitamin B_{12} given parenterally to "saturate" the tissues. Urine is collected for 24 hours. If excretion is low (less than 7 percent of administered dose excreted in 24 hours), the test is repeated with intrinsic factor. Low urinary excretion corrected by intrinsic factor indicates pernicious anemia. Low excretion not corrected by intrinsic factor suggests ileal disease or small bowel bacterial overgrowth. To distinguish between these latter two possibilities, the test should be repeated after a course of broad-spectrum antibiotics. A recently developed dual-label Schilling test may be useful in diagnosing pancreatic insufficiency [5].

The *lactose tolerance test* is performed by administering 50 gm/m^2 lactose orally with serial blood glucose measurement. Abdominal symptoms (cramps and diarrhea) and a blood glucose rise of less than 20 mg% suggest lactase deficiency. In clinical practice, the response of symptoms to a trial of a lactose-free diet is usually sufficient to make the diagnosis.

In the *bile acid breath test,* a dose of [^{14}C]glycine bile acid is given orally and [^{14}C]carbon dioxide is measured in expired breath. Small bowel bacterial overgrowth, and in some cases, ileal dysfunction, will result in increased [^{14}C]carbon dioxide excretion.

Malabsorbed carbohydrate is metabolized by intestinal bacteria with the production of hydrogen. The *hydrogen breath test* measures hydrogen in expired air after carbohydrate ingestion. Increased excretion strongly suggests carbohydrate malabsorption.

The *triolein breath test* measures [^{14}C]carbon dioxide excretion in expired air after ingestion of [^{14}C]triolein [44]. Low rates of excretion indicate fat maldigestion or malabsorption. Correction by coadministration of [^{14}C]triolein and pancreatic enzymes suggests pancreatic insufficiency.

Small bowel biopsy is done to detect mucosal pathologic conditions (e.g., sprue, Whipple's disease). *Microscopic examination of stool or small bowel fluid* may detect bacterial or parasitic pathogens.

Barium contrast radiographs of the small bowel should be obtained in most cases of malabsorption. Although the findings are usually nonspecific, they may strongly suggest a malabsorptive

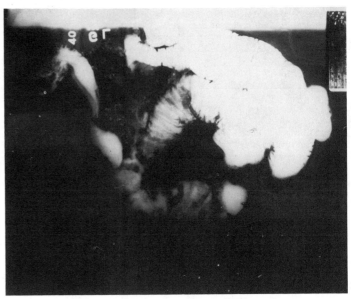

Figure 4–1. *Nontropical sprue. Malabsorption suggested by dilation of small bowel, thickening of mucosal folds, and fragmentation of barium within the bowel lumen.*

disease. Findings include dilation of the small bowel, atrophy or thickening of mucosal folds, and fragmentation of barium within the bowel lumen (Fig. 4-1).

Treatment and Prognosis

Specific treatment obviously depends on the etiology of the malabsorption and is discussed for some diseases elsewhere in this chapter (see Pancreatic Diseases, Diarrheal States, and Inflammatory Bowel Disease). Nontropical sprue responds to a gluten-free diet; tropical sprue responds to folic acid and tetracycline. Whipple's disease and bacterial overgrowth syndromes usually respond to antibiotic therapy—prolonged or repeated courses may be necessary (e.g., trimethoprim-sulfamethoxazole for 1 year). Patients with small bowel disorders for which no specific therapy is available may benefit from frequent small feedings, elemental or polymeric dietary supplements, or occasionally, total parenteral nutrition (intravenous administration of carbohydrate, protein, and fat). Symptoms of lactase deficiency will diminish with a lactose-free diet or perhaps to the use of several recently developed commercial lactase preparations.

Inflammatory Bowel Disease

Two distinct but related chronic bowel diseases are included in the term *inflammatory bowel disease*: Crohn's disease and ulcerative colitis. These diseases are of unknown etiology, affect primarily young adults, and are characterized by exacerbations and remissions. Features that serve to distinguish between the two diseases are listed in Table 4-5. Nonetheless, in some cases, features of both diseases are present, and differentiation may be impossible.

Table 4–5. *Features that Distinguish Between Crohn's Disease and Ulcerative Colitis*

Factors	Crohn's Disease	Ulcerative Colitis
Pathologic features	Transmural inflammation Deep ulcers Granulomas common	Mucosal inflammation Superficial ulcers Granulomas absent
Distribution	Mouth to anus (ileum and proximal most common)	Colon
Clinical features:		
Rectal bleeding	20–40 percent	98 percent
Fulminating episodes	Uncommon	Common
Obstruction	Common	Rare
Fistulas	Common	Rare
Perianal disease	Common	Less common
Sigmoidoscopic and radiographic findings:		
Rectal involvement	50 percent	95–100 percent
Extent	Patchy	Continuous
Ulcers	Longitudinal, deep	Shallow, collar button
Pseudopolyps	Uncommon	Common
Strictures	Common	Uncommon
Ileal involvement	Narrowed lumen with thickened wall	Dilated lumen with diminished folds but histologically normal

Crohn's Disease

Crohn's disease may affect any region of the intestinal tract [10]. Most commonly, the ileum (regional enteritis or ileitis—30 percent) or the colon (Crohn's colitis—20 percent) or both (Crohn's ileocolitis—50 percent) are involved. Grossly, the bowel wall is thickened and the lumen is narrowed. The mucosal surface is studded by ulcers varying from shallow "aphthoid" ulcers to deep linear ulcers. Involvement is also patchy with intervening normal or near normal areas. Microscopically, the disease is characterized by transmural inflammation with deep ulcers, fistulas, and occasionally, granulomas.

Diagnosis

The symptoms of Crohn's disease are variable. Diarrhea is seen in perhaps 90 percent of patients; abdominal pain is seen in 75 percent. The pain is usually steady and most often located in the right lower quadrant. With progression of disease, pain may become colicky and become associated with nausea, vomiting, and abdominal distention reflecting partial or complete bowel obstruction. Fever is seen in more than half of patients. Hematochezia is also present in about half of patients. Other symptoms include weight loss, constipation, melena, fissures, and evidence of fistulization (e.g., enterocutaneous, rectovaginal, enterovesical). Free perforation can occur, but it is rare. Malignant neoplasms of the bowel are more frequent than in the general population but less frequent than in patients with ulcerative colitis.

Symptoms vary depending on the location of the disease. Hematochezia is more common with colon involvement; intestinal obstruction is more common with ileal involvement.

The clinical course of Crohn's disease also is variable. Some patients may remain asymptomatic for long periods of time after onset. More commonly, patients experience recurrent attacks of abdominal pain, diarrhea, and fever.

Extraintestinal manifestations are common, especially if the colon is affected by the disease. Arthritis may precede symptoms of bowel disease. Large joint involvement or sacroileitis is the most common pattern. Arthritis symptoms commonly do not parallel intestinal symptoms. Eye involvement, including iritis and episcleritis, is common, as are skin manifestations such as erythema nodosum and pyoderma gangrenosum. Aphthous ulcerations of the mouth may be seen. Urinary tract involvement includes infections related to enterovesical fistulas, nephrolithiasis (oxalate stones), and amyloidosis.

Physical findings related to the preceding symptoms are often obvious. Fever, evidence of malnutrition, a palpable abdominal mass, and occult blood in the feces are especially common.

Laboratory test abnormalities are nonspecific. Leukocytosis and an elevated sedimentation rate suggest active disease. Anemia is common and usually related to iron deficiency; vitamin B_{12} malabsorption is less commonly the cause. A low serum albumin level commonly results from poor nutrition or intestinal protein loss. Abnormal liver tests may be related to fatty liver, pericholangitis, sclerosing cholangitis, or cholelithiasis, all of which are seen more frequently in patients with Crohn's disease than in the general population.

The abdominal plain film may suggest intestinal obstruction. Barium studies often demonstrate luminal narrowing, fistulizations, deep ulcerations, and strictures. Other x-ray findings that may suggest Crohn's disease include "skip areas," aphthous ulcerations, "cobblestoning," and rectal sparing.

Sigmoidoscopy or colonoscopy is frequently useful in establishing a diagnosis of Crohn's disease. Relatively specific findings include rectal sparing, "skip areas," and deep or linear ulcerations. Biopsies obtained at the time of colonoscopy also may be helpful if they demonstrate ileal involvement or granulomas.

TREATMENT AND PROGNOSIS

Abdominal cramping and diarrhea usually respond to loperamide or diphenoxylate. Analgesics may be required for pain. Symptoms of partial obstruction may require a clear liquid diet or placing the patient NPO. Complete obstruction necessitates hospitalization, nasogastric suction, and intravenous fluid administration. Malnutrition is frequent in patients with Crohn's disease. Orally administered elemental or polymeric supplements may be useful. Occasionally, total parenteral nutrition may be required to restore nutrition. The efficiency of this form of nutrition in inducing remissions in this disease is controversial.

Drug therapy aimed at suppressing inflammatory disease activity is often required. Corticosteroids, usually in high doses and for prolonged periods, are necessary in patients with severe disease. Because of dose-related side effects, attempts are made to taper the dose as rapidly as possible; long-term low-dose therapy, however, is sometimes necessary. Sulfasalazine also has been proven to be effective in suppressing disease activity, particularly with colonic Crohn's disease. Because side effects are less severe, this drug is the usual initial therapy in patients with mild to moderate symptoms. Metronidazole also has proven effective, particularly with perineal Crohn's disease; large doses for prolonged periods may be required (e.g., 20 mg/kg per day for months).

More potent immunosuppressives such as azathioprine may occasionally be employed in patients not responding to the preceding. They also may play a role in allowing reduction of steroid dosage in the steroid-dependent patient. However, serious side effects such as leukopenia and pancreatitis with both short- and long-term use of the agents limit their use.

Surgery is eventually required in most patients with Crohn's disease, but it should be deferred as long as possible in view of the high frequency of recurrences after surgery and because of the possibility of creating a short bowel syndrome. Usual indications are symptoms refractory to medical therapy and complications of the disease (e.g., obstruction or fistulization). Surgical resection with reanastomosis of the bowel is preferable; bypass operations and the creation of an ostomy may be necessary.

Although a few patients may remain asymptomatic for years after an initial attack of the disease, most will exhibit intermittent exacerbations of symptoms and will have continuous symptoms. Most will eventually require surgical resection, and the clear majority of these will develop recurrent disease, usually at the anastomotic site.

Ulcerative Colitis

Ulcerative colitis affects only the colon [7]. In general, involvement begins just proximal to the anus and extends proximally to a variable extent. If only the rectum is involved, the term *ulcerative proctitis* is used.

Grossly, the mucosal surface of the bowel is diffusely reddened, ulcerated, edematous (vascular pattern obliterated), friable (bleeds easily when touched or wiped), and granular (sandpaper appearance). Ulcers tend to be shallow. In contrast to Crohn's disease, involvement is continuous, i.e., there are no "skip areas" or intervening normal mucosa. Microscopically, the inflammation is limited to the mucosa; deep ulcers and granulomas are not present.

DIAGNOSIS

As with Crohn's disease, symptoms will vary depending on the site of the disease. With ulcerative proctitis, symptoms usually include tenesmus (the sensation of the need to defecate when the rectum is in fact empty) and frequent passage of blood and mucus. Diarrhea is not usually present. With more extensive involvement of the colon, diarrhea (usually accompanied by bleeding and abdominal cramping), fever, weight loss, and fatigue are common. Occasionally, patients may develop a more fulminant course with high fever, profuse diarrhea, intense abdominal pain, and abdominal distention (toxic megacolon). Obstruction or fistulas may occur, but they are far less common than with Crohn's disease. Free perforation may occur in fulminant disease.

Extraintestinal manifestations are common and are identical to those of Crohn's disease (see above) [22]. Physical findings vary from mild lower abdominal tenderness to severe abdominal tenderness with rebound and guarding, distention, and absent bowel sounds. Tachycardia and

dehydration may be present. Gross or occult blood is common on rectal examination. As with Crohn's disease, laboratory abnormalities are nonspecific. With disease activity, leukocytosis, an elevated sedimentation rate, and a low serum albumin level are common. Anemia, when present, is usually of the iron-deficiency type. Abnormal liver function tests may reflect the same liver abnormalities as seen with Crohn's disease, except that the prevalence of cholelithiasis is not increased. Sclerosing cholangitis is, however, more common with ulcerative colitis.

Plain abdominal films are usually normal, but they may suggest mucosal irregularity, foreshortening, or toxic megacolon (e.g., a transverse colon dilated with air). Barium studies are more sensitive, but they too may be normal, especially when disease is mild. Changes that may occur include foreshortening of the bowel, loss of distensibility, small or "collarbutton" ulcers, widening of the presacral space, and pseudopolyps (mucosal tags created by surrounding ulceration). The terminal ileum may fill with barium during the enema and appear normal, or it may show changes of "backwash ileitis," i.e., a short segment of dilated featureless ileum. This finding may help differentiate the disease from Crohn's, in which the ileum, if involved, is usually narrowed and rigid and may contain fistulas.

Sigmoidoscopy or colonoscopy is usually extremely helpful in diagnosing this disease. Visible changes usually begin at the anal verge and consist of edema (disappearance of the submucosal blood vessels), redness, granularity, friability, superficial ulcers, exudate, and pseudopolyps. Biopsies are easily obtained and may assist in making the diagnosis (see above). The gross and microscopic pictures are not specific, however; similar changes may be seen with certain infections (e.g., *Campylobacter*), radiation, and ischemia.

TREATMENT AND PROGNOSIS

Symptomatic treatment is in general identical to that of Crohn's disease. Specific drug therapy is also similar to that of Crohn's disease. Corticosteroids administered by enema, orally, or intravenously are effective in inducing remission. Sulfasalazine may be useful in treating mild to moderate disease, but it is also important because of its ability to prevent relapse once remission occurs. The benefits of metronidazole, azathioprine, and other immunosuppressives are less well documented.

The most frequent surgical indications include continuous symptoms unresponsive to medical therapy, a serious complication (e.g., perforation, massive bleeding, carcinoma), and prevention of colon carcinoma (see below). Less common indications include the need to discontinue drug therapy because of side effects (especially with steroids), growth retardation in pediatric patients, and patient dissatisfaction with the clinical course. Surgery is curative and usually consists of a total colectomy with ileostomy.

The mortality rate from the initial attack may be as high as 5 percent. If toxic megacolon devel-ops, the mortality rate may be 25 percent. After the initial attack, a small number of patients may have a prolonged remission lasting 15 years or more. As with Crohn's disease, however, most patients will have intermittent exacerbations and remissions of symptoms. Some may have continuous symptoms. Prognosis appears to vary with the severity of the first attack, those patients with the most severe attacks doing less well.

The incidence of colon carcinoma is clearly increased, especially after 7 to 10 years of disease activity [21]. In some studies this risk may rise by as much as 20 percent per decade. Factors that appear to increase the risk include total colon involvement and a history of continuous symptoms. Periodic colonoscopy with biopsies may be used to detect dysplasia, a pathologic change thought to herald an increase in carcinoma risk. Such a change requires serious consideration of "prophylactic" colectomy.

Diverticulitis

Diverticulitis occurs in perhaps 10 percent of patients with diverticulosis of the colon [1,46]. The complication is thought to arise as a result of perforation of a diverticulum and spread of inflammation to adjacent areas. The perforation and surrounding inflammation may be microscopic or large, resulting in a large abscess, extensive peritonitis, fistula formation, or obstruction.

Diagnosis

Most patients are elderly, but the disease can occur as early as the third decade. Pain and fever are the most common symptoms. The pain is usually abrupt in onset and steady. Although usually left lower quadrant in location, it may occur anywhere in the abdomen. The pain may be worsened by eating and is often partially relieved by a bowel movement. It is usually nonradiating, but it may extend to the back. The fever may be low-grade or high, and it may be preceded by a rigor. Nausea, vomiting, and diarrhea or constipation are common.

Gross rectal bleeding is uncommon. Irritation of the bladder by the adjacent inflammation may occur and lead to symptoms of dysuria and urinary frequency.

With the development of complications, additional symptoms may develop. Fistulas are usually colovesical and result in urinary tract infection, pneumaturia, or fecaluria. With a large abscess or area of peridiverticular inflammation, bowel obstruction may occur with obstipation, nausea, and vomiting.

Fever and moderate to severe tenderness, usually in the left lower quadrant, are often present. Rebound tenderness and guarding are common in the involved area. A palpable tubular mass can be present, but it may be seen in other conditions such as the irritable bowel syndrome. Rectal examination may reveal tenderness or a mass; stool may contain occult blood, but gross blood is uncommon.

Leukocytosis with a predominance of polymorphonuclear leukocytes is common. Urinalysis may show an increase in white or red blood cells if inflammation extends to the bladder or ureter.

Plain films of the abdomen are usually normal, but they may reveal nonspecific findings of paralytic ileus, mechanical obstruction, or free air. Although potentially a cause of further perforation, a "gingerly" performed barium enema is safe and can provide the most helpful and specific findings, namely, extracolonic barium, a paracolic mass, or a fistula. Ultrasound and computerized tomography of the abdomen and pelvis may reveal the presence of large abscesses. An intravenous pyelogram may be useful in excluding urinary tract involvement.

Treatment and Prognosis

Mild attacks of acute diverticulitis (mild pain, low-grade fever, mild leukocytosis) usually can be managed in the outpatient setting. Analgesics, bowel rest (liquid or low-residue diet), and antibiotics (e.g., ampicillin, tetracycline) are indicated. Patients with moderate to severe attacks (severe pain, high fever, obstruction) should be hospitalized and managed with intravenous fluids, bowel rest (NPO), analgesics, and parenteral antibiotics (e.g., ampicillin plus an aminoglycoside and clindamycin or cefoxitin alone).

Careful observation with physical examination, complete blood count, and abdominal x-rays may be needed to assess patient response to therapy.

Surgery is necessary in the acute management of perhaps 15 to 20 percent of patients hospitalized. Indications include (1) progressive disease or appearance or persistence of an abscess in spite of appropriate medical therapy, (2) generalized peritonitis, and (3) persistent obstruction. In these settings, at least a two-stage procedure is required, e.g., resection, proximal colostomy, and Hartmann's pouch or mucous fistula followed in 8 weeks by reanastomosis.

For chronic management, a high-fiber diet has been advocated by some as a means of preventing recurrent attacks, but there are no convincing data in support of this recommendation. Surgical therapy may be indicated under the following circumstances: (1) recurrent severe attacks, (2) persistent fistulas, especially a colovesical fistula, and (3) persistent narrowing of the bowel when the possibility of carcinoma cannot be excluded. In this elective setting, a one-stage procedure with resection and reanastomosis can usually be accomplished.

The recurrence rate of diverticulitis after the initial attack treated medically is probably 30 to 40 percent, with most attacks occurring in the first 5 years. Morbidity with recurrences is high.

Functional Bowel Disorders

Patients with functional bowel disorders have gastrointestinal symptoms for which no structural, biochemical, or infectious abnormality can be found after thorough investigation [37]. The irritable bowel syndrome is clearly the most common of these disorders, and this discussion will deal only with this entity [53]. This syndrome consists of a group of symptoms, the most common of which are abdominal pain and change in bowel habit.

Various electrical, hormonal, and motility abnormalities of both the small and large bowel have been described in patients with the irritable bowel syndrome, but there has been no general agreement regarding an etiology. Many patients develop symptoms during periods of stress; others relate symptoms to specific foods. Some deny any specific precipitating factors.

Diagnosis

Most patients are female (female-to-male ratio = 3:1). Onset is usually in the third and fourth decades of life, and the disease is usually chronic. Symptoms vary considerably from patient to patient and in a given patient from time to time. Abdominal pain is most common and may be located anywhere in the abdomen, although the left lower quadrant is the most common site. The pain may be steady or colicky. It is often relieved by a bowel movement or flatus and may be precipitated or worsened by meals. Alteration in bowel habit is also frequent. Diarrhea or constipation are both common, and some patients will alternate between these two symptoms. The diarrhea is frequently postprandial; the constipation is often resistant to management. Many patients will complain of increased mucus in their stools. Other complaints include "gas," bloating, eructation, and nausea. Psychological disturbances are commonly present, especially depression, anxiety, and hysteria. Symptoms not usually seen with the irritable bowel syndrome and therefore suggesting another diagnosis include gastrointestinal bleeding, weight loss, tenesmus, fever, onset of symptoms after age 50, and pain or diarrhea awakening the patient.

The physical examination is often normal. Many patients, however, will have areas of tenderness, especially in the left or right lower quadrants, and the sigmoid colon or cecum may be palpable.

Laboratory results, including a complete blood count and sedimentation rate, are normal. The finding of blood or white blood cells in the stool argues strongly *against* the diagnosis of the irritable bowel syndrome.

Various x-ray abnormalities have been described in this syndrome (e.g., exaggerated haustral markings on barium enema), but there appear to be no consistent reliable x-ray findings to aid in the diagnosis.

In general, the laboratory and x-ray studies are useful in diagnosing other conditions that may present with similar symptoms. Because there is no definitive diagnostic test for the irritable bowel syndrome, judicious use of laboratory and x-ray studies often is necessary to exclude these conditions.

Treatment and Prognosis

Management may be difficult. A close doctor-patient relationship is essential. Many of these patients have already seen other physicians, have had many tests, and have been told "there is nothing wrong" or "it's in your head." Many will have a cancerphobia. A careful history and physical examination, review of previous records and x-rays, and, on occasion, use of some diagnostic tests are required and will demonstrate to the patient the physician's interest and concern. A careful description of the nature of the motility disturbance and reassurance that nothing more serious is present are important steps in management. It is important to emphasize that this is a chronic disease and that a quick cure is impossible —the aim of therapy rather is to control symptoms as much as possible.

Additional therapy includes control or avoidance of known precipitating factors, e.g., attempts at stress-management counseling and avoidance of specific foods known to precipitate attacks. Trial of a lactose-free diet for 7 days may be useful. Many patients have fewer symptoms when on a high-roughage diet; addition of commercially prepared roughage mixtures also may be useful. Laxatives should be avoided if at all possible. Anticholinergic medications (in a dose sufficient to cause a dry mouth) also may be beneficial, especially in patients with pain. Use of antianxiety or mood-elevating drugs may occasionally be helpful in patients with psychological disturbances. Formal psychotherapy is rarely necessary.

The irritable bowel syndrome is usually a chronic condition with exacerbations and remissions. The natural history and prognosis have not been well studied. A convincing relationship to later development of diverticulosis or carcinoma has not been established.

Colorectal Adenomatous Polyps

Clinical Manifestations

Colorectal adenomatous polyps are common and increase in number with age. Polyps may be sessile or on a stalk, and they result from an accumulation of abnormally proliferating mucosal epithelial cells. Adenomatous polyps may occur anywhere in the lower bowel, but most are in the rectum and sigmoid. Histologically, approximately two-thirds of adenomatous polyps are tubular, 10 percent are villous, and the remainder are mixed tubulovillous. Large polyps, greater than 2 cm in size, tend to be villous in nature [14]. Although some polyps cause rectal bleeding or abdominal cramps, most are asymptomatic and found on a barium study or by endoscopy. The large majority of colonic polyps are visible on flexible fiberoptic sigmoidoscopy.

Adenomatous polyps are premalignant lesions. The adenoma-cancer transition is considered to be greater than 5 years and perhaps as long as 10 to 15 years. Thus removal of benign adenomas is considered to be excellent cancer prophylaxis. The malignant potential relates to both size and histologic type [42]. Overall, less than 2 percent of adenomatous polyps under 1 cm in size are malignant, whereas malignant change is found in almost 50 percent of polyps over 2 cm in size. Villous adenomas have a much higher malignant potential compared to tubular adenomas.

Treatment

Periodic screening with fiberoptic sigmoidoscopy at 3- to 5-year intervals after age 50 is advisable. Most pedunculated and small sessile polyps can be safely removed by snare cautery during colonoscopy. Even if localized malignant change is identified in the head of the polyp, most patients do not require further surgical resection. Conventional surgical resection is indicated, however, if malignancy is detected in a sessile polyp or if the malignancy involves the stock at the cautery margin. Other indications for follow-up surgery after polypectomy include an invasive malignancy of highly undifferentiated histologic type or one with demonstrable vascular or lymphatic invasion.

Colorectal Cancer

Clinical Manifestations

Colorectal cancer occurs in more than 130,000 patients and causes 65,000 deaths per year in the United States. The most overt risk factor is age. The incidence of colorectal cancer begins to rise at age 40 and accelerates markedly over age 50. Other risk factors include the presence of adenomatous polyps, heritable polypoid syndromes, ulcerative colitis beyond 7 years' duration, and a family history of colorectal cancer. Both genetic and environmental (dietary) factors are important in the etiology. In the United States, a relatively high-fat, low-fiber diet has been implicated.

All patients with a change in bowel habits or blood per rectum should be investigated promptly. Unfortunately, most symptomatic cancers are relatively far advanced. Detection of early, more curable lesions mostly depends on the conscientious use of available screening techniques. From age 40 on, patients should have a yearly rectal examination and screening of stool for occult blood. Guaiac-impregnated paper slides are inexpensive, patient-acceptable, and reliable. The finding of occult blood in the stool of an asymptomatic patient must be pursued by a flexible sigmoidoscopy and an air-contrast barium enema. Some clinicians prefer investigation with an initial colonoscopy, especially in older high-risk patients with iron-deficiency anemia. Colonoscopy, the most accurate diagnostic procedure for colon lesions, is also used to clarify any equivocal findings of the barium enema.

Treatment and Prognosis

Complete surgical removal is the only cure for colorectal cancer. The average 5-year survival rate is 40 percent, but the individual rate depends on the histologic staging of the tumor at the time of removal. Patients with cancer apparently confined to the mucosa have a better than 85 percent cure rate, while those with local lymph node involve-ment have a less than 20 percent cure rate. Peri-operative radiation therapy, especially for rectal cancer, reduces local recurrence and improves survival statistics [54]. The carcinoembryonic antigen (CEA) is of little value in the initial screen for colorectal cancer, but a rising postoperative level may be the first evidence of recurrence. Unfortunately, early diagnosis of recurrence does not often lead to prolongation of survival, since most patients have distant, nonresectable spread. Only a minority of symptomatic patients benefit from palliative chemotherapy with 5-fluorouracil (5FU).

Biliary Tract Disorders

Gallstones are present in 10 percent of the general population of the United States and in 30 percent of people over the age of 65 years. Stones are of two general types: predominantly cholesterol (90 to 95 percent of all stones) and predominantly pigment (5 to 10 percent). Cholesterol stones form when the concentration of cholesterol in bile is increased relative to bile acid and lecithin. This may result from either increased cholesterol or decreased bile acid secretion by the liver. Predisposing factors to gallstone formation are listed in Table 4-6.

Diagnosis

The majority of patients with gallstones are asymptomatic. Symptoms are usually initiated by a stone blocking the cystic duct. Biliary colic or acute cholecystitis is likely to ensue. Biliary colic is characterized by a steady (*not* colicky) pain of gradual or abrupt onset, usually but not always located in the epigastrium or right upper quadrant. Pain may last for $1/2$ to 12 hours and is frequently accompanied by nausea and vomiting. Attacks are usually self-limited, but they frequently recur at intervals of weeks to years. A gallbladder that is removed for these symptoms will usually show gallstones plus chronic signs of inflammation, cholesterolosis, or Rokitansky-Aschoff sinuses. Such patients are said to have chronic cholecystitis. In some patients, symptoms of biliary colic persist and worsen; fever and, occasionally, mild jaundice may develop. Such patients are stated to have acute cholecystitis. Although such attacks are also usually self-limited (75 percent), symptoms may persist for days to weeks and complications of infection (empyema), perforation, and fistulization may occur. If gallstones migrate into the common bile duct (15 percent of patients), back pain and jaundice are more frequent and Charcot's triad (fever, jaundice, right upper quadrant pain) may occur.

Table 4-6. Gallstones: Common Predisposing Conditions

Cholesterol stones:
  Age: Increasing prevalence with increasing age
  Sex: Female-to-male ratio = 2.5:1
  Race: Native Americans (especially)
  Obesity
  Ileal disease
  Diabetes (probably)
  Parity (probably)
  Drugs (e.g., birth control pills, clofibrate)
Pigment stones:
  Cirrhosis
  Hemolysis

With biliary colic, epigastric or right upper quadrant tenderness is usually the only finding. In acute cholecystitis, signs of acute inflammation (fever, rebound tenderness, guarding) are common, and mild jaundice may be seen. With palpation in the right upper quadrant, the patient will frequently experience increased pain with deep inspiration (Murphy's sign). With cholangitis, high fever, rigors, jaundice, and right upper quadrant tenderness are common; shock and mental confusion may be present.

Laboratory results are usually normal in patients with biliary colic. With acute cholecystitis, leukocytosis, mildly abnormal liver function tests (bilirubin up to 5 mg%), and elevated serum amylase levels may occur. With cholangitis, similar abnormalities are common and are usually more severe. Positive blood cultures are common, *E. coli, Klebsiella, Pseudomonas,* enterococci, *Proteus, Bacteroides,* and *Clostridium* being the most commonly isolated.

Plain films of the abdomen will demonstrate gallstones in 15 percent of patients. Oral cholecystography is useful in detecting gallstones (specificity and sensitivity are approximately 95 percent), but it requires a minimum of 12 hours and may be impossible in the acutely ill patient. Ultrasonography has similar specificity and sensitivity in detecting gallstones and can be performed acutely. It also will detect bile duct dilation, suggesting the presence of bile duct calculi. Abdominal CT scanning is less sensitive in detecting gallstones, but it is probably as sensitive as ultrasound in revealing bile duct dilation. Although all the preceding tests are useful in detecting gallstones, none clearly indicates that the presence of stones is responsible for the symptoms. Biliary scintigraphy (e.g., HIDA, PIPIDA scan) is especially useful in this regard. Following intravenous injection of these radionuclides, the biliary system can be imaged. If the gallbladder fails to visualize (even on a delayed film), cystic duct obstruction is highly likely. Other studies (percutaneous transhepatic cholangiography, endoscopic retrograde cholangiography) are useful in the detection of bile duct stones.

Treatment and Prognosis

Treatment of gallstone disease is still somewhat controversial. Most authorities agree that asymptomatic gallstones should not be removed surgically, except perhaps in patients with diabetes, in whom acute cholecystitis is associated with a greater morbidity and mortality. Medical dissolution of these gallstones with chenodeoxycholic acid, ursodeoxycholic acid, or a combination thereof is possible in up to 90 percent of carefully selected patients [11]. This therapeutic approach, however, may take several years and is associated with a recurrence rate of 10 percent per year after discontinuation of the bile acid regimen. Gallbladder infusion of gallstone-dissolving substances (e.g., methyl *tert*-butyl ether), shock waves, and lithotripsy are currently under study and appear promising.

Acute cholecystitis usually requires hospitalization, with use of intravenous fluids, nasogastric suction, and analgesics. Antibiotic treatment (e.g., cefoxitin or ampicillin plus an aminoglycoside) is indicated in acute cholecystitis when symptoms have been present for several days and/or symptoms of increasing fever, pain, and right upper quadrant mass indicate worsening of the disease. Surgery is indicated in acute cholecystitis, although the timing is still somewhat controversial. If symptoms appear to be worsening or if complications appear imminent, early surgery is needed. In the uncomplicated case of acute cholecystitis, most authorities also recommend early surgery for the following reasons: elimination of the possibility of complications such as perforation, surgery is at least as easily performed, and economic savings.

In cholangitis, most patients will respond to hospitalization, nasogastric suction, and antibiotics. If improvement is not apparent in 12 to 24 hours, however, immediate surgical decompression of the obstructed bile duct is indicated. In some patients this can be accomplished with endoscopic sphincterotomy; others will require a laparotomy. In those patients who do respond to medical therapy alone, elective decompression by the same technique is required.

In patients with asymptomatic gallstones, the cumulative probability of developing symptoms in one study was only 18 percent after 20 years [18]. The overall mortality rate for acute cholecystitis is about 5 percent. Higher mortality rates are present in patients with severe accompanying disease (especially diabetes mellitus and cirrhosis) and if complications are present, such as perforation, empyema, fistula, and cholangitis.

Acute Viral Hepatitis

Clinical Manifestations

There are three common types of acute viral hepatitis: hepatitis A, hepatitis B, and non-A, non-B hepatitis. The clinical manifestations of acute hepatitis vary from the usual benign, self-limited course to the infrequent chronic or fulminant fatal illness. For every recognized patient there are at least two to three subclinical cases. After exposure there is a variable incubation period followed by a prodromal illness characterized by nonspecific malaise, anorexia, and frequently, fever. Dark urine (conjugated bilirubinuria) marks the onset of the icteric phase of the illness. Fever subsides with the onset of jaundice, and constitutional symptoms usually abate within the next 2 to 4 weeks. The liver is often enlarged and somewhat tender, and the spleen may be palpable. The most characteristic biochemical finding is a 10- to 20-fold or more elevation of the serum transaminase levels (ALT/SGPT and AST/SGOT). There is usually a mild leukopenia with a relative lymphocytosis. In most patients the illness completely subsides within 6 to 12 weeks of onset.

Hepatitis A is caused by a small RNA virus. It occurs mostly in children and young adults and is the agent of most epidemics. The virus is shed in the stool, and transmission occurs via the fecal-oral route. The incubation period varies from 2 to 6 weeks. Patients are maximally contagious while still asymptomatic during the latter part of the incubation period. The clinical illness is almost always self-limited. Fatal cases are exceedingly rare, and hepatitis A does not lead to chronic liver disease or a chronic viral carrier state. The diagnosis is confirmed by demonstrating the transient acute-phase antibody (anti-HAVIgM) in the serum during the acute illness. In late convalescence, another antibody (anti-HAVIgG) predominates and confers lifelong immunity against recurrence (Fig. 4-2).

Hepatitis B is caused by a well-characterized DNA virus. Patients with acute viremia or with a chronic viral carrier state transmit disease via the overt parenteral route (blood transfusion, needle stick) or by the inapparent minute mucosal breaks such as may occur during sexual intercourse. The incubation period is 2 to 6 months. Onset of illness is often insidious, but a small number of patients present with an immune-complex-mediated urticarial rash and arthritis. Although many cases are asymptomatic, the clinically overt cases tend to be sicker and of longer duration than patients with hepatitis A. There is

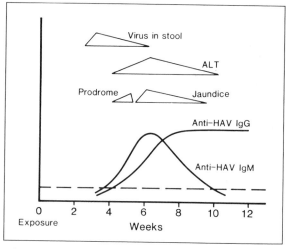

Figure 4–2. The serologic and clinical events of hepatitis A.

a greater, but still very low, incidence of fulminant hepatitis with death, and 5 to 10 percent of patients develop chronic viral infection with chronic hepatitis. Most have benign chronic persistent hepatitis, but some develop chronic active hepatitis and cirrhosis.

The diagnosis of hepatitis B is confirmed by demonstrating the new appearance of hepatitis B surface antigen (HBsAg) in the serum or the presence of acute-phase antibody to the core antigen (anti-HBc IgM). Greater than 90 percent of patients with symptomatic hepatitis B clear the surface antigen from the serum within 3 months of onset. The antibody to surface antigen (anti-HBs) then appears and confers immunity. Another antigen, hepatitis B e antigen (HBeAg) regularly circulates early in the course of acute hepatitis B. The detection of the e antigen correlates with a high concentration of circulating hepatitis B virus and indicates a high degree of infectivity. The disappearance of the e antigen or the appearance on its antibody (anti-HBe) signals a fall in concentration of circulating hepatitis B virus and reduced infectivity (Fig. 4-3). Recently, yet another viral antigen-antibody system has been found in some patients with HBsAg-positive serum. The delta antigen is a defective virus dependent on the hepatitis B virus for replication [27]. The delta antigen (HDAg) may infect patients simultaneously with acute hepatitis B or be superimposed on chronic hepatitis B illness. In either circumstance, delta-antigen infection appears to be associated with enhanced severity of the underlying hepatitis B illness. Delta infection is detected by finding the antibody (anti-HD IgM) in the serum. Currently it is found in less than 5 percent of hepatitis B patients in the United States. This infection has been termed hepatitis D.

The diagnosis of non-A, non-B hepatitis is made by serologic exclusion of other forms of acute viral hepatitis [9]. There are no serologic tests available for direct diagnosis. The epidemiology of non-A, non-B hepatitis is similar to that of hepatitis B. It accounts for more than 90 percent of posttransfusion hepatitis, but nonparenteral transmission also occurs. The acute clinical illness tends to be less severe than hepatitis B, but a prolonged course, frequently subclinical, occurs in many patients. Non-A, non-B hepatitis may lead to chronic hepatitis, cirrhosis, and a prolonged viral carrier state. The epidemiologic evidence suggests that at least two viruses cause this type of hepatitis.

Treatment

SUPPORTIVE CARE

There is no specific treatment for acute viral hepatitis, but symptomatic care at home generally suffices. Patients are encouraged to maintain adequate hydration and nutrition by frequent small feedings. Most patients seem to favor high-carbohydrate food taken early in the day. Strict bed rest is not advised, but rest periods and avoidance of exhausting activity are desirable. Unless the patient develops complications, most of the troublesome symptoms subside within 1 to 2 weeks of onset. Only a small number of patients with the most severe and protracted symptoms require hospitalization and intravenous therapy.

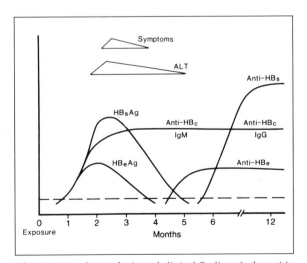

Figure 4–3. The serologic and clinical findings in hepatitis B.

IMMUNOPROPHYLAXIS

Standard immune globulin effectively prevents or attentuates the clinical illness of hepatitis A if it is given before exposure or afterwards during the early phase of the incubation period [59]. Immune globulin also may be useful after exposure to hepatitis B, but high-titer hepatitis B immune globulin (HBIG) is recommended for established high-risk exposure. Immune globulin administration provides only short-term passive protection. The currently available hepatitis B vaccine produces safe, effective, and long-term active immunization. The value of immune globulin administration for prevention of non-A, non-B hepatitis is unproven, but it is often given empirically after high-risk parental exposure.

Chronic Hepatitis

Chronic hepatitis can be diagnosed when hepatitis activity persists beyond 6 months. Chronic hepatitis encompasses a spectrum of findings with those of chronic persistent hepatitis and those of chronic active hepatitis at either end. Many patients show features intermediate between the two extremes and defy precise classification. In order to categorize patients in this spectrum of chronic hepatitis, it is necessary to integrate all the information from the history, physical examination, biochemistry, serologic data, and liver histology. The accurate assessment of an adequate specimen of liver tissue provides the most important information. Typically, chronic persistent hepatitis is a benign, nonprogressive lesion characterized by portal triaditis with mild or absent parenchymal necrosis and inflammation. A mild serum transaminase elevation is the only biochemical abnormality. Patients are asymptomatic with normal physical examination. The disease is not progressive in severity, and patients require no therapy. On the other hand, the histopathologic pattern of chronic active hepatitis includes an aggressive inflammatory necrosis of the hepatocytes adjacent to expanded portal tracts (piecemeal necrosis), diffuse parenchymal inflammation, and often a macronodular cirrhosis. The biochemical findings are grossly abnormal. Patients with chronic active hepatitis are frequently sick, and examination shows signs of chronic liver disease. The disease often progresses and leads to death from hepatic failure or complications of cirrhosis. Symptomatic patients with HBsAg-negative serum frequently benefit from steroid therapy. Benefit from antiviral therapy for patients with chronic hepatitis B infection remains to be determined.

Cirrhosis of the Liver

Cirrhosis of the liver exists when diffuse fibrous septa distort the normal hepatic architecture. Regenerative nodules often develop between fibrous bands that span between portal tracts and central veins. The two major types of cirrhosis are designated micronodular and macronodular. Micronodular cirrhosis is characterized by relatively uniform, small nodules of 2 to 3 mm in size. Virtually every portal tract and central vein is encompassed by the septating fibrosis. Micronodular cirrhosis is the most common form of cirrhosis encountered in the United States, and it usually occurs in the wake of severe alcoholic liver disease. Large nodules of variable size are seen in macronodular cirrhosis. Relatively wide bands of fibrosis traverse and distort the liver parenchyma, while adjacent parenchyma may retain normal architectural design. An important cause of macronodular cirrhosis is chronic active hepatitis. It is not uncommon to find cirrhosis of a mixed micronodular and macronodular type. The type of cirrhosis cannot always be determined from the small amount of tissue obtained by percutaneous liver biopsy.

Two interrelated processes account for the major clinical manifestations of cirrhosis. There are findings primarily related to impaired hepatocellular function, such as malaise, anorexia, jaundice, hypoalbuminemia, and prolongation of the prothrombin time. In most cases, the impaired parenchymal function is caused by a persistence of the same necroinflammatory process that has caused the cirrhosis, e.g., chronic active hepatitis or severe alcoholic hepatitis. Other findings in cirrhosis such as abdominal wall collateral veins, esophageal varices, and splenomegaly with hypersplenism are mostly related to the fibrous distortion of hepatic parenchyma causing increased resistance to portal venous blood flow and portal hypertension. Some findings such as ascites and portosystemic encephalopathy are related to an interplay of both hepatocellular dysfunction and portal hypertension. If the parenchymal injury subsides in patients with cirrhosis, the signs of hepatocellular dysfunction will improve while the portal hypertension persists or even increases in severity. This is, perhaps, best demonstrated in the occasional patient with decompensated alcoholic cirrhosis who truly abstains from alcohol.

Micronodular Cirrhosis

The most common cause of micronodular cirrhosis is alcoholic liver disease [40]. Only a minority of alcoholics develop clinically apparent liver disease. Nevertheless, it is a major cause of death in middle-aged adults in this country. Alcohol is a hepatocellular toxin, and the severity of illness largely depends on the amount and duration of alcohol abuse. The daily ingestion of alcohol equivalent to the contents of $1/2$-pint whiskey or a six-pack of beer puts one at risk. Women are more susceptible than men for similar amounts of alcohol consumed. The approximate alcohol contents of common beverages are shown in Table 4-7.

The spectrum of alcoholic liver disease ranges

Table 4–7. Approximate Alcohol Content of Common Beverages

Beverage	Amount	Alcohol Content	
		Percent	Grams
Beer	12-oz can	3.2	12
Beer	12-oz can	6	15
Natural wine	1 qt	12	100
	4-oz glass	12	14
Fortified wine	1 qt	20	150
Whiskey	1 pt	40	150
	1 shot (45 ml)	40	14

from benign fatty liver to micronodular cirrhosis. The most commonly identified syndrome between the two is alcoholic hepatitis, a toxic necroinflammatory hepatocellular lesion of variable severity. These clinical syndromes are not sharply separated, and a mixed pattern is often seen.

Fatty liver is the initial phase of alcoholic liver disease. Hepatocellular fat accumulation is an inevitable consequence of excessive alcohol metabolism. Patients are asymptomatic, but firm hepatomegaly may be present. The biochemical tests are generally normal except for alcohol-induced elevation of the gamma-glutamyl transpeptidase level and perhaps a mild, nonspecific increase in the serum alkaline phosphatase level. Histologically, the liver shows normal architectural relationships and macroglobular hepatocellular fat without inflammation or cellular necrosis. Fatty liver is reversible upon alcohol withdrawal.

With continued alcohol abuse, alcoholic hepatitis is likely to develop. The mildest form blends imperceptibly with fatty liver, except for greater disturbance of the standard liver function tests. Patients with a more severe form of disease, usually after an alcoholic binge, complain of weakness, anorexia, and dull right upper quadrant pain. They exhibit fever, jaundice, tender hepatomegaly, and often ascites with edema. Leukocytosis and markedly abnormal biochemical tests are typically found. The serum aspartate aminotransferase (AST/SGOT) level, however, seldom exceeds 10-fold elevation, but characteristically it is substantially more elevated than the alanine aminotransferase (ALT/SGPT) level. Occasionally, the serum alkaline phosphatase level is elevated greater than 10 times normal, reflecting severe intrahepatic cholestasis. In this circumstance, care must be taken to exclude distal common bile duct obstruction from associated chronic pancreatitis. Biochemical markers portending a poor prognosis include a serum bilirubin level greater than 15 mg/dl and a prothrombin time that is prolonged more than 5 seconds. In addition, a blood urea nitrogen value that is elevated or even in the upper range of normal, if not explained by intrinsic renal disease, dehydration, or gastrointestinal bleeding, might be an early indication of the hepatorenal syndrome. The histopathologic pattern shows fat, extensive hepatocellular necrosis, polymorphonuclear infiltration, and alcoholic hyaline (Mallory bodies).

The clinical course of alcoholic hepatitis is highly variable [52]. Mild forms are reversible with abstinence. Repeated episodes or prolonged low-grade alcoholic hepatitis, however, may lead to portal area fibrosis or even cirrhosis. Some patients with severe alcoholic hepatitis die of rapidly progressive liver failure or more often from complications such as gastrointestinal tract hemorrhage, aspiration, sepsis, or renal failure. Those who survive moderate to severe alcoholic hepatitis are at high risk to develop micronodular cirrhosis.

Complications of Cirrhosis
VARICEAL HEMORRHAGE
Hemorrhage from esophageal varices is a particularly fearsome complication of cirrhosis. In the alcoholic population with known esophageal varices, upper gastrointestinal tract hemorrhage occurs more often from lesions other than varices, such as erosive gastritis, peptic ulcer, and Mallory-Weiss tears. Thus urgent endoscopy is essential for accurate diagnosis. Therapy for variceal hemorrhage consists of resuscitative support and an initial trial of an intravenous infusion of vasopressin (0.1 to 0.8 µg per minute). If hemorrhage persists,

Table 4–8. Modified Child's Classification for Estimating Operative Mortality

	Class A	Class B*	Class C
Bedside findings:			
Jaundice	Absent		Present
Ascites	Absent		Present
Encephalopathy	Absent	⟶	Present
Nutrition	Good	or	Wasted
		⟵	
Laboratory values:			
Serum bilirubin	<2.0 mg%		>3.0 mg%
Serum albumin	>3.5 gm%		<3.0 gm%
Surgical mortality risk	Less than 10%		Greater than 90%

*The surgical risk for intermediate (class B) patients is widely variable and most difficult to assess. For any set of findings, the prognosis is greatly influenced by the recent trend of disease activity, i.e., deterioration toward class C or improvement toward class A parameters over the weeks or months immediately prior to evaluation.

a Sengstaken-Blakemore esophageal compression tube is placed by someone experienced in its use. This stops bleeding in most patients. If these measures fail, low-risk patients require emergency portal decompressing surgery; high-risk patients may respond to variceal sclerotherapy. The risk of operative mortality is assessed by the criteria of a modified Child's classification (Table 4-8). The early mortality rate for an episode of variceal hemorrhage exceeds 50 percent, and more than 80 percent of patients are dead within 2 years.

SPONTANEOUS BACTERIAL PERITONITIS
Spontaneous bacterial peritonitis is frequently seen in debilitated patients with alcoholic liver disease and ascites. The pathogenesis is thought to be from a prolonged bacteremia of enteric origin that seeds out in the peritoneum. E. coli is the most common pathogen; anaerobic bacteria are exceedingly rare. Patients may have typical findings of peritonitis, but more often the findings of peritoneal inflammation are subtle or even absent. The diagnosis depends on the findings on

paracentesis (see Table 4-9). The presence of more than 500 white blood cells per microliter with greater than 50 percent polymorphonuclear cells warrants empiric broad-spectrum antibiotic therapy pending the results of ascitic fluid and blood cultures. Treatment of the infection is usually successful, but patient survival is poor due to the severity of the underlying decompensated liver disease.

Portosystemic Encephalopathy

Portosystemic encephalopathy (PSE) is a neurologic syndrome often seen in patients with severe alcoholic liver disease. The diagnosis is based on clinical observation and varies from a subtle personality change to lethargy, confusion, and coma. The neurologic signs include asterixis (a nonspecific metabolic flap), hyperreflexia, clonus, and extensor plantar response. Multiple pathophysiologic causes are proposed, but shunting of toxic nitrogenous substances including ammonia from the portal venous system into the systemic circulation is best documented. Treatment is aimed at reducing the generation of nitrogenous metabolites in the lower bowel. The basic treatment regimen includes withdrawal of dietary protein and administration of oral lactulose or neomycin. Colonic bacteria degrade the nonmetabolizable lactulose into organic acids, and the lowered pH traps ammonia in the colonic lumen. Neomycin is not absorbed and reduces the colonic bacterial production of nitrogenous metabolites. For patients who develop portosystemic encephalopathy spontaneously in the course of progressive hepatocellular failure, the additional treatment options are few and prognosis is grave. The intravenous administration of branched-chain amino acids and oral bromocriptine have been used, but evidence of benefit is inconclusive. Often an event that precipitates portosystemic encephalopathy can be identified. The injudicious use of drugs (narcotics, tranquilizers, sedatives), gastrointestinal hemorrhage, and infections are common causes of this disorder in otherwise stable cirrhotic patients. Successful treatment of the pre-

cipitating event usually results in clearing of the hepatic encephalopathy.

Ascites

Ascites is one of the most common complications of cirrhosis. Large-volume ascites can be detected on physical examination by bulging flanks, shifting dullness, and fluid wave. Small amounts of peritoneal fluid are best detected by ultrasound examination.

There are many causes of ascites, but cirrhosis accounts for over 90 percent of cases. The pathogenesis of cirrhotic ascites is still debated [2]. One theory postulates a primary transudation of splanchnic and hepatic lymph leading to a hypovolemic stimulus for renal salt and water retention. An alternative hypothesis suggests an initial renal retention of salt and water with an expanded blood volume decompressing itself by ascites formation. In both instances, portal hypertension localizes the fluid retention to the peritoneal cavity. Neither theory explains all the observed findings.

A diagnostic paracentesis is useful in determining the cause of ascites. Typical findings for common causes are shown in Table 4-9. Ascitic fluid from patients with uncomplicated cirrhosis is clear, with total protein below 2.5 gm/dl, fewer than 500 white blood cells per microliter, less than 25 percent polymorphonuclear cells, and culture-negative. Recently, investigators have shown the serum-ascites albumin difference to be more reliable than total protein levels in differentiating transudative ascites (cirrhosis and congestive heart failure) from exudative ascites (peritoneal malignancy, infection, pancreatic inflammatory reaction) [48]. Patients with portal hypertension and transudative ascites have a serum-ascites albumin difference greater than 1.1 gm/dl (mean 1.6 ± 0.5 gm/dl), while patients with exudative ascites have value less than 1.1 gm/dl (mean 0.6 ± 0.4 gm/dl).

Cirrhotic ascites is generally managed with salt and occasionally fluid restriction. Ascites may subside spontaneously if the activity of the hepa-

Table 4–9. Characteristics of the Common Forms of Ascites*

Ascites	Gross Appearance	Total Protein (gm/dl)	Serum-Ascites Albumin Difference (gm/dl)	WBCs (per μl)	PMNs (%)	Other
Cirrhotic	Clear	<2.5	>1.1	<300	<25	—
Spontaneous bacterial peritonitis	Cloudy	<2.5	>1.1†	>500	>50	Positive bacterial culture
Cardiac	Clear	<2.5	>1.1	<300	<25	
Neoplastic	Clear, bloody	>2.5	<1.1	Variable	<50	Positive cytology
Pancreatic	Clear, cloudy	>3.0	<1.1	Variable	25–75	High amylase
Tuberculous	Clear, cloudy	>2.5	<1.1	Variable	<25	Positive AFB culture

*WBC = white blood cell; PMN = polymorphonuclear leukocyte; AFB = acid-fast bacilli.
†"Mixed" cause of ascites; value usually high but can be below 1.1 gm/dl.

tocellular disease improves. Large-volume paracentesis for relief of symptoms in patients with tense ascites and edema may not be as hazardous as once feared [17,29]. Recent studies show no evidence for hypovolemia or electrolyte change in such patients after a 5-liter paracentesis. Diuretic therapy, however, is still the favored method for ascites mobilization. Spironolactone alone or combined with furosemide is most often used. If the induced diuresis is too vigorous, hypovolemia and reversible prerenal azotemia may develop. This too is less likely to occur in patients with associated edema [45]. Therapy for exudative ascites is individualized according to the cause.

Primary Hepatic Tumors

Primary hepatic tumors, either benign or malignant, are not often encountered in the United States. Worldwide, however, hepatocellular carcinoma is a leading cause of death due to cancer, particularly in the Orient and Africa. Some benign hepatic tumors have increased in frequency in the past few decades with the widespread estrogen usage in birth control pills. The early and accurate diagnosis of primary hepatic tumors is crucial to appropriate treatment.

Hepatocellular Carcinoma
EPIDEMIOLOGY
Hepatocellular carcinoma (HCC) is most often found in patients with preexisting cirrhosis of the liver of varied cause. The highest incidence occurs in cirrhotic patients from chronic hepatitis B viral infection. In Asia as well as in the United States, hepatocellular carcinoma has been found in nearly half the patients dying of chronic hepatitis B liver disease. The almost 100-fold greater incidence of hepatocellular carcinoma in Asia compared to the United States is directly related to the markedly higher prevalence of chronic hepatitis B viral infection in that area of the world. In Taiwan, for example, between 15 and 20 percent of the population has HBsAg-positive serum compared to less than 0.5 percent in the United States.

DIAGNOSIS
In the United States, hepatocellular carcinoma is usually suspected when a patient with cirrhosis presents with new right upper quadrant pain, an enlarging liver, or unexplained deterioration in liver function. Occasionally, patients present with an acute abdominal crisis, a friction rub and bruit over the liver, and hemoperitoneum caused by

erosion of the hepatocellular carcinoma through the liver capsule. A disproportionately elevated serum alkaline phosphatase level and a markedly elevated serum alpha-fetoprotein level are usually present. These findings indicated a late and relatively advanced phase of the disease. At this stage, any one of the liver imaging tests is likely to show a large, solid, space-occupying lesion. The diagnosis is confirmed by liver biopsy.

In the Orient, where hepatocellular carcinoma abounds, the same scenario may exist, but prospective surveillance studies in high-risk patients have been able to detect early lesions in asymptomatic patients [32,39,57]. Ultrasonography, computed tomography, and angiography are equally sensitive, and all are superior to radioisotopic liver scanning for detection of tumors less than 3 cm in size. Magnetic resonance imaging may prove to be the most sensitive and specific test for diagnosis of early hepatocellular carcinoma, but data are not yet available. Ultrasonography is the least invasive and expensive procedure and thus is the most practical method for serial examinations. In surveillance studies, 3-month intervals have been used. The detection of a new mass combined with a rising serum alpha-fetoprotein level over 400 ng/ml is highly indicative of hepatocellular carcinoma. An alpha-fetoprotein level alone is insufficient for diagnosis. The level is often nonspecifically elevated in patients with chronic liver disease, and the level may be within the normal range in 20 to 40 percent of patients with hepatocellular carcinoma less than 3 cm in size. The diagnosis of early hepatocellular carcinoma in a suspicious mass may be confirmed by ultrasonographic guided aspiration cytology or liver biopsy. Identification of a small, asymptomatic tumor offers the best prospect for surgical cure.

TREATMENT AND PROGNOSIS

When hepatocellular carcinoma is diagnosed at an advanced stage, surgical cure is generally no longer possible and other forms of therapy, including chemotherapy, radiation, and arterial embolization, offer minimal palliation and no appreciable prolongation of life. Prognosis in these symptomatic patients from the time of diagnosis is less than 6 months. On the contrary, a good potential for resectional surgical cure exists when early, asymptomatic lesions are identified. Severe hepatic dysfunction from the often associated cirrhosis may preclude surgery or dictate the need for only a limited wedge resection. For such patients, however, who are good operative candidates, reports from the Orient in small series indicate cure rates from 50 to 90 percent. The growth rate for unresected small hepatocellular carcinoma is quite variable, and the average survival is 50 percent at 2 years after diagnosis [12].

Hepatocellular Adenoma

CLINICAL MANIFESTATIONS

Hepatocellular adenoma is an uncommon benign tumor also seen primarily in women during the childbearing years. The occurrence of this tumor has been known for many years, but the incidence has increased substantially with the advent of widespread estrogen usage in contraceptive pills [5]. From 50 to 70 percent of women with hepatocellular adenoma present with acute abdominal pain. Symptoms are caused by hemorrhagic infarction of the tumor or bleeding into the peritoneal cavity. Severe life-threatening hemorrhage may occur. A minority of patients present with an asymptomatic mass in the right upper abdominal quadrant. The tumor appears to be estrogen-responsive. In women taking estrogen supplements, the adenoma occurs more often and at a younger age, grows larger, and exhibits more hemorrhagic complications.

DIAGNOSIS

A presumptive diagnosis can often be made on gross appearance during urgent surgery for an acute bleeding event. In an elective clinical setting, the adenoma appears as a "cold" space-occupying lesion on isotopic liver scan. Ultrasonography and computed tomography often reveal a solid liver mass. A hepatic arteriogram shows a characteristic, but not diagnostically specific hypervascular pattern. The arteriogram is also useful in planning potential resectional strategy. The tumor mass is well circumscribed, often with a pseudocapsule, and symptomatic adenomas often exceed 10 cm in size. The definitive diagnosis rests with the histologic examination. The tumor is composed of nearly normal appearing hepatocytes lacking the normal columnar and lobular orientation. There are no portal tracts, and Kupfer cells are scanty or absent. On rare occasions the benign tumor harbors a focus of hepatocellular carcinoma.

TREATMENT
Surgical resection is advised for symptomatic patients to avoid the hazards of severe hemorrhage and the remote possibility of malignant transformation. A few fortuitously identified small lesions that regress promptly off estrogen may not require surgery.

Focal Nodular Hyperplasia
CLINICAL MANIFESTATIONS
Focal nodular hyperplasia is a rare benign tumor most often seen in women during their reproductive years [30]. This tumor is usually asymptomatic. It is often discovered incidentally at laparot-

omy for other reasons or as a liver mass on routine examination. Infrequently hemorrhage into the tumor or peritoneal cavity causes acute abdominal pain. There are no associated biochemical abnormalities. Evidence for estrogen responsiveness is less convincing compared to hepatocellular adenoma.

DIAGNOSIS
Imaging procedures of the liver usually detect the tumor mass, but isotopic liver scanning is variable and may show decreased, normal, or enhanced uptake of the tagged sulfur colloid. Histologic diagnosis usually requires a generous wedge biopsy, since a needle biopsy may contain too little tissue to discern the characteristic pattern likened to a focal cirrhosis. Normal-appearing hepatic tissue is septated by fibrous bands radiating from a dense, fibrous core. The fibrous septa contain many bile ducts and a chronic lymphocytic infiltration. Hepatocellular malignancy does not occur.

TREATMENT
Asymptomatic lesions require no treatment, but they should be biopsied for diagnosis. Incidentally encountered lesions found at surgery should be removed only if the resection is technically uncomplicated.

References

1. Almy, T. P., and Howell, D. A.   Diverticular disease of the colon. *N. Engl. J. Med.* 302: 324, 1980.
2. Better, O. S., and Schrier, R. W.   Disturbed volume hemostasis in patients with cirrhosis of the liver. *Kidney Int.* 23: 303, 1983.
3. Blaser, M. J., and Reller, L. B.   *Campylobacter* enteritis. *N. Engl. J. Med.* 305: 1444, 1981.
4. Blaser, M. J.   Gastric *Campylobacter*-like organisms, gastritis, and peptic ulcer disease. *Gastroenterology* 93: 371, 1987.
5. Brugge, W. R., Goff, J. S., Allen, N. C., et al.   Development of a dual label Schilling test for pancreatic insufficiency. *Gastroenterology* 78: 937, 1980.

6. Castell, D. O.   Medical therapy for reflux esophagitis: 1986 and beyond (Editorial). *Ann. Intern. Med.* 104: 112, 1986.
7. Cello, J. P.   Ulcerative Colitis. in M. H. Sleisenger and J. S. Fordtran (Eds.), *Gastrointestinal Disease*, 3d Ed. Philadelphia: Saunders, 1983. Pp. 1122–1168.
8. Cello, J. P.   Carcinoma of the Pancreas. In M. H. Sleisenger and J. S. Fordham (Eds.), *Gastrointestinal Disease*, 3d Ed. Philadelphia: Saunders, 1983. Pp. 1514–1526.
9. Dienstag, J. L.   Non-A, non-B hepatitis: I. Recognition, epidemiology and clinical features. *Gastroenterology* 85: 439, 1983.
10. Donaldson, R. M.   Crohn's Disease. In M. H. Sleis-

enger and J. S. Fordtran (Eds.), *Gastrointestinal Disease,* 3d Ed. Philadelphia: Saunders, 1983. Pp. 1088–1121.

11. DuPont, J. B., Lee, J. R., Burton, G. R., and Cohn, I. Adenocarcinoma of the stomach: Review of 1497 cases. *Cancer* 41: 941, 1978.

12. Ebara, M., Ohto, M., Schwagawa, T., Sugiura, N., Kimura, K., Matsutani, S., Moreta, M., Saisko, H., Tsuchiga, Y., and Okuda, K. Natural history of minute hepatocellular carcinoma smaller than 3 cm complicating cirrhosis. *Gastroenterology* 90: 289, 1986.

13. Ellis, F. H., Jr. Carcinoma of the esophagus. *CA* 33: 264, 1983.

14. Fenoglio-Preiser, C. M., and Hutter, R. V. P. Colorectal polyp: Pathologic diagnosis and clinical significance. *CA* 35: 322, 1985.

15. Fleischer, D. Etiology and prevalence of severe persistent upper gastrointestinal bleeding. *Gastroenterology* 84: 538, 1983.

16. Fromm, H. Gallstone dissolution therapy: Current status and future prospects. *Gastroenterology* 91: 1560, 1986.

17. Gines, P., Arroyo, V., Quintero, E., et al. Comparison of paracentesis and diuretics in the treatment of cirrhosis with tense ascites. *Gastroenterology* 93: 234, 1987.

18. Gracie, W. A., and Ransohoff, D. F. The natural history of silent gallstones. *N. Engl. J. Med.* 307: 798, 1982.

19. Gray, G. M. Maldigestion and Malabsorption. In M. H. Sleisenger and J. S. Fordtran (Eds.), *Gastrointestinal Disease,* 3d Ed. Philadelphia: Saunders, 1983. Pp. 228–256.

20. Green, P. H. R., O'Toole, K. M., Weinberg, L. M., and Goldfarb, J. P. Early gastric cancer. *Gastroenterology* 81: 247, 1981.

21. Greenstern, A. J., Sachar, D. B., Smith, H., Pucillo, A., et al. Cancer in universal and left-sided ulcerative colitis: Factors determining. *Gastroenterology* 77: 290, 1979.

22. Greenstern, A., Janowitz, H., and Sachar, D. B. The extraintestinal complication of Crohn's disease and ulcerative colitis in study of 700 patients. *Medicine* 55: 401, 1976.

23. Grendell, J. H., and Cello, J. P. Chronic Pancreatitis. In M. H. Sleisenger and J. S. Fordtran (Eds.), *Gastrointestinal Disease,* 3d Ed. Philadelphia: Saunders, 1983. Pp. 1485–1513.

24. Harney, M. R., Culane, M. D., Montgomery, R. D., et al. Evaluation of xylose absorption as measured in blood and urine: A one hour blood xylose screening test in malabsorption. *Gastroenterology* 75: 393, 1978.

25. Hawkey, C. J., and Rampton, D. S. Prostaglandins and the gastrointestinal mucosa: Are they important in its function, disease or treatment? *Gastroenterology* 89: 1162, 1985.

26. Isenberg, J. I., Peterson, W. L., Elashoff, J. D., Sandersfeld, M. A., Reedy, T. J., Ippoliti, A. F., Van Deventer, G. M., Frankl, H., Longstreth, G. F., and Anderson, D. S. Healing of benign gastric ulcer with low-dose antacid or cimetidine: A double-blind, randomized, placebo-controlled trial. *N. Engl. J. Med.* 308: 1319, 1983.

27. Jacobson, I. M., and Dienstag, J. L. The delta hepatitis agent: "Viral hepatitis, type D" (Editorial). *Gastroenterology* 86: 1614, 1984.

28. Jerzy Glass, G. B. Immunology of atrophic gastritis. *N.Y. State J. Med.* 11: 1697, 1977.

29. Kao, H. W., Rakov, N. E., Savage, E., and Reynolds, T. B. The effect of large-volume paracentesis on plasma volume: A cause of hypovolemia? *Hepatology* 5: 403, 1985.

30. Kerlin, P., Davis, G. L., McGill, D. B., Weiland, C. H., Adson, M. A., and Sheedy, P. H. Hepatic adenoma and focal nodular hyperplasia: Clinical, pathologic and radiographic features. *Gastroenterology* 84: 994, 1983.

31. Klatskin, G. Hepatic tumors: Possible relationship to use of oral contraceptives. *Gastroenterology* 73: 386, 1977.

32. Kobayashi, K., Sugimoto, T., Makino, H., Kumagai, M., Unoura, M., Tanaka, N., Kato, Y., and Hattore, N. Screening methods for early detection of hepatocellular carcinoma. *Hepatology* 5: 1100, 1985.

33. Krejs, G. J., and Fordtran, J. S. Diarrhea. In M. H. Sleisenger and J. S. Fordtran (Eds.), *Gastrointestinal Disease,* 3d Ed. Philadelphia: Saunders, 1983. Pp. 257–280.

34. Larson, D. E., and Farnell, M. B. Upper gastrointestinal hemorrhage. *Mayo Clin. Proc.* 58: 371, 1983.

35. Lauritsen, K., Rume, S. J., Bytzer, P., Kelback, H., et al. Effect of Omeprazole and cimetidine on duodenal ulcer: A double-blind comparative trial. *N. Engl. J. Med.* 312: 958, 1985.

36. Lawrence, W., Jr.   Gastric cancer. *CA* 36: 216, 1986.

37. Lennard-Jones, J. E.   Functional gastrointestinal disorders. *N. Engl. J. Med.* 308: 431, 1983.

38. Lewis, J. H.   Treatment of gastric ulcer: What is old and what is new? *Arch. Intern. Med.* 143: 264, 1983.

39. Liaw, F., Tai, D., Chic, C., Lin, D., Sheen, I., Chen, T., and Pao, C.   Early detection of hepatocellular carcinoma in patients with chronic type B hepatitis. *Gastroenterology* 90: 263, 1986.

40. Lieber, C. S.   Alcohol and the liver: 1984 update. *Hepatology* 4: 1243, 1984.

41. Lieberman, D. A., and Keeffe, E. B.   Treatment of severe reflux esophagitis with cimetidine and metoclopramide. *Ann. Intern. Med.* 104: 21, 1986.

42. Lofti, A. M., Spencer, R. J., Ilstrup, D. M., and Meton, J. M.   Colorectal polyps and the risk of subsequent carcinoma. *Mayo Clin. Proc.* 61: 337, 1986.

43. Moossa, A. R.   Diagnostic tests and procedures in acute pancreatitis. *N. Engl. J. Med.* 311: 639, 1984.

44. Newcomer, A. D., Hofman, A. F., Dimagno, E. P., Thomas, P. J., and Carlson, G. L.   Triolein breath test. *Gastroenterology* 76: 6, 1979.

45. Packros, P. J., and Reynolds, T. B.   Rapid diuresis in patients with ascites from chronic liver disease: The importance of peripheral edema. *Gastroenterology* 90: 1827, 1986.

46. Painter, N. S.   Diverticular Disease of the Colon. In S. C. Truelove and D. P. Jewell (Eds.), *Topics in Gastroenterology.* Oxford: Blas, 1973. Pp. 294–306.

47. Piper, D. W.   Drugs for the prevention of peptic ulcer recurrence. *Drugs* 26: 439, 1983.

48. Rector, W. G., and Reynolds, T. B.   Superiority of the serum-ascites albumin difference over the ascites total protein concentration in separation of "transudative" and "exudative" ascites. *Am. J. Med.* 77: 83, 1984.

49. Richter, J. E., and Costell, D. O.   Gastroesophageal reflux: Pathogenesis, diagnosis and therapy. *Ann. Intern. Med.* 97: 93, 1982.

50. Salt, W. B., II, and Schenker, S.   Amylase: Its clinical significance: A review of the literature. *Medicine* 55: 273, 1976.

51. Satterwhite, T. W., and DuPont, H. L.   The patient with acute diarrhea. *J.A.M.A.* 236: 2662, 1976.

52. Schenker, S.   Alcoholic liver disease: Evaluation of natural history and prognostic factors. *Hepatology* 4: 365, 1984.

53. Schuster, M.   Irritable Bowel Syndrome. In M. H. Sleisenger and J. S. Fordtran (Eds.), *Gastrointestinal Disease,* 3d Ed. Philadelphia: Saunders, 1983. Pp. 880–896.

54. Sischy, B., and Gunderson, L. L.   The evolving role of radiation therapy in the management of colorectal cancer. *CA* 36: 351, 1986.

55. Soergel, W.   Acute Pancreatitis. In M. H. Sleisenger and J. S. Fordtran (Eds.), *Gastrointestinal Disease,* 3d Ed. Philadelphia: Saunders, 1983. Pp. 1462–1484.

56. Somerville, K. W., and Langman, M. J. S.   Newer antisecretory agents for peptic ulcer. *Drugs* 25: 315, 1983.

57. Tong, M. J.   Diagnosis of primary hepatocellular carcinoma (Editorial). *Gastroenterology* 91: 1306, 1986.

58. Zimmer, M., Zuidema, G. D., Smith, P. L., and Mignosa, M.   The prevention of upper gastrointestinal tract bleeding in patients in an intensive care unit. *Surg. Gynecol. Obstet.* 153: 214, 1981.

59. Recommendations for protection against viral hepatitis. *Morb. Mortal. Weekly Rep.* 34: 313, 1985.

Hematology and Oncology

5

Hematology

Scot M. Sedlacek and
J. Fred Kolhouse*

Disorders of Erythrocytes

Anemia

Anemia occurs when the rate of erythrocyte loss exceeds the rate of production by the bone marrow. Since mature erythrocytes survive approximately 120 days, these cells are normally replaced by new erythrocytes (reticulocytes) such that approximately 0.8 percent of all erythrocytes at any time are reticulocytes. When survival is shortened by disease, the marrow compensates by increasing production. If marrow compensation is limited, or if the destruction occurs at a rate exceeding the ability of the healthy marrow to compensate, anemia occurs.

Anemia is usually defined by the hematocrit (or hemoglobin) concentration. The hematocrit represents the proportion of whole blood occupied by erythrocytes and adequately reflects the erythroid mass *except* when shifts in the plasma volume occur, such as in dehydration or overhydration.

DIAGNOSIS

The symptoms of anemia per se are generally quite nonspecific, consisting of lethargy, easy fatigue, and palpitations. If anemia is severe (hematocrit < 25 percent), dyspnea on exertion, syncope, palpitations, and symptoms of high-output

congestive heart failure also may be observed. Underlying vascular disease may become manifest as a result of anemia. Examples include angina or cerebral vascular symptoms when the hematocrit is below 25 to 30 percent.

The signs of anemia are also somewhat insensitive and nonspecific, and a moderately reduced hematocrit may be difficult to detect by examination of mucous membranes and nail beds for pallor. Marked changes in nail beds and mucous membranes resembling anemia may occur in other chronic diseases with little or no anemia. Some signs, however, are more specific for certain causes of anemia, and these will be discussed below.

After the decision has been made that anemia is present, the physician must begin to consider the etiology. The initial steps in this process are examination of the *peripheral blood smear* for shift macrocytes and other red cell abnormalities.

Many abnormalities may yield diagnostic information on the peripheral smear. The physician must be wary of artifacts such as erythrocytes with no central pallor and bizarre leukocyte morphology that is the result of storage in anticoagulants present in laboratory test tubes. A morphologic abnormality involving 100 percent of the erythrocytes does not occur and is always an artifact. True spherocytes will be admixed with relatively normal appearing erythrocytes. The appropriate area that minimizes artifact must be

*The authors wish to thank Drs. M. Ray Lamb and John C. Deutsch for their assistance and Susan A. Veach for preparing this chapter.

searched for on the peripheral smear. Examples of diagnostic abnormalities of erythrocytes are spherocytes, virtually always a hemolytic anemia; ecchinocytes (burr cells), pyruvate kinase deficiency and uremia; target cells, iron deficiency, hemoglobinopathies, liver disease, and after splenectomy; target cells and spherocytes, virtually diagnostic of hemoglobin C disease; sickle cells, hemoglobin S disease; and microangiopathic cells, vasculitis as in thrombotic thrombocytopenic purpura (TTP) or disseminated intravascular coagulation (DIC). Examination of leukocytes may reveal a left shift with many immature forms, such as bands, metamyelocytes, myelocytes, promyelocytes, or blasts. Hypersegmentation (right shift) where leukocytes contain more than five lobes suggests megaloblastic anemia. Vacuolation of the granulocytes in a *fresh* smear is virtually diagnostic of bacterial sepsis. Abnormalities in the size and number of platelets (see below) also may be determined. Nucleated erythrocytes always imply severe stress or hematologic disease, frequently with marrow involvement. Howell-Jolly bodies are remnants of nuclei normally present in erythrocytes following splenectomy.

The reticulocyte index (corrected reticulocyte count) is determined [52–54] by correcting the reticulocyte count for the hematocrit, assuming a normal hematocrit of 45 percent (Table 5-1). This correction is necessary because reticulocytes are enumerated per 1000 erythrocytes. For example, the absolute reticulocyte number may remain un-

changed, but the reticulocyte count will increase twofold with a decrease of the hematocrit from 50 to 25 percent. In addition, the reticulocyte count is usually corrected for maturation time of newly released erythrocytes in the peripheral blood. These erythrocytes are called shift cells and are recognized as polychromatophilic macrocytes. Under a stimulus by erythropoietin, reticulocytes that normally require 24 to 48 hours in the marrow for maturation are "shifted" into the circulation. When these cells are present, the reticulocyte count should be corrected for the hematocrit because of the maturation time of these cells [52–54]. This value is 1 when the hematocrit is 45 percent and 2.0 when the hematocrit is 30 percent (see Table 5-1). In making these two corrections, one can determine the reticulocyte index and apply the first step in the differential diagnosis of anemia by determining if the anemia is hypoproliferative (reticulocyte index less than 2) or caused by excessive destruction of erythrocytes (reticulocyte index greater than 2 and usually greater than 3). The differential diagnosis of hypoproliferative anemias is listed in Table 5-2 according to their reticulocyte index and size. Examination of the peripheral smear and other erythroid indices (especially the mean corpuscular volume, MCV) helps to further subclassify this group of anemias, which account for as many as 80 percent of all anemias.

Hypoproliferative Anemias (Reticulocyte Index < 2)

The hypoproliferative anemias may be subdivided into those with a low mean corpuscular volume (microcytic), a normal mean corpuscular volume (normocytic), and a high mean corpuscular volume (macrocytic) (see Table 5-2).

HYPOPROLIFERATIVE ANEMIAS WITH A LOW MEAN CORPUSCULAR VOLUME

The differential diagnosis of microcytic hypoproliferative anemias is shown in Table 5-2. All microcytic anemias are due to a defect in the synthesis of either heme or globin. Since heme and

Table 5–1. *Correction of the Reticulocyte Count*

$$\text{Reticulocyte index} = \text{percent reticulocytes} \times \frac{\text{observed hematocrit}}{45}$$

Correction of reticulocyte index for shift cells:

Hematocrit	Correction*
45 percent	1.0
35 percent	1.5
25 percent	2.0

*Reticulocyte index is divided by the correction factor to account for the maturation time (24 to 48 hours) of reticulocytes after release from the marrow.

Table 5–2. *Differential Diagnoses of Anemias Based on Mean Corpuscular Volume (MCV) and Reticulocyte Index (RI)*

Low MCV (RI < 2)	Normal MCV (RI < 2)	High MCV	
		Mild (100–115; RI < 2)	Mild or Severe (> 115; RI < 2)
Disorders of heme synthesis (RI < 2)	Most iron-deficiency anemia	Alcoholism	Megaloblastosis of cobalamin or folate deficiency
Iron deficiency	Anemia of chronic disorders	Liver disease	Refractory anemia, preleukemia
Anemia of chronic disorders	Renal insufficiency	Smoking	Aplastic anemias
Lead poisoning	Aplastic anemia	Hypothyroidism	
Sideroblastic anemia	Combination of macrocytic and microcytic anemias, i.e., iron deficiency and folate deficiency	Megaloblastosis of cobalamin or folate deficiency	
Disorders of globin synthesis (RI *usually* < 2):	RI > 2	RI > 2	
Alpha-thalassemias	Acute blood loss	Hemolytic anemia	
Beta-thalassemias	Hemoglobinopathies		
Other thalassemias	Hemolytic anemia		

globin synthesis are normally balanced, deficiency of synthesis in either of these parts of hemoglobin will result in decreased production of the other component.

MICROCYTIC ANEMIAS WITH DEFECTIVE
HEME SYNTHESIS

Iron Deficiency

Iron-deficiency anemia is perhaps the most common cause of anemia worldwide. Iron is important in the synthesis of heme, since conversion of protoporphyrin 9 to heme by heme synthetase involves the insertion of iron into protoporphyrin 9. When iron stores are inadequate, reduced synthesis of heme occurs, and this is followed by reduced synthesis of hemoglobin in maturing erythroid cells in the marrow. These cells probably undergo at least one extra division and thus become smaller (low mean corpuscular volume) in an abortive attempt to obtain a normal cellular hemoglobin concentration.

The most common cause for iron deficiency in developed countries is excessive blood loss, which can occur as a result of acute or chronic gastrointestinal bleeding or excessive menstrual periods [5]. Iron deficiency in females of childbearing age is almost invariably due to excessive menstrual blood loss (normally approximately 50 to 60 ml per month) or pregnancy with breast feeding (which can be associated with 900 to over 1000 mg iron loss per pregnancy) [28]. Iron deficiency in males and postmenopausal females must always be explained. Such iron deficiency in these individuals can be the initial manifestation of bleeding from an underlying occult malignancy of the gastrointestinal tract.

Iron is present in the diet at approximately 10 to 20 mg per day [79]. Between 1 and 2 mg per day is normally absorbed by a poorly understood mechanism in the duodenum [2]. This quantity of iron is usually adequate to replace insensitive losses that occur from the skin and the gastrointestinal tract in normal individuals. Once absorbed from the duodenum, iron is transported by an iron-transport protein referred to as transferrin [59]. Transferrin delivers iron to the erythroid

cells of the marrow. As erythrocytes undergo normal senescence in the blood, they are removed by the reticuloendothelial system; the heme is degraded to form bilirubin, and the iron normally is recycled by transferrin back to the erythroid precursors in the marrow. Iron is stored in the reticuloendothelial system as hemosiderin and in a more rapidly usable form as ferritin. The rate-limiting step for increases in marrow erythroid production is the mobilization of iron from the reticuloendothelial system [54].

Some signs and symptoms are unique to severe iron deficiency. The typical patient is a premenopausal female who indicates that menstrual flow is usually normal but occasionally heavy and associated with clots. Clots during the menstrual period constitute excellent evidence that menstrual flow is exceedingly heavy. In severe iron deficiency, patients develop esophageal webbs (Plummer-Vinson syndrome) with associated symptoms and spoon nails, although these are rare today. A very common characteristic feature of severe iron deficiency that will not be volunteered unless asked for is pica. Pica may be for dirt, starch, or more commonly, ice. Patient's spouses will frequently state that the patient is incessantly crunching on ice. The ice-eating pica (pagophagia) is a manifestation of iron deficiency and not a cause.

LABORATORY EVALUATION. The laboratory abnormalities in iron deficiency are related to the severity of the iron deficiency [5, 34]. Initially, when iron deficiency is present without anemia, the patient may complain of some of the preceding nonspecific symptoms but little else. At this point, the mean corpuscular volume and hematocrit are normal, the ferritin level is low, and the fasting serum iron level and iron-binding capacity (binding to transferrin) are normal. Subsequently, the serum iron level decreases, the iron-binding capacity increases, and the free erythrocyte protoporphyrin level (a reflection of disturbed porphyrin metabolism) increases prior to a decrease in the mean corpuscular volume or development of anemia. As anemia develops, the mean corpuscular volume remains normal until the hemoglobin has decreased to below 10 gm%. At this point, the mean corpuscular volume begins to decrease until the patient has the full picture of iron-deficiency anemia. It should be noted that over 90 percent of patients with anemia due to iron deficiency have a normal mean corpuscular volume. In uncomplicated iron deficiency, transferrin synthesis and serum transferrin levels begin to increase with a resultant greater total iron-binding capacity. The serum ferritin level, an indicator of iron stores, drops to below 12 ng/ml and is the earliest indicator of iron deficiency [5, 34]. In severe iron deficiency, the peripheral smear shows marked anisocytosis, and this is reflected by a very wide red cell distribution width (RDW) [9]. In contrast, in early iron-deficiency anemia, there is a mixed population of normocytic cells with hypochromic microcytic cells. The "gold standard" for body iron stores is the content of iron in the marrow, [34] since marrow iron stores disappear early in iron deficiency.

TREATMENT. If the anemia of iron deficiency is life-threatening, i.e., hemoglobin less than 5 gm% or evidence of vascular insufficiency exists, transfusion may be required to rapidly elevate the hematocrit. However, the onset of iron-deficiency anemia is usually gradual with compensation of the cardiovascular system for the decreased delivery of oxygen to tissues. In this case, iron deficiency is best and most safely treated by oral iron preparations. Table 5-3 lists the reasons for failure to respond to oral iron.

There are many iron preparations available from the pharmaceutical industry, but the simplest, most effective, and least expensive form of iron is ferrous sulfate. A 300-mg tablet of ferrous sulfate contains 60 mg elemental iron [34]. If taken three times a day, such tablets will restore

Table 5–3. *Reasons for Failure of Oral Iron Therapy*

Ineffective oral iron preparation
Malabsorption of iron
Noncompliance
Misdiagnosis or another superimposed cause for anemia
Continued blood loss

a patient's hematocrit over several months [34]. The various chemical modifications of iron salts marketed are a result of the occurrence of mid-epigastric pain and a change in bowel habits related to ingestion of ferrous sulfate. Claims that a given iron preparation does not cause these symptoms and is better tolerated may be true, but the absence of symptoms related to ingestion of oral iron is frequently a reflection of poor absorption of the iron. Poor absorption of oral ferrous sulfate also can be caused by gastrointestinal malabsorption, such as occurs after surgical procedures for ulcer disease (e.g., partial gastrectomy and gastrointestinal tract diversion procedures that bypass the duodenum). Malabsorption of iron also may occur in achlorhydria, a condition common in older individuals. Under these circumstances, acid is not available in the stomach and the patients malabsorb food iron, which is in the form of ferric iron. Adequate absorption of oral iron can be easily assessed by obtaining a fasting serum iron determination before and after ingestion of a 300-mg tablet of ferrous sulfate. The serum iron level, 4 hours later, should rise a minimum of twofold (when the fasting serum iron level is normal) to as high as fivefold when the fasting serum iron level is low [98].

Patients also fail to respond to oral iron for other reasons. One of these reasons is noncompliance because of the side effects of oral iron. A useful way to determine compliance is to ask patients if their stools have changed color. The stool always changes to a slate gray color on ingestion of iron. If the patient is noncompliant, compliance can frequently be obtained by reducing the usual dose of 300 mg ferrous sulfate three times a day to twice a day or even once a day. Alternatively, iron tablets with less quantities of elemental iron can be used, such as ferrous fumerate with 37 mg elemental iron.

Another cause of failure to respond to treatment of iron deficiency is misdiagnosis. The differential diagnosis of low mean corpuscular volume hypoproliferative anemia is shown in Table 5-2, and any of the other causes besides iron deficiency can account for failure to respond to oral iron. One expects that the reduced hematocrit and hemoglobin will be 50 percent corrected by 6 weeks after initiation of oral iron. On occasion, patients with a hypoproliferative anemia will have unrecognized thalassemia along with iron deficiency. In this situation, the anemia will correct at the appropriate rate initially but will reach a plateau below the normal level of hemoglobin. At that point, one should consider misdiagnosis. Finally, continued blood loss will negate the effect of iron replacement.

An absolute indication for parental iron therapy is malabsorption of oral iron. A relative indication for parental iron is failure to comply with the use of oral iron. The major drawback to the use of parental iron is the occasional allergic reaction associated with this therapy, and such reactions appear to occur most often in patients with underlying immunologic disorders such as systemic lupus erythematosus (SLE) and rheumatoid arthritis.

It cannot be overemphasized that the etiology of iron deficiency should be addressed in every patient. This is especially true in men and postmenopausal females, in whom the stores of iron are lost from bleeding.

Hemochromatosis

Hemochromatosis (parenchymal iron overload) may be primary (hereditary) or secondary (acquired) from a chronic transfusion requirement or excessive dietary intake of iron with alcohol (South African bantu). The primary hemochromatosis gene is closely linked to HLA-A3 and is caused by increased absorption of dietary iron by an unknown mechanism [99]. Since a total-body iron level of at least 20 gm is present prior to clinical manifestations and the abnormally increased iron absorption is 1 to 2 mg per day, 25 to 50 years are required prior to clinical disease. Hemochromatosis affects the liver, the heart, the islet cells of the pancreas (diabetes mellitus), the skin (bronzing), and the endocrine system (hypogonadism). The disease affects predominantly men. Women may, in part, be protected because of menstrual iron loss. Hemochromatosis is important to recognize because the organ dysfunction can be arrested or prevented and some of the disease may be reversible by iron removal. In these patients, the saturation of transferrin is 60 to 100 percent, the serum iron level is high, and the serum ferritin levels are typically greater than 1000 ng/ml. Removal of a unit of blood (500 ml with 250 mg iron) once each week for 2 to 3 years is effective treatment and diagnostic of hemochromatosis, since the mean corpuscular volume does not decrease and anemia does not occur even after removal of 100 to 200 units.

Anemia of Chronic Disorders

The anemia of chronic disorders is sometimes considered a wastebasket term. However, a positive diagnosis of this disorder can be established. Many of the laboratory characteristics are similar to those of iron-deficiency anemia with some exceptions. The characteristics of this anemia are that the patient's hematocrit usually does not decrease below 25 percent, and although the mean corpuscular volume may be below the normal of 80, it is rarely as low as that of severe iron deficiency [31]. Furthermore, although the serum iron level is decreased and the percent saturation of transferrin is decreased from normal as in iron deficiency, the total iron-binding capacity is reduced below normal and the serum ferritin level is normal or high. In the anemia of chronic disorders, the underlying mechanism involves a chronic inflammatory or neoplastic condition [31].

PATHOPHYSIOLOGY. The pathophysiology of this disorder is very much like that of iron deficiency, except that iron in the reticuloendothelial system is not available for mobilization for synthesis of heme by erythroid progenitors in the marrow [31]. The underlying inflammatory or neoplastic disease is frequently quite evident, but on some occasions it is unclear. The amount of effort on the part of the physician to discover a chronic inflammatory or neoplastic condition which is not evident to establish a diagnosis of anemia of chronic disorders is a matter of clinical judgment. Observation of these patients over an interval of several months to a few years will frequently provide the diagnosis.

TREATMENT. Treatment of this disorder involves treatment of the underlying disease, and oral iron therapy is ineffective and contraindicated. However, it is not at all uncommon for patients with anemia of such chronic disorders as rheumatoid arthritis to also have iron-deficiency anemia. This should be suspected when the hematocrit is reduced below the level usually considered typical for the anemia of chronic disorders. With the combination of iron deficiency and the anemia of chronic disorders, the serum iron level is low, but the total iron-binding capacity may be normal as a result of a combination of these two types of anemia. One disease (iron deficiency) tends to elevate the iron-binding capacity, and the other disease (the chronic disease) tends to decrease the iron-binding capacity.

MICROCYTIC ANEMIAS WITH DEFECTIVE GLOBIN SYNTHESIS

Adult hemoglobin consists of two alpha-globin chains and two beta-globin chains (A or A_1). In addition, a small percentage of globin consists of two alpha chains and two delta chains (A_2). In fetal and early newborn life, fetal hemoglobin is present which consists of two alpha chains and two gamma chains (F). Reduction in synthesis of either alpha chains or non-alpha chains (beta, delta, or gamma) results in thalassemia. As in all genetic disorders, thalassemia may be heterozygous or homozygous. As methods of molecular biology have improved, the number and types of genetic defects associated with thalassemia have geometrically multiplied. In general, alpha-thalassemia is associated with an absence of the gene that is responsible for synthesis of alpha chains, while in beta-thalassemia, the gene for beta chains is present but a defect exists in transcription or translation of the gene. Despite the fact that hemolysis occurs as a result of precipitation of excess beta or alpha chains, the reticulocyte index is lower than expected for a clear-cut case of hemolysis, probably because of the large component of ineffective erythropoiesis in the thalassemias [107].

Alpha-Thalassemia

In the United States, clinically significant alpha-thalassemia is a rare disorder, while in southeastern Asian populations, alpha-thalassemia is the most common form of thalassemia. Humans contain four genes for synthesis of alpha chains. Each gene appears to be responsible for approximately 25 percent of the alpha chains normally synthesized. Any combination from one to four of the alpha-chain genes may be missing. Alpha-thalassemia is clinically silent when one gene is missing, and this is referred to as alpha$_2$-thalassemia— a genetic defect present in 30 percent of black Americans [51, 107]. When two alpha genes are missing, the patient is asymptomatic but may have a low mean corpuscular volume and mildly reduced hemoglobin. This disorder is referred to as alpha$_1$-thalassemia and appears to be particularly frequent in American blacks, in whom the incidence of the genetic defect is approximately 2 percent [51, 107]. When three alpha genes are missing, the patient has the phenotype of alpha-thalassemia (beta-chain tetramers, hemoglobin H). When all four alpha genes are missing, the infant is usually stillborn with hydrops fetalis. This occurs because even fetal hemoglobin, which is the predominant hemoglobin normally present at birth, requires alpha chains in addition to gamma chains. Infants born without alpha chains have tetramers of four gamma chains of fetal hemoglobin, and this is referred to as Bart hemoglobin. Many patients with three missing alpha genes and four missing alpha genes represent double heterozygotes. Two alpha chains must be donated by each parent. Thus, in hemoglobin Bart's disease, each of the parents may be reasonably well but with the alpha-thalassemia trait from two missing alpha genes. Likewise, in patients missing three alpha genes, one parent likely has alpha$_1$-thalassemia, while the other parent has silent alpha$_2$-thalassemia. Adult patients with alpha$_1$-thalassemia (trait) have hemoglobin H, but the quantity is insufficient for detection by electrophoresis, while hemoglobin H is readily detectable as a fast-migration hemoglobin in patients missing three alpha genes.

A special type of alpha-thalassemia is that represented by alpha$_1$-thalassemia seen in the American black population. For a number of years, the fact that alpha$_1$-thalassemia was so common in the American black population combined with the observation that hydrops fetalis from hemoglobin Bart's disease was virtually unheard of in this population was a mystery [51, 107]. If the two missing alpha genes were located on the same chromosome (as in the southeastern Asian population), one would expect a significant incidence of offspring with hydrops fetalis born to parents who each have alpha$_1$-thalassemia. Further investigations by molecular biologic techniques have shown that although two genes are frequently missing in the American black population, they are missing on separate chromosomes virtually 100 percent of the time [51, 107]. Thus each black child gets at least one alpha gene from each parent and therefore never has a disease worse than alpha$_1$-thalassemia.

The diagnosis of alpha$_1$-thalassemia and alpha$_2$-thalassemia have, in the past, been made by exclusion of beta-thalassemia. Thus an American black patient or an Asian patient with a low mean corpuscular volume and a normal or mildly reduced hemoglobin level is presumed to have alpha$_1$-thalassemia if criteria (see below) for beta-thalassemia are not present. Patients with three alpha chains missing have hemoglobin H disease diagnosed on electrophoresis, but a precise diagnosis of the number of missing alpha genes can be determined by using a cDNA probe in hybridization studies [51, 82, 107].

Beta-Thalassemia
Beta-thalassemia is a disorder that predominantly arises from the Mediterranean population. In this disorder, insufficient beta chains are synthesized, although usually normal beta genes are present.

As a result of the inadequate synthesis of beta chains, alpha chains form tetramers and inclusions of this hemoglobin attached to the plasma membranes of erythrocytes result in hemolytic anemia much as occurs in alpha-thalassemia. Patients with homozygous beta-thalassemia have a severe anemia and a low mean corpuscular volume and their anemia requires transfusion. Major complications arise from excessive accumulation of iron and toxicity of iron to tissues from the large numbers of transfusions required to maintain a hemoglobin compatible with life. These patients are rarely seen in the United States, compared to the large number of heterozygous beta-thalassemias seen by hematologists in the United States. Heterozygous beta-thalassemia is associated with a moderate decrease in the hemoglobin and hematocrit and a marked decrease in the mean corpuscular volume. It is important to recognize so that it may be differentiated from iron-deficiency anemia. In these patients, the serum iron level, iron-binding capacity, and ferritin level are entirely normal unless the patient has superimposed iron-deficiency anemia. The physician should be suspicious that heterozygous beta-thalassemia is present when the hemoglobin level is greater than 10 gm% yet the mean corpuscular volume is markedly reduced. As pointed out earlier, reduction of the mean corpuscular volume is unusual in iron deficiency unless the hemoglobin has dropped below 10 gm%. In addition, the red cell distribution width (degree of anisocytosis) is normal in heterozygous thalassemia. If patients with combined iron deficiency and beta-thalassemia are treated with iron, their hemoglobin rises at the expected rate, but it reaches a plateau at approximately 10 gm% and does not rise further. If a hemoglobin electrophoresis is performed at this point, it is usually diagnostic of heterozygous beta-thalassemia.

The diagnosis of beta-thalassemia is made by hemoglobin electrophoresis. Because alpha-chain synthesis is not interfered with, the other hemoglobins present in adults, including hemoglobin A$_2$ and hemoglobin F, are compensatorily increased. Thus the patient with heterozygous beta-thalassemia would typically have an elevated hemoglobin A_2 or F level. It should be pointed out that for reasons that are unclear, hemoglobin A_2 synthesis is decreased in patients with iron deficiency. Thus the patient with a combination of heterozygous beta-thalassemia and iron deficiency will have a low hemoglobin A_2 level in the iron-deficient state, while after repletion of iron at a time when the hematocrit has reached a plateau at a subnormal level, the hemoglobin A_2 level will be abnormally high. The prenatal diagnosis of homozygous beta-thalassemia utilizes restriction-fragment-length polymorphisms on amniotic cells [83].

NORMOCYTIC ANEMIAS

As pointed out earlier, a major cause of normocytic anemia in the United States is mild iron-deficiency anemia. Another major cause of normocytic anemia is acute blood loss. In acute blood loss, plasma and erythrocytes are initially lost in the proportion that existed in the circulation. Therefore, initially the hematocrit does not change; it only begins to decrease after the plasma volume is reexpanded toward normal. The rate of decrease of the hematocrit after an acute episode of bleeding is directly related to the rate at which the plasma volume is restored. This usually requires a minimum of 48 to 72 hours, and therefore, the nadir of the hematocrit is not reached after an acute bleed until at least 48 to 72 hours. If bleeding is severe, the hematocrit may have been restored to some extent by transfusion. If the hematocrit is not restored, the reticulocyte index will rise above 2. Thus the anemia of acute blood loss may appear to be hypoproliferative or hyperproliferative (see Table 5-2). These patients should be given sufficient iron after they are discharged from the hospital to allow them to restore a normal hematocrit and replete their iron stores (500 to 1000 mg).

Another major cause of normocytic normochromic anemias is failure of the marrow to produce erythrocytes. This can occur as a result of damage resulting in aplastic anemia or an autoimmune disease in which antibodies are directed against erythrocyte precursors (pure red cell aplasia). Pure red cell aplasia is recognized by a complete absence of erythroid precursors in the marrow, while other marrow elements, including myeloid cells and megakaryocytes, are normal [21, 58]. This disease has a high association with other autoimmune diseases, including myasthenia gravis and the presence of a thymoma [21, 58]. Pure red cell aplasia is treated by immunosuppressive therapy and transfusions as required, [21, 58] but it may eventually progress to aplasia of the other two cell lines (myeloid or megakaryocyte).

Aplastic anemia is due to a heterogeneous group of etiologies [26, 27]. In some patients the marrow has been damaged by chemicals such as benzene, chloramphenicol, or quinidine, while in others the disease appears to be based on autoimmune phenomenon. Recent studies have incriminated the T-lymphocyte populations as etiologic factors mediating aplastic anemia in a significant proportion of patients [26, 27, 42]. These patients may respond to the conditioning regimen used for marrow transplantation, since the cells that recover in the marrow are sometimes not from the donor but are from the patient's cells [26, 27, 42]. The diagnosis of aplastic anemia is established by noting a peripheral *pancytopenia* and a marrow that is less than 10 percent cellular. It has been suggested, since random sampling is a problem in marrow biopsies, that at least two marrow biopsies from different sites with less than 10 percent cellularity be obtained prior to confirming the diagnosis of aplastic anemia. Furthermore, it should be noted that the mean corpuscular volume may be increased in some cases, presumably as a result of a high percentage of relatively young erythrocytes that are not reticulocytes, since the absolute reticulocyte number is low.

The treatment of aplastic anemia depends on the age of the patient and whether or not an HLA-compatible donor can be found in the patient's family. If the patient is less than 30 years old and an HLA-compatible donor can be found, marrow transplantation is the treatment of choice [26,

42]. In these patients it is important to minimize the number of platelet and erythrocyte transfusions used prior to the marrow transplantation, which should be undertaken within the first month or two of diagnosis, if possible [26, 42]. In patients over the age of 30 in whom graft versus host disease is frequent and has a high mortality or in patients under 30 for whom no HLA-compatible donor exists, the treatment of choice is antithymocyte globulin (ATG) [19, 35]. Although little is known about the mechanism of action of antithymocyte globulin in these patients, approximately 50 percent have a partial or complete response to this treatment. A significant percentage of patients also will respond to a second course of this treatment, even if the first course was unsuccessful. Because antithymocyte globulin is obtained from horses, these patients must be monitored very carefully for severe allergic reactions and are predicted to get serum sickness during the course of treatment.

The mortality rate in unsuccessfully treated aplastic anemia is high. With severe pancytopenia, especially after hepatitis [42], mortality rates as high as 90 percent in 2 years have been observed.

Patients with chronic renal insufficiency regularly have a normocytic anemia that is roughly proportional to the degree of renal insufficiency [32]. Although a portion of their anemia is thought to be based on shortened erythrocyte survival as a result of elevation of substances (spermine) in the blood with renal insufficiency, the predominant cause of anemia in these patients is lack of erythropoietin, which is synthesized by the kidney. It should be noted that even though chronic renal insufficiency is in fact a chronic disease, the anemia is not at all like the anemia of chronic disorders (see above). These patients typically have hemoglobin levels between 7 and 8 gm%, and since it is a chronic anemia, it is usually well tolerated. However, in some older patients with underlying vascular disease, this degree of anemia is unacceptable. These patients usually require transfusions to maintain their hemoglobin at a level at which they do not have symptoms of

angina or cerebrovascular insufficiency. In recent studies, the fact that much of the anemia of chronic renal insufficiency is due to inadequate erythropoietin has been confirmed, and these studies have further suggested a form of treatment for this anemia. Using recombinant human erythropoietin, investigators have shown that administration of erythropoietin restores the hemoglobin level and hematocrit to normal in many patients with chronic renal insufficiency [33]. Human recombinant erythropoietin will undoubtedly become the treatment of choice for at least some selected patients with the anemia of chronic renal insufficiency. In the meantime, all other factors that could be deficient and contributing to the anemia in patients with chronic renal insufficiency should be investigated. Since these patients have gastrointestinal blood loss, iron deficiency should be searched for when the anemia is more severe than usual. Furthermore, since folate is dialyzable, these patients will become folate-deficient unless they are provided extra folate in their diet.

Macrocytic (High Mean Corpuscular Volume) Anemias

The differential diagnosis of high mean corpuscular volume anemias is shown in Table 5-2. The symptoms and signs of these anemias differ little from those encountered in chronic anemia of any etiology. These patients, however, have some of the most severe anemias known, and frequently, the severity of the anemia is belied by the paucity of symptoms and signs. This occurs because of the chronic, slowly progressive manner in which the disease presents, thus allowing maximum expression of cardiopulmonary compensatory factors. Characteristic of these anemias are abnormalities of other blood elements (leukocytes and platelets) and the frequent association with a hypercellular (packed) marrow. When progenitors of erythrocytes in the marrow are increased despite anemia and a low reticulocyte index, the abnormality is referred to as *ineffective erythropoiesis* (thalassemia is another example). Associated with this picture are marked cytologic abnormalities of the precursor cells in the marrow (dys-myelopoiesis).

Megaloblastic Anemias

This group of macrocytic anemias is secondary to vitamin B_{12} (cobalamin) or folate deficiency. From a hematologic standpoint, the manifestations of deficiencies of these two vitamins cannot be distinguished. This likely occurs because the hematologic manifestations are a result of reduced activity of methionine synthetase, an enzyme that uses folate as a substrate and cobalamin (Cbl) as a necessary coenzyme [6]. Deficient activity of the other human cobalamin-dependent enzyme, methylmalonyl-CoA mutase, requires only cobalamin and probably accounts for the neurologic manifestations unique to cobalamin deficiency. The manifestations that occur as a result of cobalamin deficiency may occur *without hematologic abnormalities* [7]. The neurologic manifestations consist of a spectrum that ranges from decreased mentation to frank dementia in the central nervous system and from peripheral neuropathy to subacute combined degeneration of the spinal cord in the peripheral nervous system and on occasion involvement of the corticospinal tracts. Subacute combined degeneration involves the posterolateral columns of the spinal cord, where fibers for vibratory and position sense to the lower extremities are contained, and is the classic neurologic presentation of cobalamin deficiency. The hematologic changes [7] of either cobalamin or folate deficiency include frequent panocytopenia. On peripheral smear, the erythrocytes are large macro-ovalocytes, and there is considerable anisocytosis (as reflected by the wide red cell distribution width). Megaloblastic-appearing (see below) nucleated erythrocytes also may be present along with giant bands and metamyelocytes.

Abnormalities of Cobalamin Metabolism

Megaloblastic anemia as a result of cobalamin deficiency or abnormal metabolism of cobalamin can occur at any of the steps listed in Table 5-4. Dietary lack of cobalamin occurs in *true vegetari-*

ans and requires 15 years to develop because of the large stores of cobalamin in the liver. *Achlorhydria* results in inadequate release of cobalamin from food whether or not intrinsic factor (IF) is present. Intrinsic factor may be absent, may have reduced affinity for cobalamin, or may be rapidly degraded [3, 111]. In pancreatic insufficiency, the R-type cobalamin-binding protein present in gastric juice is not degraded; thus cobalamin is not transferred to intrinsic factor, a step required for ileal absorption. Bacterial overgrowth in a segment of blind loop in the intestine or infestation with a fish tape worm may result in cobalamin deficiency from utilization by these organisms. Absence of the ileal receptor for intrinsic factor, (Immerslund-Grasbock syndrome) results in failure of gastrointestinal absorption of cobalamin. Defects in plasma transport of cobalamin result from abnormalities or absence of transcobalamin II. The other transcobalamins (I and III) are R-type proteins, and the absence of these proteins does not result in signs of cobalamin deficiency. However, because 80 percent of the cobalamin in plasma is bound to transcobalamin I and 20 percent is bound to transcobalamin II, deficiency of transcobalamin II is associated with a normal serum cobalamin level while deficiency of R protein is associated with a low serum cobalamin level despite the absence of tissue cobalamin deficiency [18]. Inherited defects in intracellular cobalamin metabolism result in megaloblastic anemia and neurologic disease shortly after birth [6, 7].

Folate deficiency may result from inadequate absorption or excess utilization. An inadequate dietary supply of folate results in a megaloblastic anemia within 4 months [50]. Such dietary insufficiency is commonly observed in alcoholics, but the hematologic picture is complicated by the effects of alcohol on the marrow, including suppression of erythropoiesis [75]. Ingestion of alcohol results in a mild macrocytosis with or without liver disease, and liver disease from any cause also can result in macrocytosis. Dietary intake of folate may be adequate, but absorption may be impaired by diseases affecting the small

Table 5–4. *Steps in Absorption and Transportation of Cobalamin*

Cobalamin metabolism	Causes of deficiency
I. Dietary intake: animal protein	1. True vegetarians

II. Stomach:
  A. Release from food binders
  B. Binds to R-type protein but not to intrinsic factor
  C. Secretion of intrinsic factor
	1. Gastrectomy
	2. Achlorhydria
	3. Absent intrinsic factor
	4. Abnormal intrinsic factor

III. Duodenum:
  A. Influx of cobalamin from bile
  B. Influx of cobalamin–R-type cobalamin-binding protein complex along with intrinsic factor from stomach
  C. Degradation of R-type protein by pancreatic enzymes and transfer of cobalamin to intrinsic factor
	1. Pancreatic exocrine insufficiency
	2. Bacterial overgrowth
	3. Other parasites

IV. Distal ileum:
  A. Binding of intrinsic factor–cobalamin complex to specific ideal receptors
  B. Release of cobalamin into portal blood
	1. Ileal resection
	2. Abnormal intrinsic factor receptor

V. Plasma:
  A. Binding to transcobalamin I, II, and III. Transcobalamin I and III are R-type proteins, and their functional significance is unknown
  B. Transcobalamin II–cobalamin complex binds to specific cell surface receptors and enters cells by receptor-mediated endocytosis.
	1. Abnormal or absent transcobalamin II

VI. Cellular:
  A. Cobalamin is released in the lysosomes and enters the cytosol, where it becomes bound to methylmalonyl CoA mutase and methionine synthetase
  B. A portion of cobalamin leaves cells and is again bound to transcobalamin II in plasma
	1. Abnormal or absent methylmalonyl CoA mutase and methionine synthetase
	2. Abnormal cobalamin coenzyme synthesis

intestine. These include tropical and nontropical sprue and inflammatory bowel disease. Tropical sprue appears to be specifically corrected by administration of folate. Excessive utilization of folate occurs in chronic hemolytic anemias as well as in pregnancy and skin diseases such as psoriasis.

Diagnosis of Cobalamin and Folate Deficiency
The diagnosis of cobalamin deficiency is usually made from a low serum cobalamin assay. These assays were once insensitive, but they have been improved in recent years [70]. The serum folate assay is used to screen for folate deficiency. This test is poor and is more a reflection of recent dietary ingestion of folate than of the tissue stores of folate. The erythrocyte folate level is a more accurate reflection of folate deficiency, but the test is technically more difficult to perform. Other

tests that measure the metabolic consequences of cobalamin and folate deficiency have been reported. Methylmalonicaciduria occurs in cobalamin deficiency, while the Figlu excretion test is abnormal in folate deficiency [6, 7, 101, 102]. However, these tests require the collection of urine and are cumbersome. Recent studies have shown that methylmalonicacidemia and homocystinemia occur in the serum in cobalamin deficiency, while only homocystinemia occurs in folate deficiency. These metabolic substrates are rapidly quantified in serum using gas chromatographic/mass spectroscopy methods [101, 102].

BONE MARROW ABNORMALITIES. The characteristic marrow changes of cobalamin or folate deficiency consist of a markedly hypercellular marrow (90 to 95 percent) that can easily be mistaken for acute leukemia on core biopsy. Cytologically, an increase in the number of erythroid and myeloid elements is seen. Giant bands and metamyelo-cytes as well as hypersegmented polymorphonu-clear leukocytes are seen. Hypersegmentation is the earliest morphologic change in folate defi-ciency [7] and the last to correct after treatment. The characteristic change in the erythroids is *nu-clear-cytoplasmic dissociation.* The cytoplasmic mat-uration of the erythroids is normal, while the nu-cleus remains immature.

ABNORMALITIES IN SERUM CHEMISTRY. Elevations in the indirect bilirubin and lactate dehydrogenase (LDH) levels are reflections of the death of ery-throid precursors in the marrow. Hypouricemia accompanies the ineffective synthesis of DNA.

SCHILLING TEST. In this test, radioactive coba-lamin is administered by mouth as crystalline cobalamin or cobalamin bound to intrinsic factor. A large dose of parenteral nonradioactive coba-lamin is administered so that radioactive coba-lamin absorbed from the small intestine will be excreted in the urine rather than bound by the transcobalamins. The Schilling test is used to de-termine the absorption of cobalamin and the mechanism of deficiency—not deficiency per se. If the Schilling test is normal and the intrinsic fac-tor system is intact, the cobalamin deficiency may have occurred from inadequate dietary intake or failure to release cobalamin from food. The for-mer can be established from the history, while the latter is usually associated with old age and ach-lorhydia. Failure to absorb cobalamin from food can be measured by employing a special form of the Schilling test where the radioactive cobalamin is incorporated into food protein [29].

MEASUREMENT OF AUTOANTIBODIES. The most com-monly recognized form of cobalamin deficiency in the United States is *pernicious anemia.* This disor-der is an autoimmune disease that has been suc-cessfully treated by immunosuppression with ste-roids. Autoantibodies are directed against gastric parietal cells and intrinsic factor. The anti-intrin-sic factor antibodies may be of the precipitating or blocking types. Although anti-intrinsic factor blocking antibodies are not thought to be in-volved in the pathogenesis, they are present in the

great majority of the cases [7]. Because of anti-parietal antibodies, patients typically demonstrate histamine-fast achlorhydria and an inability to absorb crystalline cobalamin normally while cob-alamin given with intrinsic factor is absorbed nor-mally. Pernicious anemia is an important form of cobalamin deficiency to distinguish because it is associated with other autoimmune disorders such as thyroiditis (hypothyroidism), diabetic mellitus, and rarely, Addison's disease and it may have a hereditary component.

THERAPEUTIC TRIALS. In the final analysis, either cobalamin or folate deficiency is best diagnosed after a response to treatment is observed. In the absence of complicating factors, a reticulocyte re-sponse is observed within a week and is propor-tional to the severity of the anemia at presenta-tion.

Treatment of Megaloblastic Anemias

Treatment of cobalamin deficiency involves life-long parenteral administration of cobalamin, while treatment of folate deficiency involves the use of oral or parenteral folic acid. The marrow begins to change toward normal within 24 hours after specific therapy is instituted. During this pe-riod, profound hypokalemia may develop and should be guarded against [73].

Occasionally, patients present with severe ane-mia and cardiopulmonary compromise (high-output failure). Occasionally, lactic acidosis is present, and this may be precipitated by a super-imposed stress such as bacterial sepsis. Although transfusions can usually be avoided in these cir-cumstances, an immediate increase in the hema-tocrit may be necessary. Transfusions should consist of packed erythrocytes and should be un-dertaken with great caution to avoid precipitation or further worsening of the circulatory overload. Exchange transfusion may be necessary if such overload cannot be avoided. Until the specific de-ficiency is diagnosed, both cobalamin and folate should be given. Folate given to a patient with cobalamin deficiency will produce a hematologic response (and vice versa) [6, 7]. Furthermore, the neurologic disease of cobalamin deficiency may be precipitated [6, 7, 62] or masked by this treatment.

Megaloblastic Anemia Unresponsive to Cobalamin or Folate: Refractory Anemia

Refractory anemias are a heterogeneous group of disorders that morphologically superficially resemble megaloblastic anemia of cobalamin or folate deficiency but do not respond to replacement of the vitamins. The mean corpuscular volume may be low (as in sideroblastic anemia), normal, or high. The peripheral blood usually reveals a pancytopenia with variable erythrocyte size and hemoglobin content. Sideroblastic anemias typically have a dimorphic population of erythrocytes with normochromic and hypochromic erythrocytes [88]. The marrow ranges from normal cellularity to hypercellular with features suggestive of megaloblastosis (megaloid changes). Occasionally, multinucleate erythroid precursors are observed, and iron stain reveals increased iron with *ringed sideroblasts.* The marrow cellularity is virtually always less than the marked hypercellularity of cobalamin or folate megaloblastosis, and this reduced cellularity is an important clue to the correct diagnosis. The serum cobalamin and folate levels are normal, and no response to the administration of these vitamins is observed.

Many studies of chromosomal abnormalities in refractory anemia have been performed. Several translocations have been reported, but the outcome of the disease cannot be reliably predicted by chromosomal studies. A characteristic syndrome of 5q− refractory anemia [38, 40, 57, 69, 92, 110] appears to differ from the other syndromes in that the platelet count is normal or elevated. Some of these patients will ultimately develop a picture of acute nonlymphocytic leukemia, while others improve and others have a persistent transfusion requirement. No method is currently available to diagnose "preleukemia," and preleukemia remains a retrospective diagnosis. Various forms of treatment have been tried with minimal success.

Hyperproliferative Anemias (Reticulocyte Index > 2)

ACUTE BLOOD LOSS

Anemia associated with acute blood loss was discussed earlier. With acute bleeding, the reticulocyte index will increase, with iron mobilization being the rate limiting step.

NUTRIENT REPLACEMENT

Occasionally, anemia is first observed during replacement of iron, cobalamin, or folate, at which time a high reticulocyte index will be observed along with the residual anemia. These patients may be mistakenly thought to have a hemolytic anemia. Observation and a careful history will usually resolve this question.

HEMOLYTIC ANEMIA

Hemolytic anemia is the term used to describe anemia in which the primary process involves shortened erythrocyte survival in the circulation with maximum marrow compensation. Hemolysis should be strongly suspected when the hemoglobin level falls by greater than 1 to 1.5 gm% per week in the absence of external or internal blood loss. Because iron can readily be recycled in these diseases, the reticulocyte count may exceed 50 percent of the total erythrocyte population. In the history it is important to determine if the patient ever had a normal hematocrit to establish if the hemolytic process is inherited (lifelong) or acquired. Frequently, autoimmune hemolytic anemias are associated with a recent infection. Both congenital and acquired hemolytic anemias can be exacerbated by exposure to drugs and by infection. Occasionally, the drug is a primary cause of the disease. The physical examination may reveal icterus from indirect hyperbilirubinemia or lymphadenopathy and splenomegaly from a lymphoproliferative disorder. The morphology of the erythrocytes on the peripheral smear may be normal or misshapen (microangiopathia, sickle cell disease), or they may have abnormal localization of hemoglobin (hemoglobin C) or be spherocytes. Greater than 5 to 10 percent spherocytes may or

Table 5–5. *Some Hemolytic Disorders Associated with the Three Major Components of Erythrocytes*

I. Membrane
   A. Intrinsic (inherited):
      1. Hereditary spherocytosis
      2. Hereditary elliptocytosis
      3. Paroxysmal nocturnal hemoglobinuria
         (acquired)
   B. Extrinsic (acquired):
      1. Autoimmune hemolytic anemias
      2. Microangiopathic hemolytic anemias
II. Hemoglobin:
   A. Sickling hemoglobins: S- , S-C- , S-thalassemia
   B. Other hemoglobinopathies: unstable hemoglobins, methemoglobins
III. Cytosolic enzymes:
   A. Decreased reduction of normally produced methemoglobin (Fe^{3+} hemoglobin):
      1. Glucose-6-phosphate dehydrogenase deficiency
      2. Methemoglobin reductase deficiency
   B. Decreased ATP production:
      1. Pyruvate kinase deficiency
      2. Deficiency of other enzymes in anaerobic glycolysis

may not be present in hemolytic anemias, but when present, they are diagnostic of hemolytic anemia of some variety.

The differential diagnosis of hemolytic anemias centers around the three main parts of erythrocytes: the plasma membrane, the hemoglobin, and the cytosolic enzymes. Table 5-5 lists the hemolytic anemias, inherited and acquired, grouped by the part of the erythrocyte involved.

Plasma Membrane

HEREDITARY SPHEROCYTOSIS AND HEREDITARY ELLIPTOCYTOSIS. Studies of erythrocytes in these conditions have revealed significant heterogeneity. The abnormalities are in spectrin, ankyrin, and other membrane proteins (protein 4.1) [84]. This heterogeneity may account, in part, for the clinical presentation that varies from severe anemia to incidentally discovered disease in asymptomatic individuals. In hereditary spherocytosis, the peripheral smear reveals a high percentage of spherocytes (cells without central pallor *and* deeply staining hemoglobin, i.e., *high mean corpuscular hemoglobin concentration*) or elliptocytes. These anemias are chronic and associated with reticulocytosis, increased indirect bilirubin, increased lactate dehydrogenase, bilirubinate gallstones, and splenomegaly. Hereditary spherocytosis is the only nonartifactual cause for an elevated mean corpuscular hemoglobin concentration in medicine. This elevation occurs because of the high percentage of spherocytes. If the percentage of spherocytes is low or there is a superimposed disease that causes a low mean corpuscular hemoglobin concentration (iron deficiency or thalassemia), the mean corpuscular hemoglobin concentration will be normal in hereditary spherocytosis.

ACQUIRED AUTOIMMUNE HEMOLYTIC ANEMIA. In this disorder autoantibodies are produced that are directed against erythrocyte membrane antigens. The disease may be idiopathic or occur secondary to an immune disorder such as systemic lupus erythematosus, a lymphoproliferative disease, or a drug reaction. The onset of anemia may be explosive or subtle. Two general classes of antibodies are involved. Antibody with a maximal thermal amplitude at 37°C causes warm acquired autoimmune hemolytic anemia, while antibody with a maximal thermal amplitude at a temperature lower than 37°C causes the cold-mediated form. Warm antibodies are usually IgG, whereas cold antibodies are usually IgM. In the warm form of this disease, IgG or rarely IgA attaches to erythrocytes and may or may not fix complement, while in the cold-mediated form, IgM attaches to erythrocytes in the cooler (32°C) periphery, fixes complement (C), and then the IgM dissociates at 37°C [39].

The presence of abnormal quantities of proteins (antibodies and complement) bound to the erythrocytes is detected by the *direct Coomb's test,* which can reveal IgG alone, IgG plus complement, or rarely, complement alone in the warm form, while in the cold form only complement is detected [20, 63]. IgM antibody usually has specificity directed against the I antigen present on all adult erythrocytes, while IgG has specificity for a variety of erythrocyte antigens. Thus the antibodies are considered panagglutinins and result in great difficulty in crossmatching of blood. The *indirect Coombs' test* measures antibody that is free in the serum. This antibody may represent free autoantibody or an alloantibody from prior transfusions or pregnancy. The indirect Coombs' test has little pathophysiologic significance and is mainly a blood-banking problem.

The peripheral smear in acquired autoimmune hemolytic anemia usually reveals *microspherocytes* and *rouleaux* (in the cold-mediated form). Occasionally, thrombocytopenia may be associated with this anemia (Evan's syndrome). At other times, the reticulocyte index may be low in this anemia as well as in other chronic hemolytic states because of an aplastic crisis induced by infection or folate deficiency, as well as an antibody directed against antigens present on reticulocytes or earlier erythrocyte progenitors. The differential diagnosis of warm- and cold-mediated acquired autoimmune hemolytic anemia is shown in Table 5-6. Acquired autoimmune hemolytic anemia caused by infections usually results from a polyclonal antibody, while that caused by lymphoproliferative diseases has a monoclonal antibody. Three distinct types of this anemia occur with different classes of drugs. Methyldopa (Aldomet) in large doses for several months results in a positive direct Coombs' test with IgG alone [109]. However, clinical acquired autoimmune hemolytic anemia is uncommon and will disappear several months after discontinuation of the drug [109]. Quinidine results in an immune-complex type of acquired autoimmune hemolytic anemia with complement fixation, while penicillin in high doses results in a hapten type of acquired autoimmune hemolytic anemia [109].

Acute management consists of initiation of prednisone at doses of 1 to 3 mg/kg. However, this therapy usually requires 1 to 3 weeks for improvement to occur. Replacement of folate and any other deficiencies also should be instituted to support marrow compensation. Even under these conditions, the anemia may become life-threatening, and close cooperation with a major blood bank is required. Since the antibody is a panagglutinin, obtaining crossmatched erythrocytes to avoid a major transfusion reaction is virtually impossible [78]. An in vivo crossmatch using 25 to 50 ml of the "most compatible" units of donor erythrocytes can be performed by ^{51}Cr labeling of injected cells. The half-life of these cells will be shortened by the panagglutinin, but units with the largest fraction of surviving cells can be obtained to support the hematocrit. One also can examine the serum for increases in free hemoglobin, indirect bilirubin, and lactate dehydrogenase that will occur if there is a transfusion reaction after infusion of a small fraction of a unit. Chronic management consists of control of the hemolysis by prednisone. Steroids are successful in the majority of cases, but if relapse occurs on tapering of prednisone, splenectomy is indicated. In many instances in acquired autoimmune hemolytic anemia secondary to an underlying disease or drug, removal of the drug or treatment of the underlying disease results in improvement or disappearance of the anemia. This is especially true for the cold-mediated form, which is usually less severe than the warm-mediated form and may be secondary to an underlying infection such as *Myco-*

Table 5–6. *Autoimmune Hemolytic Diseases*

Warm-mediated	Cold-mediated

Primary:
  Idiopathic
	Primary:
	  Idiopathic

Secondary:
  Systemic lupus erythematosus, lymphoproliferative
    disorders, and drugs
	Secondary:
	  Infections: *Mycoplasma,* infectious mononucleosis,
	    others such as viral infection or syphilis may
	    cause paroxysmal cold hemoglobinuria

plasma, infectious mononucleosis, or a treatable lymphoproliferative disease. Cold-mediated acquired autoimmune hemolytic anemia may respond poorly to steroids and splenectomy, and the latter should be undertaken with extreme caution. Immunosuppression may be useful in refractory cases of either form of this anemia.

The prognosis of acquired autoimmune hemolytic anemia is largely dependent on the underlying disease process [4]. Cases that appear to be idiopathic at presentation will frequently eventually present with an underlying disease [4]. Patients with this and other types of hemolytic anemia have a high incidence of thromboembolism [4] which may result in death. Other patients die of uncontrolled hemolysis (uncommon) or their underlying disease (very common).

Acquired hemolytic anemias also can be due to a vast array of other disorders, including vascular (see thrombotic thrombocytopenic purpura and disseminated intravascular coagulation below) disorders resulting in microangiopathic erythrocytes or metabolic disease such as liver disease [24].

Deficiency of Cytosolic Enzymes
Deficiency of any of the enzymes of the pathway of anaerobic glycolysis or of other erythrocyte enzymes such as methemoglobin reductase may result in an acute or chronic hemolytic anemia. These hemolytic disorders are referred to as congenital nonspherocytic hemolytic anemias. This is an unfortunate name because it implies that spherocytes are not seen on the peripheral smear. While the hemolysis in this group of disorders may or may not be associated with spherocytes, it is true that spherocytes are less commonly observed than in hereditary spherocytosis. However, *severe* hemolysis in glucose-6-phosphate dehydrogenase deficiency, for example, may be associated with spherocytes. The term *nonspherocytic* originates from past days when two types of congenital hemolytic anemias were known: those due to hereditary spherocytosis and those due to other hereditary defects which, at the time, were not characterized.

The prototype of these enzyme deficiencies is glucose-6-phosphate dehydrogenase (G-6-PD) deficiency, which is normally responsible for the production of reducing equivalents in erythrocytes. A large number of variants of the defective enzyme have been described [11]. While most patients have episodic hemolytic anemia, rarely some patients have a chronic hemolytic anemia. Upon oxidant stress, as in ingestion of drugs such as primaquine, an acute hemolytic anemia occurs. At low doses of the oxidant, only the older erythrocytes with the lowest levels of glucose-6-phosphate dehydrogenase are hemolyzed [11]. As the dose of the oxidant is increased, younger erythrocytes are hemolyzed. The mechanism of hemolysis is incompletely understood, but it involves the inability to reduce oxidized iron in hemoglobin (methemoglobin) [11]. Glucose-6-phosphate dehydrogenase deficiency is an X-linked recessive trait that occurs in 10 percent of black American males [11]. Since the X chromosome is randomly inactivated in females, the glucose-6-phosphate dehydrogenase level usually averages 50 percent in females, who are rarely clinically affected. The reticulocyte index is increased during glucose-6-phosphate dehydrogenase hemolysis, and reticulocytes contain supranormal levels of the enzyme. Thus a "normal" glucose-6-phosphate dehydrogenase level in the face of reticulocytosis suggests deficiency. It is more reliable to determine the glucose-6-phosphate dehydrogenase level after the hemolysis has subsided (i.e., after the offending oxidant has been removed). The peripheral smear of patients with glucose-6-phosphate dehydrogenase deficiency is remarkable only for increased polychromatophilic macrocytes (reticulocytes) and, if the hemolysis is brisk, spherocytes.

In pyruvate kinase (PK) deficiency (the second most common erythrocyte enzyme deficiency), the erythrocytes may be misshapen and are referred to as burr cells—a condition reproduced by depletion of ATP. This enzyme is involved in the production of 2 mol ATP from glucose late in the anaerobic glycolytic pathway. Thus erythrocytes from pyruvate kinase-deficient patients have insufficient ATP to support energy-requiring steps such as Na-K ATPase. The hemolytic anemia is chronic and usually present from birth.

Treatment of glucose-6-phosphate dehydrogenase deficiency involves avoidance of the offending oxidant; splenectomy is of no value [11]. Pyruvate kinase deficiency is treated by transfusions, and approximately 20 percent of patients are improved by splenectomy [12].

Hemoglobinopathies

While thalassemias involve a quantitative reduction in globin-chain synthesis, hemoglobinopathies result from production of abnormal globin chains from genetic defects resulting in substitutions in alpha and beta chains. The most commonly recognized clinically significant hemoglobinopathy is sickle-cell disease (SCD), which results from a substitution of valine for glutamic acid in one *(heterozygous/trait)* beta chain or both beta chains *(homozygous/disease)*. The diagnosis can be established by hemoglobin electrophoresis. The peripheral smear does not reveal sickle cells in heterozygous disease, but it will reveal classic sickle cells in homozygous disease. Screening tests for the presence of hemoglobin S depend on the relative insolubility of S hemoglobin on reduction of the oxygen tension. Pathophysiologically, the reduced solubility of hemoglobin S with reduced oxygen tension results in crystallization of hemoglobin S, which in turn results in the characteristic misshapen erythrocyte—the sickle cell [16]. This defect results in a marked increase in blood viscosity which is partly offset by the anemia resulting from the shortened erythrocyte survival. The increased viscosity and rigidity of sickle erythrocytes result in the occlusion of small vessels, which produces pain or infarction in organs. Splenic infarction is so common that by adulthood the spleen is very small. Small-vessel occlusion in other organ systems leads to CNS infarction, repetitive pulmonary infarctions, renal infarctions, and bone infarctions. Because sickle-cell disease is a chronic hemolytic anemia, as re-

Table 5–7. *Types of Crises in Sickle-Cell Disease**

A. Painful: Most common; due to sludging of erythrocytes with infarction

B. Splenic sequestration and dactylitis: Usually in children; rarely in adults

C. Aplastic: Uncommon; associated with even mild infections; low reticulocyte index

D. Megaloblastic: Low reticulocyte index secondary to folate deficiency

E. Hemolytic: Rare

*C, D, and E may occur in the setting of any chronic hemolytic disorder, while A and B are unique to sickle-cell disorders.

flected by a high reticulocyte index, the marrow shows marked erythroid hyperplasia.

Many types of crises can occur in sickle-cell anemia patients, as shown in Table 5-7. By far the most common crisis resulting in symptoms is the painful crisis. Painful crisis is usually associated with fever and leukocytosis. Since patients with sickle-cell disease more commonly acquire severe infections (osteomyelitis, sepsis, etc.), the leukocytosis associated with a painful crisis may strongly suggest infection. In this setting, the history of previous painful crises is important, since painful crises tend to occur repetitively in the same location and with a similar complex of symptoms, signs, and time duration. Aplastic crises can be due to either folate deficiency (megaloblastic marrow) or interrecurrent infection. In aplastic crises, the hematocrit falls rapidly, since the hemolysis is ongoing and the reticulocyte index is low. Crisis secondary to splenic sequestration of erythrocytes is rare in adults, since the spleen is usually quite small. The hand-foot syndrome (dactylitis) is also found only in the pediatric age group.

Sickle-cell crises frequently present as a pulmonary syndrome. Patients usually complain of pleuritic chest pain, fever, and shortness of breath. An infiltrate is present on the chest x-ray, and it is unclear whether the infiltrate represents infection or infarction of a portion of lung. Patients are usually cultured and given broad antimicrobial coverage. Repeated episodes of pulmonary vascular occlusion may lead to pulmonary hypertension and right ventricular failure.

Other Hemoglobinopathies

Other hemoglobinopathies or thalassemias may be associated with hemoglobin S. Hemoglobin S–C disease is similar to sickle-cell disease except that the hematocrit is higher and the blood viscosity is greater, resulting in a higher incidence of aseptic necrosis of the femoral head and retinopathy [16]. The retinopathy of sickle-cell disease and hemoglobin S–C disease is peripheral in the retina. This characteristic lesion may lead to blindness.

SICKLE–BETA-THALASSEMIA. When hemoglobin S is associated with no beta-chain production *(beta-thal⁰)* from the allelic gene, the disease cannot be clinically distinguished from sickle-cell disease. When a small amount of beta chain is produced *(beta-thal⁺)*, the disease is less severe than sickle-cell disease.

The treatment of an acute sickle pain crises involves hydration, adequate pain relief, and treatment of any underlying infection. Most clinicians also use nasal oxygen, although its use is controversial. It is important to correct factors such as ambient cold, acidosis, and dehydration that are known to precipitate crises. As a last resort, transfusion or exchange transfusion of erythrocytes will rapidly improve the crises. Transfusion must be undertaken with the usual precautions for transfusion reactions and volume overload as well as the risk of rapidly increasing the blood viscosity—thus possibly worsening the crises.

No completely satisfactory method of preventing chronic crises is known other than avoiding precipitating factors. A program of prophylactic regular exchange transfusions may be used in the experimental setting in patients with frequent crises. The dangers of such a program involve difficulty with crossmatching and iron overload as well as the risk of hepatitis and other infections. The ability of iron chelating agents to prevent iron overload in this setting is under trial.

Polycythemia

Polycythemia refers to a condition in which the erythrocyte mass is increased. This is usually manifested by an hematocrit of greater than 55 percent in males and 50 percent in females. It should be noted that the hematocrit can be abnormally high when the erythrocyte mass is normal but the plasma volume is reduced. This disease is referred to as *Gaisböck's syndrome* and is usually present with many other cardiovascular risk factors, such as type A personality, hypertension, and smoking. In Gaisböck's syndrome, the measured erythrocyte mass is normal and the measured plasma volume is contracted.

In "smokers polycythemia," the hemoglobin is converted to carboxyhemoglobin, which is irreversibly unable to carry oxygen. This disease is associated with a combination of increased erythrocyte mass and reduced plasma volume.

In true polycythemia, the erythrocyte mass accounts for the high hematocrit, while the plasma volume is normal or near normal. True polycythemia may result from autonomous production of erythrocytes by the marrow, autonomous erythropoietin production by tumors, or appropriate erythropoietin production from hypoxia secondary to cardiopulmonary etiologies or abnormal hemoglobins (rare) that have an abnormally high affinity for O_2 (resulting in tissue hypoxia).

AUTONOMOUS PRODUCTION OF ERYTHROCYTES
Polycythemia Rubra Vera (PRV)

This disorder is a clonal malignancy that involves all the marrow cell lines (erythrocytes, granulocytes, and platelets). Polycythemia rubra vera is part of a spectrum of diseases that range from predominantly excess erythrocytes (polycythemia rubra vera) to predominantly excess granulocytes (chronic granulocytic leukemia) or to predominantly excess platelets (essential thrombocythemia) [80]. Erythropoietin production is markedly reduced in polycythemia rubra vera. This disease is differentiated from diseases that cause polycythemia from excess erythropoietin by evidence that all cell lines are affected in this disease, while excess erythropoietin causes abnormalities only in the erythrocyte line. Thus hepatosplenomegaly as well as trilinear hyperplasia of the marrow occur in polycythemia rubra vera in contrast to polycythemia due to excess erythropoietin. Differential diagnostic criteria have recently been published [8]. Except for increased granulocytes and platelets, the peripheral smear is usually normal. Occasionally, patients with polycythemia rubra vera present with evidence of iron deficiency (low mean corpuscular volume) usually from occult gastrointestinal bleeding. In addition, peptic ulcer disease and gout occur with increased frequency in polycythemia rubra vera.

TREATMENT. Urgency of treatment depends on the degree of erythrocytosis and symptoms of vascular insufficiency (from blood hyperviscosity). The two major forms of treatment include phlebotomy to create iron deficiency and marrow suppression with either chemotherapy or ^{32}P. Phlebotomy alone is usually used as initial therapy in patients younger than age 50 [8]. This therapy has the advantage of a lower incidence of subsequent development of acute leukemia compared to chemotherapy or ^{32}P. Although phlebotomy lowers the hematocrit (by creating iron deficiency), the red blood cell count may become very high. Thus patients have a high red blood cell count and a low mean corpuscular volume, giving a normal hematocrit—a situation similar to that observed in heterozygous thalassemias. In these patients, the blood viscosity may remain high, and little to reduce vascular insufficiency has been gained by phlebotomy. Furthermore, the platelet count may rise to over 1 million, and although randomized trials have not demonstrated increased thrombosis, most hematologists institute marrow-suppressive therapy when the platelet count is 1 million or more. Various types of marrow suppression can be used, and early results suggest a lower incidence of leukemic conversion using hydroxyurea compared to ^{32}P or alkylating agents [8, 80]. Marrow-suppressive

therapy is regularly used in patients over age 70, since several years usually pass prior to conversion to leukemia. It should be noted that thrombosis and bleeding occur with *great frequency* following general surgery in patients with uncontrolled polycythemia vera. Elective surgery should be postponed until several months after the polycythemia has been controlled.

Secondary Polycythemia

In contrast to polycythemia vera, this common group of disorders involves an appropriate or inappropriate increase in erythropoietin. Only the erythrocyte line is affected, and no evidence of a generalized myeloproliferative process is found (e.g., hepatosplenomegaly or panhyperplasia of the marrow). An appropriate excess of erythropoietin occurs when the hemoglobin-oxygen saturation falls below 92 percent, as in lung disease or right to left cardiac shunts. An appropriate excess of erythropoietin also may occur with a normal calculated hemoglobin-oxygen saturation while direct measurement of hemoglobin saturation is low, as in smoker's polycythemia, where carboxyhemoglobin accounts for a significant percentage of the total hemoglobin. Rarely, certain hemoglobinopathies occur in which the abnormal hemoglobin binds oxygen with higher than normal affinity producing tissue hypoxia. These hemoglobins are diagnosed by their abnormal P50—the partial pressure of oxygen required to give 50 percent saturation of hemoglobin. In approximately 50 percent of these patients, the hemoglobin electrophoresis is abnormal. Situations with an inappropriate excess of erythropoietin also occur and are usually secondary to tumors, such as renal cell carcinoma, uterine myomas, or hepatomas, or to structural abnormalities of the kidney, such as cysts, hydronephrosis, and acute graft versus host rejection. In all these conditions, erythropoietin is produced without regard to tissue oxygenation. A scheme for the evaluation of secondary polycythemias is given in Table 5-8.

Table 5–8. Polycythemias

I. Stress erythrocytosis: Due to a contracted plasma volume; erythrocyte mass is normal
II. True polycythemia: Increased erythrocyte mass with normal or contracted plasma volume:
   A. Autonomous production of erythrocytes (polycythemia rubra vera), a clonal malignancy involving all cell lines in the marrow
   B. Secondary polycythemia:
     1. Autonomous production of erythropoietin: hepatic, renal, and uterine tumors and benign renal disorders, e.g., cysts, renal artery stenosis
     2. Appropriate production of erythropoietin:
       a. Hypoxia
       b. High oxygen-affinity hemoglobinopathies

Agnogenic Myeloid Metaplasia (Myelofibrosis)

Myelofibrosis (MF) is frequently idiopathic and occasionally associated late in the course of polycythemia rubra vera. The disorder is chronic, and the patient may present with early satiety from a massively enlarged spleen or symptoms of anemia [106]. The peripheral smear [106] shows leukoerythroblastosis with immature myeloids, basophils, and nucleated erythrocytes. Nonnucleated erythrocytes are typically teardrop-shaped. The marrow is replaced by fibrous tissue, and the bones themselves become sclerotic [106]. Myelofibrosis is chronic, and the course is frequently 20 years. Eventually, the spleen may have to be removed because of painful splenic infarcts or hypersplenism that result in an increased transfusion requirement. Splenectomy should be performed with caution and only under conditions in which the platelet count is controlled. Splenectomy usually results in an increasing liver size due to extramedullary hematopoiesis, which can occur in any organ, including the skin, lymph nodes, brain, pericardium, and pleurae.

Disorders of Leukocytes

Leukocytosis and leukopenia should be further classified as to the abnormal leukocyte involved. For example, leukopenia may result from granulocytopenia, lymphopenia, or both. The disorders that result in these types of abnormal leukocyte counts can be found in standard hematology textbooks.

Acute Leukemias

Acute leukemias are first classified as to their cell of origin as lymphocytic or nonlymphocytic—including monocytic, myelomonocytic, myelocytic, and erythroleukemic. The common leukemias were classified by the French, American, and British (FAB) classification [43]. This classification is of use in the study setting; however, since the different nonlymphocytic leukemias are treated with the same drugs, little practical utility derives from the FAB classification. The acute lymphocytic leukemias (ALL) are more commonly observed in children and are important to recognize because of the improved prognosis in adults as well as children. Null-cell acute lymphocytic leukemias and acute lymphocytic leukemias with T- or B-cell markers have a worse prognosis than common acute lymphocytic leukemia antigen-positive (CALLA) leukemias [55]. Recently, much information has been acquired as to the markers present during T- and B-cell development, and malignancy at many of the developmental stages has been observed [38, 40, 105, 110]. T-cell malignancies have a predilection for skin involvement (mycosis fungoides and Sezary's syndrome). Monocytic leukemias have a predilection for involvement of tissues (chloromas) such as gums, bones, and spinal cord (compression).

DIAGNOSIS

Bleeding from various mucous membranes, infection, and weakness from anemia are the usual presenting features. The physical examination in acute leukemia may range from essentially normal to pallor, petechiae, and organomegaly, including hepatosplenomegaly and adenopathy. The hemoglobin, white blood cell count, and platelet count may be normal or low or the white blood cell count may be increased. Typically, the peripheral smear reveals numerous immature (blast) forms together with mature granulocytes creating the typical leukemic hiatus [49]. In nonlymphocytic acute leukemia, the blasts usually contain granules, and these may coalase to form Auer rods—a finding diagnostic of acute myeloid or monocytic leukemias. When the marrow is packed, nucleated erythrocytes also may be observed in the peripheral blood smear. It is very important to recognize acute promyelocytic leukemia (APL), since lysis of these cells during induction treatment may lead to disseminated intravascular coagulation and death. Heparin is usually added to the initial treatment of acute promyelocytic leukemia to avoid this complication.

A variety of chromosomal abnormalities [57, 69, 92, 95] occur in acute leukemia, and some are typical of different types. The 15 : 17 translocation can assist in the diagnosis of acute promyelocytic leukemia, especially the hypogranular form. Other chromosomal abnormalities occur, such as 8 : 21 translocation in acute myeloblastic leukemia, but it is unknown for certain whether these abnormalities are a primary part of the disease (reflection of oncogene expression) or a secondary manifestation of the leukemic process.

TREATMENT

For treatment to produce a complete remission in acute nonlymphocytic leukemia (defined as less than 5 percent blasts in the marrow), transient aplasia of the marrow must be achieved. With such aplasia, both normal and leukemic cells are eliminated, and when marrow repopulation occurs, this is usually with the normal cell line. This result suggests that normal marrow progenitors have a shorter cell cycle than leukemia progenitors. The drugs usually used to produce marrow aplasia are cytosine arabinoside in various combinations with anthracyclines. Typically, the patient relapses in 12 to 18 months, and complete remission becomes progressively more difficult to obtain. Approximately 20 percent of adults with acute nonlymphocytic leukemia have long-term (more than 3 years) disease-free survival [43], and many of these may be cures, since late relapse is infrequent (although it does occur). It is imperative that the patient be supported with erythrocytes, platelets, and antibiotics during the aplastic phase of induction. During this period, patients are at high risk for bleeding and infection, especially from the mouth and anus. Invasive procedures involving these areas should be minimized. The risk of mortality during induction may be as high as 20 percent, even in facilities with access to unlimited support.

Because of the high risk of relapse, many strategies have been tried, such as consolidation and late intensification chemotherapy while patients are in a complete remission. Marrow transplantation in younger patients also has been studied. At this time, all these strategies are considered experimental and are used only in a protocol setting. Patients with acute lymphocytic leukemia or acute nonlymphocytic leukemia tend to relapse in sanctuary sites such as the meninges and gonads. Treatment to the central nervous system is usually given prophylactically in acute lymphocytic leukemia, but this treatment is controversial in acute nonlymphocytic leukemia.

Chronic Leukemias

CHRONIC LYMPHOCYTIC LEUKEMIA

Chronic lymphocytic leukemia (CLL) is a disease of older adults that is characterized by an increase in absolute mature lymphocytes in the peripheral blood to greater than 4000/mm³. Typically, chronic lymphocytic leukemia is associated with lymphadenopathy (sometimes massive) and infiltration of the marrow, liver, spleen, and other organs. The architecture of the lymph node is effaced with lymphocytes and is indistinguishable from well-differentiated lymphocytic lymphoma, diffuse (see below).

Diagnosis

The diagnosis is usually established by physical examination and examination of the peripheral blood. Marrow examination may not be necessary, but it is usually performed to confirm the diagnosis.

Chronic lymphocytic leukemia is a malignancy of B-lymphocytes. Rarely, it may be a malignancy of T-lymphocytes with marked skin disease (cutaneous T-cell lymphomas). Frequent infections and hypogammaglobulinemia are observed. Late in the disease, anemia and thrombocytopenia occur. These manifestations may be related to replacement of the marrow with malignant lymphocytes or autoimmune phenomena. Autoimmune hemolytic anemia with a positive direct Coombs' test is common. Occasionally, anemia and thrombocytopenia are manifestations of massive splenomegaly. Although splenectomy may improve cytopenia due to autoimmune disorders or hypersplenism, general surgery must be undertaken with caution because of the risk of infection.

Treatment

Chronic lymphocytic leukemia in most patients is an indolent disease, and many years may pass before the preceding manifestations occur. Usually treatment is withheld until a specific indication occurs, such as anemia, thrombocytopenia, massive adenopathy, or splenomegaly. Treatment usually involves long-term exposure to an alkylating agent in association with steroids.

Chronic Myelogenous Leukemia

Chronic myelogenous leukemia (CML) is a disease in which myeloid hyperplasia predominates [45]. A less prominent increase in platelets also is observed along with other evidence of a myeloproliferative disorder. Hepatosplenomegaly and hypercellular marrow are typical presenting features. Chronic myelogenous leukemia is a malignant clonal disease that is associated with a deletion of the long arm of chromosome 22 in over 90 percent of patients (the Philadelphia chromosome) [92].

Diagnosis

At presentation, patients may be asymptomatic and may be found to have a high absolute granulocyte count with a marked left shift. Bands, metamyelocytes, promyelocytes, and a small percentage (< 5 percent) of blasts may be observed. Physical findings may be limited to hepatosplenomegaly and a tender sternum (from the packed marrow). Chronic myelogenous leukemia must be differentiated from granulocytic leukemoid reactions. The presence of significant increases in absolute basophil and eosinophil counts is virtually diagnostic of chronic myelogenous leukemia. It is important to think in terms of absolute counts, since 1 to 2 percent basophils may not seem significant. However, if the total white blood cell count is 200,000, a 2 percent basophil count represents 4000 basophils, or a 20-fold increase above normal. Differentiation from a granulocytic leukemoid reaction also is accomplished by demonstration of a low leukocyte alkaline phosphatase (LAP) level (< 5) in chronic myelogenous leukemia. The prognosis is worse in the presence of greater than 5 percent blasts, greater than 15 percent eosinophils and basophils, a platelet count greater than 700,000, and anemia. Chronic myelogenous leukemia usually develops into a "blast crisis" within 1 to 3 years when these poor prognostic factors are present. In blast crises, the white blood cell count rises rapidly over a few days and may be associated with bleeding from thrombocytopenia and fever along with severe bone pain. Blast transformation may be myelocytic or lymphocytic. The terminal deoxytransferase (TdT) is positive in lymphocytic transformation and negative in myelocytic transformation.

Treatment

Treatment for the chronic phase is aimed at controlling the white blood cell count and the size of the spleen. The spleen may become symptomatic with pain and early satiety. Treatment usually consists of an alkylating drug or hydroxyurea given in doses sufficient to lower the white blood cell count but avoid severe cytopenias. During the blast phase, no treatment has been found to significantly prolong survival. The lymphocytic transformation has been treated with palliation using vincristine and prednisone, while the myeloid transformation is treated as acute nonlymphocytic leukemia. Occasionally, patients present in the blast phase with marked increases in blast counts (80,000 to 100,000) accompanied by leukostasis. Symptoms of leukostasis occur as a result of occlusion of small vessels in the brain and pulmonary vascular beds. This complication must be treated with a rapid-acting drug with or without leukopheresis to lower the blast count. This is usually accomplished using large doses of hydroxyurea. The time to development of blast transformation usually ranges from 1 to 3 years, but rarely it occurs sooner or later than this range. After development of blast transformation, survival is usually limited to a few months.

HAIRY-CELL LEUKEMIA (HCL)

This disorder usually presents in adults and is associated with splenomegaly and pancytopenia [46, 47]. Lymphadenopathy is not a prominent feature. Recent evidence [91] suggests that some hairy-cell leukemias are associated with HTLV II viral infection. The marrow usually cannot be aspirated, and unless the abnormal lymphocytes with their cytoplasmic projections are appreciated on the peripheral blood smear, the disease may be confused with aplastic anemia or myelofibrosis (see above). However, splenomegaly is extremely rare in aplastic anemia at presentation, and the marrow core biopsy provides ready distinction between hairy-cell leukemia and these other disorders. In addition, the lymphocytes in hairy-cell leukemia have a tartarate-resistant acid phosphatase (TRAP) that is virtually diagnostic of the disease in the appropriate clinical setting [46, 47]. Rarely, other benign and malignant lymphocyte disorders have a tartarate-resistant acid phosphatase. Hairy-cell leukemia usually follows an indolent course [46, 47], but ultimately, treatment will be required because of infection and bleeding as a result of the pancytopenia. Standard myelosuppressive chemotherapy is frequently poorly tolerated in hairy-cell leukemia, and these agents should be used as a last resort. The treatment sequence should be splenectomy followed by interferon or deoxycoformycin. The latter two agents are still experimental, but they are very effective in hairy-cell leukemia. If the pancytopenia is not controlled, survival is measured in months to a few years.

ACUTE MYELOFIBROSIS (ACUTE MEGAKARYOCYTIC LEUKEMIA)

A syndrome of rapid development of pancytopenia and subsequently increased megakaryoblasts and fibrosis in the marrow has been described [49]. Acute myelofibrosis and acute megakaryocytic leukemia may be separate entities, but they share many morphologic features. These diseases are fatal, treated or untreated, in a few months.

EOSINOPHIL LEUKEMIAS (HYPEREOSINOPHILIC SYNDROMES)

Marked elevations of the absolute eosinophil counts (10,000 to 100,000 or more) are rarely reactive (i.e., secondary). Eosinophilic leukemia may resemble chronic myelogenous leukemia or be more acute in presentation. Patients may complain of allergic-like symptoms (bronchospasm or pruritus) or symptoms related to thrombosis and cardiac fibroelastosis, both of which are common in this rare disease [49]. The most effective treatment is with hydroxyurea, although refractory disease may have to be treated like acute nonlymphocytic leukemia.

SMOLDERING LEUKEMIA (PRELEUKEMIA)

This diverse group of disorders [69], which includes refractory anemia with excess blasts and sideroblastic anemias, is brought together under the designation myelodysplastic disorders (see above). These patients have a variety of chromosomal abnormalities, and some will develop frank leukemia while others have only a transfusion requirement. Rarely, the disease may spontaneously remit. Several agents, including vitamins and low-dose cytosine arabinoside, have been tried, but none is of proven benefit.

Malignant Lymphomas

The nomenclature for neoplasms of the immune system has become increasingly complex in response to the expanding classification schemes that have become available as a result of new immunologic technology [57]. Various lymphocytic cell lines are separated into different levels of maturation and are correlated with their malignant counterparts [40]. The malignancies of the immune system can be simplified into three basic groups: neoplasms associated with B-lymphocytes, neoplasms associated with T-lymphocytes, and neoplasms whose etiologies are currently not clearly defined. An example of the latter is the Sternberg-Reed cell of Hodgkin's disease, which is currently thought to be a reticulum cell found in the interfollicular area of lymph nodes, but significant controversy as to the point of origin still exists.

HODGKIN'S DISEASE

Approximately 25 percent of all lymphomas diagnosed in 1985 were Hodgkin's disease. In most economically developed countries there is a bimodal incidence curve of Hodgkin's disease with respect to age at diagnosis. The histologic morphology in the first age peak of Hodgkin's disease is predominantly the nodular sclerosing morphology, while the second age peak has no predominant morphology. The pattern of spread in Hodgkin's disease is different from that of non-Hodgkin's lymphoma. Hodgkin's disease spreads by lymphatic channels to contiguous lymphatic structures in 90 percent of patients, whereas non-Hodgkin's lymphoma is multicentric in the majority of the patients. This is an important point for treatment planning, since radiation therapy can cure local disease (as occurs frequently in Hodgkin's disease).

Diagnosis

Clinical manifestations range from asymptomatic (A) lymph node enlargement to symptoms (B) of fever, night sweats, and loss of greater than 10 percent of ideal body weight. Symptoms, regardless of the anatomic stage of disease, are always associated with a worse prognosis.

Treatment

The treatment of Hodgkin's disease is with curative intent and involves either local treatment with radiotherapy or systemic treatment with chemotherapy. Since doses of radiotherapy of 4000 rads (tumor dose) are required to have a greater than 90 percent likelihood of sterilizing the tumor in the radiation field containing Hodgkin's disease, and since such doses given to the total body are lethal, the choice of the preceding two modalities (radiotherapy or chemotherapy) depends on the stage of the disease at presentation. (The staging of Hodgkin's disease is shown in Table 5-9.) Generally, stage I and some stage II

Table 5–9. *Stages of Hodgkin's Disease*

Stage I: Node involvement in a single area or involvement of a single extralymphatic organ

Stage II: Nodal involvement on one side of the diaphragm in more than one area, e.g., neck and mediastinum or both sides of neck

Stage III: Nodal involvement on both sides of diaphragm (the spleen is considered as a lymph node):
　　Stage III_1: Upper abdominal nodes
　　Stage III_2: Lower abdominal nodes

Stage IV: Involvement outside of nodes, e.g., marrow, liver, lung:

Stage modifiers:
　A. No symptoms
　B. Fever, night sweats, and loss of greater than 10 percent of ideal body weight in 6 months

and III disease is treated with radiotherapy, whereas some stage II, III, and all stage IV disease is treated with chemotherapy. For any given clinical anatomic stage, the presence of symptoms (B) implies an actual higher stage. For example, many clinical stage IIA patients can be shown to be the pathologic stage IIA, while many stage IIB patients will be shown to be stage III or IV. Although the cure rate with radiotherapy of stage IA is greater than 95 percent, the physician must be wary of the correct stage in patients considered to be stage IB. True stage IB probably does not exist even in the very small numbers of patients reported to be stage IB in some large series of Hodgkin's disease. An exception to the use of radiotherapy in stage II is a large mediastinal mass, where chemotherapy must be employed [17]. Choice of treatment modalities is important in patients with Hodgkin's disease. Since many of these patients are young and will be cured, strong consideration must be given to the long-term side effects of the curative therapy [85]. The incidence (0.5 to 1 percent per year) of acute nonlymphocytic leukemia is higher in patients treated with chemotherapy or chemotherapy plus radiotherapy compared to radiotherapy alone [22, 85]. Although it was recently believed that chemotherapy with MOPP resulted in a higher incidence of acute leukemia than with other agents, it is clear that any chemotherapy is associated with a higher risk of development of leukemia early (within 10 years) after treatment. Although radiotherapy does not appear to increase the early risk of leukemia, it may be associated with an increased risk of solid tumors developing in the port of radiation late (greater than 15 years) after treatment. The lack of leukemogenesis after radiotherapy use in Hodgkin's disease may be related to technical advances in the radiotherapy method, since treatment of ankylosing spondylitis with vertebral radiotherapy [25] and exposure to the atomic bomb in World War II were clearly associated with a marked increase in leukemia [13] as well as other tumors. Another disadvantage of radiotherapy that depends on the total area irradiated is destruction of marrow reserves. This becomes important in patients who relapse after initial curative radiotherapy and in whom salvage is attempted with chemotherapy. Forty percent of adult marrow is in the pelvis, whereas 50 percent is in the vertebral column and rib cage and 10 percent is in the skull. Thus patients with large areas of irradiated marrow may have their marrow reserves reduced so as to compromise effective doses of chemotherapy.

Another consideration for choice of therapy, especially in young patients, is the issue of sterility. Chemotherapy results in temporary or permanent sterility in the majority of patients (men more than women) [17]. Patients must be informed of this probability, and men may elect to bank sperm. Occasionally, therefore, treatment choice is dictated primarily by the issue of probability of sterility. Studies are currently underway to determine methods to provide "gonadal protection" using manipulations of hormones and hormone analogues.

A frequently asked question in the evaluation of Hodgkin's disease is when to perform a laparotomy for accurate stage assessment. The answer to this question is when the laparotomy would make a difference in the treatment modality. Although all stages (including IA) of Hodgkin's disease can be successfully treated with chemotherapy, the relatively high incidence of leukemia and the morbidity of this therapy dictate that most patients with stage IA and IIA disease (exceptions listed above) be treated with radiotherapy alone, while stage IIIB, IVA, and IVB disease should be treated with chemotherapy alone. Controversy exists between radiotherapy and chemotherapy in stage IIB and IIIA disease. With outstanding radiotherapy, stage IIIA disease with high abdominal lymph node involvement (stage $IIIA_1$) has a good prognosis, while stage IIIA disease with low abdominal lymph node involvement (stage $IIIA_2$) has a poor prognosis [17]. Furthermore, many oncologists believe that stage IIB disease should be treated with chemotherapy as the primary treatment modality.

Laparotomy will increase the accuracy of staging, and the degree of increased accuracy depends on the diagnostic expertise, e.g., the radiology department, in a given institution. Expertise in performance and interpretation of marrow biopsy specimens, lymphangiograms, and abdominal CT scans leads to decreased requirements for surgical staging. The administration of chemotherapy, usually MOPP or ABVD (adriamycin, bleomycin, vinblastine, and dacarbazine), should be done by those with expertise, since maximum dosages increase the chance of cure.

In summary, Hodgkin's disease is a curable disease in 70 percent of all patients. The likelihood of cure depends heavily on the expertise in histology (e.g., the pathology department), in diagnostic staging (e.g., the radiology and surgery departments), and treatment (e.g., the radiotherapy and oncology departments).

NON-HODGKIN'S LYMPHOMA

The biology of non-Hodgkin's lymphomas (NHL) is usually markedly different from Hodgkin's lymphoma in that non-Hodgkin's lymphoma tends to be multicentric at the time of diagnosis. True stage IA disease, especially high-grade lymphomas such as diffuse large-cell lymphomas, tend to be curable using radiotherapy alone. However, stage I non-Hodgkin's lymphoma is uncommon, and 90 percent of non-Hodgkin's lymphomas are widespread at time of diagnosis. Because of this fact, radiotherapy is rarely the primary treatment, and the mode of treatment is usually chemotherapy. Radiotherapy is particularly useful in non-Hodgkin's lymphoma for local palliation such as epidural spinal cord compression or local bone or soft-tissue masses that produce pain or obstruction.

Of the non-Hodgkin's lymphomas, 40 percent are of the follicular morphology, with an equal percentage of the large-cell morphology. Non-Hodgkin's lymphomas are clonal neoplasms of the lymphocytic system involving either the B- or T-cell lines [97]. Many chromosomal abnormalities and immunoglobulin gene rearrangements (monoclonality) have been described [100]. The popular Rappaport classification system, which was used for many years, is being replaced by the National Cancer Institute working formulation [81] in an attempt to give increased clinical relevance to the major classifications. To be noted is the fact that over time, non-Hodgkin's lymphoma may change morphologic features from follicular (nodular) to diffuse. In addition, changes in the cell type have commonly been demonstrated. Non-Hodgkin's lymphomas are two to three times as common as Hodgkin's disease, and although they tend to appear at a median age of 55 (approximately 10 to 15 years older than the median age of patients with Hodgkin's disease), they can occur at any age. However, non-Hodgkin's lymphomas are rare below the age of 2, and they are seen with increasing frequency with increasing age. Recently, an increased incidence in adult T-cell lymphoma has been reported, and the etiology of this variant of non-Hodgkin's lymphoma has been ascribed to the human T-cell lymphotrophic virus type I (HTLV I), the endogenous areas of which are found in the southern islands of Japan, the Caribbean islands, southeastern United States, and New York City [14, 15, 64]. These T-cell malignancies have been reported with immunodeficiency syndromes, both genetic and acquired, including ataxia telangectasia, Wiskott-Aldrich syndrome, congenital sex-linked agammaglobulinemia, Chédiak-Higashai syndrome, renal transplant patients, and in association with the acquired immunodeficiency syndrome (AIDS) [14, 15, 64].

Diagnosis

Non-Hodgkin's lymphoma presents in a manner similar to Hodgkin's disease (see above) and is differentiated from Hodgkin's disease mainly by lymph node histology. Non-Hodgkin's lymphomas are subdivided by the Rappaport system and have recently been further classified as to lymphocyte cell of origin. Prognostically, non-Hodgkin's lymphomas are classified as to grade. Low-grade disease is comprised of nodular lymphomas or diffuse well-differentiated lymphomas [81]. Individuals with low-grade non-Hodgkin's lymphoma have long (5 years or more) median survivals, and it is unclear whether treatment has changed the outlook in these patients. On the other hand, high-grade lymphomas have a short (less than 2 years) median survival, and cures are increased by chemotherapeutic treatment [58, 87].

The physician should be aware of some special forms of non-Hodgkin's lymphoma that have unusual presentations. Lymphoma involving the skin (e.g., mycosis fungoides) is frequently a T-cell variety [14, 15, 96]. HTLV I lymphomas (see above) involve skin and bone and are associated with hypercalcemia [14, 15]. Burkitt's lymphoma is a B-lymphocytic lymphoma that is a rapidly growing tumor, and treatment may result in a lethal disorder referred to as the tumor lysis syndrome. Non-Hodgkin's lymphoma involves the brain and central nervous system more often than Hodgkin's disease, especially when the marrow is involved.

Angioimmunoblastic lymphadenopathy (AIL) is an uncommon disorder that appears reactive with polyclonal hyperglobulinemia, but it may progress to malignant lymphoma [41].

Plasma Cell Disorders

Disorders of plasma cells comprise a number of syndromes, including multiple myeloma, macroglobulinemia of Waldenström, heavy-chain disease, monoclonal gammopathy of undetermined significance (MGUS), and primary amyloidosis. The specific proteins secreted in each of these disorders are immunologically and electrophoretically homogeneous, thus leading to the classification. The abnormal proteins are immunoglobulins found in the gamma fraction of a protein electrophoresis and are broken into five major classifications: IgG, IgM, IgA, IgD, and IgE. These immunoglobulins are analogous to the normal antibodies, but they are produced by an abnormal clone of malignant lymphoid cells. The abnormal proteins correspond to their normally occurring counterparts with a basic structure of two heavy chains and two light chains joined by disulfide bridges and containing both constant

and variable regions on each heavy and light chain. Based on differences in constant regions, the heavy chains are divided into gamma, alpha, mu, delta, and epsilon. The light chains consist of either kappa or lambda chains. All but IgM are secreted as monomers, with IgA having a J protein added at a later time. IgM is secreted as a pentamer that has a very high molecular weight. These homogeneous immunoglobulins give a sharp elevation in the gamma zone of a protein electrophoresis and are collectively referred to as M proteins (for monoclonal proteins). Once found, the M protein is characterized further through the use of immunoelectrophoresis into its specific heavy-chain and light-chain components. Sometimes the plasma cell disorder will secrete excess quantities of light chains, which are filtered and excreted by the kidneys and are known as Bence-Jones proteins. The urine protein electrophoresis can help classify these diseases and is useful, along with the serum protein electrophoresis, in following patients to determine the clinical course of their disease with treatment.

MULTIPLE MYELOMA

Multiple myeloma is a plasma cell disorder characterized by an M-protein spike, lytic bone lesions, and the presence of an increased number of plasma cells in the marrow. It is associated with anemia, renal failure, hypercalcemia, skeletal destruction, and increased susceptibility to infections. The M-protein level is proportional to the mass of the malignant cell line.

The myeloma cell mass follows a Gompertzian growth curve in terms of growth kinetics [94]. Specifically, at a low cell mass, the doubling time can be measured in days, but as a cell mass increases, the doubling time slows and is measured in months. Multiple myeloma can be diagnosed with a cell mass as low as 0.5 kg, roughly 0.5×10^{12} cells. At the time of extensive cell mass, there is generally over 3 kg of myeloma cells, roughly greater than 3×10^{12} cells, and the patient is close to death.

Besides the M protein made by the myeloma

cells, which leads to an elevated viscosity of the patients' blood (as evidenced by rouleaux formation and an elevated erythrocyte sedimentation rate), plasma cells secrete other substances, of which the best characterized is osteoclast-activating factor (OAF). Osteoclast-activating factor stimulates bone resorption by a selective activation of osteoclasts while inhibiting osteoblast activity. For this reason, radiolabeled bone scans are not helpful in multiple myeloma, since the radiolabel is generally absorbed by the osteoblast and not the osteoclast. Osteoclast-activating factor leads to lytic bone lesions as well as generalized osteoporosis. The lytic bone lesions appear as "punched out" lesions best seen in x-rays of long bones, vertebra, or lateral skull films.

Diagnosis

Bone pain is the most common presenting symptom in patients with multiple myeloma. Pain usually involves the back or ribs and can be commonly mistaken for the chronic low-back pain secondary to strain or stress. This pain is worse with motion or exertion and is poorly palliated by rest or over-the-counter medications. The lysis of the bone matrix also leads to an elevation of calcium in the blood and urine which may be associated with changes in mental status, headache, fatigue, lethargy, constipation, and nausea.

The next most common problem is that of the increased susceptibility to bacterial infections, most notably of the common encapsulated organisms and other organisms found commonly in the urinary tract. The reason for the increased susceptibility is secondary to the diffuse hypogammaglobulinemia of other uninvolved immunoglobulins.

Signs and symptoms of renal failure are observed in 25 percent of patients with myeloma, and occasionally, myeloma presents with renal failure. Renal failure is usually caused by Bence-Jones proteins, but contributory factors are high calcium and uric acid, urinary tract infections, and urolithiasis. Approximately 1 percent of patients with multiple myeloma have nonsecretory

myeloma. Also, patients with light-chain myeloma (20 percent) and the rare patients with IgD or IgE do not have an M protein in their sera. All but those with nonsecretory myeloma and some plasmacytomas (see below) have urinary light chains, however. Diagnosis can be made in the absence of lytic bone lesions if the M protein progressively increases over time or extramedullary mass lesions develop which on biopsy are plasma cells.

It should be noted that variations (see below) of myeloma include solitary bone plasmacytomas and extramedullary plasmacytomas, which are more commonly seen in younger individuals, and only 25 to 30 percent of these patients have an M protein. The solitary bone plasmacytoma is a single lytic lesion seen inside the medullary sections, most commonly the long bones. Extramedullary plasmacytomas more often involve the mucosal lymphoid tissue of the nasopharyngeal or paranasal sinuses and do not involve the medullary portion of the bone.

The most common state which is mistaken for multiple myeloma is monoclonal gammopathy of uncertain significance (MGUS). This disorder is 100 times more common than myeloma and is seen in 1 percent of the population over age 50 and 3 percent of the population over age 70. In a longitudinal study of a large series of patients with this disorder, it was shown that 2 percent per year develop a B-cell neoplasm [72]. The beta-2 microglobulin correlates closely with disease activity and is normal in monoclonal gammopathy of uncertain significance [10]. Patients with this disorder usually have no lytic bone lesions, no renal failure, no hypercalcemia, and generally no anemia. Their marrow contains less than 10 percent plasma cells, the M-protein level is usually less than 2 gm/dl, and no urinary Bence-Jones protein is present. It should be noted that the dipsticks for detecting proteinuria are unreliable for the detection of the urinary light chains, and a negative dipstick for protein with a positive sulfosalycylic acid precipitation test is presumptive evidence of light chains in the urine.

Treatment and Prognosis

The treatment of myeloma is generally divided into systemic therapy with or without radiotherapy and supportive care to treat the complications of the disease. In general, all symptomatic patients should be considered as candidates for treatment because less than 10 percent of patients with myeloma have an indolent course (not requiring antitumor therapy). Patients with solitary bone plasmacytomas and extramedullary plasmacytomas have a better disease-free survival using treatment consisting of radiotherapy alone compared to patients with more systemic involvement of their myeloma [68].

The standard treatment of myeloma is systemic chemotherapy, which consists of intermittent pulses of an alkylating agent and steroids given every 4 to 6 weeks. While there is no doubt that this form of therapy does improve the quality of life in the myeloma patient, it does not increase survival. Currently, there are multiple experimental protocols using a variety of other systemic chemotherapeutic agents with and without marrow transplants. Although these protocols seem to give a higher disease-free survival, they demonstrate increased toxicity and morbidity.

After the initiation of systemic chemotherapy, patients generally respond with prompt relief of the bone pain, reversal of the signs and symptoms associated with hypercalcemia, and frequently a sense of improved well-being. However, the healing of osteolytic lesions and improvement in the quantity of M protein (used to follow the patient) take a longer period of time. The rate of fall in the serum M-protein concentration or the urinary light-chain excretion depends both on the rate of kill of the myeloma cells and the metabolism rate of the protein. Approximately half the patients will achieve a plateau in the level of their M protein, and additional chemotherapy during this time has not been demonstrated to prolong survival. Most myeloma patients have approximately one log of tumor regression with chemotherapy and can remain in "remission" for approximately 1 to 3 years before they relapse as manifested by

a rising M-protein level or new symptoms. The median survival ranges from greater than 60 months for early-stage patients to less than 15 months for late-stage patients [30].

Supportive Care

The hypercalcemia generally responds well to corticosteroid therapy, hydration, and natriuresis. Allopurinol is used to prevent hyperuricemia and hyperuricosuria. For hypercalcemia refractory to hydration and diuresis, the use of oral phosphates, calcitonin, or mithramyicin should be entertained.

One of the major causes of morbidity is spinal cord compression, which can occur from a compression fracture secondary to osteoporosis and/or from lytic bone lesions from the myeloma. Investigation through the use of myelograms and magnetic resonance imaging (MRI) scans and initiation of radiotherapy and neurosurgery should be instigated. Any delay in diagnosis or treatment can lead to irreversible paralysis.

The use of prophylactic gamma globulin over a 2- to 3-week interval has not been proven to be of benefit in decreasing infections. Prophylactic use of antibiotics has decreased the incidence of skin infections, but it has not shown to benefit in the prevention of any life-threatening septic episodes. When a patient does have a major septic episode (frequently with pneumococcus), appropriate antibiotics must be administered in adequate dosages. However, avoiding nephrotoxic antibiotics should be attempted so as to prevent any additional renal impairment.

VARIANT FORMS OF MYELOMA

There appears to be a small subset (less than 10 percent) of myeloma patients who have localized plasmacytomas of bone or an indolent variety of multiple myeloma in whom careful long-term follow-up without any systemic chemotherapy is justified. These patients are asymptomatic due to the low tumor mass. Once the patient shows an elevation of Bence-Jones proteins, disease progression occurs within 1 to 2 years. There is no evidence that delay in the initiation of systemic therapy in this subset of patients until proven evidence of tumor progression occurs has any adverse effect on the long-term outcome.

Waldenström's macroglobulinemia is a malignancy of a plasma cell line that secretes IgM, in contrast to myeloma. Also different from myeloma is the fact that Waldenström's macroglobulinemia is usually associated with lymphadenopathy and hepatosplenomegaly with increased frequency of the hyperviscosity syndrome. In contrast to multiple myeloma, osteolytic bone lesions, renal impairment, and amyloidosis are all quite rare in the macroglobulinemia.

Clinically, macroglobulinemia has a slow and insidious progression with symptoms of weakness, fatigue, and bleeding abnormalities as the main manifestations. Patients generally are asymptomatic in terms of bone pain, but they can have recurrent infections, visual difficulties (secondary to hyperviscosity syndrome), and other neurologic complaints. Examination will reveal peripheral lymphadenopathy and hepatosplenomegaly, with the funduscopic examination revealing venous dilatation and vascular segmentation of retinal veins ("sausage links"). The sludging of the blood flow secondary to hyperviscosity also leads to bleeding and oozing from mucous membranes.

To diagnose Waldenström's macroglobulinemia, the presence of IgM levels of greater than 3 gm/dl and histologic evidence of lymphocytoid plasmacytosis are required.

The treatment of macroglobulinemia is divided into symptomatic and chemotherapeutic modalities, with plasmapheresis for the hyperviscosity syndrome. This is effective treatment, since some 80 to 90 percent of IgM is intravascular. The use of alkylating agents as in myeloma controls the IgM level. Survival rates for patients with macroglobulinemia are similar to those for patients with multiple myeloma; however, there are patients with indolent disease who may survive for 10 years or more.

Amyloidosis

Amyloidosis is a collection of syndromes related to each other by the fact that all result in the deposition of a homogeneous eosinophilic substance into body tissues. Amyloid is a fibrillar substance when viewed by electron microscopy with a characteristic beta-pleated sheet when seen by x-ray diffraction; an additional characteristic is its staining property of green birefringence with Congo red and under polarized light. In spite of its rather uniform appearance, the existence of many different types of amyloid has been demonstrated by biochemical and immunologic studies of the amyloid proteins. Amyloidosis is generally categorized into primary amyloidosis and secondary amyloidosis [61].

In primary amyloidosis, a clear relationship has been shown to exist between the amyloid fibrillar deposits and Bence-Jones proteins, which are related to multiple myeloma and other plasma cell dyscrasias. Primary amyloid protein (AL) has been shown to have amino acid sequence homogeneous with the variable region of the light-chain sequence of paraproteins. Deposition of a second type of amyloid protein which is unrelated to any known immunoglobulin results in secondary amyloidosis. The secondary protein (AA) is seen with chronic diseases such as rheumatoid arthritis. A third protein, known as AF, is observed in familial Mediterranean fever.

The signs and symptoms of amyloidosis [71] are a result of infiltration of tissues by the amyloid protein. The amyloid deposition causes swelling of tissues and decreased compliance, and these affect the individual mainly in terms of the organ systems most infiltrated. The symptoms associated with amyloidosis most commonly are weakness, weight loss, fullness of the tongue, pedal edema, and orthostatic symptoms. Physical findings also are correlated with the involved organ systems. Involvement of the skin leads to soft-tissue thickening and plaques. Purpura occurs secondary to vascular involvement. A common finding is periorbital purpura ("racoon eyes") after a sustained Valsalva maneuver. Cardiac involvement leads to an enlarged heart with signs and symptoms of congestive heart failure that is generally refractory to therapy. Involvement of the autonomic nervous system may lead to orthostatic hypotension. Ankle edema also is associated with renal involvement, which is usually the nephrotic syndrome with a nonspecific proteinuria. Involvement of the joints can lead to findings similar to that of rheumatoid arthritis. Involvement of the cardiac and renal systems occurs most commonly, and together they comprise the leading cause of mortality [71].

Laboratory Findings
The majority of patients with amyloidosis (both primary and secondary) have proteinuria, with approximately half having a mild to moderate anemia with evidence of renal failure. Of the patients with amyloidosis, approximately one-half to three-fourths will have an M-protein spike on serum protein electrophoresis—the higher percentage associated with patients with primary amyloidosis. The majority of patients have light chains in serum and urine.

Diagnosis
The diagnosis of amyloidosis is made by biopsy with its pathognomic properties (see above). The location of the biopsy should initially be the rec-

tum or oral mucosa, with additional sites selected depending on specific symptoms or findings on physical examination. Patients with amyloidosis tend to bleed profusely after biopsy.

Treatment
There is no good form of therapy to remove the amyloid deposition. Treatment of an associated disease process should be paramount. A number of attempts to control amyloidosis using alkylating agents, mitotic inhibitors, or steroids have shown little promise. Efforts to control the symptomatology should include measures to support the cardiac and renal systems. However, without control of the underlying disease process, the benefits of palliation are brief in duration.

The prognosis [71] of patients with systemic amyloidosis is poor. However, the average survival is dependent on whether the patient has a secondary cause of the amyloidosis or a primary amyloidosis most commonly associated with myeloma. Patients with primary amyloidosis have a median survival of approximately 3 to 4 months and comprise some 20 percent of the cases. The average survival for patients without underlying myeloma (secondary amyloidosis) is better, but still is only approximately 15 months.

Disorders of Hemostasis

Hemostasis is a delicately designed state that rapidly arrests bleeding from vessels that have undergone a break in their integrity without compromising the fluidity of the normal circulation. Disorders of hemostasis result in excessive bleeding or clotting.

Abnormalities in the hemostatic mechanism result from interference in one of three broad categories: those affecting platelets, those affecting soluble factors, and those affecting the blood vessel. Although many diseases fall into a single cat-

egory, such as low platelets in idiopathic thrombocytopenic purpura (ITP) or low factor VIII levels in hemophilia A, some result from disorders in a combination of categories, such as the combined platelet disorder and abnormal factor VIII complex in von Willibrand's disease or thrombocytopenia with decreased soluble factors in disseminated intravascular coagulation. Disorders can be either quantitative or qualitative. Figure 5-1 (See Appendix) presents a schematic diagram of the hemostatic mechanism.

Evaluation of a Suspected Bleeding Disorder

The history is very important in bleeding disorders, with particular attention to five major questions. (1) Did past bleeding occur from one site or from multiple sites? One-site bleeding is less likely to represent a coagulation problem. (2) Is the bleeding lifelong or recent onset? Specific inquiry should be made about bleeding episodes requiring physician visits or transfusions after minor surgical procedures such as tooth extractions, circumcision, or minor trauma. (3) Does the type of bleeding suggest an etiology? Platelet problems often result in petechiae or mucosal oozing, while soluble-factor abnormalities result in giant ecchymoses or hemarthroses. (4) What drugs have been ingested? Ask about alcohol history, aspirin use, recent antibiotics, quinidine, gold, and the thiazides. (5) Is there a family history of bleeding? Even with a negative history, some patients with a congenital coagulation disorder will present with severe bleeding after a major provocation.

The physical examination should be thorough, but in particular, one should first assess the volume status and signs of ongoing bleeding. The skin and mucous membranes should be examined for petechiae, oozing, or ecchymosis. Intravenous sites and sites of recent blood draws should be examined. The skin also should be checked carefully for signs of liver disease, such as spiders or jaundice. Organ systems should be examined, looking for evidence of neoplasia that could infiltrate the marrow, especially carcinoma of the breast and prostate. The abdomen should be examined to assess both liver and spleen size. The stool should be checked for occult blood. Joints should be checked for evidence of old or new hemarthrosis, and attention should be paid to the retroperitoneal areas.

The general laboratory assessment includes tests of liver function, kidney function, and blood glucose. A complete blood count and smear should be done in all patients to examine both red cell and white cell morphology. The more specific workup of an initial bleeding disorder involves four tests: (1) the platelet count and blood smear, (2) the bleeding time, (3) the prothrombin time (PT), and (4) the partial thromboplastin time (PTT). Almost all significant bleeding disorders will have an abnormality in one of these tests.

Evaluation of the blood smear is important in assessing quantitative platelet abnormalities. Between 10 and 20 platelets should be seen per normal oil-immersion field. Platelet morphology is useful in that states of excessive destruction often have large platelets, whereas states of underproduction often have small platelets [65].

Qualitative disorders of platelet function should be examined by use of the bleeding time, which measures platelet function and small-vessel integrity. This test is useful when the platelet count is normal. However, in thrombocytopenic states, the bleeding time will be abnormal without a qualitative defect in platelets [48, 74].

The prothrombin time involves activation of factor VII with tissue thromboplastin to measure the extrinsic system of the soluble clotting factors. It is the most sensitive screening test for abnormalities of the vitamin K-dependent factors and tends to be more affected by liver disease, since these factors are produced by the liver.

The partial thromboplastin time measures the intrinsic system starting with activation of factor XII (see Fig. 5-1, Appendix). This test is usually more sensitive to the effects of heparin than the prothrombin time and is abnormal in factor VIII and IX deficiencies (the hemophilias).

Other useful tests include (1) the thrombin time, which specifically tests the ability to convert fibrinogen to fibrin monomers, (2) the reptilase time, which checks the ability of a snake enzyme with thrombin-like activity to clot human fibrinogen, (3) the fibrinogen levels, and (4) fibrin split products and fibrin monomers. If a positive bleeding history is obtained and the preceding tests are normal, the euglobulin lysis time and the urea clot stabilization test should be ordered. The euglobulin lysis time measures the ability of serum to dissolve clots, a normal part of hemostasis. This may be the only defect found in patients with alpha-2 antiplasmin deficiency. The urea clot stabilization test checks the integrity of a clot and is abnormal in factor XIII deficiency, while all other clotting tests are normal.

After finding an abnormality, particularly in the prothrombin time or partial thromboplastin time, a repeat test should be obtained, since these tests are subject to artifact, particularly with heparin contamination. Then, if either the prothrombin time or partial thromboplastin time is longer than normal, a 50 : 50 mix with incubation should be done with normal plasma. Normally, 50 percent of a cofactor will result in a normal prothrombin time or partial thromboplastin time. In the face of an inhibitor, a 50 : 50 mix will prolong both. If the mix normalizes both, a deficiency state is diagnosed and specific factor assays can be obtained. If an inhibitor is found, one can further classify it at the factor level.

Quantitative platelet problems are best evaluated by obtaining marrow biopsy and aspirate. This evaluates the source of production and can separate these patients into mechanisms of underproduction versus excess destruction of platelets. If qualitative platelet problems are found, one should exclude acquired causes such as drugs, antibodies, or sepsis, then test for von Willibrand's disease, and perform specific tests of platelet aggregation.

Platelet Disorders

DISEASES OF UNDERPRODUCTION

The most common of these illnesses are aplastic anemia, marrow infiltration by tumor (including leukemia), and drug-related disorders. Other processes include alcohol, viral infections, vitamin B_{12} and folate deficiency, and radiation. Examination of the marrow biopsy is useful in the differential diagnosis: panhypoplasia of aplastic anemia, marrow infiltration by tumor or infection, and the megaloblastic changes of vitamin B_{12} and folate deficiency. It is very important to obtain both a red blood cell folate level and a serum B_{12} level in cases without an obvious diagnosis, since the treatments for vitamin B_{12} and folate deficiencies are simple, safe, and effective. In all the un-

derproductive states, severe bleeding can occur when the platelet count is below 20,000. Platelet transfusions should be used for evidence of acute bleeding with a platelet count of less than 50,000 or prophylactically with a platelet count of less than 15,000. Prophylaxis is not used in cases of long-term aplasia, where recovery is not expected, or when transplantation is being considered, as in aplastic anemia. Invasive procedures should be covered with platelet transfusions for platelet counts of less than 50,000.

DISEASES OF EXCESSIVE DESTRUCTION

The marrow in these patients shows excessive megakaryocytes. These patients tend not to bleed unless the platelet count is less than 5000 to 10,000. Platelet transfusions are not usually helpful unless active bleeding is occurring. Nonimmune causes of excessive platelet destruction include infections (including gram-negative sepsis), disseminated intravascular coagulation (DIC), thrombotic thrombocytopenic purpura (TTP), and hemolytic uremic syndrome (HUS).

Disseminated intravascular coagulation is diagnosed on both a clinical and a laboratory basis. The patient usually has precipitating events such as sepsis or eclampsia. Oozing is noted from various sources. The prothrombin time and partial thromboplastin time tend to be elevated, and the platelet count is low. Useful confirmation includes falling fibrinogen levels, rising levels of fibrin split products, and the presence of fibrin monomers. The blood smear may reveal a microangiopathic picture. The treatment of disseminated intravascular coagulation is directed at the underlying cause. The control of bleeding in this disorder is somewhat controversial, but most authors would use fresh-frozen plasma, cryoprecipitate, and platelets as needed, depending on the clinical circumstance. Heparin use is controversial and usually not needed, particularly in disease associated with sepsis. Heparin is useful in cases of disseminated intravascular coagulation with promyelocytic leukemia, where low doses are used and the fibrinogen level is monitored.

Thrombotic thrombocytopenic purpura is an

uncommon disease of unknown etiology that can be rapidly fatal. This disease is classically seen in young to middle-aged women. The diagnosis is suggested on a clinical basis with renal and central nervous system involvement, a microangiopathic hemolytic anemia with a blood smear showing fragmentation of red cells, thrombocytopenia, and fever. Hemolytic uremic syndrome tends to have more prominent renal failure and no neurologic symptoms. The prothrombin time and partial thromboplastin time are usually normal in both these diseases, helping to separate it from disseminated intravascular coagulation. The treatment consists of large-volume plasma exchanges of 50 to 100 ml/kg per day. This can salvage up to 70 percent of these patients. Other therapies include high-dose corticosteroids, antiplatelet drugs, vincristine, and splenectomy. Platelet transfusion should be avoided.

Acquired immune causes of thrombocytopenia are usually either secondary to a drug or a disease state such as lupus or of unknown cause, in which case it is called idiopathic. The most important part of the diagnosis and treatment of immune thrombocytopenic states is to discontinue any potentially offending drug. The most commonly incriminated drugs include quinidine, gold, and heparin, but almost any drug can be implicated. Antiplatelet antibodies may be useful in the diagnosis of an immune state of platelet destruction [66].

Idiopathic thrombocytopenic purpura (ITP) is usually diagnosed after discontinuing all drugs and excluding all other disorders. It can be either acute, which is less than 6 month's duration and often remits spontaneously, or chronic. These patients tend not to bleed unless the platelet counts are severely depressed. If the disease is stable and the platelet count is greater than 50,000, no immediate treatment is usually required. The therapy of idiopathic thrombocytopenic purpura is often effective. For the acute case with bleeding, the patient can be given gamma globulin infusions of 300 to 400 mg/kg followed by 5 to 10 units of platelets [36]. Prednisone in doses of 1 to 2 mg/kg per day should be added. The gamma globulin infusions are usually continued for 3 to 5 days. In patients without ongoing bleeding, prednisone alone should be started. If no response is seen after 1 to 3 weeks of prednisone, intolerable steroid side effects occur, or thrombocytopenia relapses during reduction of the steroid dose, splenectomy is recommended. In patients failing to respond to splenectomy, vincristine or danazol [1] can be used. Splenectomy is effective in up to 50 percent of patients, and even if it isn't effective, it will frequently decrease the steroid requirement. After splenectomy, a rebound thrombocytosis often occurs.

QUALITATIVE PLATELET DISORDERS

Qualitative platelet disorders may be either congenital or acquired [89]. The congenital disorders are very uncommon, except for von Willibrand's disease. Von Willibrand's disease is caused by an abnormality of part of the factor VIII complex [112]. Normally, factor VIII, which consists of both a von Willibrand's portion and the antihemophilia factor, forms multimers while in the circulation. The large multimers assist the platelets in aggregation through a platelet receptor. Defects in von Willibrand's disease range from a deficiency of the normal von Willibrand's protein to abnormal proteins that may fail to form multimers or fail to interact with platelets. Abnormalities are seen in both the partial thromboplastin time and the bleeding time, but these fluctuate and can be normal. Several types of von Willibrand's disease are described (Table 5-10). The common types are type I, which consists of an absolute deficiency of a normal von Willibrand's protein; type IIA, which consists of the production of an abnormal von Willibrand's protein that fails to form large multimers in both platelets and in plasma; and type IIB, which has abnormal plasma multimers but active multimer formation on the surface of platelets. Ristocetin is an antibiotic that has been shown to clump normal platelets in the presence of normal von Willibrand's factor. Plasma from von Willibrand's patients will not clump normal platelets in the presence of ristocetin and is virtually diagnostic of von

Table 5–10. Von Willibrand's Disease

Type	Ristocetin cofactor (von Willibrand's plasma with normal platelets, then aggregation with ristocetin)	Ristocetin-induced platelet aggregation (von Willibrand's platelet aggregation from concentrated specimen with ristocetin)	Von Willibrand antigen	Electrophoresis
I	Decreased	Decreased	Low	Diffuse
IIA	Decreased	Decreased	Low or normal	No large multimers
IIB	Decreased	Increased	Low or normal	No large multimers

Willibrand's disease. To separate the different types of von Willibrand's disease, either electrophoresis can be done to examine the multimer pattern or activity versus antigenicity of the factor VIII complex can be measured along with the ability of ristocetin to aggregate platelet concentrates of the patient in question. Von Willibrand's disease type I responds well to dDAVP, a synthetic form of antidiuretic hormone. The dose used is 0.3 μg/kg given 30 minutes before invasive procedures or with bleeding. dDAVP increases the endothelial release of von Willibrand's factor and often will normalize the coagulopathy. Effects on the bleeding time last from 3 to 6 hours. dDAVP can be repeated at 24- to 48-hour intervals and the bleeding time can be followed for effect. Von Willibrand's type IIB has hyperaggregatable platelets, and severe thrombocytopenia can occur with the administration of dDAVP [56]. For type IIA and IIB von Willibrand's disease and failures of dDAVP in the other von Willibrand's disease cases, cryoprecipitate at 1 unit per 10 kg every day is the treatment of choice. The risk of non-A, non-B hepatitis with these preparations is great, and patients should be monitored for hepatitis and vaccinated against hepatitis B.

ACQUIRED QUALITATIVE PLATELET DISORDERS

Acquired qualitative platelet disorders are relatively common. The most common causes are drugs such as aspirin or other nonsteroidal anti-inflammatory agents, uremia, myeloproliferative disorders, and dysproteinemias. It is very impor-

tant when discovering a prolonged bleeding time in a patient to take a careful drug history and remove any potentially offending drugs. If treatment is needed in cases of acquired qualitative platelet disorders such as uremia, dDAVP can be administered [76]. Approximately 50 percent of patients will respond. If no response is noted, particularly in acute situations, both platelet transfusions and cryoprecipitate can be given to control bleeding. It should be noted that in some myeloproliferative disorders there is often a platelet dysfunction despite a grossly elevated platelet count. It is important both to measure and to normalize the bleeding time in these patients prior to invasive procedures, using dDAVP or platelet transfusion in addition to cryoprecipitate.

Disorders of the Soluble Factors of Coagulation

Congenital disorders in the soluble factors of coagulation are relatively common. Both quantitative and qualitative abnormalities of all the clotting factors have been described. The two most common diseases associated with these factors are hemophilia A and hemophilia B. Both these are sex-linked disorders that can be mild to very severe.

Hemophilia A is a deficiency of factor VIII activity. The severity of the illness is correlated with the amount of factor VIII activity measurable in plasma. In severe cases, the activity is less than 1 percent. These patients are characterized by life-long bleeding tendencies, especially spontaneous bleeds into joints. Hemophilia A is usually diagnosed by the typical family history and a prolonged partial thromboplastin time, and the diagnosis is confirmed by low factor VIII activity. The antigenic levels of factor VIII can be normal, but usually they are decreased. Treatment is given either in acute situations such as active bleeding or as prophylaxis for surgical procedures. For mild hemophilia A with greater than 5 percent activity, DDAVP can be infused, but an adequate response must be documented. For emergencies, factor VIII concentrates should be given, as shown in Table 5-11. If factor VIII concentrate is not available, cryoprecipitate contains approximately 100 units of factor VIII per bag and should be given in doses similar to that for factor VIII concentrates. A severe complication of hemophilia is the development of inhibitors to factor VIII (see below). During the early 1980s, human immunodeficiency virus (HIV) was common in these products, but now the factors are heat-treated. Because of past contamination, there is a high frequency of positivity of HIV antibodies in patients with hemophilia.

Hemophilia B, or lack of factor IX, otherwise known as Christmas disease, is less common than hemophilia A, but it is very similar in clinical presentation. Treatment is with a specific factor IX concentrate or fresh-frozen plasma, which contains 1 unit of activity per milliliter. Cryoprecipitate is not useful in factor IX deficiency (see Table 5-11 for dosages).

Table 5–11. *Treatment of Hemophilia*

Hemophilia A bolus: Weight in kg × 50 = units of factor VIII needed for 100 percent activity. Repeat every 12 hours.

For surgery or life-threatening hemorrhage, continual infusion of 2 units/kg/per hour is given after the bolus. Cryoprecipitate = 100 units factor VIII per unit.

Hemophilia B Bolus: Weight in kg × 100 = units of factor IX activity needed for 100 percent activity. Repeat every 24 hours.

Owing to instability of factor IX concentrates, continuous infusion is not used. Fresh-frozen plasma = 1 unit factor IX per milliliter.

ACQUIRED DISORDERS OF SOLUBLE CLOTTING FACTORS

Acquired disorders of soluble clotting factors are relatively common, usually being due to either liver disease, drugs, or disseminated intravascular coagulation. Severe liver disease can present with a profound bleeding disorder due not only to mechanical problems such as varices, but also to thrombocytopenia resulting from hypersplenism and deficiency of all clotting factors, except factor VIII, which is produced in endothelial cells. The diagnosis is usually obvious after a history, physical examination, and screening laboratory tests. The treatment of bleeding with liver disease is difficult, but it can be done through the judicious use of factor replacement with fresh-frozen plasma or cryoprecipitate and platelets as needed. Each unit of fresh-frozen plasma contains about 3 percent of the vitamin K-dependent factors for a 70-kg adult. For patients presenting with a long prothrombin time, a trial of vitamin K, 10 mg subcutaneously every day times 3, is indicated.

A difficult problem in the patient with chronic liver disease is separating the coagulopathy due to liver disease from disseminated intravascular coagulation. In disseminated intravascular coagulation the factor VIII level should be decreased due to consumption, whereas it is often elevated in liver disease.

Another clinical presentation of vitamin K deficiency occurs in postoperative patients who have been on nasogastric suction and antibiotics that depress the intestinal bacterial flora that produce vitamin K. About 10 days of this treatment is required before evidence of depletion of vitamin K-dependent factors becomes apparent.

Bleeding from anticoagulants represents a special problem because generally there is some other medical condition that requires the anticoagulated state. Heparin with its short half-life is reversed by stopping the infusion or, if needed, protamine will rapidly reverse its effects. Warfarin with its long half-life will respond to vitamin K replacement. Acutely, fresh-frozen plasma is indicated. In patients in whom continued anticoagulation is needed, such as those with prosthetic heart valves, plasma replacement alone can be given while continuing with anticoagulation. This bypasses the problem of repleting vitamin K stores, which makes anticoagulation with coumadin more difficult after resolution of the acute event.

CIRCULATING INHIBITORS

Circulating inhibitors are detected when the patient is discovered to have a long partial thromboplastin time or prothrombin time, and this laboratory abnormality does not correct with a 1 : 1 mix with normal plasma. Normally, both the prothrombin time and the partial thromboplastin time are insensitive enough (see above) that a 50 percent deficiency will continue to give normal values. If the patient's plasma increases or does not decrease either the prothrombin time or the partial thromboplastin time when mixed with normal plasma, an inhibitor to coagulation is diagnosed. The most common inhibitor is heparin contamination, which can be excluded with a combination of a normal reptilase time and an abnormal thrombin time. Significant acquired inhibitors [37, 108] with bleeding are found in approximately 10 percent of hemophiliacs. The level of inhibition is measured in Bethesda units, where 1 Bethesda unit will remove 50 percent of factor VIII activity from 1 ml normal plasma in 2 hours. The significance of inhibitors varies somewhat in the clinical situation. Those acquired in hemophilia A and B tend to be very tightly bound and have a very strong amnestic response, often rising to extremely high titers after exposure to the antigen in blood products. Those acquired in nonhemophiliacs and in other conditions, such as postpartum, tend to be lower and not to have this amnestic response.

The treatment of hemophiliacs with inhibitors consists of the infusion of activated complexes that bypass the need for factor VIII activity. These include the use of factor IX concentrate, Autoplex, or FEIBA in doses of 50 to 75 units/kg. There is no good laboratory test to measure the effect. In life-threatening hemorrhages, patients with an inhibitor titer of less than 10 Bethesda units can be given massive doses of factor VIII; however, an amnestic response will be expected. More recently, porcine factor VIII has become available, and this tends to have less affinity for the anti-factor VIII antibody produced by hemophiliacs and in conjunction with plasmapheresis is sometimes useful in acute situations. The nonhemophiliac who develops spontaneous inhibitors to factor VIII can often be treated with steroids and porcine factor VIII, in an attempt to overwhelm the inhibitor. If this treatment is not successful, then plasmapheresis with porcine factor VIII and factor VIII bypass products can be used. These patients often have spontaneous remissions over time.

A relatively common inhibitor is the lupus anticoagulant [86, 103]. This inhibitor appears to be an antibody directed against the phospholipids used in the prothrombin time and partial thromboplastin time. Despite laboratory evidence of prolongation of both these tests, these patients are often hypercoagulable and present with clotting and spontaneous abortions rather than bleeding. Bleeding is only a problem if they have a specific anti-factor II antibody or an associated platelet abnormality (common). The diagnosis of a lupus inhibitor is made by correction of the prothrombin time and partial thromboplastin time using excessive phospholipids from normal platelets to absorb the inhibitor. Treatment of patients with lupus inhibitors depends on the clinical situation, but a good response is often obtained from steroids and anticoagulation with coumadin. Paradoxically, these patients rarely have other manifestations of systemic lupus erythematosus.

VASCULAR DISORDERS

Generalized vascular disorders are an uncommon cause of significant bleeding, but often they present with ecchymoses. It is important in these patients to search for an underlying platelet function abnormality that can occur in hereditary diseases of connective tissue, such as Ehlers-Danlos syndrome, and to think about treatable systemic illnesses associated with a vascular fragility, such as Cushing's syndrome, vasculitis, and scurvy.

Hypercoagulopathies

Thrombotic disorders are very common in clinical practice. Unfortunately, understanding of thrombotic tendencies lags behind understanding of hemorrhagic disorders. Often no underlying abnormalities of hemostasis are discovered, but rather associated conditions, such as bed rest, heart failure, recent abdominal surgery, or estrogen use, are found.

The history is critical. Patients with congenital thrombotic disorders often have a family history of hypercoagulability [23, 90]. The patient should be questioned about associated illnesses, dehydration, bed rest, intravenous catheterizations, drug use, tobacco use, and weight loss. The physical examination will often point toward the associated illness or signs of past thrombosis, but often it is normal. One should look closely for an underlying malignancy [93].

The laboratory assessment of the hypercoagulable state should include tests of renal function, complete blood count with morphology, a prothrombin time, partial thromboplastin time, and special tests of hypercoagulability, such as antithrombin III levels, the protein which normally inhibits the action of thrombin, protein C and its associated cofactor protein S (which are normal inactivators of factors V and VIII), and the euglobulin lysis time, which may be markedly prolonged with abnormal plasminogens.

PLATELET DISORDERS ASSOCIATED WITH HYPERCOAGULABLE STATES

Paroxysmal nocturnal hemoglobinuria is associated with thrombosis. The diagnosis is based on evidence of hemolysis in the face of thrombocytopenia with thrombosis. Further investigations, such as the Coomb's test and the Ham's test, confirm the diagnosis. Coumadin and antiplatelet drugs can be used with variable success. Heparin-associated thrombocytopenia presents as a severe thrombosis in the face of heparin anti-coagulation [67]. It is important to discontinue the administration of heparin in these patients.

Fibrinolytic therapy may be used in the acute thrombotic situation and has been suggested to decrease the incidence of the postphlebitic syndrome in deep venous thrombosis [77, 104].

The thrombocytopathic states, particularly polycythemia vera and essential thrombocythemia, are associated with thrombosis or bleeding. Control of the underlying process with drugs such as hydroxyurea is of benefit. Antiplatelet drugs are of questionable use in these conditions because of both the bleeding and the clotting tendencies.

SOLUBLE FACTORS ASSOCIATED WITH THROMBOSIS

The best-defined biochemical conditions associated with thrombosis are antithrombin III deficiency, protein C deficiency, and protein S deficiency [44, 90]. Antithrombin III deficiency is a relatively common disorder that can be inherited as an autosomal-dominant trait or acquired, as in the nephrotic syndrome. Patients present with deep venous or arterial thrombosis. The diagnosis is made by measuring the activity of antithrombin III in plasma. It should be noted that heparin may decrease levels of antithrombin III by 30 percent in the first 24 to 48 hours, and extensive thrombosis will cause levels to fall. Timing is important in the measurement of these tests. Lifelong coumadin therapy is recommended to those with a history of thrombosis, but the treatment of asymptomatic patients is controversial.

Protein C and its enhancer, protein S, are both vitamin K-dependent factors that inhibit the activity of factor VIII and factor V. Deficiency can result in severe thrombosis. In congenital homozygous protein C deficiency, death in utero or in the neonatal period due to massive thrombosis occurs.

Decreased levels of proteins S and C are also found in liver disease and during coumadin therapy, since they are vitamin K-dependent. Since protein C has a very short half-life, treatment with coumadin can cause early thrombosis, particularly the syndrome of coumadin-induced skin necrosis. For protein C and S deficiencies with thrombosis, several options are available. If no history of problems with coumadin anticoagulation is obtained despite past use, coumadin can be given during standard heparin administration as outlined below. Otherwise, fresh-frozen plasma can be administered while coumadinizing the patient on heparin, or outpatient subcutaneous heparin can be given.

The procoagulant activity associated with cancer is poorly defined, but there may be a soluble factor that activates the clotting cascade. Thrombosis is commonly seen in association with adenocarcinomas [93]. Treatment is with either coumadin or subcutaneous heparin, along with treatment of the underlying disease process.

DISORDERS OF VESSELS AND BLOOD FLOW

Abnormalities of the blood vessels and flow are by far the most common categories associated with thrombosis, particularly in atherosclerotic disease and conditions of venous stasis. Treatment of an acute thrombotic event varies depending on the vessel involved and the symptoms. For acute arterial thrombosis, fibrinolytic agents such as streptokinase, urokinase, or tissue plasminogen activator can be used [104]. For larger arterial thrombi, embolectomy may be carried out. Acute heparin anticoagulation and chronic anticoagulation with heparin and coumadin also can be used.

A very common problem in medicine is deep venous thrombosis. Treatment by anticoagulation can prevent potentially fatal pulmonary embolus.

Standard therapy consists of an intravenous heparin bolus of 5000 to 10,000 units and a continuous infusion of 15 to 20 units/kg per hour. The partial thromboplastin time and platelet count should be checked prior to and 4 to 6 hours into therapy to prolong the partial thromboplastin time to 1.5 times normal [60]. Heparin should be continued for 7 to 10 days. Coumadin, a vitamin K antagonist with a long half-life, should be started 2 or 3 days after heparin anticoagulation is started with a 5-day overlap. Loading doses are not necessary on this schedule. The prothrombin time should be prolonged to 1.5 times control. Patients should avoid medications that potentiate coumadin effects or that interfere with other aspects of hemostasis. The duration of anticoagulation is controversial, but it is usually continued for 3 to 6 months after the first thrombotic episode.

Fibrinolytic therapy with streptokinase or urokinase can be used in deep venous thrombosis of less than 7 days' duration. Contraindications include allergy, recent surgery, cerebrovascular accidents, older age, or other problems where fibrinolysis could cause severe bleeding [77]. The thrombin time is monitored for indirect evidence of attainment of a fibrinolytic state.

Streptokinase is given as a 200,000-unit intravenous bolus and then 100,000 units per hour for up to 72 hours before switching to heparin. For patients resistant to streptokinase, urokinase, a 4400 units/kg bolus and then 4400 units/kg per hour, can be given for 12 hours. During such treatment, blood draws and other invasive procedures should be kept at a minimum.

References

1. Ahn, Y. S., Harrington, W. J., Seinon, S. R., Mylvaganaru, R., Pall, L. M., and So, A. G.   Danazol for the treatment of idiopathic thrombocytopenic purpura. *N. Engl. J. Med.* 308: 1396, 1983.
2. Aisen, P.   Current concepts in iron metabolism. *Clin. Haematol.* 11: 241, 1982.
3. Allen, R. H.   Cobalamin (vitamin B$_{12}$) absorption and malabsorption. *Viewpoints Dig. Dis.* 14: 17, 1982.
4. Allgood, J. W., and Chaplin, H., Jr.   Idiopathic acquired autoimmune hemolytic anemia: A review of 47 cases treated from 1955 through 1965. *Am. J. Med.* 43: 254, 1967.
5. Beck, W. S.   Hypochromic Anemias. In W. S. Beck (Ed.), *Hematology,* 3d Ed. Cambridge, Mass.: MIT Press, 1982. Pp. 97–117.
6. Beck, W. W.   Metabolic Aspects of Vitamin B$_{12}$ and Folic Acid. In W. J. Williams, E. Beutler, A. J. Erslev, and M. A. Lichtman (Eds.), *Hematology,* 3d Ed. New York: McGraw-Hill, 1983. Pp. 311–331.

7. Beck, W. W. The Megaloblastic Anemias. In W. J. Williams, E. Beutler, A. J. Erslev, and M. A. Lichtman (Eds.), *Hematology,* 3d Ed. New York: McGraw-Hill, 1983. Pp. 434–463.

8. Berk, P. D., Goldberg, J. D., Donovan, P. B., Fruchtman, S. M., Berlin, N. I., and Wassermen, L. R. Therapeutic recommendations in polycythemia vera based on Polycythemia Vera Study Group protocols. *Semin. Hematol.* 23: 132, 1986.

9. Bessman, J. D., Gilmer, P. R., Jr., and Gardner, F. H. Improved classification of anemias by MCV and RDW. *Am. J. Clin. Pathol.* 80: 322, 1983.

10. Betaille, R., Grenier, J., and Sany, J. Beta-2-microglobulin in myeloma: Optimal use for staging, prognosis and treatment—A prospective study of 160 patients. *Blood* 63: 468, 1984.

11. Beutler, E. Glucose-6-Phosphate Deficiency. In W. J. Williams, E. Beutler, A. J. Erslev, and M. A. Lichtman (Eds.), *Hematology,* 3d Ed. New York: McGraw-Hill, 1983. Pp. 561.

12. Beutler, E. Hereditary Nonspherocytic Hemolytic Anemia—Pyruvate Kinase and Other Abnormalities. In W. J. Williams, E. Beutler, A. J. Erslev, and M. A. Lichtman (Eds.), *Hematology,* 3d Ed. New York: McGraw-Hill, 1983. Pp. 573.

13. Brill, A. B., Tomonga, M., and Heyssel, R. M. Leukemia in man following ionizing radiation: Summary of findings in Hiroshima and Nagasaki and comparison to other human experience. *Ann. Intern. Med.* 56: 590, 1962.

14. Broder, S., and Bunn, P. A., Jr. Cutaneous T-cell lymphomas. *Semin. Oncol.* 7: 310, 1980.

15. Broder, S., Bunn, P. A., Jr., Jaffe, E. S., Blattner, W., Gallo, R. C., Wong-Staal, E., Waldmann, T. A., and DeVita, V. T., Jr. T-cell lymphoproliferative syndrome associated with human T-cell leukemia/lymphoma virus. *Ann. Intern. Med.* 100: 543, 1984.

16. Bunn, H. F. Hemoglobin II. Sickle Cell Anemia and Other Hemoglobinopathies. In W. S. Beck (Ed.), *Hematology,* 3d Ed. Cambridge, Mass.: MIT Press, 1981. Pp. 141.

17. Canellos, G. P., Come, S. E., and Skarin, A. T. Chemotherapy in the treatment of Hodgkin's disease. *Semin. Hematol.* 20: 1, 1983.

18. Carmel, R., and Herbert, V. Deficiency of vitamin B_{12}-binding alpha globulin in two brothers. *Blood* 33: 1, 1969.

19. Champlin, R., Ho, W., and Gale, R. P. Antithymocyte globulin treatment in patients with aplastic anemia: A prospective randomized trial. *N. Engl. J. Med.* 308: 113, 1983.

20. Chaplin, H. Clinical usefulness of specific antiglobulin reagents in autoimmune hemolytic anemias. *Prog. Hematol.* 8: 25, 1973.

21. Clark, D. A., Dessypris, E. N., and Krantz, S. B. Studies on pure red cell aplasia. *Blood* 63: 277, 1984.

22. Coleman, C. N., Burke, J. S., and Varghese, A. Secondary Leukemia and Non-Hodgkin's Lymphoma in Patients Treated for Hodgkin's Disease. In H. S. Kaplan and S. A. Rosenberg (Eds.), *Malignant Lymphomas: Etiology, Immunology, Pathology, Treatment,* Vol. 3. Orlando, Fla.: Academic Press, 1982.

23. Comp, P. C. Hereditary disorders predisposing to thrombosis. *Prog. Thromb. Hemost.* 8: 71, 1986.

24. Cooper, R. A. Hemolytic syndromes and red cell membrane abnormalities in liver disease. *Semin. Hematol.* 17: 103, 1980.

25. Court-Brown, W. M., and Doll, R. Mortality from cancer and other causes after radiotherapy for ankylosing spondylitis. *Br. J. Med.* 4: 1327, 1965.

26. Curitta, B. M., Staub, R., and Thomas, E. D. Aplastic anemia: Pathogenesis, diagnosis, treatment and prognosis. *N. Engl. J. Med.* 306: 645, 1982.

27. Curitta, B. M., Staub, R., and Thomas, E. D. Aplastic anemia: Pathogenesis, diagnosis, treatment and prognosis. *N. Engl. J. Med.* 306: 712, 1982.

28. DeLeouw, N. K., Lowenstein, L., and Hsieh, Y. Iron deficiency and hydremia in normal pregnancy. *Medicine* 45: 291, 1966.

29. Doscherholman, H., and Swaime, W. R. Impaired assimilation of egg ^{57}Co-vitamin B_{12} in patients with hypochlorhydria and achlorhydria and after gastric resection. *Gastroenterology* 64: 913, 1973.

30. Durie, B. G. M., and Salmon, S. E. A clinical staging system for multiple myeloma. Correlation of measured myeloma cell mass with presenting clinical features, response to treatment and survival. *Cancer* 36: 842, 1975.

31. Erslev, A. Anemia of Chronic Disorders. In W. J. Williams, E. Beutler, A. J. Erslev, and R. W. Rundles (Eds.), *Hematology.* New York: McGraw-Hill, 1972. Pp. 371–377.

32. Erslev, A. J., and Shapiro, S. S. Hematologic As-

pects of Renal Failure. In L. E. Earley and C. W. Gottschalk (Eds.), *Diseases of the Kidney,* 4th Ed. Boston: Little, Brown, 1988. Pp. 3019.

33. Eschbach, J. W., Egrie, J. C., Downing, M. R., Browne, J. K., and Adamson, J. W. Correction of the anemia of end-stage renal disease with recombinant human erythropoietin. *N. Engl. J. Med.* 316: 73, 1987.

34. Fairbanks, V. F., and Beutler, E. Iron Deficiency. In W. J. Williams, E. Beutler, A. Erslev, and M. A. Lichtman (Eds.), *Hematology,* 3d Ed. New York: McGraw-Hill, 1983. Pp. 466–493.

35. Fairhead, S. M., Chipping, P. M., and Gordon-Smith, E. C. Treatment of aplastic anemia with antithymocyte globulin (ALG). *Br. J. Haematol.* 55: 7, 1983.

36. Fehr, J., Holmann, V., and Kappeler, U. Transient reversal of thrombocytopenia in idiopathic thrombocytopenic purpura by high-dose intravenous gamma globulin. *N. Engl. J. Med.* 306: 1254, 1982.

37. Feinstein, D. I. Acquired Inhibitors Against Factor VIII and Other Clotting Proteins. In R. W. Colman, J. Hirsh, V. J. Marder, and E. W. Salzman (Eds.), *Hemostasis and Thrombosis: Basic Principles and Clinical Practice,* 2d Ed. Philadelphia: Lippincott, 1987.

38. Foon, K. A., Gale, R. P., and Todd, R. F. III. Recent advances in the immunologic classification of leukemia. *Semin. Hematol.* 23: 257, 1986.

39. Frank, M. M., Schreiber, A. D., Atkinson, J. P., and Jaffee, C. J. Pathophysiology of immune hemolytic anemia. *Ann. Intern. Med.* 87: 210, 1977.

40. Freedman, A. S., and Nadler, L. M. Cell surface markers in hematologic malignancies. *Semin. Oncology* 14: 193, 1987.

41. Frizera, G., Moran, E. M., and Rapaport, H. Angioimmunoblastic lymphadenopathy: Diagnosis and clinical course. *Am. J. Med.* 59: 803, 1975.

42. Gale, R. P., Champlin, R. E., Feig, S. A., and Fitchen, J. H. Aplastic anemia: Biology and treatment. *Ann. Intern. Med.* 95: 477, 1981.

43. Gale, R. P., and Foon, K. A. Therapy of acute myelogenous leukemia. *Semin. Hematol.* 24: 40, 1987.

44. Gardiner, H. E., and Griffin, J. H. Human protein C and thromboembolic disease. *Prog. Hematol.* 13: 265, 1983.

45. Goldman, J. M., and Lu, Dao-Pei. New approaches in chronic granulocytic leukemia: Ori-

gin, prognosis and treatment. *Semin. Hematol.* 19: 241, 1982.

46. Golomb, H. M. Hairy-cell leukemia: The importance of accurate diagnosis and sequential management. *Adv. Intern. Med.* 29: 245, 1984.

47. Golomb, H. M., Catovaky, D., and Golde, D. W. Hairy-cell leukemia: A 5-year update on 71 patients. *Ann. Intern. Med.* 99: 485, 1983.

48. Harker, L., and Slichter, S. The bleeding time as a screening test for evaluation of platelet function. *N. Engl. J. Med.* 287: 155, 1972.

49. Henderson, E. S. Acute Myelogenous Leukemia. In W. J. Williams, E. Beutler, A. J. Erslev, and M. A. Lichman (Eds.), *Hematology,* 3d Ed. New York: McGraw-Hill, 1983. Pp. 243–244.

50. Herbert, V. Minimum daily adult folate requirement. *Arch. Intern. Med.* 110: 649, 1962.

51. Higgs, D. R., and Weatherall, D. J. Alpha-thalassemia. *Curr. Top. Hematol.* 4: 37, 1983.

52. Hillman, R. S., and Finch, C. A. Erythropoiesis: Normal and abnormal. *Semin. Hematol.* 4: 327, 1967.

53. Hillman, R. S. Characteristics of marrow production and reticulocyte maturation in normal man in response to anemia. *J. Clin. Invest.* 48: 443, 1969.

54. Hillman, R. S. Acute Blood Loss Anemia. In W. J. Williams, E. Beutler, A. J. Erslev, and M. A. Lichtman (Eds.), *Hematology,* 3d Ed. New York: McGraw-Hill, 1983. Pp. 667–671.

55. Hoelzer, D., and Gale, R. P. Acute lymphoblastic leukemia in adults: Recent progress, further directions. *Semin. Hematol.* 24: 27, 1987.

56. Hohnberg, L., Nilsson, I. M., Borge, L., Gunnorsson, M., and Sjorin, E. Platelet aggregation induced by 1-desamino-8-D-arginine vasopressin (DDAVP) *N. Engl. J. Med.* 309: 816, 1983.

57. Holt, J. T., Morton, C. C., Nienhuis, A. W., and Leder, P. Molecular Mechanisms of Hematologic Neoplasms. In G. Stamatoyannopoulos, A. W. Nienhuis, P. Leder, and P. W. Majerus (Eds.), *The Molecular Basis of Blood Diseases.* Philadelphia: Saunders, 1987. Pp. 347.

58. Horwich, A., and Peckham, M. "Bad-risk" non-Hodgkin's lymphomas. *Semin. Hematol.* 20: 35, 1983.

59. Hueberg, H. A., and Finch, C. A. Transferrin: Physiologic behavior and clinical implications. *Blood* 64: 763, 1984.

60. Hull, R., Hirsh, J., Jay, R., Carter, C., England, C.,

Gent, M., Turpie, A. G. G., McLaughlin, D., Dodd, P., Thomas, M., Raskob, G., and Ockelford, P. Different intensities of oral anticoagulant therapy in the treatment of proximal-vein thrombosis. *N. Engl. J. Med.* 307: 1676, 1982.

61. Isobe, T., and Osserman, E. Patterns of amyloidosis and their association with plasma cell dyscrasias, monoclonal gammaglobulins and Bence-Jones proteins. *N. Engl. J. Med.* 290: 473, 1974.

62. Israels, M. C. G., and Wilkinson, J. F. Risk of neurological complications in pernicious anemia treated with folic acid. *Br. Med. J.* 2: 1072, 1949.

63. Issitt, P. D. Serological Diagnosis and Characterization of the Causative Autoantibodies. In H. Chaplin (Ed.), *Immune Hemolytic Anemias.* New York: Churchill-Livingstone, 1985. Pp. 1–46.

64. Jaffe, E. S., Blattner, W. A., Blaymey, D. W., et al. The pathologic spectrum of HTLV-associated leukemia/lymphoma in the United States. *Am. J. Surg. Pathol.* 8: 263, 1984.

65. Karpatkin, S. Autoimmune thrombocytopenic purpura. *Semin. Hematol.* 22: 260, 1985.

66. Kelton, J. G., Powers, P. J., and Carter, C. J. A prospective study of the usefulness of the measurement of platelet-bound IgG for the diagnosis of idiopathic thrombocytopenic purpura. *Blood* 60: 1050, 1982.

67. King, D. J., and Kelton, J. G. Heparin-associated thrombocytopenia. *Ann. Intern. Med.* 100: 535, 1984.

68. Knowling, M., Harwood, A., and Bergsagel, D. E. A comparison of extramedullary plasmacytomas with multiple and solitary plasma cell tumors of bone. *J. Clin. Oncol.* 1: 255, 1983.

69. Koeffler, H. P. Myelodysplastic syndromes. *Semin. Hematol.* 23: 284, 1986.

70. Kolhouse, J. F., Kondo, H., Allen, N. C., Podell, E., and Allen, R. H. Cobalamin analogues are present in human plasma and can mask cobalamin deficiency because current radioisotope dilution assays are not specific for true cobalamin. *N. Engl. J. Med.* 299: 785, 1978.

71. Kyle, R. A., and Bayrd, E. D. Amyloidosis: Review of 236 cases. *Medicine* 54: 271, 1975.

72. Kyle, R. A. Monoclonal gammopathy of undetermined significance (MGUS): A review. *Clin. Haematol.* 11: 123, 1982.

73. Lawson, D. H., Murray, R. M., Parker, J. L. W., and Hay, G. Hypokalemia in megaloblastic anemias. *Lancet* 2: 588, 1970.

74. Lind, S. E. Prolonged bleeding time. *Ann. Intern. Med.* 77: 305, 1984.

75. Lindenbaum, J., and Lieber, C. S. Hematologic effects of alcohol in man in the absence of nutritional deficiency. *N. Engl. J. Med.* 281: 333, 1969.

76. Mannacci, P. M., Remuzzi, G., Pusineri, F., Lombardi, R., Valsecchi, C., Mecca, G., and Zimmerman, T. S. Deamino-8-arginine vasopressin shortens the bleeding time in uremia. *N. Engl. J. Med.* 308: 8, 1983.

77. Marder, V. J. The use of thrombolytic agents: Choice of patient, drug administration, laboratory monitoring. *Ann. Intern. Med.* 90: 802, 1979.

78. Masouredis, S. P., and Chaplin, H. Transfusion Management of Autoimmune Hemolytic Anemia. In H. Chaplin (Ed.), *Immune Hemolytic Anemias.* New York: Churchill-Livingstone, 1985. Pp. 177–206.

79. Moore, C. V. Iron nutrition and requirements. *Semin. Haematol.* 6: 1, 1965.

80. Murphy, S., Iland, H., Rosenthal, D., and Laszlo, J. Essential thrombocythemia: An interim report from the polycythemia vera study group. *Semin. Hematol.* 23: 177, 1986.

81. National Cancer Institute Sponsored Study of Classifications of Non-Hodgkin's Lymphomas. Summary and description of a working formulation for clinical usage. *Cancer* 49: 2112, 1982.

82. Nienhuis, A. W., Anagnau, N. P., and Ley, T. J. Advances in thalassemia research. *Blood* 63: 738, 1984.

83. Orkin, S. H., Kazazian, H., Jr., and Antonarakis, S. E. Linkage of beta-thalassemia mutations and beta-globin gene polymorphisms in human beta-globin gene cluster. *Nature* 296: 627, 1982.

84. Palek, J., and Lux, S. E. Red cell membrane skeletal defects in hereditary and acquired hemolytic anemias. *Semin. Hematol.* 20: 189, 1983.

85. Pedersen-Bjergaard, J., and Larsen, S. Evidence of acute nonlymphoblastic leukemia, preleukemia and acute myeloproliferative syndrome up to 10 years after treatment of Hodgkin's disease. *N. Engl. J. Med.* 307: 965, 1982.

86. Petri, M., Rheinschmidt, M., Quin, W. O., Helbuan, D., and Carash, L. The frequency of lupus anticoagulant in systemic lupus erythematosus. *Ann. Intern. Med.* 106: 524, 1987.

87. Portlock, C. S. "Good-risk" non-Hodgkin's lymphomas: Approaches to management. *Semin. Hematol.* 20: 25, 1983.

88. Rapaport, S. I. Anemias Due to Failure of Erythropoiesis. In S. I. Rapaport (Ed.), *Introduction to Hematology,* 2d Ed. Philadelphia: Lippincott, 1987. Pp. 167–184.

89. Rapaport, S. I. In S. I. Rapaport (Ed.), *Introduction to Hematology,* 2d Ed. Philadelphia: Lippincott, 1987. Pp. 505–526.

90. Rosenberg, R. D., and Rosenberg, J. S. Natural anticoagulant mechanisms. *J. Clin. Invest.* 74: 1, 1984.

91. Rosenblatt, J. D., Golde, D. W., Wachsman, W., Giorge, J. V., Jacobs, A., Schmidt, G. M., Quan, S., Gasson, J. C., and Chen, I. S. Y. A second isolate of HTLV II associated with atypical hairy-cell leukemia. *N. Engl. J. Med.* 315: 372, 1987.

92. Rowley, J. D. Biological implications of consistent chromosome rearrangements in leukemia and lymphoma. *Cancer Res.* 44: 3159, 1984.

93. Sack, G. H., Levin, J., and Bell, W. R. Trousseau's syndrome and other manifestations of chronic disseminated coagulopathy in patients with neoplasms. *Medicine* 56: 1, 1977.

94. Salmon, S. E. Immunoglobulin synthesis and tumor kinetics of multiple myeloma. *Semin. Hematol.* 10: 135, 1973.

95. Sandberg, A. A. The chromosomes in human leukemia. *Semin. Hematol.* 23: 201, 1986.

96. Schein, P. S., MacDonald, J. S., and Edelson, R. Cutaneous T-cell lymphoma. *Cancer* 38: 1859, 1976.

97. Seligman, P. A., Steiner, L. L., and Allen, R. H. Studies of a patient with megaloblastic anemia and an abnormal transcobalamin II. *N. Engl. J. Med.* 303: 1209, 1980.

98. Seligman, A., Caskey, J. H., Frazier, J. L., Zuker, R. M., Podell, E. R., and Allen, R. H. Measurements of iron absorption from prenatal multivitamin-mineral supplements. *Obstet. Gynecol.* 61: 356, 1983.

99. Seligman, P. A., Klausner, R. D., and Hereberg, H. A. Molecular Mechanisms of Iron Metabolism. In G. Stamatoyannopoulos, A. W. Nienhuis, P. Leder, and P. W. Majerus (Eds.), *The Molecular Basis of Blood Diseases.* Philadelphia: Saunders, 1987. Pp. 235.

100. Showe, L. C., and Croce, C. M. Chromosome translocations in B and T cell neoplasms. *Semin. Hematol.* 23: 237, 1986.

101. Stabler, S. P., Marcell, P. D., Podell, E. R., Allen, R. H., and Lindenbaum, J. Assay of methylmalonic acid in the serum of patients with cobalamin deficiency using capillary gas chromatography-mass spectrometry. *J. Clin. Invest.* 77: 1606, 1987.

102. Stabler, S. P., Marcell, P. D., Podell, E. R., and Allen, R. H. Quantitation of total homocysteine, total cysteine and methionine in normal serum and urine using capillary gas chromatography—mass spectrometry. *Anal. Biochem.* 162: 185, 1987.

103. Thiagarajan, P., and Shapiro, S. S. Lupus Anticoagulants. In R. W. Colman (Ed.), *Disorders of Thrombin Formulation.* New York: Churchill-Livingstone, 1983.

104. Vande Werf, E., Ludbrook, P. A., Bergmann, S. R., Tiefenbrunn, A. J., Fox, K. A. A., deGeest, H., Verstraete, M., Collen, D., and Sobel, B. Coronary thrombolysis with tissue-type plasminogen activator in patients with evolving myocardial infarction. *N. Engl. J. Med.* 310: 609, 1984.

105. Wachsman, W., Golde, D. W., and Chen, I. S. Y. HTLV and human leukemia: Perspectives 1986. *Semin. Hematol.* 23: 245, 1986.

106. Ward, H. P., and Block, M. H. The natural history of agnogenic myeloid metaplasia (AMM) and a critical evaluation of its relationship with the myeloproliferative syndrome. *Medicine* 50: 357, 1971.

107. Weatherall, D. J. The Thalassemias. In W. J. Williams, E. Beuther, et al. (Eds.), *Hematology,* 3d Ed. New York: McGraw-Hill, 1983. Pp. 493–521.

108. White, G. C., II, McMillan, C. W., Blatt, P. M., and Roberts, H. R. Factor VIII inhibitors: A clinical overview. *Am. J. Hematol.* 13: 335, 1982.

109. Worlledge, S. M. Immune drug-induced hemolytic anemias. *Semin. Hematol.* 10: 327, 1973.

110. Wyke, J. Principles of viral leukemogenesis. *Semin. Hematol.* 23: 189, 1986.

111. Yang, Y. M., Ducos, R., Rosenberg, A. J., Catrou, P. G., Levine, J. S., Podell, E. R., and Allen, R. N. Cobalamin malabsorption in three siblings due to an abnormal intrinsic factor that is markedly susceptible to acid and proteolysis. *J. Clin. Invest.* 76: 2057, 1985.

112. Zimmerman, T. S., Ruggeri, A. M., and Fulcher, C. A. Factor VIII–von Willebrand factor. *Prog. Hematol.* 13: 279, 1983.

Section II

Oncology

Scot M. Sedlacek and
J. Fred Kolhouse

Management of the patient with cancer has changed dramatically during the past two decades. Great strides have been made with individual therapies, although some of the greatest achievements have involved the integration of the therapeutic modalities (surgery, radiation, and chemotherapy) into a multidisciplinary approach to the cancer patient.

Optimal care of the patient with cancer requires accurate and timely diagnosis and staging, appropriate primary therapy, intensive supportive care, and proper recognition and management of attendant complications. The type of therapeutic modalities chosen to treat a patient with a malignancy depends to a great extent on the biologic behavior of that particular histologic type. Certain malignancies such as squamous cell cancers of the head and neck are by and large local/regional invasive cancers that require appropriate aggressive local therapy. This entails primary surgical resection followed by local irradiation. Other malignancies have a much greater potential for systemic spread such that at presentation virtually all patients have metastatic disease. Small-cell carcinoma of the lung is a systemic disease at presen-

tation in 98 percent of patients, thus rendering primary surgical resection or irradiation, which are strictly local modalities, unable to prevent disease recurrence and therefore exposing the patient to potential morbidity and mortality from the procedures but without anticipated benefits.

Other factors utilized in determining types of therapy for cancer patients include the general physical condition of the patient (performance status), nutritional status, associated preexisting medical conditions, types of anticipated adverse side effects, modality availability, and more recently, cost. Obviously, a patient in otherwise excellent health and entirely asymptomatic despite having a malignancy will have a higher chance for responding to or tolerating a particular type of treatment and therefore a longer survival and ultimately a greater chance for cure than a bedridden, nutritionally depleted, cachetic patient with cancer.

Only when all the factors are taken into account, along with the most important of factors, the patient's wishes, can optimal, appropriate care be offered to the cancer patient.

Lung Cancer

Cancer of the lung is the number one cancer killer of both men and women in the United States. The death rate from lung cancer in men has risen 15-fold since 1925 (Fig. 5-2, Appendix), while the corresponding number for women is 6-fold since 1960 (Fig. 5-3, Appendix). Currently, the incidence of lung cancer in women in the United States is rising approximately 10 percent per year. It is estimated that 150,000 newly diagnosed cases of lung cancer will be seen in 1987 and 136,000 people will die from lung cancer.

There are four main histologic subtypes of carcinoma of the lung. The most frequent is squamous cell carcinoma, making up approximately 40 percent of diagnoses, followed by adenocarcinoma, which makes up 25 percent, small cell (oat-cell) carcinoma, comprising 25 percent, and large cell carcinoma, making up approximately 10 percent of diagnosed cases. All the different histologic subtypes have tobacco smoking as a major risk factor, but adenocarcinoma is the most common histologic type diagnosed in nonsmokers [14]. Squamous cell carcinoma of the lung tends to be centrally located and locally invasive. Adenocarcinoma of the lung tends to be peripheral and smaller in size. Small cell carcinomas, which are thought to arise from neuroectodermal cells, tend to be centrally located and are the most likely histologic types to have distant metastases at presentation. Large cell carcinoma of the lung can be either peripheral or central and is frequently bulky in size.

Diagnosis

Patients with lung cancer can present with a variety of symptoms, such as recent onset of a cough or an increase in a chronic cough, hemoptysis, hoarseness, pain in the chest, or weight loss. Nearly 90 percent of all patients with lung cancer have a history of smoking in the past [14]. Other significant risk factors include exposure to uranium, and more recently, studies have shown the hazards of passive smoking (a nonsmoker breathing air contaminated by cigarette smoke). The risk for developing lung cancer after cigarette smoking cessation drops rapidly in the first 5 years and after 15 years is close to the baseline risk for the population that has never smoked.

The physical examination of a patient with lung cancer may reveal signs of consolidation in the lungs due to an obstructed bronchus with subsequent collapse of the pulmonary segment or lobe with or without postobstructive pneumonia. There may be signs of a pleural effusion with decreased breath sounds and dullness in the bases. In patients with hoarseness there may be involvement of the left recurrent laryngeal nerve that courses down through the aortopulmonary (AP) window on the left which when involved by lung cancer can cause paralysis of the left vocal cord as seen on laryngoscopy. Cancers presenting in the apex of the lung (Pancoast tumor) may cause a brachial plexopathy or a unilateral Horner's syndrome (unilateral ptosis, miosis, and anhidrosis) due to involvement of the sympathetic fibers that course near the apex. Some patients with cancer of the lung may manifest the disease first as a paraneoplastic syndrome such as (1) hypertrophic pulmonary osteoarthropathy, i.e., clubbing of the finger and toes and periostitis of the long bones, (2) Trousseau's syndrome, i.e., migratory thrombophlebitis, or (3) Eaton-Lambert syndrome, i.e., proximal muscle weakness which improves with exercise.

The laboratory tests that are abnormal in lung cancer are most commonly due to paraneoplastic syndromes or metastatic spread of the tumor to other organs. Hyponatremia is a common paraneoplastic syndrome seen with small cell carcinoma of the lung, with approximately 10 percent of patients having the clinical syndrome of inappropriate secretion of antidiuretic hormone (SIADH) with a serum sodium level less than 130 mEq/liter. Subclinical syndrome of inappropriate secretion of antidiuretic hormone can be brought out by administering a free water load in 50 to 60 percent of small cell lung cancer patients [9]. Hypercalcemia can be due to either metastatic disease to the bone or to a paraneoplastic syndrome caused by the secretion of a parathyroid hormone-like substance from the cancer. The most common histologic subtype to cause this latter syndrome is squamous cell carcinoma. The laboratory tests used in the staging of lung cancer include liver function tests to help evaluate for hepatic metastases, complete blood count (CBC) to help evaluate for marrow metastases, and alkaline phosphatase determinations to evaluate for cortical bone involvement.

The chest x-ray is usually the first study that suggests the presence of lung cancer and frequently gives the first clue as to the histologic subtype by its location and presentation. As mentioned earlier, squamous cell and small cell cancers tend to present centrally, whereas adenocarcinoma more frequently presents as a peripheral lesion and also can develop in old scars of the lung. Other findings on chest x-ray include a pleural effusion which can be either a sympathetic effusion due to an obstructive pneumonia or a frankly malignant effusion. Other findings on chest x-ray include involvement of the hilar and/or mediastinal lymph nodes. In the staging of lung cancer, nuclear medicine and computerized tomography (CT) scans play a vital role [30]. For patients with neurologic signs and symptoms, a CT scan of the head is the best modality to evaluate for brain metastases. Liver metastases should be looked for in patients with hepatomegaly and/or abnormal liver function tests. The liver can be evaluated in one of three ways, including a nuclear medicine liver/spleen scan, abdominal ultrasound, or a CT scan of the abdomen, which provides other information such as enlargement of the adrenal glands and periaortic lymph nodes. Bony metastases are best evaluated by the nuclear medicine bone scan with abnormal areas corroborated by plain x-rays.

Treatment: Acute Management

For the patient with non-small cell carcinoma of the lung, the best chance for long-term survival or cure is for complete surgical resection of the cancer [39]. Tests used to evaluate for potential resectability of patients with lung cancer include pulmonary function tests with the minimum residual FEV_1 following the anticipated resection (lobectomy, pneumonectomy) of approximately 800 to 1000 ml. Also, the arterial blood gas is used to help determine a patient's potential for resectability, with minimum requirements being a room-air $PO_2 \geqslant 55$ mmHg and a $PCO_2 \leqslant 45$ mmHg. It is very unlikely that a patient on continuous oxygen supplementation would be a candidate for resection. Because of the significant morbidity and possible mortality associated with the surgical resection, it is important to exclude those patients who would not benefit from such a procedure. Patients to exclude are those with distant metastases, those who are physiologically poor candidates, and those with locally advanced disease precluding complete resection, such as mediastinal lymph node involvement. Mediastinoscopy is a frequently performed staging procedure in patients who do not have distant metastases [28]. The paratracheal and subcarinal lymph nodes can be reached with the mediastinoscope and biopsied to determine cancer involvement that would preclude surgical resection. Mediastinoscopy also can be used as a therapeutic trial for patients with borderline pulmonary function tests. If a patient has difficulty being extubated following the procedure, it is unlikely he or she would tolerate a surgical resection of the lung. For patients with left-sided cancers, there may be enlargement of the lymph nodes in the aortopulmonary (AP) window, which cannot be reached with a mediastinoscope. These patients can have the aortopulmonary window examined with a Chamberlain procedure (left minithoracotomy) to evaluate for cancer involvement.

The surgical procedures most commonly employed include pneumonectomy and lobectomy. Subsegmental and wedge resections are currently being investigated to determine if they can be performed in patients with small primary lung cancers.

For the patient with small cell cancer of the lung, primary surgical resection is rarely utilized. As mentioned earlier, up to 98 percent of patients with small cell carcinoma of the lung have overt distant metastases or microscopic metastases not detectable on screening tests. Because of the overwhelming likelihood of distant metastases at the time of presentation, systemic treatment with chemotherapy is the mainstay of acute management for small cell carcinoma of the lung. Cyclophosphamide, doxorubicin, vincristine, and most recently VP-16 and *cis*-platinum are the most active chemotherapeutic agents in small cell carcinoma of the lung. Response rates to combination chemotherapy range from 50 to 95 percent, with median survivals of 6 to 9 months for those patients with disseminated disease and 11 to 15 months for those patients with disease limited to one hemithorax at presentation. Response rates to combination chemotherapy are high and of rapid onset such that patients who present with superior vena caval obstruction can receive chemotherapy as their initial therapeutic modality [41].

Radiotherapy is used in the acute management of non-small cell lung cancer when it presents with a centrally obstructing lesion and a postobstructive pneumonia. Also, patients with non-small cell lung cancer and extensive anterior mediastinal involvement causing superior vena caval obstruction are best treated with radiotherapy. In patients with disease limited to the chest who, because of poor pulmonary function or locally advanced disease, are not considered candidates for surgical resection, radiotherapy also can be used to treat the primary lesion.

Treatment: Chronic Management

The chronic management of patients with non-small cell cancer of the lung is typically for metastatic disease requiring systemic chemotherapy. The most active agents in this disease include *cis*-platinum, VP-16, vinblastine, mitomycin C, and most recently vindesine. As opposed to the previously mentioned high response rates in small cell carcinoma of the lung, only 20 to 25 percent of patients with non-small cell cancer will respond to combination chemotherapy. Radiation therapy is also used in the chronic management of patients with lung cancer, most frequently for patients who have symptomatic bone metastases.

Prognosis

In small cell cancer of the lung, where patients have a 6- to 12-week median survival when untreated, combination chemotherapy has produced meaningful prolongation of survival, yet only 10 to 15 percent of patients with limited disease and 2 percent with metastatic disease are alive at 2 to 3 years. For patients with non-small cell cancer of the lung, overall 5-year survival rate for all patients is still less than 10 percent. For those patients who are surgically resected, this rate may be as high as 20 to 40 percent. Long-term survival in these patients is heavily dependent on the stage of disease.

Breast Cancer

Cancer of the female breast remains the number one cancer among women in the United States, making up 27 percent of all cancers diagnosed. In 1987 it is estimated there will be 130,000 newly diagnosed women and 41,000 women who will die from their breast cancer. Factors that predispose women to breast cancer development include (1) family history, most notably in a sister and/or mother, especially if either was premenopausal and/or had bilateral disease, (2) age (the risk of developing breast cancer increases markedly with advancing age, with less than 1.5 percent of all breast cancers occurring in women younger than age 30), (3) proliferative breast disease, i.e., ductal or lobular hyperplasia with atypia, (4) long periods of unopposed estrogenic stimulation (this includes a woman who had an early menarche, late menopause, and/or first pregnancy after the age of 30), and (5) diet (high-fat diets increase the risk for breast cancer) [43]. There are two major distinctions in histologic types of breast carcinoma, namely, invasive and in situ carcinoma. There are also two major types of invasive carcinoma that have indistinguishable clinical presentations and prognoses: (1) infiltrating ductal carcinoma, which is the most common, and (2) infiltrating lobular carcinoma. In situ carcinoma has two histologic subtypes with differing characteristics. Ductal carcinoma in situ has approximately a 30 to 35 percent chance of developing into invasive carcinoma and will be associated with axillary lymph node involvement in 1 to 4 percent of patients. Lobular carcinoma in situ (most recently named lobular neoplasia) is a disease that is multifocal in the ipsilateral breast in 50 to 67 percent, and in 33 to 50 percent of patients it will be bilateral. A woman with lobular neoplasia has a 20 to 30 percent chance of developing subsequent invasive carcinoma which can be either invasive lobular or invasive ductal carcinoma and can involve either breast with equal frequency.

Diagnosis

The typical presentation of breast cancer is that of a lump in the breast most commonly noted by the patient. On average, the lump is a 2.5 cm in size, painless, and typically in a woman over the age of 30. The differential diagnosis includes a fibroadenoma, which is a hard, painless, easily movable mass in the breast sometimes referred to as "feeling like a marble." The other differential diagnostic possibility is fibrocystic changes in the breast. The term *fibrocystic disease* is a poor name that refers to many different pathologic changes, and perhaps the process should not be called a disease, since up to 90 percent of women may

have such changes in their breasts [29]. Fibrocystic changes can present as a lumpy-bumpy breast to palpation which may fluctuate as the woman progresses through her menstrual cycle. Typically, the lumps may get larger and more tender the week prior to the initiation of menstrual flow.

Breast cancer typically presents as a hard mass in the breast which may cause dimpling of the overlying skin, inversion of the nipple, bloody or clear discharge from the nipple, enlarged axillary lymph nodes due to metastatic spread, and in the subset termed inflammatory carcinoma, erythema, warmth, and direct skin involvement termed peau d'orange.

There are currently no blood tests available that are helpful in making the diagnosis of breast cancer. The presence of metastases to the bone and liver can be screened with measurements of the serum alkaline phosphatase, lactate dehydrogenase, SGOT, and total bilirubin levels. Breast cancer is known to be one of the hormonally responsive cancers, in which hormone receptors have been shown to be of great value. The estrogen and progesterone receptor levels should be obtained on all breast cancers whether primary or metastatic for importance in both prognosis and therapeutic strategies. Most recently, DNA flow cytometry, which can determine if a cancer has a normal complement of DNA or has a large fraction of cells in a proliferative phase, is becoming an important prognostic indicator as well.

Mammography (breast x-rays) has become the single best modality available for diagnosing breast cancer. Up to 91 percent of all cancers may be seen on the mammogram, whereas only 58 percent may be palpated by an examiner [2]. The different patterns that suggest malignancy include an asymmetrical density, dominant mass, cluster of microcalcifications, and thickening or dimpling of the skin. While mammography may be the single best modality in detecting cancer of the breast, it is not infallible. Any women over the age of 25 years with a palpable breast mass and a negative mammogram should have a breast biopsy to exclude carcinoma. Other radiographic studies are performed to detect evidence of metastatic disease. The chest x-ray may show a malignant pleural effusion or parenchymal pulmonary metastases, which may present as discrete nodules or as diffuse lymphangitic spread. Liver/spleen scan or CT scan of the abdomen are utilized to search for liver metastases. Bone scans are obtained to look for bony metastases, and a CT scan of the head is done to detect brain metastases when clinically indicated (new neurologic signs and/or symptoms such as headaches, personality changes, or motor or sensory dysfunctions).

Treatment: Acute Management

The acute management of breast cancer is primarily surgical. Surgical procedures used to extirpate the tumor include radical mastectomy, modified radical mastectomy, and most recently, lumpectomy [15]. Radical mastectomy, which included resection of the pectoralis major muscle, has largely been replaced since the late 1970s by the modified radical mastectomy, which leaves the pectoralis major muscle intact. Lumpectomy consists of an excisional biopsy in which the tumor is resected with a rim of normal tissue surrounding it. All three types of surgery include an axillary dissection to search for spread of the cancer to the axillary lymph nodes.

Adjuvant chemotherapy has been employed in an attempt to eradicate microscopic metastases in patients at risk for disease recurrence. The patient population that has received the most benefit from adjuvant chemotherapy is comprised of premenopausal, lymph node-positive women [5].

Adjuvant hormone therapy, again, is a prophylactic treatment for patients who are thought to have micrometastases following primary surgical resection. The most commonly used hormonal therapy is the antiestrogen tamoxifen. The patients most likely to benefit from adjuvant hormonal therapy are the postmenopausal women with axillary lymph node involvement who also have the estrogen receptor present in their cancer [34].

Adjuvant radiotherapy is a localized treatment that will decrease local recurrence rates but has not been shown to increase overall survival rates. It is now employed routinely in patients who have undergone lumpectomy, decreasing their chance for local recurrence in the breast from approximately 30 to 8 percent.

Treatment: Chronic Management

Chemotherapy for metastatic disease involves numerous chemotherapeutic agents used singly or in combinations. Patients who should be treated with chemotherapy include those patients having potentially life-threatening disease (brain, lung, or liver involvement) or those who are estrogen receptor/progesterone receptor negative. Most commonly used combinations include cyclophosphamide, methotrexate, and 5FU (CMF); cyclophosphamide, Adriamycin/doxorubicin, and 5FU (CAF); and mitomycin C with vinblastine.

Hormonal therapy for metastatic disease is typically utilized in patients with non-life-threatening disease (bone, soft-tissue, pleural effusion) who are hormone receptor-positive. Patients who have both the estrogen and progesterone receptors in their cancer have approximately a 70 percent chance of responding to some type of hormonal therapy [42]. Those patients with just one positive hormone receptor have a 33 percent chance of responding, and those patients with both receptors absent from their cancer have only a 10 percent chance of responding to some type of hormonal therapy. There are many different types of hormonal therapies, including additive hormones and antagonistic hormones along with ablative therapy. The most commonly used hormonal therapy in the United States is the antiestrogen tamoxifen. Progestational agents include megestrol acetate and medroxyprogesterone acetate. Estrogens such as diethylstilbestrol and androgens such as fluoxymesterone have been used extensively for the treatment of metastatic disease. Aminoglutethimide is an aromatase inhibitor that produces a medical adrenalectomy. Ablative hormonal therapy for metastatic disease includes oophorectomy, which typically has been reserved for the premenopausal patient. Most recently, tamoxifen has been shown to be equally effective as oophorectomy and may replace it as primary therapy for the premenopausal patient. Other ablative therapies include bilateral adrenalectomy, which has been replaced by aminoglutethimide and hypophysectomy, which currently is rarely employed for the therapy of metastatic disease.

Prognosis

The most important prognostic factors include, (1) number of axillary lymph nodes involved at the time of primary surgery, (2) hormone receptors on the primary cancer, and (3) DNA flow cytometry to determine if there is an aneuploid population or a rapidly proliferating cancer. Stage, tumor size, menopausal status, and age are no longer considered independent variables for prognosis in breast cancer.

Gastrointestinal Malignancies

Colorectal Cancer

Cancer of the colon and rectum together constitute the second most commonly diagnosed cancer in the combined male and female populations in the United States. There will be 145,000 newly diagnosed cases in 1987, with 60,000 patients dying from their disease. The risk of developing colon cancer has been related to high-fat, low-fiber diets and the presence of adenomatous polyps.

DIAGNOSIS

Patients who have adenocarcinomas of the right colon tend to have large exophytic tumors, but because of the large diameter of the cecum and ascending colon and the fact that the contents are mainly liquid, patients do not commonly present with bowel obstruction. The most common symptoms are those of abdominal pain, weight loss, and bleeding leading to iron-deficiency anemia. Cancers of the left colon tend to present with symptoms of bowel obstruction, change in bowel habit, and/or decrease in stool caliber. This is due to the semisolid to solid nature of the stool contents in the left colon as well as to the smaller diameter of the descending and sigmoid colon. Patients with colonic carcinoma tend to be older than 40 years of age. They can present with occult or gross blood in their stool as either melena, hematochezia, or bright red blood per rectum.

Digital examination of the rectum remains an essential tool for diagnosing colorectal carcinoma. A mass may be palpable on rectal examination, or stool Hemoccult testing may show the presence of an occult colonic lesion. Further examination of the colon can be performed with either a rigid proctosigmoidoscopy, a flexible sigmoidoscopy (which can reach the splenic flexure), or a colonoscopy to evaluate the whole colon and rectum. A mass can rarely be palpated in the abdomen, and this is more frequent with right-sided colonic lesions. Other physical findings are usually due to metastatic disease, such as an enlarged nodular, firm liver due to liver metastases or an enlarged left supraclavicular (Virchow's) node.

A frequent laboratory abnormality seen with right colonic carcinomas is anemia due to blood loss (iron deficiency). The carcinoembryonic antigen (CEA) level may be elevated in patients with adenocarcinoma of the colon, and this correlates with tumor bulk and the presence of metastatic disease, thus having prognostic importance [31]. While important prognostically, the carcinoembryonic antigen level cannot be utilized as a screening test for colorectal cancers because it may be elevated in other nonmalignant disorders (e.g., hepatitis, ulcerative colitis).

Traditional single-contrast barium enemas have been shown to miss 20 to 25 percent of all documented colonic carcinomas and up to 40 percent of all polyps. Double-contrast (air and barium) studies, though, have been shown to be as good as colonoscopy in detecting polyps and colonic carcinomas. Other studies that should be performed are specifically directed at detecting metastatic disease, with the most common site being the liver. This can be evaluated with either a nuclear medicine liver/spleen scan, abdominal ultrasound, or CT scan of the liver and abdomen.

TREATMENT: ACUTE MANAGEMENT

The primary management of colorectal carcinoma is almost exclusively surgical, with nearly 95 percent of lesions being resectable. Despite the fact that 25 percent of patients with colorectal carcinoma have distant metastases at time of presentation, most are considered for surgical resection to prevent colonic obstruction and/or continued gastrointestinal blood loss. Lesions presenting in the cecum and ascending colon are treated by right hemicolectomy, whereas lesions of the transverse colon down to the sigmoid colon are typically treated by left hemicolectomy. Rectal adenocarcinomas are treated by either a low anterior resection or an abdominal-perineal resection. For those cancers which present 12 cm or more from the anal verge, a low anterior resection can be performed with primary anastamosis. For those cancers which are within 8 cm of the anal verge, the abdominal-perineal resection is the preferred surgical procedure, and this leaves the patient with a colostomy. Lesions that are between these two distances can undergo either surgery depending on factors such as pelvic size, size of the lesion, and tumor differentiation. A good general rule is that any lesion that can be easily palpable by an examining finger on rectal examination should be treated with an abdominal-perineal resection. Preoperative or postoperative radiation therapy for rectal adenocarcinomas has been shown to decrease local recurrence rates, and most recently, postoperative radiation therapy combined with chemotherapy has been shown to decrease local recurrence rates and also to increase overall survival rates [17]. The role of adjuvant therapy for adenocarcinomas of the colon is actively being investigated, but adjuvant therapy cannot be considered standard therapy.

TREATMENT: CHRONIC MANAGEMENT

For patients who develop local recurrences, such as at the anastamotic site, surgical resection may be the cure. Also, patients who develop isolated liver metastases (up to three in number) may undergo surgical excision, with documented prolongation of survival and some patients cured (up to 40 percent) despite the presence of metastatic disease [25]. As mentioned previously, the most common sites for metastases from colorectal cancer are the liver, the lungs, and bone.

Chemotherapy for metastatic colorectal adenocarcinoma has only a 15 to 20 percent response rate. The most active agents in this disease are 5FU, mitomycin C, and the nitrosoureas (BCNU, CCNU, methyl-CCNU). The response duration with these drugs, although short, averages 2 to 5 months. There is no known benefit to combination chemotherapy in this disorder. Patients with liver metastases who are not considered candidates for resection (more than three in number or involving both lobes of the liver) and have disease confined to their liver may be treated with intraarterial hepatic perfusion. When perfusing the liver with chemotherapeutic agents, drugs are utilized which are extracted and metabolized by the liver, thus decreasing the systemic adverse reactions. These include 5FU and 5-FUDR (experimental). There have been some promising results in multiple trials with increased response rates with intraarterial chemotherapy. Survival has not been prolonged due to the occurrence and progression of extrahepatic metastases.

Radiotherapy has a limited role for metastatic colorectal carcinoma except for palliation of pelvic recurrences or other bony metastases in patients who have received no prior radiation therapy to the involved area.

PROGNOSIS

The most important determinant of prognosis for patients with colorectal carcinoma is the stage of the disease. The most commonly employed staging system is the Astler-Coller modification of the Duke's system (as modified again by Turnbull). Table 5-12 outlines the surgical staging system

Table 5–12. Colon Cancer Staging
System and Survival at 5 Years

Stage	Involvement	Percent Alive
O	Carcinoma in situ	
A	Limited to mucosa	81
B₁	Into muscularis propria but not beyond	} 64
B₂	Extending through bowel wall with complete penetration of muscularis propria	
C₁	Limited to bowel wall but with involved lymph nodes	} 27
C₂	Through all layers of bowel wall with involved lymph nodes	
D	Any invasion of bowel wall with or without lymph node metastases but with distant metastases	14

and the expected 5-year survival rates for each stage of disease. Other prognostic factors besides surgical stage include histologic tumor grade, preoperative carcinoembryonic antigen and lactate dehydrogenase levels, and performance status.

Pancreatic Carcinoma

Pancreatic cancer is the number two gastrointestinal malignancy, with 26,200 newly diagnosed cases and 24,300 deaths predicted for 1987. Death rates per 100,000 population have nearly doubled since 1930 in women and nearly tripled in men during the same period. The etiology of this rise is not definite, although it has been reported to correlate with cigarette smoking and parallels the rise of lung cancer.

DIAGNOSIS

For carcinomas that arise in the head of the pancreas near the confluence of the common bile duct and pancreatic duct, a common triad observed is progressive jaundice, pain, and weight loss. Cancers in the body and tail of the pancreas are less likely to cause biliary obstruction due to

their location. As many as 10 percent of patients with pancreatic carcinoma present with symptoms of depression.

As mentioned earlier, carcinomas of the pancreatic head are likely to cause jaundice, whereas tumors of the tail and body are able to reach much larger dimensions prior to discovery and may even be palpable as an epigastric or left upper quadrant mass. Later in the course of disease the presence of ascites may be demonstrated.

The jaundiced patient will have elevated bilirubin and serum alkaline phosphatase levels. As with any gastrointestinal malignancy, the carcinoembryonic antigen (CEA) level will be elevated at some time in the majority of patients. Alphafetoprotein (AFP) is less commonly elevated. At presentation, 20 to 40 percent of patients will have elevated fasting glucose levels diagnostic of diabetes mellitus.

A variety of pancreatic imaging techniques have been employed over the years [47]. The upper gastrointestinal x-ray is frequently obtained because of symptoms of epigastric pain, and it may reveal pyloric or duodenal obstruction, narrowing of the first and second portions of the duodenum, widening or indentation of the duodenal loop, or irregularity of the duodenal mucosa due to direct tumor invasion. Upper endoscopy with retrograde cholangiopancreatography has shown to be 95 percent accurate in diagnosing pancreatic cancer. With the addition of endoscopic aspiration cytology, cytologic confirmation may be obtained in 55 to 90 percent of patients. Abdominal ultrasound is unable to detect small lesions in the pancreas, but it is good at demonstrating large lesions and also dilatation of the biliary tree. The presence of liver metastases also may be demonstrable with this modality. CT scans may be the single best noninvasive means to detect pancreatic masses. CT scans also can be used to evaluate the extent of involvement (liver, stomach, retroperitoneal lymph nodes) and resectability. CT-guided fine-needle percutaneous aspirations may obtain cytologic confirmations in up to 90 percent of patients. Angiography as a diagnostic study has largely been replaced by the above-mentioned modalities, but it still has a role in demonstrating vascular supply to tumors and in assisting in the estimation of resectability.

TREATMENT: ACUTE MANAGEMENT

Surgical therapy is a modality most commonly employed as initial therapy. An exploratory laparotomy may be required to make the diagnosis, and in the majority of patients, a curative surgical resection is not feasible due to extensive local spread or metastatic disease, most frequently to the liver. Patients who present with obstructive symptoms, either biliary or duodenal, require palliative bypass procedures. A choledochojejunostomy or cholecystojejunostomy may be performed to relieve obstructive jaundice, and a gastrojejunostomy should be performed for duodenal obstruction. For tumors of the head of the pancreas which are deemed resectable, a radical pancreaticoduodenectomy (Whipple procedure) is the preferred surgical operation. This extensive operation should be reserved for good-prognosis patients (age less than 70, good performance status, small tumors ≤ 3 cm in maximum diameter) and be performed by experienced surgeons because of the high morbidity and mortality rates of the procedure [1]. For unresectable, locally advanced carcinomas, the combination of radiotherapy plus chemotherapy has been shown to prolong survival by approximately 6 to 8 months.

TREATMENT: CHRONIC MANAGEMENT

Metastatic disease is managed with chemotherapy, with the most active agents being 5FU, mitomycin C, and streptozocin, with response rates of 28, 21, and 17 percent, respectively. Combination chemotherapy has gained wide usage, particularly the FAM regimen (5FU, Adriamycin/doxorubicin, and mitomycin C). The overall response rates, however, are not much better than with 5FU alone, and there are more toxic side effects and added expense [10].

PROGNOSIS

Carcinoma of the pancreas carries a dismal prognosis, with an almost universal fatal outcome. With less than 20 percent of patients being candidates for curative resections, only 4 percent of resected patients are alive at 5 years and potentially cured.

Gastric Carcinoma

Carcinoma of the stomach has shown the most rapid decline in incidence rates in the United States of any cancer, falling from 29 per 100,000 population in 1930 to only 7 per 100,000 population in 1966. The reasons for this decline are largely unknown. Japan has the highest incidence of gastric carcinoma in the world, with dietary factors thought to play a major etiologic role (dried or salted fish, pickled vegetables).

DIAGNOSIS

The most common presenting symptom in patients with gastric carcinoma is a vague epigastric discomfort, along with early satiety, anorexia, weight loss, dysphagia, or obstructive symptoms.

Physical findings in patients with carcinoma of the stomach are few and nonspecific, thus rarely leading the examiner to a definitive diagnosis by examination. They include (1) palpable epigastric mass, (2) palpable left supraclavicular lymph node (Virchow's node), and (3) palpable umbilical nodule (Sister Mary Joseph's node).

There are no specific diagnostic serum or blood tests for gastric carcinoma. As with the physical examination, blood tests are nonspecific. Patients may have an iron-deficiency anemia due either to chronic blood loss from the cancer and/or to decreased iron absorption secondary to an underlying atrophic gastritis, which may predispose patients to the development of gastric carcinoma. While the carcinoembryonic antigen is not as well studied as in colorectal cancer, it may prove to be useful as a follow-up test after surgery in these patients.

Since introduction of the flexible upper endo-

Table 5-13. *Differential Between Benign and Malignant Gastric Ulcers*

	Benign	Malignant
Mucosal folds	Radiate outward from the crater center	Do not radiate toward the center, maintain usual contour
Size	Less frequently > 1 cm	Usually > 1 cm
Extension	May extend beyond stomach wall	Does not extend beyond stomach wall but lies in tumor mass
Air/fluid level	No air/fluid level in crater	May have air/fluid level in ulcer crater

scope, the diagnosis of gastric carcinoma has been greatly facilitated [50]. The diagnostic accuracy of endoscopic biopsy may reach 85 percent and possibly as high as 99 percent when combined with endoscopic cytologic examination. The barium swallow with an upper gastrointestinal x-ray has for years been the foundation for diagnostic studies in gastric carcinoma [37]. Characteristic findings include filling defects in the gastric contour, decreased or complete loss of distensibility (seen best by the person performing the study), and/or gastric ulceration. Gastric ulcers are much more frequently associated with malignancy than duodenal or pyloric channel ulcers. Factors that help differentiate benign from malignant gastric ulcers are presented in Table 5-13. The abdominal CT scan with oral and IV contrast may be able to demonstrate a large gastric tumor, but it is more commonly employed to document local tumor spread into the liver, spleen, and/or surrounding lymph nodes.

TREATMENT: ACUTE MANAGEMENT
The only known successful curative treatment for gastric carcinoma is surgical resection. The type of surgical procedure depends on the size and location of the cancer. Curative resections mandate a 6-cm margin of normal tissue on either side of the cancer. The Billroth I procedure is a partial gastrectomy with gastroduodenostomy reconstruction, whereas the more commonly utilized Billroth II procedure is a reconstruction by gastrojejunostomy. Patients with larger tumors that require total gastrectomy have intestinal continuity

established most commonly by an end-to-side esophageal-jejunal anastomosis with a jejunal Roux-en-Y for pancreatic and biliary secretions. Approximately 85 to 95 percent of patients are surgical candidates, with approximately 50 percent potentially resected for cure. For unresectable, locally advanced cancers, limited palliation may be obtained with a combination of radiotherapy and chemotherapy with 5FU.

TREATMENT: CHRONIC MANAGEMENT
Chemotherapy is the mainstay of treatment of metastatic disease, but it has limited benefits. The most active single agents include 5FU, adriamycin/doxorubicin, and mitomycin C. More recently, *cis*-platinum has been shown to be an active single agent. As in pancreatic carcinoma, the FAM regimen (5FU, Adriamycin/doxorubicin, mitomycin C) has gained in popularity but with minimal advantage over single-agent 5FU [10].

PROGNOSIS
As in pancreatic carcinoma, the long-term outcome in gastric cancer remains grim, with only a 5 to 10 percent 5-year survival rate. Even patients with the smallest tumors, which can be resected by a Billroth I subtotal gastrectomy, only have a 22 to 33 percent chance of 5-year survival.

Esophageal Cancer
Cancer of the esophagus represents the cancer with most dramatic regional fluctuations in incidence around the world. A mountainous region

in Hunan Province, China has an incidence of 139 per 100,000 population, whereas not far from that region an incidence of only 1.4 per 100,000 population was found [13]. In the United States, esophageal cancer is the twenty-first most common malignancy, with only 10,000 newly diagnosed cancers per year and nearly 9000 deaths. The male-to-female ratio is 4 : 1. The incidence of esophageal cancer has more than doubled among black men in the United States over the last 30 years. The etiologic factors include tobacco use, alcohol consumption, and preexisting Barrett's esophagus (columnar epithelium in the distal esophagus due to chronic gastric reflux) [44]. Esophageal cancer includes squamous cell carcinoma of the esophagus, adenocarcinoma arising in Barrett's epithelium, and adenocarcinoma arising in the gastroesophageal junction.

DIAGNOSIS

The vast majority of patients present with dysphagia (difficulty swallowing). The dysphagia typically is an insidious process initially noted with solid foods but progressing to include liquids. As the ability to swallow foods worsens, weight loss is a frequent complaint, being present in 90 percent of afflicted patients. Pain with swallowing (odynophagia) will be seen in up to 50 percent of patients.

Specific abnormal physical findings are unusual in esophageal cancer. Thus the clinician must depend heavily on the history to suggest the diagnosis.

Patients with esophageal cancer may have chronic bleeding leading to iron-deficiency anemia or an acute bleed leading to volume-loss anemia. Up to 25 percent of patients may exhibit a paraneoplastic syndrome of hypercalcemia due to the secretion of a parathyroid hormone-like hormone (squamous cell carcinoma variety).

The barium swallow remains the most important diagnostic tool in the evaluation of a patient with dysphagia. The typical pattern seen is an irregular, ragged mucosal lesion with narrowing of the lumen. The histologic diagnosis is made on upper endoscopy with biopsy of the abnormal mucosal lesion. Other diagnostic studies that should be performed include bronchoscopy to determine if there is involvement of the tracheobronchial tree and, more recently, CT scans of the chest and abdomen to determine extent of local spread of the cancer.

TREATMENT: ACUTE MANAGEMENT

Surgical resection for esophageal and gastroesophageal junction carcinomas has been the mainstay of treatment since the first successful esophageal resection in 1913 [11]. For lesions below the aortic arch, an esophagogastrectomy (partial esophagectomy and partial gastrectomy) with esophagogastrostomy is performed, whereas higher lesions require esophagectomy with a colonic interposition (i.e., transposing a portion of the large bowel with its vascular supply intact into the esophageal position to reestablish esophageal continuity). Operative mortality for surgical resections remains high in these patients (10 to 20 percent) due to the radical nature of the surgery and the general debility of the patients, who frequently exhibit weight loss, malnutrition, and associated heart and lung disease. Because of these factors, along with local and distant spread of the malignancy, up to 50 percent of patients are not resectable surgically, and these patients are typically treated with radiation therapy. Attempts to improve resectability rates along with overall survival rates have been undertaken with neoadjuvant (prior to surgery) chemotherapy and radiotherapy; this remains an experimental course of action [36].

TREATMENT: CHRONIC MANAGEMENT

Metastatic and locally advanced disease can be treated with chemotherapy, with a variety of agents having a 15 to 27 percent response rate when administered singly. Combination chemotherapy (5FU plus *cis*-platinum) has improved on these results, with response rates of 50 to 60 percent, but such therapy has not been shown to prolong survival.

PROGNOSIS

As with the other upper gastrointestinal malignancies (gastric and pancreatic carcinomas), the overall 5-year survival rate for patients with esophageal carcinoma remains dismal at less than 10 percent. Median survival is 10 to 12 months for all patients. Even for those patients who are able to undergo potentially curative resections, the 5-year survival rate remains only 15 to 20 percent.

Hepatocellular Carcinoma

Primary cancer of the liver (hepatoma, hepatocellular carcinoma) is an uncommon malignancy in the United States, with only 2500 newly diagnosed cases a year, yet it is believed to be the most common cancer worldwide due to the endemic presence of hepatitis B in southeast Asia and Africa. Recently, the connection between the hepatitis B virus and hepatocellular carcinoma has been strengthened [4]. By using recombinant DNA technology, the hepatitis B viral genome has been demonstrated to be present in the cells of patients with hepatoma, even in patients with underlying alcoholic cirrhosis as the predisposing lesion [6].

DIAGNOSIS

Patients with hepatocellular carcinoma may present with nonspecific symptoms of abdominal fullness or pain, along with abdominal distension, weight loss, fever, and fatigue. Other patients may have a more dramatic presentation with massive hemorrhage from esophageal varices, rapidly developing ascites, or intraperitoneal hemorrhage. In any patient with a known history of cirrhosis who takes an unexplained turn for the worse, the diagnosis of hepatoma should be entertained.

Primary cancer of the liver may present with jaundice, abdominal distension with or without demonstrable ascites, hepatomegaly, and marked cachexia. Also, the other signs of chronic liver disease may be present (spider angiomata, palmar erythema, testicular atrophy, gynecomastia).

An elevated serum bilirubin level along with other elevated liver function tests is common. Alpha-fetoprotein (AFP) has been used as a tumor marker in hepatocellular carcinoma, being elevated in up to 90 percent of patients. Markers for hepatitis B are very common in these patients (HBsAg, antibodies to hepatitis B, DNA viral genome) and possibly may be universal when using recombinant DNA technology. An acquired dysfibrinogenemia can be found in approximately 50 percent of patients, causing prolonged prothrombin, thrombin, and reptilase times [19]. Recently, 91 percent of biopsy-confirmed hepatocellular carcinoma patients possessed an abnormal prothrombin molecule called des-gamma-carboxy prothrombin which may prove to be useful along with the alpha-fetoprotein level in diagnosing this malignancy [27].

Abdominal CT scanning has become an invaluable tool in the diagnosis of hepatic lesions, although histologic confirmation is still necessary. Abdominal ultrasound and nuclear medicine scanning are also useful techniques in diagnosing hepatocellular carcinoma, but they may not be as sensitive in documenting the extent of disease in the abdomen. Angiography may be helpful in the diagnosis of hepatic lesions, but its major role remains as a preoperative study to evaluate for the possibility of surgical resection. Histologic confirmation of hepatocellular carcinoma can be achieved by either percutaneous needle biopsy, laparoscopic needle biopsy, or even an exploratory laparotomy with open liver biopsy.

TREATMENT: ACUTE MANAGEMENT

Surgery remains the only possibility for cure in this disease, but owing to extensive intrahepatic and extrahepatic involvement, few patients are even offered surgical resection. For patients with unresectable tumors, liver transplantation has been attempted, but long-term survival has been shown to be less than 20 percent. Disease tends to recur within 2 years of transplantation.

TREATMENT: CHRONIC MANAGEMENT

For the vast majority of patients who have unresectable or metastatic disease, systemic chemotherapy is offered. Doxorubicin is the most active agent, with only a 15 to 25 percent response rate. Results with administration of chemotherapy regionally via the hepatic artery (either 5FU or 5-FUDR) have shown modest improvements in response rates (30 to 40 percent) and possibly survival.

PROGNOSIS

The median survival for patients with hepatocellular carcinoma is 1 to 3 months. The only patients alive at 5 years are those who have been completely resected surgically. Patients responding to systemic chemotherapy have a median duration of survival of approximately 7 to 9 months.

Genitourinary Malignancies

Prostate Cancer

Adenocarcinoma of the prostate is a disease mainly of elderly males. Causative or etiologic factors for the development of carcinoma of the prostate are not known. American black men have the highest incidence rate for prostate cancer in the world, having risen from 31 per 100,000 population in 1937 to 78 per 100,000 population in 1971. The true incidence of adenocarcinoma of the prostate is dramatically higher than reported incidence rates due to the occult nature of the disease. In autopsy series, up to 40 percent of men over the age of 70 years have histologically diagnosed prostate cancer.

DIAGNOSIS

Prostate cancer in its early stages presents without any symptoms. The most common symptoms are those referable to the ever-present benign prostatic hypertrophy (BPH) that causes urinary voiding complaints. Patients with metastatic disease (stage D), which is most commonly to the bones, present with bone pain, vertebral body compression fractures, or pathologic fractures of bones.

Early-stage prostate cancer is seen as an incidental finding during a transurethral resection of the prostate (TURP) for bladder outlet obstruction from benign prostatic hypertrophy (stage A) or as a nodule on rectal examination (stage B). Fifty percent of all prostatic nodules are found to be malignant when biopsied. Local extension of the cancer (stage C) involves the periprostatic region and seminal vesicles, which can be evaluated on rectal examination.

The serum acid phosphatase level has been widely utilized in the evaluation of patients with carcinoma of the prostate [16]. Up to 85 percent of patients with bone metastases will have an elevated acid phosphatase level, whereas only 5 percent with a malignant prostatic nodule will have an abnormal test. More recently, the prostatic acid phosphatase level (radioimmunoassay) or prostate-specific antigen level has been touted as a more sensitive test that also can be utilized as a screening test for prostate cancer. Unfortunately, because approximately 6 percent of patients with benign prostatic hypertrophy and no demonstrable cancer can have an abnormal prostatic acid phosphatase level, and since the incidence of benign prostatic hypertrophy in the elderly male population is nearly universal, the positive predictive value of the test is meaningless (< 0.5 percent) for diagnosing asymptomatic cancer [49]. The serum alkaline phosphatase level is another marker for bony metastases.

To determine if a palpable nodule is malignant, either a transrectal or transperineal biopsy is performed. If the patient also has urinary obstructive symptoms, then a transurethral resection of the prostate may be performed to alleviate the obstruction, but also to possibly demonstrate cancer in the resected prostatic specimen. The intravenous pyelogram (IVP) is performed to evaluate the distal ureters for obstruction, which usually signifies locally advanced (at least stage C) disease.

The CT scan has become more commonly utilized to help evaluate the pelvic retroperitoneal lymph nodes, which, if they are found to be enlarged, can be biopsied by CT-guided fine-needle aspiration.

The nuclear medicine bone scan is the most sensitive technique to diagnose metastatic spread to the bones. Plain x-rays of positive areas show the typical blastic bone involvement by prostatic carcinoma. Transrectal prostatic ultrasound is now being investigated as a possible diagnostic tool in the asymptomatic patient.

TREATMENT: ACUTE MANAGEMENT

For patients with localized disease, either radical prostatectomy or radiation therapy has been the treatment of choice [35]. Because of the inherent elderly population of men afflicted by this disease, many may not be candidates for surgical resection and thus are treated with radiation to the prostate and pelvis with either external beam and/or radioactive implants. For those patients who are considered candidates for surgery, the procedure performed is a radical prostatectomy. In recent years, as the importance of pelvic lymph node metastases has become recognized, patients are more routinely undergoing pelvic lymph node dissections prior to definitive local therapy. While pelvic lymph node dissection will identify a patient who will not benefit from local therapy to the prostate, it is unclear whether it actually has changed overall survival rates in these patients.

TREATMENT: CHRONIC MANAGEMENT

Patients with asymptomatic spread to the bones are not known to receive benefit from any form of therapy, and therefore, the institution of treatment is delayed until symptoms arise [7]. Prostate cancer is a hormonally responsive cancer in males, being driven by the male hormone testosterone. Bilateral orchiectomy, which can be performed under local anesthesia, remains the procedure of choice to eliminate testosterone production. Results are rapid, with some patients showing improvement in a matter of days. In those patients who are not candidates for bilateral orchiectomy, oral medication can be administered to decrease testosterone levels to those seen in castrated patients. The two agents utilized are estrogens (diethylstilbestrol, DES) and the gonadotropin-releasing hormone agonist leuprolide [26]. Both function via the hypothalamic-pituitary axis to ultimately decrease luteinizing hormone (LH) secretion by the pituitary and thus reduce production of testosterone by the testes. Estrogens have adverse side effects such as thromboembolic events and myocardial infarction and thus are not appropriate for patients with preexisting cardiovascular disease. In patients who fail one type of hormonal therapy, there is little utility in trying another hormonal therapy.

For patients who have progressive disease despite hormonal therapy, chemotherapy has been employed but with very limited success. 5FU, cyclophosphamide, methotrexate, and doxorubicin are the agents with the best, yet marginal (approximately 20 percent response rate) activity in adenocarcinoma of the prostate. Combination chemotherapy may have a slightly better response rate of 20 to 30 percent.

PROGNOSIS

The prognosis for patients with prostate cancer varies greatly with the stage of disease. A patient with an incidentally found focal, well-differentiated adenocarcinoma on a transurethral resection of the prostate has a survival similar to an age-matched control population. Nearly 60 percent of patients, though, present with stage D (metastatic to pelvic lymph nodes or bones) disease. Patients with stage D_1 disease (metastases to pelvic lymph nodes) have approximately a 3- to 5-year median survival, with two-thirds of them developing distant metastases in 2 to 3 years. Patients with stage D_2 disease (usually metastases to the bone) have a median survival of approximately $1\frac{1}{2}$ to $2\frac{1}{2}$ years.

Bladder Cancer

Carcinoma of the bladder is the fifth most common cancer in the United States, with over 45,000 newly diagnosed cases in 1987 and nearly 11,000 deaths. There is a male-to-female ratio of nearly 3 : 1. Here in the United States, transitional cell carcinoma makes up 90 to 95 percent of histologic subtypes, followed by squamous cell carcinoma at 5 to 10 percent and true adenocarcinoma at 2 to 3 percent. In countries where schistosomiasis is endemic, such as Egypt, the proportion of squamous cell carcinomas is greatly increased. Risk factors for developing transitional cell carcinoma of the bladder are smoking and a variety of occupational carcinogens.

DIAGNOSIS

Hematuria is the presenting symptom in approximately three-quarters of all patients with bladder cancer. The second most common symptom is bladder irritability, which occurs in about a quarter of patients. Another less common presentation is a urinary tract infection in a male in whom urethritis and prostatitis have been excluded as etiologic possibilities.

The only physical findings in patients with bladder carcinoma are seen in those patients who present with clinically evident metastatic disease (less than 10 percent).

Urinalysis reveals hematuria, either gross or microscopic, in nearly all bladder cancer patients. Cytologic examination of the urine can support a diagnosis of cancer, but it does not reveal the site or the invasiveness of the lesion [32]. There is also a 20 percent false-negative rate with urine cytology, thus limiting the overall usefulness of this test in diagnosing bladder cancer and in screening programs to detect asymptomatic bladder cancer patients.

The definitive diagnostic study for detecting cancer of the bladder is cytoscopic examination. The accuracy of cystoscopy is nearly 100 percent. Biopsies of the suspected areas along with bladder mapping (biopsies of the whole bladder) are crucial in the diagnosis and staging of bladder cancer. A bimanual examination performed under anesthesia is also an important staging procedure to evaluate for a palpable tumor mass and for extent of local spread.

An intravenous pyelogram (IVP) should be performed in all bladder cancer patients, since approximately 10 percent of them will have a second, synchronous primary cancer elsewhere in the urinary tract. Also, complete visualization of the upper urinary tracts will be important both for staging (70 percent of patients with hydronephrosis have a deeply invasive tumor) and subsequent surgical resection and reconstruction if needed.

CT scanning of the pelvis may be helpful in evaluating extension of the bladder cancer to surrounding structures and for involvement of pelvic lymph nodes. CT-guided fine-needle aspiration of enlarged lymph nodes may provide cytologic proof of regional spread.

TREATMENT: ACUTE MANAGEMENT

Transurethral resection of bladder cancers (TURB) is the treatment of choice for noninvasive lesions. In patients in whom there are too many small cancers to resect, fulguration can be utilized. For the 25 to 30 percent of patients who present with invasive tumors, radical cystectomy with urinary diversion remains the standard method of treatment. In the few patients (less than 8 percent) who present with a lesion confined to the dome of the bladder without other areas of carcinoma in situ, segmental resection (partial cystectomy) can be employed with similar results as radical cystectomy.

Carcinoma in situ of the bladder is a multifocal process that is typically too widespread for limited surgical resection or fulguration. Intravesical chemotherapy with agents such as mitomycin C, bacillus Calmette-Guérin, and doxorubicin can reverse the atypical cytologic changes seen in carcinoma in situ. For patients who fail this approach, radical cystectomy is performed.

TREATMENT: CHRONIC MANAGEMENT

To prevent the recurrence of bladder cancer following transurethral resection, intravesical chemotherapy has been shown to be effective. Thiotepa, mitomycin C, doxorubicin, and BCG are the most commonly used agents. For patients with metastatic disease, chemotherapy has been shown to prolong survival. Active single agents include *cis*-platinum, cyclophosphamide, doxorubicin, methotrexate, and vinblastine. Combination chemotherapy has yielded response rates as high as 60 to 70 percent (e.g., MVAC: methotrexate, vinblastine, Adriamycin/doxorubicin, *cis*-platinum) [45].

PROGNOSIS

Overall 5-year survival rates for noninvasive bladder cancer are relatively good (65 to 80 percent), but tumor recurrence is frequent, with 70 to 85 percent of patients developing a recurrent cancer. Patients with invasive cancers have a 25 to 30 percent 5-year survival rate when treated by radical cystectomy. Median survivals for nonresponding patients with metastatic disease treated with chemotherapy is 2 to 4 months, whereas patients responding to combination chemotherapy have a 9- to 11-month median survival.

Renal Cell Carcinoma

Adenocarcinoma of the kidney, which is also called hypernephroma and renal cell carcinoma, affects adults in the fifth through seventh decades, with a male-to-female ratio of 3 : 1. Risk factors are few, but they include cigarette smoking, von Hippel-Lindau's disease, and polycystic kidney disease. It affects nearly 22,000 people per year, with over 9000 dying from the malignancy.

DIAGNOSIS

The classic triad of hematuria, abdominal mass, and flank pain is no longer a common presentation in patients with renal cell carcinoma (less than 10 percent), although pain still is the most frequent symptom noted in 45 percent of these patients. Other complaints include weight loss and fever, which may be due to the presence of metastatic disease or a paraneoplastic syndrome.

A palpable abdominal mass can be found in 45 percent of patients with renal cell carcinoma from a series reported in 1971. Today, no doubt, this figure would be smaller. The sudden onset of a varicocele may be the only physical finding noted.

Renal cell carcinoma is well known for its many paraneoplastic syndromes, which include erythrocytosis, hypercalcemia, hypertension, and Stauffer's syndrome (Table 5-14). Stauffer's syndrome (nephrogenic hepatic dysfunction syndrome) is seen in 7 to 15 percent of patients with renal cell carcinoma and is manifested by fever, weight loss, hepatomegaly, and splenomegaly, with abnormal liver function tests (bilirubin, SGOT, alkaline phosphatase, bromsulphalein clearance), along with hepatic synthetic dysfunction (decreased serum albumin and increased prothrombin time) in the absence of liver metastases [46]. Following radical nephrectomy, the preceding abnormalities typically revert back to normal. Hematuria is a frequent finding seen in 60 percent of patients.

Technical advances in diagnostic radiology have changed our approach to the patient with a

Table 5–14. Paraneoplastic Syndromes in Renal Cell Carcinoma

Disorder	Cause	Frequency
Hypercalcemia	Parathyroid hormone-like hormone	3 percent
Hypertension	Renin	15–40 percent
Erythrocytosis	Erythropoietin	3 percent
Stauffer's syndrome	Unknown	7–15 percent

suspected renal mass. Previously, an intravenous pyelogram with tomograms followed by arteriography was the standard approach. In recent years, computerized tomography (CT scan) has become the main or sole diagnostic study performed to evaluate these patients in some centers. Information concerning structure (cystic versus solid mass), renal vein, or vena caval involvement, local extension, and regional lymph node involvement can all be obtained by the CT scan. The CT scan also can be used to direct a fine-needle aspiration of the lesion for cytologic confirmation of the suspected renal cell carcinoma.

TREATMENT: ACUTE MANAGEMENT
Surgical resection remains the mainstay of treatment for patients who do not have distant metastases. Radical nephrectomy is performed that includes Gerota's fascia and its contents (kidney plus adrenal gland).

TREATMENT: CHRONIC MANAGEMENT
Nearly 50 percent of patients with renal cell carcinoma will have metastatic disease at presentation, thus making radical nephrectomy of very limited value in patients with severe local symptoms such as pain and/or hemorrhage. Chemotherapy has been used in patients with metastatic disease but with extremely poor results. The only agent with any hope of inducing a tumor regression has been vinblastine, which has a 15 to 25 percent response rate. Hormonal therapies with megestrol acetate or tamoxifen have a 5 to 10 percent response rate with minimal toxicity. Most recently, interleukin-2 with lymphokine-activated killer (LAK) cells has been shown to have a 33 percent rate of disease regression in renal cell carcinoma, but not without significant potential for toxicity [40].

PROGNOSIS
For patients with disease confined to the kidney (stage 1) who undergo a radical nephrectomy, median 5-year survival rates are from 65 to 75 percent. The median survival for patients with metastatic disease is 6 to 9 months, but there is a wide variation in survival rates despite metastatic disease, with some patients living as long as 6 years.

Testicular Cancer
Cancer of the testes receives more attention than its incidence can justify. Testicular cancer is the twenty-fifth most common cancer in the United States, with only 5500 cases in 1987. The reason for the attention is the dramatic reversal of outcomes in this malignancy, which in 1971 was 90 percent fatal and now is more than 90 percent curable. Testicular cancer represents one of the modern-day triumphs of combination chemotherapy. Some researchers have even made the statement that no patient with testicular cancer should ever die of his disease. Tumors of germ-cell origin make up approximately 95 percent of all neoplasms of the testes. The six main histologic subtypes of testicular cancer are seminoma, embryonal carcinoma, teratoma, teratocarcinoma, choriocarcinoma, and yolk-sac tumors. The remaining 5 percent of cancers are of gonadal stromal origin. The only known etiologic factors are cryptorchidism and gonadal dysgenesis, which increase a patient's risk by 10 to 40 times that of the general population.

DIAGNOSIS
The most frequent complaint (75 to 90 percent) is that of swelling or heaviness in the scrotum. Trauma may be elicited as an inciting event, but it simply has drawn attention to the preexisting disorder. Between 15 and 50 percent of patients have associated mild testicular pain which is not acute in onset. Another 5 to 15 percent have symptoms referable to metastatic disease at the time of presentation.

An enlarged hemiscrotum is the most frequent physical finding, and this must be differentiated from an infectious/inflammatory process. Rarely, retroperitoneal lymph nodes can be palpated as an abdominal mass.

Table 5–15. *Tumor Markers in Testicular Carcinoma*

Histologic type	Alpha-fetoprotein (%)	Human chorionic gonadotropin (%)	Alpha-fetoprotein and/or human chorionic gonadotropin (%)
Seminoma	0	9	9
Teratoma	37.5	25	43.7
Embryonal carcinoma	70.3	60	87.5
Teratocarcinoma	64.2	57	85.7
Choriocarcinoma	0	100	100
Yolk-sac tumor	75	25	75

Tumor markers are of central importance in the diagnosis and management of patients with testicular cancer [24] (Table 5-15). The beta subunit of human chorionic gonadotropin (HCG) is secreted by trophoblastic elements in testicular cancers; thus 100 percent of choriocarcinomas have an elevated level. Alpha-fetoprotein (AFP) occurs in adults only in pathologic states such as embryonal cell carcinoma and yolk-sac tumors. Lactate dehydrogenase (LDH) is a ubiquitous intracellular enzyme that also can be used as a nonspecific tumor marker in testicular cancer patients. Tumor marker values should be obtained prior to surgical intervention in any patient suspected of having testicular cancer.

In patients in whom it may be difficult to differentiate between a testicular mass and an infectious/inflammatory process involving the hemiscrotum, an ultrasound may be helpful. Any suspected testicular tumor should be explored surgically through an inguinal approach rather than transscrotally. Other diagnostic studies are performed in an attempt to determine metastatic sites in proven cases of malignancy. CT scanning of the abdomen has become the most important tool in staging patients with testicular cancers, largely replacing the intravenous pyelogram and the lymphangiogram. Chest x-rays should be performed to evaluate for mediastinal and pulmonary involvement. Full-lung tomography or CT scans of the chest are more accurate methods of assessing the chest cavity for metastatic spread.

TREATMENT: ACUTE MANAGEMENT

To make the diagnosis of a germ cell testicular cancer, a radical inguinal orchiectomy is performed as the initial step. Tumor markers should return to normal after orchiectomy if the patient has disease confined to the testes (stage A). In patients found to have a seminoma, this is followed by radiation therapy in all patients but those with bulky retroperitoneal disease (stage B$_3$) or mediastinal involvement (stage C). In patients found to have nonseminomatous malignancy, the orchiectomy is followed by a retroperitoneal lymph node dissection, except in those with stage B$_3$ or stage C disease. Approximately 60 to 70 percent of nonseminomatous testicular tumor patients will have lymph node involvement in the retroperitoneum at presentation. In those patients found to have lymph node involvement, combination chemotherapy is given in the adjuvant setting to decrease the chance for disease recurrence.

TREATMENT: CHRONIC MANAGEMENT

In patients with stage B$_3$ or C seminoma, nonseminomatous stage B$_3$ or C disease, and recurrent metastatic disease, combination chemotherapy is employed with great success (80 to 95 percent response rates) [12]. Active agents include *cis*-platinum, VP-16, cyclophosphamide, bleomycin, vinblastine, actinomycin D, and ifosfamide. Combination regimens include PVB (*cis*-platinum, vinblastine, bleomycin), VAB-6 (cyclophosphamide, bleomycin, actinomycin D, vinblastine, *cis*-

platinum), and *cis*-platinum/VP-16. After three or four cycles of chemotherapy, patients whose tumor markers have normalized but who have residual tumor masses should undergo surgical resection of the lesions. The resected specimens will contain only fibrosis in a third of patients, mature teratoma in another third, and persistent carcinoma in another third. Germ cell tumors of the testes are one of the only malignancies where therapy may be determined solely by the serum level of the beta subunit of human chorionic gonadotropin or alpha-fetoprotein.

PROGNOSIS

As mentioned earlier, testicular carcinoma is a highly curable malignancy, with greater than 90 percent of afflicted patients cured of their cancers. Only 400 people are expected to die in the United States in 1987 from testicular cancer.

Gynecologic Malignancies

Endometrial Carcinoma

Carcinoma of the endometrium is the fourth most frequent malignancy in women in the United States. Most cases occur in women in the sixth and seventh decades. The incidence has been shown to rise in recent years, possibly related to the increased use of supplemental estrogen. There is a strong association between estrogen replacement therapy in postmenopausal women and the development of endometrial carcinoma [22]. The risk increases with increasing duration of use and higher doses of estrogens, rising four to eight times that of the normal, non-estrogen-taking population. Combination estrogen and progesterone oral contraceptives have been shown to be protective for the development of endometrial carcinoma, reducing the risk by approximately 50 percent [23]. Other risk factors include obesity, hypertension, diabetes, and Stein-Leventhal syndrome (polycystic ovary syndrome with hyperestrogenism). Adenocarcinoma makes up over 90 percent of the malignancies arising in the uterus.

DIAGNOSIS

Postmenopausal vaginal bleeding is the most frequent complaint in the older population, whereas prolonged and/or excessive menstrual bleeding (menometrorrhagia) is most common in the premenopausal age group. Eighty percent of patients with endometrial carcinoma are postmenopausal. Some patients also may complain of a yellowish or serosanguineous vaginal discharge.

The only physical findings typically seen are uterine bleeding and possibly an enlarged uterus. Five to 10 percent of patients will have extension into the endocervical canal which may be seen on pelvic examination. Less than 10 percent of patients will present with advanced disease manifested by ascites, jaundice, or bowel obstruction.

Approximately 15 to 20 percent of patients are asymptomatic with negative physical findings but are detected by an abnormal Papanicolaou (PAP) smear for adenocarcinoma. Otherwise there are no specific laboratory tests for endometrial carcinoma.

Every postmenopausal female with vaginal bleeding requires an investigation as to the cause. Techniques to cytologically evaluate cells from the lining of the uterus have varying sensitivities from 50 to 95 percent. The most accurate are saline irrigation, endometrial brush, and the jet washer techniques. Histologic confirmation can be obtained by endometrial biopsy, Vabra aspiration, or uterine curettage. Once the diagnosis has been made, staging is carried out by cystoscopy, sigmoidoscopy, intravenous pyelogram, barium enema, and chest x-rays to evaluate for local spread and distant metastases.

TREATMENT: ACUTE MANAGEMENT

For patients with disease confined to the corpus of the uterus, primary treatment includes an exploratory laparotomy with total abdominal hysterectomy and bilateral salpingo-oophorectomy

(TAH/BSO). It is unclear whether a pelvic lymph node dissection is of benefit to these patients, but it may determine the need for subsequent radiation therapy. Patients with poorly differentiated malignancies should receive preoperative radiation therapy prior to total abdominal hysterectomy and bilateral salpingo-oophorectomy. Patients with extensions to the cervix (stage II), outside the uterus but confined to the true pelvis (stage III), and outside the true pelvis (stage IVA) typically receive combination therapy with either preoperative or postoperative radiation therapy with a total abdominal hysterectomy and bilateral salpingo-oophorectomy. Patients with distant metastases (stage IVB) should receive radiation therapy, chemotherapy (or hormonal therapy), followed by an attempted surgical resection.

TREATMENT: CHRONIC MANAGEMENT
It is not known whether adjuvant therapy in patients at high risk for relapse is of benefit. Adjuvant progestational therapy has been utilized, but it is known that the progesterone receptor-positive tumors are the most likely tumors to benefit from progestin therapy yet are the least likely to recur, while, on the other hand, the progesterone receptor-negative tumors are most likely to recur yet are the least responsive to progestin therapy. For patients with metastatic disease, progestational therapy can be employed in hormone receptor-positive tumors (a 70 percent response rate) and/or in well-differentiated tumors when the hormone receptor status is not known [38]. Otherwise, chemotherapy has been utilized in these patients. Active agents are *cis*-platinum, doxorubicin, 5FU, and cyclophosphamide, with response rates of 20 to 40 percent. It is not known whether combination chemotherapy is of added benefit over single-agent therapy in this disorder.

PROGNOSIS
With the increased usage of supplemental estrogens in postmenopausal females, the associated rise in cases of endometrial carcinoma have been largely of early-stage disease, with over 90 percent of cases being stage I or stage II. Therefore,

while we are diagnosing more cases of endometrial carcinoma, they are very treatable and curable malignancies. Despite 35,000 newly diagnosed cases in 1987, less than 3000 deaths are expected from this malignancy.

Ovarian Cancer
Cancer of the ovary is the fifth most common cause of cancer deaths in women in the United States, with 19,000 newly diagnosed cases in 1987 and 11,700 deaths. It has been estimated that a woman in the United States has a 1 in 70 chance of developing cancer of the ovary in her lifetime. Nearly two-thirds of ovarian malignancies occur between the ages of 40 and 65 years. Eighty-five to 90 percent of malignant ovarian tumors are of epithelial origin, with the remaining 10 percent being germ cell and sex cord-stromal tumors. Risk factors include nulliparity, late age at menopause, and prolonged intervals of ovulation. Oral contraceptives have been shown to decrease the risk for developing ovarian cancer [8].

DIAGNOSIS
Cancer of the ovary tends to manifest itself as nonspecific complaints at an advanced stage of disease. Patients may complain of increasing abdominal girth due to malignant ascites and/or vague abdominal/pelvic pain or discomfort.

The presence of a pelvic or adnexal mass may be the only physical finding in the 30 to 40 percent of patients who present with early-stage disease confined to the pelvis (stage I, i.e., confined to the ovary, and stage II, i.e., confined to the pelvis). Other abnormalities include ascites, pleural effusions, and/or enlarged supraclavicular lymph nodes, all indicative of advanced disease.

A murine monoclonal antibody called CA-125 has been developed, which detects an antigen in the serum of approximately 80 percent of patients with ovarian cancer [3]. Prior to its introduction in 1983, there were no other blood tests useful in the diagnosis of ovarian malignancies.

Pelvic ultrasonography is frequently utilized in

patients to evaluate pelvic masses. Carcinoma typically presents as a solid or complex mass which is differentiated from benign simple ovarian cysts. Ovarian cancer's pattern of spread is along the pelvic and abdominal peritoneal surfaces; therefore, preoperative evaluation of bowel and ureteral involvement can be accomplished by barium enema, an upper gastrointestinal series with small bowel follow-through, and an intravenous pyelogram. The chest x-ray is performed to exclude the presence of parenchymal pulmonary metastases and pleural effusions which may or may not contain malignant cells. Preoperatively, abdominal CT scans may be useful to evaluate the extent of disease, including the retroperitoneum and liver.

TREATMENT: ACUTE MANAGEMENT

Surgical exploration is nearly always undertaken irrespective of preoperative imaging modalities in patients with suspected ovarian cancer. Once the diagnosis of ovarian carcinoma is made, an extensive surgical exploration is undertaken with removal of as much gross tumor as possible and sampling of the omentum, both hemidiaphragms, paracolic gutters, retroperitoneal lymph nodes, and peritoneal washings for cytologic examination [21]. Such debulking procedures may even require resecting portions of the bowel. Patients have the best survival when the residual tumor diameter is less than 2 cm in maximum dimension. A total abdominal hysterectomy and bilateral salpingo-oophorectomy is performed in peri- and postmenopausal females, whereas a unilateral salpingo-oophorectomy may be performed in selected women in the childbearing years.

TREATMENT: CHRONIC MANAGEMENT

Patients with advanced disease (stages III or IV) are treated with postoperative chemotherapy. Active single agents include melphalan, cyclophosphamide, thiotepa, chlorambucil, doxorubicin, hexamethylmelamine, methotrexate, 5FU, and cis-platinum, all with approximately a 25 to 50 percent response rates. Combination chemotherapy with such regimens as hexaCAF (hexamethylmelamine, cyclophosphamide, methotrexate, 5FU) and CAP (cyclophosphamide, Adriamycin/doxorubicin, cis-platinum) have a 60 to 80 percent response rate. Following 10 to 12 cycles of combination chemotherapy, a second-look operation is typically undertaken in patients with no obvious residual tumor in an attempt to document pathologically those patients who were clinical complete responders [18]. Those patients who are pathologic complete remissions can have their therapy discontinued, whereas those with documented residual disease can have their therapy changed. Adjuvant whole abdominal radiation therapy may be of benefit in stages I and II and microscopic stage III patients (disease outside the pelvis).

PROGNOSIS

With nearly 60 percent of women with ovarian cancer presenting with advanced disease (stage III or stage IV, i.e., distant metastases), the overall 5-year survival for all patients is therefore disappointingly low at approximately 30 percent. Death rates for ovarian cancer have not been shown to change in the last 50 years.

Cancer of the Uterine Cervix

Cervical cancer has shown the second greatest decline in cancer death rates over the past 30 years, with over a 50 percent reduction among women in the United States. Risk factors for the development of cervical cancer include early sexual activity, multiple sexual partners, and prior venereal diseases. Viral agents such as the herpes simplex virus and the papilloma virus have been strongly associated with the development of cervical cancer and are thought to play an important etiologic role. Ninety percent of cervical carcinomas are of the squamous cell variety. The mean age at diagnosis is approximately 45 years.

DIAGNOSIS

With over 80 percent of cancers of the cervix detected in the preinvasive phase, most women have no symptoms referable to their carcinoma.

In patients with more advanced, invasive lesions, bleeding or a vaginal discharge may be noted by the patient.

Preinvasive carcinomas typically present without abnormal physical findings at the time of visualization and palpation of the uterine cervix. Those preinvasive lesions which are visible and invasive carcinomas present as a thickened, whitish, and irregular epithelium which may only be appreciated with the aid of a colposcope.

There currently are no blood tests helpful in the diagnosis of cervical carcinoma. Patients with metastatic spread to the bones may have an elevated alkaline phosphatase level. Patients with direct extension of the tumor to involve the bladder may have hematuria noted on urinalysis.

The dramatic decline in deaths due to cancer of the cervix is largely credited to the widespread use of the Papanicolaou (PAP) smears (Table 5-16). This technique permits cytologic examination of the cervix and endocervical canal and can diagnose both preinvasive (dysplasia and carcinoma in situ) and invasive lesions [33]. Ninety to 95 percent of preinvasive lesions and 85 to 90 percent of invasive cancers are diagnosed by the PAP smear. Patients with a class III, IV, or V PAP smear must undergo a cervical biopsy to confirm the presence of neoplasia. Visible lesions can be easily biopsied, whereas a colposcope may be used in cases where there is no visible lesion. If there is any question concerning the PAP smear and biopsy results, or if there is an endocervical tumor, a cervical conization is performed to obtain more tissue for histologic examination to correctly identify the severity of the malignant process. Once the diagnosis of invasive cervical carcinoma has been made, pretreatment staging procedures are carried out, which include an intravenous pyelogram and chest x-ray.

TREATMENT: ACUTE MANAGEMENT

Those patients with dysplasia are effectively treated by a cervical conization. In patients wishing not to risk the possible loss of fertility by injury to the internal cervical sphincter, regular follow-up but with repeated PAP smears performed every 3 months is acceptable. Carcinoma in situ (also called stage 0) is effectively treated by total abdominal hysterectomy. In the reliable patient desiring to have children, cryotherapy to the lesion followed by PAP smears every 3 months is a viable alternative. Invasive cancers entirely confined to the cervix (stage I) are effectively treated by total abdominal hysterectomy. Pelvic lymph node dissection is added for patients with invasion extending 3 to 5 mm or more below the basement membrane. When the malignancy extends to the upper third of the vagina and/or the pericervical soft tissue (stage II), treatment can be effected either by radical hysterectomy and pelvic lymph node dissection or by radiation therapy. Cervical carcinoma that extends to the lower third of the vagina or the pelvic sidewall (stage III) is treated with radiation therapy by both the external beam and intracavitary routes. Tumors that involve the bladder or rectum (stage IVA) are treated with either pelvic exenteration, aggressive radiation therapy, or a combination of the two modalities.

TREATMENT: CHRONIC MANAGEMENT

Patients who have metastatic disease at time of presentation (stage IVB) or develop recurrent metastatic spread following primary surgical or radiation therapy are treated with chemotherapy. Active agents include methotrexate, *cis*-platinum, 5FU, cyclophosphamide, doxorubicin, mitomycin C, and bleomycin. While combination chemotherapy may exhibit a higher response rate than single agents, the duration of response is unfortunately short (3 to 6 months).

Table 5–16. Cervical Cancer: PAP Smear Classification

Class	Description
I	Normal
II	Atypical, suspicious
III	Dysplasia
IV	Carcinoma in situ
V	Invasive carcinoma

PROGNOSIS

It can be argued that if every woman underwent screening for cervical carcinoma with periodic (yearly) PAP smears, practically no patient should ever die from this malignancy. Despite the proven efficacy of PAP smears, only 60 percent of women over the age of 20 obtain smears on a regular basis in the United States. Overall survival rates show 56 percent of patients with invasive cervical carcinoma still alive at 5 years.

Malignant Melanoma

Malignant melanoma currently represents the tenth most common cancer in the United States, with nearly 26,000 newly diagnosed cases in 1987. The incidence of malignant melanoma has shown the most rapid rise of any cancer in recent years (excepting lung cancer in women), doubling every decade. At the present rate of increase, it is estimated that by the year 2000, 1 of every 100 to 150 Caucasians in the United States will develop malignant melanoma. The most important etiologic factor for the development of malignant melanoma is exposure to solar radiation. Other factors relate to a person's genetic composition, with fair-haired, light-eyed (blue is the most common) persons who have difficulty or are unable to suntan but easily burn when exposed to the sun being most likely to develop malignant melanoma. Families who carry the dysplastic nevus syndrome, which is an autosomal-dominant trait, have a 50 to 100 percent chance of developing malignant melanoma in their lifetime [20].

Diagnosis

Patients with malignant melanoma typically state that a preexisting mole has shown a change in color, size, or shape or has become nodular, pruritic, ulcerated, or subject to bleeding episodes.

The same changes noted by the patient are the typical physical findings noted by the examiner, along with possible enlargement of the respective draining lymph nodes.

Blood tests are only of value in the staging of patients with malignant melanoma to determine if there may be metastatic disease to the bones and/or liver.

An excisional biopsy that includes a portion of subcutaneous tissue should be performed on suspected nevi. If lesions are quite large, an incisional biopsy that includes adjacent normal skin can be performed. A chest x-ray should be performed to evaluate for possible pulmonary metastases, while liver, bone, and brain scans in patients with disease confined to the skin (stage I) who do not have clinical or laboratory evidence of metastases should not be performed routinely.

Treatment: Acute Management

The only known effective therapy for primary malignant melanoma is surgical resection. A wide surgical excision is carried out with a 2.5- to 5.0-cm margin depending on the location of the primary lesion, and the depth of the resection should include the underlying fascia of the muscle. Frequently, split-thickness skin grafts are required to cover an excision site. For patients with clinically suspicious or pathologically involved regional lymph nodes, a regional lymph node dissection is indicated. The routine performance of lymph node dissection is not warranted. The use of adjuvant immunotherapy, chemotherapy, or combination therapies in patients thought to be at high risk for relapse (positive lymph nodes and deeply invasive lesions) has been unsuccessful [48].

Treatment: Chronic Management

Patients who relapse in regional lymph nodes after surgical excision of their primary melanoma are treated by lymph node dissection. Those patients with distant metastases have been treated with chemotherapy but with discouraging overall results. DTIC is the most commonly utilized agent, with a 15 to 25 percent response rate. Combination chemotherapy regimens have not been shown to be superior to single-agent dacarbazine (DTIC). More recently, recombinant interferon has been shown to have a 10 to 20 percent response rate in the treatment of patients with metastatic malignant melanoma.

Prognosis

The single most predictive factor for overall survival is the depth of invasion of the primary lesion at the time of diagnosis. As a general rule, lesions invading less than 0.76 mm rarely metastasize, whereas those with greater than 1.7 mm depth of invasion frequently metastasize. Other factors that significantly affect prognosis are sex (female better than male) and location of primary site (extremity better than trunk).

References

1. Andren-Sandberg, A., and Ihse, I. Factors influencing survival after total pancreatectomy in patients with pancreatic cancer. *Ann. Surg.* 198: 605, 1983.
2. Baker, L. H. Breast cancer detection demonstration project: Five-year summary report. *CA* 32: 194, 1982.
3. Bast, R. C., Jr., Klug, T. L., St. John, E., et al. A radioimmunoassay using a monoclonal antibody to monitor the course of epithelial ovarian cancer. *N. Engl. J. Med.* 309: 883, 1983.
4. Beasley, R. P., Lin, C. C., Hwang, L. Y., et al. Hepatocellular carcinoma and hepatitis B virus: A prospective study of 22707 men in Taiwan. *Lancet* 2: 1129, 1981.
5. Bonadonna, G., Brusamolino, E., Valaqussa, P., et al. Combination chemotherapy as an adjuvant treatment in operable breast cancer. *N. Engl. J. Med.* 294: 405, 1976.
6. Brechot, C., Nalpas, B., Courouce, A. M., et al. Evidence that hepatitis B virus has a role in liver-cell carcinoma in alcoholic liver disease. *N. Engl. J. Med.* 306: 1384, 1982.
7. Byar, D. P. The Veterans Administration Cooperative Urological Research Group studies of cancer of the prostate. *Cancer* 32: 1126, 1973.
8. Cancer and Steroid Hormone Study of the Centers for Disease Control and the National Institute of Child Health and Human Development. The reduction of risk of ovarian cancer associated with oral-contraceptive use. *N. Engl. J. Med.* 316: 650, 1987.
9. Comis, R. L., Miller, M., and Ginsberg, S. J. Abnormalities in water homeostasis in small cell anaplastic lung cancer. *Cancer* 45: 2414, 1980.
10. Cullinan, S. A., Moertel, C. G., Fleming, T. R., et al. A comparison of three chemotherapeutic regimens in the treatment of advanced pancreatic and gastric carcinoma. Fluorouracil vs. fluorouracil and doxorubicin vs. fluorouracil, doxorubicin, and mitomycin. *J.A.M.A.* 253: 2061, 1985.
11. Earlam, R., and Cunha-Melo, J. R. Oesophageal squamous cell carcinoma: I. A critical review of surgery. *Br. J. Surg.* 67: 381, 1980.
12. Einhorn, L. H., and Williams, S. D. Chemotherapy of disseminated testicular cancer: A random prospective study. *Cancer* 46: 1339, 1980.
13. Ellis, F. H., Jr. Carcinoma of the esophagus. *CA* 33: 264, 1983.
14. Fielding, J. E. Smoking: Health effects and control. Part I. *N. Engl. J. Med.* 313: 491, 1985.
15. Fisher, B., Bauer, M., Margolese, R., et al. Five-year results of a randomized clinical trial comparing total mastectomy and segmental mastectomy with or without radiation in the treatment of breast cancer. *N. Engl. J. Med.* 312: 665, 1985.
16. Foti, A. G., Cooper, J. F., Herschman, H., and Malvaez, R. R. Detection of prostatic cancer by solid-phase radioimmunoassay of serum prostatic acid phosphatase. *N. Engl. J. Med.* 297: 1357, 1977.
17. Gastrointestinal Tumor Study Group. Prolongation of the disease-free interval in surgically treated rectal carcinoma. *N. Engl. J. Med.* 312: 1465, 1985.
18. Gershenson, D. M., Copeland, L. J., Wharton, J. T., et al. Prognosis of surgically determined complete responders in advanced ovarian cancer. *Cancer* 55: 1129, 1985.
19. Gralnick, H. R., Givelber, H., and Abrams, E.

Dysfibrinogenemia associated with hepatoma: Increased carbohydrate content of the fibrinogen molecule. *N. Engl. J. Med.* 299: 221, 1978.

20. Green, M. H., Clark, W. H., Jr., Tucker, M. A., et al. High risk of malignant melanoma in melanoma-prone families with dysplastic nevi. *Ann. Intern. Med.* 102: 458, 1985.

21. Hacker, N. F., Berek, J. S., Lagasse, L. D., et al. Primary cytoreductive surgery for epithelial ovarian cancer. *Obstet. Gynecol.* 61: 413, 1983.

22. Horwitz, R. I., and Feinstein, A. R. Estrogens and endometrial cancer: Responses to arguments and current status of an epidemiologic controversy. *Am. J. Med.* 81: 503, 1986.

23. Hulka, B. S., Chambless, L. E., Kaufman, D. G., et al. Protection against endometrial carcinoma by combination-product oral contraceptives. *J.A.M.A.* 247: 475, 1982.

24. Javadpour, N. Germ cell tumor of the testis. *CA* 30: 242, 1980.

25. Kortz, W. J., Meyers, W. C., Hanks, J. B., et al. Hepatic resection for metastatic cancer. *Ann. Surg.* 199: 182, 1984.

26. Leuprolide Study Group. Leuprolide versus diethylstilbestrol for metastatic prostate cancer. *N. Engl. J. Med.* 311: 1281, 1984.

27. Liebman, H. A., Furie, B. C., Tong, M. J., et al. Des-gamma-carboxy (abnormal) prothrombin as a serum marker of primary hepatocellular carcinoma. *N. Engl. J. Med.* 310: 1427, 1984.

28. Little, A. G., DeMeester, T. R., and MacMahon, H. The staging of lung cancer. *Semin. Oncol.* 10: 56, 1983.

29. Love, S. M., Gelman, R. S., and Silen, W. Fibrocystic "disease" of the breast—A nondisease? *N. Engl. J. Med.* 307: 1010, 1982.

30. MacMahon, H., Courtney, J. V., and Little, A. G. Diagnostic methods in lung cancer. *Semin. Oncol.* 10: 20, 1983.

31. Moertel, C. G., O'Fallon, J. R., Go, V. L. W., et al. The preoperative carcinoembryonic antigen test in the diagnosis, staging and prognosis of colorectal cancer. *Cancer* 58: 603, 1986.

32. National Bladder Cancer Collaborative Group A. Cytology and histopathology of bladder cancer cases in a prospective longitudinal study. *Cancer Res.* 37: 2911, 1977.

33. Nelson, J. H., Jr., Averette, H. E., and Richart, R. M. Dysplasia, carcinoma in situ, and early invasive cervical carcinoma. *CA* 34: 306, 1984.

34. Novadex Adjuvant Trial Organization. Controlled trial of tamoxifen as single adjuvant agent in management of early breast cancer. *Lancet* 1: 836, 1985.

35. Paulson, D. F., Lin, G. H., Hinshaw, W., et al. Radical surgery versus radiotherapy for adenocarcinoma of the prostate. *J. Urol.* 128: 502, 1982.

36. Poplin, E., Fleming, T., Leichman, L., et al. Combined therapies for squamous-cell carcinoma of the esophagus: a Southwest Oncology Group study (SWOG-8037). *J. Clin. Oncol.* 5: 622, 1987.

37. Ramming, K. P., and Haskell, C. M. Stomach Cancer. In C. M. Haskell (Ed.), *Cancer Treatment*, 2d Ed. Philadelphia: Saunders, 1985. Pp. 259.

38. Rao, B. R., and Weist, W. G. Receptors for progesterone. *Gynecol. Oncol.* 2: 239, 1974.

39. Rizk, N. W. Selection of patients with non-small-cell lung carcinoma for surgical resection. *West. J. Med.* 143: 636, 1985.

40. Rosenberg, S. A., Lotze, M. T., Muul, L. M., et al. A progress report on the treatment of 157 patients with advanced cancer using lymphokine-activated killer cells in interlenkin-2 or high-dose interlenkin-2 alone. *N. Engl. J. Med.* 316: 889, 1987.

41. Sculier, J. P., Evans, W. K., Feld, R., et al. Superior vena caval obstruction syndrome in small cell lung cancers. *Cancer* 57: 847, 1986.

42. Sedlacek, S. M., and Horwitz, K. B. The role of progestins and progesterone receptors in the treatment of breast cancer. *Steroids* 44: 467, 1984.

43. Seidman, H., Stellman, S. D., and Mushinski, M. H. A different perspective on breast cancer risk factors: Some implications of the nonattributable risk. *CA* 32: 301, 1982.

44. Spechler, S. J., and Goyal, R. K. Barrett's esophagus. *N. Engl. J. Med.* 315: 362, 1986.

45. Sternberg, C. N., Yagoda, A., Scher, H. I., et al. Preliminary results of M-VAC (methotrexate, vinblastine, doxorubicin and cisplatin) for transitional cell carcinoma of the urothelium. *J. Urol.* 133: 403, 1985.

46. Strickland, R. C., and Schenker, S. The nephrogenic hepatic dysfunction syndrome: A review. *Dig. Dis.* 22: 49, 1977.

47. VanDyke, J. A., Stanley, R. J., and Berland, L. L. Pancreatic imaging. *Ann. Intern. Med.* 102: 212, 1985.

48. Veronesi, U., Adamus, J., Aubert, C., et al. A randomized trial of adjuvant chemotherapy and immunotherapy in cutaneous melanoma. *N. Engl. J. Med.* 307: 913, 1982.

49. Watson, R. A., and Tang, D. B. The predictive value of prostatic acid phosphatase as a screening test for prostatic cancer. *N. Engl. J. Med.* 303: 497, 1980.

50. Winawer, S. J., Melamed, M., and Sherlock, P. Potential of endoscopy, biopsy, and cytology in the diagnosis and management of patients with cancer. *Clin. Gastroenterol.* 5: 575, 1976.

6

Infectious Diseases

John M. Douglas, William F. Ehni,
Richard T. Ellison, Laurel A. Miller, and
J. Joseph Marr

Use of Antimicrobial Agents

The cardinal concept in the use of antimicrobial agents is that no drug, whether bacteriostatic or bactericidal, will be curative in and of itself. All therapy must be chosen after due consideration of the nature of the infecting organism, its rate of multiplication, and the status of the host's defense mechanisms. The physician's evaluation of these considerations, through initial clinical and laboratory assessments of the patient, is of major importance in the subsequent management of an infectious disease.

Clinical Evaluation

There is no substitute for a complete history and physical examination in the evaluation of any patient. This is of particular importance in determining the nature of an infectious process. Since many diseases are a result of interactions with the environment, details of the occupational or travel history may be important as will information regarding other diseases in the family or community. A history of recurring infections may lead to the discovery of an underlying malignant process or deficiency in one of the natural host defense mechanisms (e.g., a skull fracture or chronic sinusitis in recurring bacterial meningitis).

The careful physical examination is an often overlooked valuable source of clues. When an infectious process is under consideration, there should be an emphasis on cutaneous manifestations of bacteremia or viral infections, careful inspection of the fundi for evidence of bacteremia, percussion of the paranasal sinuses, examination of the teeth as sources of bacteria in endocarditis or aspiration pneumonia, percussion of the liver for abscess, careful palpation of the abdomen, and thorough pelvic examination for occult sources of infection, such as perirectal abscess.

The usual laboratory tests are often helpful, but the use of laboratory testing without specific clues to a disease process is generally without value. This applies equally to serologic studies and the various noninvasive radiographic procedures.

The data gleaned from the history, physical examination, and simple laboratory tests generally will be the only information available when a diagnosis must be made and therapy initiated. Microbiologic testing will yield results only after a delay of many hours or days. A knowledge of the most probable organisms associated with common disease processes is helpful. A list of these agents is given in Table 6-1. This is not meant to be inclusive nor to serve as a substitute for careful patient evaluation.

There is a plethora of antimicrobial agents from which to choose. There also is a tendency to select the newer agents which receive publicity or to

Table 6–1. Microorganisms Commonly Isolated from Acute Adult Infection

Skin and subcutaneous tissues:
  Staphylococcus aureus
  Streptococcus pyogenes (group A)
Decubitus ulcers:
  S. aureus
  Gram-negative organisms
Paranasal sinuses:
  S. pneumoniae
  H. influenzae
  Anaerobic organisms
  S. aureus
Lungs:
  S. pneumoniae
  Mycoplasma pneumoniae
  Respiratory viruses
  Gram-negative organisms (hospital-acquired aspiration
    pneumonia)
	Urinary tract:
	  Escherichia coli
	  Other gram-negative organisms
	  S. aureus (after surgery)
	Meninges:
	  S. pneumoniae
	  Neisseria meningitidis
	  Hemophilus influenzae
	  S. aureus (after neurosurgery or trauma)
	  Gram-negative organisms (bacteremia, urinary tract
	    infections)
	Bones (osteomyelitis):
	  S. aureus
	Joints:
	  S. aureus
	  N. gonorrhoeae

employ the broadest-spectrum agents in the mistaken impression that this will be the best choice for the patient. In general, the narrowest-spectrum agent should be chosen, except for the immunocompromised host, in order to minimize the alterations in the host's normal flora, which inevitably lead to superinfection or other complications. A list of the appropriate antimicrobials is given in Table 6-2.

Determination of Infecting Organism
Insofar as possible, therapy should be initiated only after determination of the etiologic agent. Initially, this determination is based primarily on clinical information, but confirmatory laboratory data should always be sought.

GRAM'S STAIN
In the hospital, the major immediate laboratory aid is Gram's stain. Common errors in the use of this method are overdecolorization and misinterpretation of precipitated stain as gram-positive cocci. Much of this may be avoided by smearing a small amount of gingival scrapings on the slide to be heat-fixed and stained along with the material in question. Since the mouth contains large numbers of gram-positive and gram-negative organisms, the finding of both in this control section

assures the physician that the slide is properly stained.

CULTURE
Since the staining characteristics of an organism provide only a general indication as to its identity, adequate culture methods must be used as well. Methods of culturing peculiar to particular disease processes will be discussed in later sections; however, a few general rules will be stated here:

1. When bacteremia is suspected, two or three sets of blood cultures are sufficient.
2. Saliva should not be cultured. If the material that has been obtained from an expectorated specimen does not show leukocytes, then it will be as likely to yield erroneous information as useful information.
3. Body fluids obtained for culture should be taken directly to the laboratory and not allowed to stand. A delay may allow fastidious organisms to die and contaminating organisms to overgrow the pathogen.
4. It is usually best to keep specimens at 37°C during transport.
5. When the possibility of infection by anaerobic organisms exists, the specimen must be cultured under anaerobic conditions as rapidly as possible. A delay of more than 30 minutes may allow fastidious organisms to die.

Table 6–2. *Antimicrobial Agents of Choice*

Organism	Antimicrobial of choice	Alternative agents
Gram-positive cocci:		
Staphylococcus aureus:		
Non-penicillinase producing	Penicillin	A cephalosporin,* vancomycin, clindamycin, erythromycin
Penicillinase producing	A penicillinase-resistant penicillin†	A cephalosporin,* vancomycin, clindamycin, erythromycin
β-Streptococci (groups A,B,C,G)	Penicillin	A cephalosporin,* erythromycin
α-Streptococci (*Streptococcus viridans*)	Penicillin	A cephalosporin,* vancomycin, erythromycin
Streptococcus bovis	Penicillin	A cephalosporin,* vancomycin, erythromycin
Enterococci:		
Endocarditis or other serious infection	Penicillin (or ampicillin) plus gentamicin or streptomycin	Vancomycin plus gentamicin or streptomycin
Uncomplicated urinary tract infection	Ampicillin or amoxicillin	Erythromycin, nitrofurantoin
Streptococcus pneumoniae	Penicillin	A cephalosporin,* erythromycin, chloramphenicol
Gram-negative cocci:		
Neisseria meningitidis	Penicillin	Chloramphenicol, a sulfonamide
Neisseria gonorrhoeae	Ampicillin	Spectinomycin, ceftriaxone
Gram-negative bacilli:		
Acinetobacter spp. (*Mima, Herellea*)	Tobramycin or kanamycin (± carbenicillin)	Sulfisoxazole, trimethoprim-sulfamethoxazole, ± ticarcillin, mezlocillin, piperacillin, doxycycline
Brucella spp.	Tetracycline (± streptomycin)	Chloramphenicol (± streptomycin)
Campylobacter spp.	Erythromycin	Tetracycline, chloramphenicol, gentamicin
Enterobacter spp.	Gentamicin or tobramycin	Carbenicillin, ticarcillin, piperacillin, netilmicin, amikacin, cefotaxime
Escherichia coli:		
Uncomplicated urinary tract infection	Ampicillin, amoxicillin or sulfisoxazole	A cephalosporin,* a tetracycline
Systemic infection	Gentamicin or tobramycin	Ampicillin, a cephalosporin,* ticarcillin, kanamycin, amikacin
Francisella tularensis	Streptomycin	Tetracycline, chloramphenicol
Hemophilus influenzae:		
Meningitis	Chloramphenicol, cefotaxime, or moxalactam	Ampicillin
Other infections	Ampicillin	Trimethoprim-sulfamethoxazole,‡ chloramphenicol, tetracycline, cefamandole

Table 6–2 (continued)

Organism	Antimicrobial of choice	Alternative agents
Klebsiella pneumoniae	Gentamicin or tobramycin	A cephalosporin,* cefotaxime, cefoxitin, cefuroxime, amikacin, chloramphenicol, trimethoprim-sulfamethoxazole‡
Legionella spp.	Erythromycin	Rifampin plus erythromycin
Proteus mirabilis	Ampicillin	Gentamicin or tobramycin, a cephalosporin*
Other *Proteus* spp. (*P. rettgeri*, *M. morganii*, *P. vulgaris*)	Gentamicin or tobramycin	Cefotaxime, ticarcillin, piperacillin, amikacin, kanamycin
Providencia spp.	Gentamicin or tobramycin	Cefotaxime, moxalactam, amikacin, kanamycin, netilmicin, carbenicillin, ticarcillin, mezlocillin, piperacillin
Pseudomonas aeruginosa	Tobramycin or gentamicin, ± ticarcillin, azlocillin, or piperacillin	Amikacin, a polymyxin
Salmonella spp.	Chloramphenicol	Ampicillin or amoxicillin, trimethoprim-sulfamethoxazole‡
Serratia marcescens	Gentamicin or amikacin	Cefotaxime, ticarcillin, tobramycin
Shigella spp.	Trimethoprim-sulfamethoxazole‡	Ampicillin, chloramphenicol
Yersinia pestis	Streptomycin	Tetracycline, chloramphenicol
Anaerobes:		
Anaerobic streptococci	Penicillin	Clindamycin, erythromycin, chloramphenicol
Bacteroides spp.:		
Oropharyngeal strains	Penicillin	Clindamycin, chloramphenicol, metronidazole, cefoxitin
Gastrointestinal strains	Clindamycin	Chloramphenicol, metronidazole, cefoxitin, ticarcillin, piperacillin
Clostridium spp.	Penicillin	Chloramphenicol, clindamycin, metronidazole

*The term *cephalosporin* refers to the first-generation cephalosporins: cephalothin, cefazolin, cephapirin, cephradine, cephalexin, cefactor, cefadroxil.
± Methicillin, nafcillin.
‡Not approved for this indication by the U.S. Food and Drug Administration.
Source: Modified from Mandell, G. L., Douglas, R. G., and Bennett, J.E. *Principles and Practice of Infectious Diseases.* New York: Wiley. 1985. P. 155. Used with permission.

Antibiotic Susceptibility Testing of Isolated Organisms

The importance of sensitivity testing of organisms known for their innate ability to develop resistance cannot be overemphasized. Disk testing, however, does not give information about the concentration of drug necessary for killing the microorganism either in vitro or in vivo; it serves merely as a guide in the choice of an appropriate agent. In serious infections, e.g., subacute bacterial endocarditis, serial dilutions of the patient's serum should be assayed against a standard inoculum of the patient's organism. The highest dilution which kills the inoculum is the minimal bactericidal concentration (MBC). Infection is usually controlled by titers of 1 : 16 or higher. Table 6-3 lists the approximate serum and urine concentrations that may be expected following the administration of the usual doses of antibiotics.

Knowledge of the Susceptibility Patterns of Local Organisms

Since the results of culture and sensitivity tests require 2 or 3 days to be reported, it is usually necessary to treat with an antibiotic that is effective

Table 6–3. *Expected Antimicrobial Concentrations in Adults with Normal Renal Function**

Antimicrobial	Dose and route of administration (adults)	Usual peak serum concentration (μg/ml) 1 h after dose	Usual peak urine concentration (μg/ml)
Amikacin	7.5 mg/kg IM	25	700
Ampicillin	2 gm IV	20	1,600
Amoxicillin	500 mg PO	7	1,500
Ceftazidime	2 gm IV	120	10,000
Cefazolin	1 gm IV	75	4,000
Cefotaxime	2 gm IV	120	5,000
Cefoxitin	2 gm IV	100	5,000
Ceftriaxone	1 gm IV	120	1,000
Cephalexin	500 mg PO	20	1,500
Cephapirin	2 gm IV	50	4,000
Chloramphenicol	1 gm IV	10	200
Clindamycin	600 mg IV	10	20
Dicloxacillin	500 mg PO	10	500
Erythromycin	500 mg PO	1.5	40
Gentamicin	1.5 mg/kg IM or IV	8	150
Imipenem	500 mg IV	40	100
Metronidazole	500 mg PO or IV	15	300
Mezlocillin	3 gm IV	250	3,000
Nafcillin	2 gm IV	30	1,000
Norfloxacin	400 mg PO	1.6	480
Penicillin G	4 million units IV	20	700
Piperacillin	4 gm IV	350	10,000
Sulfadiazine	2 gm PO	100	High
Sulfamethoxazole	1.6 gm PO	100	High
Ticarcillin	3 gm IV	250	3,000
Tobramycin	1.5 mg/kg IM or IV	8	150
Trimethoprim	100 mg PO	1	100
Vancomycin	1 gm IV	30	800

*Note: Actual concentrations vary from patient to patient and depend on multiple factors, including rate of infusion, age, weight, and renal function. The above values are estimates only.

against the organism suspected to be the causative agent. Lists of microorganisms and their antibiotic susceptibilities usually are published by the clinical microbiology laboratory. The physician therefore should be familiar with the susceptibilities of the microorganisms in the hospital in which he or she practices. These may differ from data published in the literature. The initiation of therapy based on probabilities is not a pledge to continue. If testing indicates that the organism is different or has susceptibilities other than expected, therapy should be altered appropriately. As a rule, the most specific (narrowest-spectrum) agent should be selected.

Rate of Growth of the Infecting Agent
Infection by indolent organisms which are metabolizing slowly (subacute bacterial endocarditis abscesses) will require long periods of chemotherapy. Treatment failures in these types of infections usually are not due to an inability to attain the minimal bactericidal concentration in the serum, but rather to early discontinuation of therapy.

Status of the Host's Defense Mechanisms
The physiologic status of the patient will have obvious importance in the choice of therapy, its route of administration, the rapidity with which treatment is initiated, and the possibilities of drug toxicity due to associated disease (e.g., renal failure).

CHOICE OF THERAPY
In a patient with an immunologic deficiency or an infection with an organism that is capable of rapid growth (streptococcal cellulitis) or is virulent either by virtue of its locus of infection (meningitis) or the toxic substances it produces (gas gangrene), the agent of choice is one that is bactericidal.

ROUTE OF ADMINISTRATION
In serious infections and in any situation in which hypotension exists, antimicrobial agents should be given intravenously (IV). In less demanding

circumstances, intramuscular (IM) or oral therapy may be used, but when appropriate, oral therapy is preferred. The physician should ask these questions before using the oral route: (1) Does predictable absorption of the drug occur? (2) Is the patient taking anything else that might interfere with the absorption of the drug? (3) Can blood levels of the antibiotic equivalent to those secured by the parenteral route be obtained orally? The last question incorporates the others, and if it can be answered affirmatively, oral therapy will be adequate.

THE RAPIDITY WITH WHICH THERAPY IS INSTITUTED
This depends entirely on the clinical situation. In many cases the following question may be asked: Is the risk of withholding therapy greater than that involved in starting it? If the answer is affirmative, treatment should be instituted. If not, there may be much to gain by withholding treatment until a definitive diagnosis can be made. If the decision is to treat, therapy should be as complete as possible; partial therapy or temporizing is never indicated.

ASSOCIATED DISEASES INFLUENCING THE CHOICE OR DOSAGE OF A DRUG
Bactericidal agents should be used in patients with impaired host defense mechanisms (e.g., those with leukemias, lymphomas, receiving corticosteroids or antimetabolites, the elderly). Factors influencing the dosage of an antibiotic usually are associated liver or renal disease and the pharmacology of the agent. For example, agents used to treat biliary tract infections should be excreted by the liver; however, in the presence of cirrhosis, drugs metabolized and excreted primarily by the kidney should be used.

A major management problem on the medical ward is the patient with renal insufficiency. The dosages of antibiotics used in such a patient are generally reduced in parallel with the creatinine clearance. Hemodialysis and peritoneal dialysis may further alter the regimen. A general list of antimicrobials and their modifications in renal failure is given in Table 6-4.

Table 6–4. Antimicrobial Use in Patients
with Varying Degrees of Impaired Renal Function

Antimicrobial agents requiring no dosage change
    regardless of renal function:
  Erythromycin, clindamycin, chloramphenicol,
    doxycycline, cefoperazone, oxacillin, cloxacillin,
    dicloxacillin, nafcillin, nalidixic acid, rifampin,
    amphotericin B,* sulfadimidine
Antimicrobial agents requiring dosage change only with
    severe renal failure:
  Penicillin G, amoxicillin, ampicillin, methicillin,
    cephalothin, cephalexin, cefamandole, cefoxitin,
    cefotaxime, ceftizoxime, piperacillin, lincomycin,
    isoniazid, ethambutol, trimethoprim-sulfamethoxazole
Antimicrobial agents requiring dosage change with
    impaired renal function:
  Carbenicillin, ticarcillin, cefazolin, moxalactam,
    streptomycin, kanamycin, gentamicin, tobramycin,
    sisomicin, amikacin, nefilmicin, polymyin B, colistin,
    vancomycin, flucytosine
Antimicrobial agents contraindicated in renal failure:
  Tetracyclines (except doxycycline and possibly
    minocycline), nitrofurantoin, cephaloridine, long-
    acting sulfonamides, methenamine, *para*-
    aminosalicyclic acid

*Even though amphotericin B is excreted primarily by
nonrenal means, this drug must be used with caution in
patient with impaired renal function because of its nephrotoxicity.
Source: Reprinted from Mandell, G. L., Douglas, R. G.,
and Bennett, J. E. *Principles and Practice of Infectious Diseases.* New York: Wiley, 1985. P. 157. Used with permission.

Drug Interactions, Toxicity, and Allergy

In current hospital practice, the patient who is taking more than one drug is the rule rather than the exception. The possibility of drug interactions should be considered by the physician each time he or she prescribes. Since approximately one-third of the patients in any general hospital are receiving antimicrobial agents at any given time,

the potential for toxic and allergic side effects is substantial. The physician must decide on the basis of the risk-benefit ratio of the drug and select accordingly. The need for an aminoglycoside must outweigh its tendency to cause renal failure; the accumulation of any antimicrobial in the presence of renal or hepatic failure must be considered.

Allergic reactions occur in about 5 percent of persons who receive an antimicrobial. There are four major types: type I is IgE-mediated anaphylaxis, type II is an IgG- or IgM-mediated cytotoxicity, type III is an IgG- or IgM-mediated immune complex disease, and type IV is a T-cell-mediated delayed hypersensitivity. If a patient gives a history of an allergic reaction, he or she should be questioned carefully regarding symptoms of the previous episode. Most persons who claim allergy will not have one, and labeling a patient as hypersensitive to an antimicrobial, penicillin being the most common example, may be detrimental to future medical care.

Failure to Respond to Therapy

At times a patient will not respond to the appropriate agent, in which case the reasons for selecting the current therapy must be reconsidered. If no obvious changes are indicated, then the following questions should be asked: (1) Is a previously unsuspected abscess present? (2) Is the fever due to a drug reaction? (3) Has the organism developed resistance? (4) Is the antibiotic penetrating the body space in which the infection is located? (5) Is a superinfection present? (6) Is the isolated organism really the etiologic agent?

Fever of Unknown Origin (FUO)

Prolonged fever without a known etiology can be a difficult problem for both patients and physicians. The large number of possible causes and the myriad tests and procedures available with which to pursue them can be quite a challenge to the physician. Persistence of symptoms without a di-

agnosis despite prolonged hospitalization and testing is frustrating for the patient. The evaluation of fever of unknown origin requires a logical approach, but it must be individualized for each patient.

Fever is a complex biological phenomenon.

Current theory [16] holds that mononuclear phagocytic cells release interleukin I (IL-I) in response to a variety of stimuli. These include microorganisms (via phagocytosis or endotoxin release), antigen-antibody complexes, circulating antigens, and cell-mediated immunity—the latter presumably due to lymphokine release from lymphocytes. IL-I, probably by the local release of prostaglandins in the hypothalamus, activates thermoregulatory neurons. Hypothalamic activity then results in the familiar clinical phenomena of shivering, vasoconstriction, and tachycardia.

There is a circadian periodicity to body temperature. Late afternoon temperatures average 0.8°C higher than early morning temperatures. Further, average daily temperature can vary from as low as 36°C to as high as 38°C. Temperature readings also vary with the site from which they are taken. Axillary temperatures are 1°C cooler and rectal temperatures are 0.5 to 1.0°C higher than oral temperatures. Thus a single reading is of little value, and multiple daily readings from the same site are necessary to document fever.

The standard definition of fever of unknown origin is that of Petersdorf and Beeson [63]. Illness must be of at least 3 weeks' duration with at least 1 week of in-hospital evaluation and multiple documented temperatures of greater than 38.3°C. Although arbitrary, these criteria eliminate low-grade "fevers" which may arise from exaggerated circadian temperature variations, postovulation exercise, pregnancy, meals, or smoking. Also, brief self-limited febrile illnesses, presumably viral, and illnesses easily diagnosed after a thorough history, physical examination, and basic laboratory tests are excluded. Most authors do not include immunosuppressed individuals. Patients meeting the definition for fever of unknown origin then fall into two groups. Some have no evidence for disease other than fever and nonspecific symptoms such as myalgias, arthralgias, malaise, fatigue, and weight loss. Others have historical data, focal physical findings, or specific laboratory abnormalities that suggest certain diagnoses. In the former group it is important

to rule out benign causes with a careful history and physical examination, basic laboratory tests, and daily temperature record. Exaggerated diurnal temperature variations, drug fever, occupational exposures, factitious fever, hereditary periodic fevers (familial Mediterranean fever), and disorders of temperature regulation are examples [88]. A normal sedimentation rate in such a patient who appears well and has a stable weight should limit extensive workup in favor of reassurance and clinical observation.

Evaluation of a Patient with Fever

Documentation of fever is a crucial first step in the evaluation of fever of unknown origin. It is most efficient to allow a relatively well outpatient to measure and record his or her own temperature regularly, although this cannot exclude factitious fevers. Full documentation requires that the patient be observed throughout the temperature-taking process. Absence of peripheral manifestations of fever such as shivering, vasoconstriction, diaphoresis, or tachycardia should raise the question of factitious fever. Pulse rates normally increase 10 to 15 beats per minute for each degree centigrade of fever. A relative bradycardia should suggest typhoid fever, drug fever, and factitious fever.

HISTORY

Although extensive, the differential diagnosis of fever of unknown origin should be kept in mind during the performance of a thorough history and physical examination. If clues are missed here, there will be a delay in reaching the correct diagnosis and the patient may be exposed to unnecessary or even harmful tests. Most causes of fever of unknown origin will be found in three groups of diseases: infectious, neoplastic, and collagen-vascular diseases. They will account for 40, 29, and 15 percent, respectively, of the ultimate diagnoses [15]. The balance will comprise a group of miscellaneous illnesses, and 5 percent will remain undiagnosed. As shown in Table 6-5, the

Table 6–5. *Etiologies of Fevers of Unknown Origin*

Local infection:
    Abscess (abdominal, dental)
    Endocarditis or other intravascular infection
    Hepatobiliary system (hepatic abscess, cholecystitis, cholangitis, empyema of the gallbladder)
    Osteomyelitis
    Genitourinary tract (renal or perinephric abscess, ureteral obstruction with infection, prostatic abscess, pelvic abscess)
    Sinusitis
    Wound infection
    Catheter-associated infection
Systemic infection:
    Bacteria:
        Brucellosis
        Salmonella (typhoid fever)
        Listeriosis
        Disseminated gonococcemia
        Disseminated meningococcemia
        Tularemia
        Rat-bite fever
        Nocardiosis
    Mycobacteria:
        Tuberculosis
        Mycobacterium avium-intracellulare
    Spirochetes:
        Syphilis
        Leptospirosis
    Rickettsia:
        Q Fever
    Chlamydia:
        Psittacosis
    Viral:
        HIV
        Cytomegalovirus
        Epstein-Barr virus
    Hepatitis (A; B; non-A, non-B)
    Fungal:
        Disseminated histoplasmosis
        Cryptococcus
        Candida albicans
        Coccidiomycosis
        Blastomycosis
    Parasitic:
        Malaria
        Toxoplasmosis
        Trichinosis
        Amebic liver abscess
    Other:
        Cat scratch fever

cause of a fever of unknown origin is most often an unusual manifestation of a common disease rather than a rare disorder.

Important aspects of the history include age, race and ancestry, a history of repeated febrile episodes, occupation, travel history, pets, animal contact, insect exposures, eating habits, sexual activity and preference, blood transfusions, intravenous drug abuse, exposures to tuberculosis, and the results of previous skin tests. Past medical history should include previous surgeries and endoscopies because of their risk of abscesses; dental work that can be associated with abscesses, osteomyelitis, and endocarditis; rheumatic fever, and the implantation of any prosthetic devices. Medication history and family history may provide clues to drug fever, heritable disorders, or common exposures. Social history should include a quantitation of alcohol use.

FEVER PATTERN

Fever tends to have a particular pattern. The types usually observed are *sustained* or *continuous* fever with little or no variation throughout the day, *remittent* fever with greater than one degree variation during the day but with the temperature remaining above normal, *intermittent* or *quotidian* fever with daily elevations but with the temperature returning to normal each day, and *relapsing* or *recurrent* fever characterized by a day or more of fever interspersed with one or more days of normal temperature.

The pattern of the patient's fever may be of diagnostic significance as long as it is not altered by antipyretic agents. For this reason, in the evaluation of the patient with fever, one of the most important diagnostic measures is to eliminate antipyretics. This usually causes little discomfort to the patient, as long as the fever is below 40°C, and the information gained from the pattern may be useful. The intermittent fever curve is the most common, and for this reason, it is of limited diagnostic value. If the curve is hectic or septic with wide swings in temperature one or more times a day, a pyogenic infection, usually with abscess formation, should be suspected. Septicemia also may produce this pattern. The double quotidian fever is one that spikes twice in a 24-hour period and returns to the baseline between peaks. In this country the most common disease to cause this is miliary tuberculosis. It also may be caused by gonococcal endocarditis and injudicious antipyretic therapy. Those conditions causing a sustained or continuous fever include injury to the central nervous system, typhoid fever, and rickettsial disease. A relapsing or recurrent fever, sustained for several days before returning to normal, is seen in Hodgkin's disease. In association with this disease it is known as Pel-Ebstein fever. It also may occur in some unusual infections, such as tuberculosis, brucellosis, relapsing fever, and malaria. The periodic use of antipyretic therapy may convert a continuous fever to a relapsing type. A remittent pattern may be seen in brucellosis or typhoid fever and in drug fevers.

PHYSICAL EXAMINATION

Physical examination must be done meticulously and repeatedly, since new findings may appear during the course of the evaluation. Particular attention should be given to skin lesions. A maculopapular rash, petechiae, pustules, splinter hemorrhages, Janeway lesions, Osler's nodes, plaquelike sarcoid lesions, purplish Kaposi's lesions, telangiectasias, or erythema nodosum may be seen in conditions associated with fever of unknown origin. Careful examination of any wounds and indwelling catheters may be helpful. Head and neck examination should include palpation of the temporal arteries, percussion of the sinuses, and careful evaluation of the oropharynx. Thorough auscultation of the heart for murmurs, examination of the abdomen for organomegaly and masses, bimanual pelvic examination, and rectal examination are important. A search for lymphadenopathy, palpation of the spine and bones, and a good neurologic examination must not be omitted.

LABORATORY TESTS

Initial laboratory tests may include a complete blood count with differential, sedimentation rate, biochemical profile, urinalysis, a VDRL test, antinuclear antibody titer (ANA), rheumatoid factor, three sets of blood cultures for aerobic and anaerobic incubation, chest x-ray, and electrocardiogram. Cultures should be held at least 21 days to permit detection of slow-growing organisms. Between 5 and 10 ml serum should be saved to be paired with later samples for subsequent serologic testing. A purified-protein derivative skin test and controls should be placed, although as many as 25 percent of patients with fever of unknown origin may be anergic.

Subsequent Evaluation

All nonessential medications should be discontinued, and appropriate substitutions should be made for any essential medications with a high risk of drug fever [45]. Table 6-6 lists those medications frequently implicated in drug fever.

Table 6–6. Medications Implicated in Drug Fever

Allopurinol	Isoniazid
Amphotericin B	6-Mercaptopurine
Antihistamines	Methyldopa
L-Asparaginase	Nitrofurantoin
Azothioprine	*Para*-aminosalicylic acid
Barbiturates	Penicillins
Bleomycin	Phenytoin sodium
Cephalosporins	Rifampin
Chlorambucil	Quinidine sulfate
Cimetidine	Salicylates
Hydralazine	Streptomycin
Ibuprofen	Sulfonamides
Iodides	Vancomycin

Sources: Compiled from Dinarello, C. A., and Wolff, S. M. Fever of Unknown Origin. In G. L. Mandell, R. G. Douglas, J. E. Bennett (Eds.), *Principles and Practice of Infectious Diseases*, 2d Ed. New York: Wiley, 1985. Pp. 339–347; and Lipsky, B. A., and Hirschmann, J. V. Drug fever. *J.A.M.A.*, 245:851, 1981.

Any suspicion of Epstein-Barr virus or human immunodeficiency virus (HIV) should prompt appropriate antibody determinations. Central neurologic findings require computed tomographic (CT) scanning of the head and a lumbar puncture. Besides routine tests such as cell counts, chemistries, and bacterial culture, one should consider a VDRL test, an india ink preparation, a cryptococcal antigen titer, an acid-fast bacillus (AFB) smear and culture, and fungal culture. Appropriate travel history should lead to examination of peripheral blood smears for malaria, *Borrelia,* and trypanosomes. Any suspicion of sinus, ocular, or neoplastic disease should prompt the performance of sinus films, slit-lamp examination, and serum protein electrophoresis, respectively.

Lymphadenopathy or skin lesions demand early biopsy. Tissue specimens should have a portion sent to the microbiology laboratory for aerobic and anaerobic bacterial, fungal, and mycobacterial cultures and a portion sent to pathology for routine stains, silver stains for fungi, and Ziehl-Neelsen or auramine O stains for mycobacteria. Immunofluorescent staining may be useful in toxoplasmosis, chlamydial infections, vasculitis, and lymphomas.

Complaints or physical findings related to bones demand an x-ray and perhaps a bone scan or CT scan. A new heart murmur may warrant extra blood cultures and an echocardiogram. Suspicion of urinary tract infection or the presence of hematuria may require an intravenous pyelogram, cystoscopy, and/or renal biopsy. Multiple pulmonary emboli can often be diagnosed with a ventilation-perfusion scan, but they may require pulmonary artery angiography.

Evidence of an abdominal process can be pursued with a number of different tests depending on what organ or area of the abdomen is implicated. Upper gastrointestinal series with small bowel follow-through, barium enema, upper and lower endoscopies, oral cholecystogram, ultrasound, CT scan, and liver-spleen scan may be employed. A lower gastrointestinal evaluation in young patients with fever of unknown origin should be considered early in the evaluation, since inflammatory bowel disease presenting solely with fever is not uncommon.

For a number of infectious agents, serology may be the only diagnostic test available. Typhoid fever, hepatitis A and B, brucellosis, Epstein-Barr virus, HIV, toxoplasmosis, *Mycoplasma,* leptospirosis, Q fever, psittacosis, tularemia, *Yersinia,* amebic liver abscess, and some parasitic infections may be diagnosed serologically.

Extensive and Invasive Diagnostic Methods

If the diagnosis has not been made by the foregoing procedures, then the probability of obtaining a diagnosis in a given hospitalization becomes relatively low. There is a tendency to turn to the more expensive or invasive methods to secure a diagnosis. At this point, the patient's record and course should be reviewed and a clinical determination made as to whether further testing should be done or if the patient should be simply observed for several weeks or months to allow the correct diagnosis to declare itself. Further diagnostic procedures should be implemented very circumspectly.

A gallium scan may be done, but in the absence of signs of localized infection, the likelihood of a false-positive or false-negative result outweighs the probability of a successful result; thus it generally is not indicated. The sole exception may be its use in persons infected with HIV in whom a gallium scan of the lungs may be positive and indicate subclinical infection with *Pneumocystis carinii.* Another option is marrow biopsy, which is a relatively innocuous procedure with a 5 to 15 percent diagnostic yield. It may be useful in brucellosis, typhoid fever, tuberculosis, fungal infections (especially histoplasmosis), lymphoma, aleukemic leukemia, and disseminated cancer. Liver biopsy has a similar diagnostic yield but some increased risk, especially in patients with coagulopathies. Mitchell et al. [58] showed that the yield was higher in patients with hepatomegaly and elevated liver function tests.

Table 6–7. Yield of Diagnostic
Procedures in Fevers of Unknown Origin

Laparotomy	30–80 percent
Biopsy	20–35 percent
Clinical course	10–25 percent
Culture	5–15 percent
Radiology	5–10 percent
Autopsy	10 percent
Serology	5–10 percent
Response to empiric therapy	0–10 percent

Sources: Compiled from Petersdorf, R. G., and Beeson, P. B. Fever of unexplained origin: Report on 100 cases. *Medicine* 40: 1, 1961; and Larson, E. B., Featherstone, H. J., and Petersdorf, R. G. Fever of undetermined origin: Diagnosis and follow-up of 105 cases, 1970–1980. *Medicine* 61: 269, 1980.

Several other tests are available to exclude specific diagnoses, such as lymphangiogram for lymphoma and other abdominal tumors, pulmonary arteriography for multiple pulmonary emboli, abdominal arteriography for tumors and polyarteritis nodosa, temporal artery biopsy for temporal arteritis, and directed biopsies of other organs such as kidney and spleen.

The final decision point in the workup is often whether to perform exploratory laparotomy, initiate a therapeutic trial, or observe the patient over time. In general, the marked improvements in noninvasive methods, such as the CT scan, magnetic resonance imaging (MRI) techniques, and ultrasound, have greatly diminished the need for exploratory laparotomy. The yield of laparotomy is 30 to 80 percent in various older studies. Given the morbidity and mortality of the procedure, especially in chronically ill patients, laparotomy is generally recommended only after all noninvasive testing is complete and *only in those patients with indications of an abdominal source for their fever.* Individuals with marked weight loss or with clinical evidence of deterioration or profound illness should be considered for earlier laparotomy, whereas those who are more stable clinically may be observed for a time. Table 6-7 shows the approximate yield of various procedures in

the studies by Petersdorf and Beeson [63] and Larson et al. [41]. The average number of biopsies prior to diagnosis was four.

Therapeutic Trial

The therapeutic trial as a diagnostic measure remains controversial. It should be considered when all other diagnostic measures, except laparotomy, have proven unsuccessful. Too often therapeutic trials are substituted before a thorough investigation of the patient's illness, and these trials do more harm than good. In managing a patient with a fever of unknown origin, the basic principle is *simplify the problem,* and a therapeutic trial may complicate it. For example, a patient with a hidden liver abscess may improve when given corticosteroids. If clinical judgment indicates that none of the organ systems is being seriously impaired by the underlying process, there is no reason to rush into a therapeutic trial. Fever alone is no cause for alarm. Many times a wait of several months will reveal the cause, and this should be considered seriously in anyone who is not clinically ill.

On the other hand, a rapidly advancing life-threatening disease clearly demands a therapeutic trial, especially when the cause of a serious illness has been narrowed to one or two possibilities and the general health of the patient does not permit further investigation, e.g., a person with severe cardiopulmonary disease who has either disseminated tuberculosis or metastatic carcinoma. The administration of antituberculous therapy would be a reasonable course of action in the latter circumstance.

Summary

The majority of patients who continue to have fever despite a thorough diagnostic workup will do well. Of such patients, less than 10 percent die of diseases ultimately related to their fever and 10 to 40 percent may eventually have a diagnosis made. Most either defervesce or continue to have fevers and yet remain clinically stable. The diagnoses in prolonged fevers of unknown origin (greater than 6 to 12 months in duration) are shown in Table 6-8 [1]. In general, the longer the duration of a fever of unknown origin, the less the chance it has an infectious or neoplastic etiology.

Symptomatic therapy after adequate documentation of fever can include acetaminophen, aspirin, or nonsteroidal anti-inflammatory agents. Corticosteroids should be avoided because of the risk of exacerbating an underlying infection.

Table 6–8. *Causes of Prolonged Fevers of Unknown Origin*

Exaggerated circadian temperature variation	27 percent
Uncertain	19 percent
Miscellaneous	13 percent
Factitious	9 percent
Granulomatous hepatitis	8 percent
Neoplasm	7 percent
Still's disease	6 percent
Infection	6 percent
Collagen-vascular disease	4 percent
Familial Mediterranean fever	3 percent

Source: Compiled from Aduan, R. P., Fauci, A. S., and Dale, D. C. Prolonged fever of unknown origin. *Clin. Res.* 26:558A, 1978.

Septicemia

Septicemia is a syndrome characterized by hemodynamic instability and increased vascular permeability which occurs when microorganisms are present in the bloodstream in sufficient numbers that their cell-wall products can exert a pharmacologic effect. The syndrome is associated with viral, rickettsial, and bacterial infections, but it usually refers to the latter. Although gram-positive organisms and *Candida* can produce the syndrome, gram-negative rods are the more common cause, and their presence in the bloodstream generally is associated with some defect in the host defense system.

The syndrome is characterized by fever, hyperventilation, confusion, hypotension, oliguria, acidosis, pulmonary edema, and a bleeding diathesis. Not all elements are present initially, but they are more likely to develop as the disease increases in severity and duration. When hypotension is a significant component, the term *septic shock* is employed.

Epidemiology
Gram-negative sepsis was uncommon prior to antimicrobial chemotherapy. In the last 30 years its frequency has increased steadily [37]. Factors

contributing to this increase include more severe underlying disease, increasing patient age, more frequent and extensive surgery and invasive procedures, greater numbers of catheters, and increasing use of antibiotics, corticosteroids, and immunosuppressive agents. The organisms responsible for gram-negative sepsis are shown in Table 6-9. Patients with *Pseudomonas* bacteremia have the highest mortality rate and those with *E.*

Table 6–9. *Etiologic Agents of Gram-Negative Bacteremia*

Organism	Frequency of isolation (%)
E. coli	31
Klebsiella spp.	12
Pseudomonas spp.	10
Proteus spp.	8
Enterobacter spp.	8
Bacteroides spp.	7
Other	8
Polymicrobial	16

Source: Adapted from Kreger, B. E., Craven, D. E., and McCabe, W. R. Gram-negative bacteremia: IV. Reevaluation of clinical features and treatment of 612 patients. *Am. J. Med.* 68: 344, 1980.

Table 6–10. Sources of Gram-Negative Bacteremia

Site	Frequency of involvement (%)
Urinary tract	34
Gastrointestinal tract	14
Respiratory tract	9
Skin and soft tissue	7
Other known sites	6
Unknown site	30

Source: Adapted from Kreger, B. E., Craven, D. E., and McCabe, W. R. Gram-negative bacteremia: IV. Reevaluation of clinical features and treatment of 612 patients. *Am. J. Med.* 68: 344, 1980.

coli bacteremia have the lowest mortality rate. When mortality rates are analyzed with respect to the severity of the underlying illness, however, these differences are not seen. This implies that *Pseudomonas* infection occurs most commonly in severely ill patients, such as those with extensive burns or neutropenia, whereas *E. coli* sepsis is seen more commonly in less severely ill patients. Most *E. coli* bacteremia originates from urinary or gastrointestinal sources, most *Proteus* bacteremia originates from the urinary tract, and most *B. fragilis* bacteremia comes from the gastrointestinal tract (Table 6-10). The urinary and gastrointestinal tracts make up 70 percent of the identifiable sources of bacteremia; with addition of the respiratory tract, skin, and soft tissues, one can account for over 90 percent. Thus it should be possible to identify a primary site of infection in over 90 percent of septic episodes.

Pathophysiology

Gram-negative bacteremia is the end result of a sequence of events. The first is the presence of gram-negative rods in the local flora. They may be part of the normal flora or colonize a site where they normally are not present. Examples of the latter include the oropharynx in hospitalized patients, as facilitated by debilitation, antibiotics, and factors that reduce salivary flow; the

skin, due to exposure to fecal flora and antibiotics; and the urinary tract, from exposure to fecal flora.

The second event is the establishment of local infection through the loss of normal barriers to microbial invasion. In the gastrointestinal tract this may include ulceration due to trauma, tumor, chemotherapy, surgery, inflammation, and obstruction. In the urinary tract decreased urinary flow, anatomic abnormalities or obstruction, and indwelling catheters are important etiologic factors. Depressed gag and cough reflexes with aspiration of oral material, decreased mucociliary clearance secondary to smoking and/or viral infections, and obstruction contribute to pulmonary infection. Percutaneous catheters, ulcerations, and other wounds interrupt the integrity of the skin to allow local infection. Microbial factors are also important at this stage.

The third step requires persistence of the local infection with subsequent dissemination via the bloodstream. Dissemination is favored by resistance to phagocytosis, which is mediated by the unique capsular composition of certain gram-negative rods. Serum resistance is the ability of certain bacteria to resist the nonspecific killing activity of normal human serum which is mediated by complement. Most bacteremic gram-negative isolates are serum-resistant. Host factors such as dysfunctional neutrophils, neutropenia, hypo- or agammaglobulinemia, and hypocomplementemia limit the host's ability to contain local infection.

Once infection disseminates, the syndrome of septicemia will occur if the microorganisms can persist for a sufficient period in relatively large numbers. The syndrome is apparently due to the presence of the lipopolysaccharide endotoxin in the cell walls of these bacteria and specifically to the lipid A component with its associated proteins. This agent activates Hageman factor (XIII), which, in turn, activates the clotting system, the complement system, and the fibrinolytic system, generates bradykinin, and causes the release of endorphins and catecholamines. Antibody directed against lipid A has been shown to protect animals and humans from sepsis during gram-negative rod bacteremia [101].

The initial hypotension associated with the syndrome is due primarily to the generation of bradykinin, the most powerful vasodilating agent present in the body. In sepsis it can be present at concentrations 100-fold greater than normal. The hypotension may be abetted by the release of endorphins, which are present in all forms of shock. This release can be prevented by the use of corticosteroids and may be one of the reasons why these agents are sometimes useful in the management of shock. The vasodilation causes an increase in the cardiac output, which nevertheless is associated with a decrease in the peripheral arterial pressure and diminished perfusion of the microvascular bed. It is this hypoperfusion which may result in lactic acidosis and the augmented response to catecholamines which also characterize this syndrome.

As the syndrome progresses, the elaboration of catecholamines may cause a progressive tightening of the precapillary sphincters and shunt blood through the metarterioles and away from the capillary bed. This stage is characterized by an increasing peripheral arteriolar resistance, a continually decreasing tissue perfusion, and progressive acidosis. All organ systems are affected by this sequence, but the kidney is one of the most responsive. For this reason, a decreasing urinary output is one of the cardinal signs of progressive septic shock. Since the brain and cardiac vasculature dilate in response to acidosis, the functions of these two organs may appear to be relatively normal when assessed clinically even though acidosis is present. For this same reason, when the ability of these two systems to function begins to deteriorate, it is a grave prognostic sign; they are among the last of the vascular beds to decompensate. This latter response to progressive lactic acidosis is usually irreversible.

The activation of the complement system usually occurs at sites where lipid A has accumulated. The most important of these are the endothelium and the alveolar cells. The generation of C5a at these membranes serves as a chemoattractant for neutrophils, which appear to release oxygen radicals that cause lipid peroxidation and a lessening of membrane integrity. This inability to retain fluid within the vascular system may be worsened by the release of certain prostaglandins as well as by the generation of thromboxane, which can promote local clotting. The sequence occurs throughout the body but is manifest most strikingly in the lungs as pulmonary edema and is given the clinical designation of the adult respiratory distress syndrome (ARDS).

The clotting can worsen by the recruitment of more neutrophils from the marrow, and these young forms can further activate the clotting system and cause disseminated intravascular coagulation, which is a not infrequent concomitant of severe septic shock.

In summary, the syndrome of septicemia is one of vascular instability due to the pharmacologic effects of bacterial endotoxin. It is worsened by the local acidosis due to hypoperfusion, and this acidosis may become generalized as the liver becomes a net producer of lactic acid and the pH of the plasma decreases. The neutrophils participate in the phagocytosis of the endotoxin on the membrane surfaces and appear to damage the membranes in the process. This process worsens the transudation of fluid and results in pulmonary edema. For these reasons, treatment is directed primarily toward the cardiovascular effects of endotoxin and secondarily toward the causative organism.

Clinical Manifestations

The earliest symptoms of sepsis include fever, rigors, malaise, dyspnea, lethargy, and confusion. There also may be tachypnea, tachycardia, and, in more severe or prolonged sepsis, hypotension. Physical examination may show evidence of the local infection responsible for sepsis, usually on abdominal, pulmonary, or skin examination. Evidence for bacteremia includes pustules, vesicles, or bullae, and a bleeding diathesis may be manifest as petechiae or ecchymoses.

Laboratory evaluation will show an initial leu-

Table 6–11. Coagulation Abnormalities
in Gram-negative Bacteremia

Finding	Frequency observed (%)
Thrombocytopenia	56
Other clotting abnormalities*	31
Isolated thrombocytopenia	30
Disseminated intravascular coagulation	11
No clotting abnormalities	36

*Exclusive of thrombocytopenia and disseminated intravascular coagulation.
Source: Adapted from Kreger, B. E., Craven, D. E., and McCabe, W. R. Gram-negative bacteremia: IV. Reevaluation of clinical features and treatment of 612 patients. *Am. J. Med.* 68: 344, 1980.

kopenia that may progress to leukocytosis with a left shift. Thrombocytopenia is seen in 50 percent of patients and is due to disseminated thrombosis and bleeding. A respiratory alkalosis is seen initially and is then complicated by a metabolic acidosis when tissue ischemia occurs. Coagulation abnormalities occur in two-thirds of patients (Table 6-11) and are more frequent among those with more severe underlying disorders. Patients with disseminated intravascular coagulation have a higher rate of shock and death than those with other coagulation abnormalities or a normal coagulation status [39]. Renal insufficiency is common and is accompanied by oliguria; acute tubular necrosis can occur. Abnormalities of liver function are common and may present as cholestasis, hepatocellular damage, or a mixed pattern. Blood cultures are positive in the majority of patients not previously treated with antibiotics. While not all cultures are positive, presumably due to an intermittent bacteremia, three separate blood cultures have at least 90 percent yield. Of these positive cultures, 90 percent become positive in the first 72 hours [99].

Aggressive hemodynamic monitoring is crucial for patients with hypotension, oliguria, or bleeding. About 40 percent of patients with gram-negative rod sepsis will develop shock [39]. Despite this hypotension, initially the extremities are warm because of vasodilation. Cardiac output will be increased, central venous pressure and systemic vascular resistance will be decreased, and a respiratory alkalosis will predominate. As tissue ischemia progresses, patients develop vasoconstriction with cold, pale extremities. Cardiac output will fall as the systemic vascular resistance increases, central venous pressure will remain low, and progressive metabolic acidosis appears. Refractory hypotension and metabolic acidosis indicate a poor prognosis. Death is due to intractable hypotension, hypoxia from pulmonary edema, arrhythmias, uncontrolled bleeding from disseminated intravascular coagulation, and cerebral anoxia.

Prognosis

The mortality from gram-negative sepsis varies from 20 to 80 percent. Prognosis is worse with increasing severity of the underlying disease, granulocytopenia, age greater than 60 years, prior treatment with antibiotics or corticosteroids, preexisting diabetes or congestive heart failure, nosocomial infection, inability to mount a fever in the first 24 hours, polymicrobial bacteremia, development of renal insufficiency or shock, and inappropriate antibiotic treatment [39, 99].

Diagnosis

The diagnosis of sepsis should be suspected in any patient with fever, rigors, tachypnea, tachycardia, or confusion who has developed leukocytosis. Deteriorating renal or clotting function, hypotension, or acidosis should always suggest the possibility of sepsis. Elderly patients may be more difficult to diagnose due to the absence of fever, rigors, and leukocytosis. Patients receiving corticosteroids may have a blunted febrile response and a leukocytosis secondary to the medication. Appropriate cultures and institution of empiric therapy are essential when sepsis is suspected.

Therapy

Treatment consists of supportive measures to maintain circulation, respiration, and coagulation in addition to irradiation of the underlying infection. Mild sepsis usually can be managed by control of the infection. If hypotension is present, intravenous fluids are crucial to support intravascular volume. Appropriate hemodynamic monitoring is necessary to determine pulmonary capillary wedge pressure, cardiac output, systemic vascular resistance, and accurate blood pressure. Pulmonary capillary wedge pressure should be kept at a level sufficient to maintain blood pressure, but levels greater than 20 mmHg may increase the risk of pulmonary edema in patients already predisposed to adult respiratory distress syndrome. Vasopressors are needed if fluids alone cannot reverse hypotension. Dopamine is a good initial choice because it preserves renal perfusion at lower doses than other vasoconstrictors. Higher doses of dopamine or more potent vasoconstrictors may be necessary on occasion. Close monitoring of urine output, acid-base status, arterial oxygen concentration, hematocrit, electrolytes, renal function, and clotting studies is important. Maintaining an appropriate arterial oxygen concentration and circulating red cell mass will limit tissue hypoxia. Reversal of coagulation abnormalities should be attempted when bleeding occurs; administration of vitamin K, fresh-frozen plasma, and platelets may be helpful. The use of heparin in disseminated intravascular coagulation is controversial and may aggravate bleeding. Control of fever with antipyretics and cooling blankets is not necessary unless temperature exceeds 40°C or the patient is uncomfortable.

Successful treatment of the underlying infection may require a combination of antibiotics, drainage of any abscesses, removal of foreign bodies, discontinuation of steroid and cytotoxic medications, elimination of anatomic abnormalities and obstruction, and reconstitution of the immune system. Unless appropriate bacteriologic information is already available, empiric antibiotic therapy must be begun. The advantages of combinations of two drugs against potential gram-negative pathogens include a wider spectrum of coverage, the potential for synergy, and less chance for an organism to have or to develop resistance to both agents. Disadvantages of combination therapy include greater costs and increased risk of toxicity. Therapy with two agents has been proven to be more effective than a single agent only in neutropenic patients. Given the small margin for error in patients with severe sepsis, however, the use of two drugs is prudent. In most situations, a combination of a first-generation cephalosporin and an aminoglycoside given in maximal doses is appropriate. This regimen does not provide optimal coverage for methicillin-resistant staphylococci, enterococci, *H. influenzae, B. fragilis,* or *Pseudomonas aeruginosa.* The choice of aminoglycoside depends on local resistance patterns. An antipseudomonal penicillin (piperacillin) or an antipseudomonal third-generation cephalosporin (ceftazidime) may be substituted if the patient is neutropenic, severely ill, or otherwise at high risk for *Pseudomonas* infection. A third-generation cephalosporin alone may be used in patients who are less ill. Anaerobic coverage with metronidazole, clindamycin, imipenem, cefoxitin, or chloramphenicol should be employed in infections originating in the gastrointestinal or female genital tracts (e.g., septic pelvic thrombophlebitis) in which anaerobes are considered to be important causes of infection. Anaerobic bacteria are important in aspiration pneumonia, but they are much less likely to produce penicillinase and may be successfully treated with penicillins or clindamycin.

Control of blood sugar levels to less than 200 μg/dl will improve neutrophil function in diabetes mellitus. Gamma globulin replacement in the hypo- or agammaglobulinemic patient is worthwhile.

The use of corticosteroids in septic shock is controversial, and studies exist that show benefit, no effect, and even increased mortality in patients so treated. Theoretically, corticosteroids may stabilize endothelial membranes, block the release of beta-endorphins, and interfere with complement activation. Given the lack of solid clinical data, however, their use cannot be advocated [77].

Naloxone, an opiate antagonist, has been shown to ameliorate endotoxin-induced hypotension in humans, presumably by antagonizing the effect of endogenous opiates (beta-endorphin) [62]. The effect is seen within minutes but wanes in 20 to 45 minutes, so continuous administration is required. The effect is blocked by corticosteroids and requires an intact hypothalamic-pituitary axis.

Treatment of gram-negative sepsis in humans with antibodies to lipid A has been shown to increase survival in sepsis and septic shock [101]. While this is an encouraging development, mortality was still 44 percent in septic shock and 22 percent in sepsis overall despite antibody treatment. This form of therapy is not widely available at present.

Granulocytopenia

Neutropenic patients are defined as those with fewer than 1000 neutrophils per cubic millimeter of circulating blood. This condition is seen most frequently in patients treated for malignancies with chemotherapeutic agents. These patients are predisposed to infection with bacterial and fungal organisms. Broad-spectrum empiric antibiotic coverage must be initiated immediately after a febrile episode because of the high mortality associated with a delay in therapy while awaiting culture results [72]. Antibiotics must be continued until the neutrophil count exceeds 1000/mm^3. Patients with fever unresponsive to antibiotics for 1 week should receive empiric amphotericin B therapy [8]. Granulocyte transfusions have not been of consistent benefit in clinical studies and carry the risk of cytomegalovirus infection and pulmonary damage. They are not used in most clinical situations.

Cutaneous Infections

Cutaneous infections may be either primary infections of the skin and subcutaneous tissues or manifestations of more generalized diseases such as bacteremia, viremia, endocarditis, and disseminated fungal infections. The important cutaneous manifestations of systemic infections or other diseases are described in the respective sections. Although there are many primary dermal infections, which vary in their etiologies from one geographic region to another, there are some common themes. These few can be grouped under the headings of staphylococcal and streptococcal infections. They are of most importance to the practitioner of medicine.

Pathophysiology

The intact skin is a very effective barrier against invasion by microorganisms. Few have the innate ability to penetrate the skin and must gain access by some physical means, e.g., an arthropod vector, trauma, the surgical knife, an intravenous catheter. The papovavirus (warts) is an exception. The antimicrobial properties of the skin are poorly understood, but it is clear that the dryness, the mild acidity (pH 5 to 6), and the normal skin flora act in concert to prohibit infection. Inflamed skin is more permeable to water, and if the skin is covered by an occlusive dressing, its humidity can become quite high enough to encourage the growth of gram-negative rods and Candida. Oily skin also may retard the evaporation of water and encourage similar overgrowth.

Mucous membranes support a larger number of microorganisms but also offer mechanical resistance and are bathed in antimicrobial secretions. Cervical mucus, prostatic fluid, and tears are toxic to many microorganisms by virtue of the presence of lysozymes (especially active against gram-positive organisms) and specific immunoglobulins, especially IgG and IgA. The latter blocks attachment of some organisms.

Manifestations of Cutaneous Infections

Infections that enter the skin from without will usually provoke an acute inflammatory response with the formation of pus which may be contained in a small area or which may spread along fascial planes. In areas where the skin is bound tightly to the underlying tissues, ischemia may occur from the increased tissue pressure. Bacteria which appear in the skin from a bacteremia caused by infection at another site also will provoke an inflammatory response, but this may be muted by the presence of antibodies which have appeared as the distant infection developed. These infected cutaneous sites are more contained, as, for example, in the cutaneous manifestations of endocarditis.

Infections that are normally controlled by the cell-mediated immune response will excite an acute inflammatory reaction in the skin when they appear for the first time. Thus inoculation tuberculosis or blastomycosis will be associated with a slowly spreading infection and lymphangitis until it is brought under control by the immune response. The same diseases, when reactivated later in life from a previously dormant pulmonary focus may metastasize to the skin, but there will be little or no inflammatory response.

Most cutaneous infections, either in normal or newly damaged skin, are caused by streptococci and staphylococci. Gram-positive organisms can resist the dryness of normal skin; gram-negative bacilli cannot. In chronically damaged skin, such as burns or decubitus ulcers, the wetness and exposure to other microbial flora result in superinfections by anaerobes and gram-negative rods. For this same reason, swimmer's ear, an otitis externa usually caused by *Pseudomonas* or other gram-negative rod, occurs only when the skin of the external canal remains chronically wet.

Staphylococcal Infections

Staphylococcal infections often are contained in a relatively small area as a folliculitis or a furuncle. They also can manifest as a spectrum from furuncles to severe disease such as carbuncles and nec-rotizing fasciitis or produce a cellulitis that resembles streptococcal disease. These infections are caused by organisms which are part of the normal flora and have gained entrance due to a break in the skin. Elek demonstrated, about 50 years ago, that it was necessary to place about 100,000 staphylococci on the unbroken skin in order to cause an infection, whereas if the organisms were placed on a suture and passed through the skin, then 100 would suffice. Surgical infections and intravenous catheter-induced phlebitis are excellent examples of this principle. Furuncles are so commonly caused by staphylococci that the etiology can be presumed on the appearance of the lesion alone. Carbuncles develop when the infection extends along fascial planes, creating a larger abscess with draining fistulas. They are usually located in the intertriginous areas, scalp, face, upper back, or posterior neck because of their origin in hair follicles.

Staphylococci frequently are associated with group A streptococci as causes of impetigo (see below). They also can cause other syndromes which are more typically assigned to streptococci, such as lymphangitis, staphylococcal scarlet fever (a toxin-induced disease), erysipelas, and fasciitis.

Although treatment must be individualized, there are some generalizations. Staphylococci should be considered resistant to penicillin G until proven otherwise. A beta-lactamase-resistant semisynthetic penicillin, such as dicloxacillin, oxacillin, or nafcillin, is the drug of choice. Cephalosporins are alternatives, but those which are more likely to be effective against staphylococci, such as the first- or second-generation drugs, should be chosen. Minor infections will respond to erythromycin, which is considerably less expensive than semisynthetic penicillins or cephalosporins. While oral therapy is adequate for minor infections, parenteral treatment is indicated for infections which are more severe or in which the extent of disease is not certain. Because of the propensity of these organisms to form abscesses, therapy may be required for prolonged periods or surgical drainage may be needed. The latter should be considered when the patient is first seen or if the infection does not resolve within an appropriate period.

Streptococcal Infections

Group A streptococcal infections characteristically spread rapidly along lymphatics and fascial planes. Organisms in a small wound in the finger can move to the axillary lymphatics in several hours. A rapidly spreading fasciitis often will require extensive surgery to debride the area and prevent ischemic necrosis from the edema—especially when the infection occurs in a tightly constrained compartment such as the hand or forearm.

Impetigo begins insidiously and follows a protracted course. Small vesicles form initially, usually on the face, and develop into pustules with crusting. Regional adenopathy is common. Although group A streptococci are the primary cause, *S. aureus* superinfects most lesions. These infections persist for about 2 weeks in the absence of antibiotic therapy; treatment shortens the course substantially. Penicillin is adequate, since group A streptococci remain very sensitive. If healing is not evident within a few days, then therapy may have to be changed to erythromycin or a semisynthetic penicillin to treat penicillinase-producing staphylococci which are present. Generally, penicillin is adequate. This infection is easily spread by scratching to other parts of the body and to other persons who touch the lesions.

Lymphangitis is a seemingly minor consequence of a local streptococcal infection. It should be treated early and watched carefully, however, since this complication can progress to sepsis and death or to an extensive fasciitis in a matter of hours. Penicillin is the drug of choice. Fasciitis is often more extensive than is appreciated by observation. The infection spreads along superficial and deep fascial planes and may be preceded by a rapidly advancing red margin. The edema is generally extensive. Treatment requires immediate parenteral penicillin and thorough surgical debridement.

Decubitus Ulcers and Diabetic Foot Ulcers

While the majority of cutaneous infections are caused by streptococci and staphylococci, decubitus ulcers are generally infected with gram-negative rods and anaerobic organisms. These are mixed bacterial infections which reflect the normal flora of the skin in that area. They may be indolent, but they can progress rapidly. The clinical spectrum includes uncomplicated ulcers without soft-tissue inflammation, cellulitis with or without abscesses, necrotizing fasciitis, cellulitis with gas formation in the soft tissues, and osteomyelitis as complications. Septicemia is not uncommon with more severe infections.

Ulcers in the diabetic foot often penetrate into the inner tissue compartments and progress to cellulitis or osteomyelitis. Since these infections begin at the surface and enter the deeper tissues, they are polymicrobial and contain both aerobes and anaerobes. The host response is compromised by microangiopathy and neuropathy. As a result, the individual often does not know the extent of the infection and seeks medical attention late in its course. Healing is compromised by the decreased blood supply, and therapy is correspondingly protracted. If osteomyelitis is present, it frequently is not possible to cure the infection medically, and surgical intervention is required. The amount of surgical debridement will be governed by the extent of the infection and the degree of vascular and neurologic compromise.

Treatment for each of these ulcers must be individualized and will depend on the extent of the ulcer, the degree of cellulitis, and the presence of underlying osteomyelitis. Often surgical debridement of the infected areas is necessary, particularly in the case of the diabetic foot, and measures to prevent pressure on the infected areas should be implemented. Broad-spectrum antibiotic treatment usually is necessary in the treatment of the diabetic foot. This may include an aminoglycoside with another agent. This can be clindamycin or an extended-spectrum penicillin or a second-generation cephalosporin. Cefoxitin may be effective as a single agent because of its relatively broad coverage of anaerobes and aerobes. Imipenem alone provides treatment for most of the organisms associated with diabetic foot infections. Definitive therapy depends on the results of cultures.

Decubitus ulcers usually require debridement and little or no antibiotic therapy unless there is an underlying cellulitis or osteomyelitis.

Lower Respiratory Tract Infections

Bronchitis

Acute bronchitis is an inflammation of the major airways caused primarily by *Mycoplasma pneumoniae* and the respiratory viruses. These include rhinoviruses, coronaviruses, parainfluenza viruses, influenza viruses, and adenoviruses. Very rarely, a bacterial superinfection with *S. pneumoniae* or *H. influenzae* may develop. The major clinical manifestations are hoarseness, low-grade fever, and a nonproductive cough. The development of high fever and a productive cough suggests either pneumonia or bacterial superinfection. Physical examination and laboratory studies, including the peripheral white blood cell (WBC) count and chest roentgenogram, are typically unremarkable. Only symptomatic therapy is indicated unless bacterial infection is suspected by clinical findings and a sputum Gram stain showing polymorphonuclear leukocytes and a single predominant bacterial organism. Either ampicillin (250 to 500 mg orally every 6 hours) or trimethoprim-sulfamethoxazole (80–400 mg every 12 hours) is effective.

Chronic bronchitis, a daily productive cough for at least 3 months at a time for 2 or more years, occurs predominantly in individuals with chronic airway damage from tobacco abuse. It also can arise from alteration of the mucociliary transport system of the bronchi due to other inhaled irritants, inherited ciliary abnormalities, or IgA deficiency. In contrast to normal individuals, the major airways of the chronic bronchitic are chronically colonized with oral bacteria including *S. pneumoniae* and *H. influenzae*. Individuals with chronic bronchitis may suffer from acute exacerbations manifest by changes in sputum color, consistency, and amount and associated with worsened pulmonary function. In most instances, the exacerbations are related to respiratory virus or *M. pneumoniae* infection. The potential contribution of bacterial pathogens to these exacerbations remains undefined, and the role of antibiotics is controversial. The primary therapy for these exacerbations is the more intensive use of bronchodilators and corticosteroids. In moderately ill patients with acute exacerbations, prospective randomized trials have not demonstrated any benefit of antibiotics [61]. However, with severe exacerbations it is probably not unreasonable to add an oral antibiotic to the more intensive bronchodilator therapy. Tetracyclines, ampicillin, or trimethoprim-sulfamethoxazole are used in this setting.

Pneumonia

Acute pneumonia remains a leading cause of morbidity and mortality as both a common community-acquired illness and a major nosocomial infection. While relatively few pathogens cause the majority of community-acquired disease, a large number of pathogens can occasionally be implicated (Table 6-12). In adolescents and adults, the influenza viruses, *S. pneumoniae,* and *Mycoplasma pneumoniae* have been the most frequently recognized community-acquired pathogens, with mycoplasmal disease predominating in the younger population [59]. *Streptococcus pneumoniae* is the most common agent in patients requiring hospitalization; mixed anaerobic bacteria and gram-negative bacilli, including *H. influenzae* and *Klebsiella pneumoniae,* are additional important pathogens in the elderly and individuals

Table 6–12. Pathogens of Community-Acquired Pneumonia

Viral:
    Influenza A and B
    Parainfluenza
    Adenovirus
    Varicella
    Measles
    Cytomegalovirus
Bacterial:
    Streptococcus pneumoniae
    Hemophilus influenzae
    Mixed oral aerobic and
        anaerobic species
    Legionella pneumophila
    Legionella species
    Staphylococcus aureus
    Neisseria meningitidis
    Streptococcus pyogenes
    Streptococcus viridans
    Branhamella catarrhalis
    Escherichia coli
    Klebsiella pneumoniae
    Acinetobacter species
    Francisella tularensis
    Yersinia pestis
    Nocardia asteroides
    Actinomyces israelii

Mycobacterial:
    Mycobacterium tuberculosis
    Mycobacterium kansasii
    Mycobacterium avium-
        intracellulare
Mycoplasmal:
    Mycoplasma pneumoniae
Chlamydial:
    Chlamydia psittaci
    TWAR strain
    Chlamydia trachomatis
Rickettsial:
    Coxiella burnetti (Q fever)
Fungal:
    Histoplasma capsulatum
    Coccidioides immitis
    Aspergillus species
    Cryptococcus neoformans
    Blastomyces dermatitidis

compromised by chronic alcohol consumption. Recently, *Legionella pneumophila* and the TWAR strain of *Chlamydia psittaci* have been recognized as causes of community-acquired pneumonia, but their relative importance is still to be defined [100, 26]. With nosocomial pneumonia, the most frequent single pathogen is again *S. pneumoniae,* but in this setting enteric gram-negative bacilli, *S. aureus,* mixed anaerobes, and *L. pneumophila* are also frequent pathogens [4]. Immunocompromised individuals may develop pneumonia due to a wide spectrum of unusual microorganisms, the nature of which will depend on the clinical setting. Community-acquired pneumonia usually presents as one of three patterns: acute lobar pneumonia, atypical generalized pneumonia, or aspiration pneumonia. Lobar pneumonia primarily develops in middle-aged or elderly patients with underlying chronic medical disease and oc-

curs during the winter or early spring following an upper respiratory tract viral infection. The predominant pathogens include *S. pneumoniae, H. influenzae,* and *L. pneumophila.* It begins with the abrupt onset of high fever and shaking chills, accompanied by a cough productive of yellow-green to rusty sputum. Pleuritic pain over the involved lung is common; tachypnea and tachycardia are present. Physical examination finds percussion dullness, increased tactile and vocal fremitus, and bronchovesicular breath sounds with crepitant inspiratory rales. The chest roentgenogram reveals dense lobar consolidation of one or more lobes (Fig. 6-1). Pleural effusions are not uncommon. The peripheral white blood cell count shows a neutrophil predominance and a shift to immature forms, whereas the total white blood cell count is usually elevated; a count less than 5000 in this setting is a poor prognostic finding suggesting fulminant infection.

Atypical pneumonia is usually seen in adolescents or young adults and presents with a 3- to 4-day prodrome of malaise, myalagias, coryza, headache, nonproductive cough, and low-grade fever. *Mycoplasma pneumoniae* is the most common agent, although the TWAR species of *C. psittaci* and the less common agents of psittacosis, coccidioidomycosis, and histoplasmosis produce the same syndrome. Physical examination may reveal some localized crackles, but other chest findings are not impressive. Chest roentgenograms reveal diffuse, patchy infiltrates that are often out of proportion to the physical findings (Fig. 6-2). Lower lobe involvement is common, and pleural effusions are unusual. The white blood cell count is normal or only mildly elevated with a normal differential.

Aspiration pneumonia occurs in patients with depressed gag and cough reflexes due to underlying neurologic disease or to the use of CNS depressants such as alcohol. The findings depend on the material aspirated [32]. The aspiration of gastric acid may produce an immediate intense chemical pneumonitis; the aspiration of particulate material can occlude airways and produce

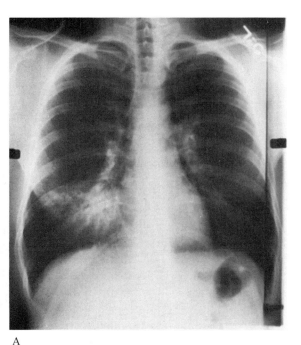

A

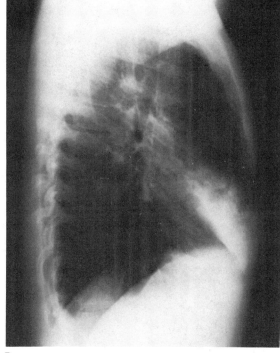

B

Figure 6–1. Chest roentgenogram of a patient with a right middle lobe pneumococcal pneumonia. (A) Posteroanterior view. (B) Lateral view.

atelectasis and recurrent localized infection. More commonly, the aspiration of large amounts of oropharyngeal secretions causes an indolent pneumonia due to mixed aerobic and anaerobic oral flora. Fever, chills, anorexia, weight loss, and a cough productive of foul-smelling sputum gradually develops over a 1- to 2-week period. The process is characteristically localized to gravitationally dependent lobes, and pleural involvement is common. The peripheral white blood cell count is usually elevated. If aspiration pneumonia is not recognized early, it will frequently progress to the development of a lung abscess.

DIAGNOSIS

While the clinical presentation suggests probable pathogens, in severely ill patients blood cultures and lower respiratory tract secretions should be studied. An expectorated sputum sample should be observed for amount, purulence, color, and odor, and a representative portion of mucopurulent material should be examined with a Gram-stained smear. The presence of more than 25 polymorphonuclear leukocytes or columnar epithelial cells and fewer than 10 squamous epithelial cells per $100\times$ field is indicative of lower respiratory tract material with little oropharyngeal contamination [60]. Since the sputum sample is contaminated with oropharyngeal flora, the culture results should be used only to corroborate the presence of an organism identified by Gram-stained smear and should be ignored if they do not correlate with the microscopic findings. In a severely ill patient who cannot spontaneously produce sputum, lower respiratory secretions should be obtained by nasotracheal suctioning, fiberoptic flexible bronchoscopy, or transtracheal

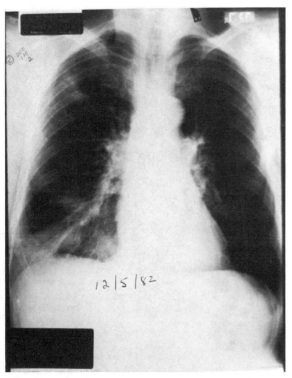

Figure 6–2. *Posteroanterior chest roentgenogram of a patient with mycoplasmal pneumonia and patchy right lower lobe and right upper lobe and left lower lobe infiltrates.*

aspiration. Any pleural effusion associated with a pneumonic process should be aspirated for diagnosis. In the immunocompromised patient it is particularly important to consider these additional approaches, since the potential causes are so diverse [80]. If a diagnosis is not established by these techniques in the immunocompromised patient, an open lung biopsy should be considered.

Pulmonary embolism, atelectasis, congestive heart failure, neoplasia, hypersensitivity pneumonitis, collagen-vascular diseases, sarcoidosis, tuberculosis, and lipoid pneumonia are other diagnostic considerations in the evaluation of a pulmonary infiltrate, and these should be investigated by appropriate studies.

TREATMENT

The management of pneumonia depends on the clinical setting. Young individuals without underlying illness who develop uncomplicated pneumonia can be managed as outpatients. Most other patients should be hospitalized. For outpatient treatment, pneumococcal pneumonia can be treated effectively with procaine penicillin (300,000 to 600,000 units IM twice a day for 7 to 10 days) or phenoxymethyl penicillin V (250 mg orally four times a day for 7 to 10 days). Penicillin-allergic patients can receive erythromycin (500 mg orally every 6 hours) or trimethoprim-sulfamethoxazole (160-800 mg orally every 12 hours for 7 to 10 days). Presumed mycoplasmal or TWAR pneumonia can be treated with erythromycin (500 mg orally every 6 hours) or tetracycline (500 mg orally four times a day) for 7 to 10 days.

For patients requiring hospitalization, the initial antibiotic therapy should be based on the clinical presentation and examination of the sputum Gram stain. Patients with presumed pneumococcal disease can be treated with intravenous penicillin G. As infections with relatively resistant *S. pneumoniae* are being increasingly noted, seriously ill patients should initially receive 1 to 2 million units every 4 hours until results of susceptibility testing are available; susceptible strains can then be treated with 600,000 units penicillin G intravenously every 6 hours. Ampicillin (1 to 2 gm intravenously every 4 hours) or trimethoprim-sulfamethoxazole (160-800 mg intravenously every 12 hours) is appropriate for patients with either mixed flora or small coccobacillary gram-negative bacteria on Gram's stain.

Presumed aspiration pneumonia can be managed initially with aqueous penicillin G (1.5 to 2 million units intravenously every 4 hours) or clindamycin (600 to 900 mg intravenously every 8 hours) with intravenous therapy continued for 7 to 10 days and oral treatment continued until the chest roentgenogram stabilizes.

Treatment of nosocomial pneumonia should be

guided by both the sputum Gram stain and knowledge of the predominant nosocomial flora. Frequently, intensive care units become colonized with highly resistant bacteria, and therapy should be directed against these pathogens. Where this is not a problem, therapy should be guided by the sputum Gram stain. If the sputum is nondiagnostic, a first-generation cephalosporin and an aminoglycoside or a third-generation cephalosporin (such as cefotaxime, ceftizoxime, or ceftriaxone) could be used. Therapy for the immunocompromised patient with fever and pulmonary infiltrates depends on the underlying predisposing condition and should be guided by the results of specific diagnostic studies.

PREVENTION

Prevention of pneumonia should be considered in the elderly and chronically ill. Immunization against influenza with a killed-virus vaccine is 70 to 80 percent effective. It should be considered for individuals with chronic cardiovascular or pulmonary disorders, residents of nursing homes or long-term care facilities, persons older than 65 years, and individuals with chronic metabolic diseases, renal failure, anemia, immunosuppression, or asthma severe enough to require regular follow-up. To prevent spread within a hospital, all hospital personnel working with patients in high-risk groups should be vaccinated. Additionally, amantidine (200 mg per day orally) is an effective prophylactic agent for influenza A and can be used to protect nonimmunized high-risk individuals during epidemics with this virus.

The efficacy of polyvalent vaccine against *S. pneumoniae* remains controversial [9]. However, the vaccine is relatively nontoxic and should be considered for the same patient populations as for influenza vaccine. Since the majority of patients who develop pneumococcal disease have been hospitalized recently, an effective vaccination strategy is to immunize all high-risk patients upon discharge from the hospital.

Empyema

Contiguous parapneumonic sympathetic pleural effusions may develop in association with pneumonia due to *S. pneumoniae*, *H. influenzae* type B, *S. aureus*, group A *Streptococcus pyogenes*, or mixed anaerobes. Less commonly, bacterial empyema occurs. This usually presents as new or continued fever in a patient with pneumonia and may or may not be associated with pleuritic pain. With empyema there may be an elevated peripheral white blood cell count with a shift to immature forms, and the chest roentgenogram may demonstrate loculated pleural fluid. The most important diagnostic study is an examination of the pleural fluid by thoracentesis. Typically, these effusions are exudates rather than transudates, meeting one of the following criteria: LDH > 200 units, LDH ratio > 0.6, or pleural fluid–blood protein ratio > 0.5. The finding of gross pus or bacteria on pleural fluid Gram stain or culture confirms a diagnosis of empyema. An exudative effusion with a pleural fluid pH less than 7.0 or a pleural fluid glucose level less than 40 mg/dl also indicates an empyema [44]. Pleural fluid cell counts are not diagnostically discriminatory, although a predominance of mononuclear cells is atypical in this setting and suggestive of another disease process.

Uncomplicated parapneumonic effusions often can be managed expectantly with systemic antibiotic therapy alone. If the effusion does not resolve over the course of several days, chest tube drainage should be employed. Bacterial empyema requires both appropriate antibiotic therapy and immediate chest tube drainage, although complicated empyemas may eventually require a pleural decortication.

Infective Endocarditis

The manifestations of bacterial endocarditis range from an indolent, nonspecific febrile illness that may go undiagnosed for prolonged periods of time to a fulminant disease with sepsis and rapid cardiac decompensation. Bacterial endocarditis is defined as an infection on one of the cardiac valves or the endocardium, such as the chordae tendineae, papillary muscles, or mural surface of the ventricle. Bacterial endarteritis, infection of an arterial wall, conceptually is identical. This occurs on the pulmonary artery with patent ductus arteriosus, on the aorta in the presence of a coarctation, and in prosthetic arterial graft infections.

Pathophysiology

Blood flowing from a high-pressure to a low-pressure area through an orifice causes turbulence and promotes infection on the low-pressure side [89]. For example, in aortic insufficiency, turbulence occurs on the ventricular side of the valve and a jet of blood streams through the chamber during diastole to strike the chordae tendineae. The turbulence and jet flow cause endothelial damage and expose the underlying collagen framework. Platelet aggregates form over this defect, and fibrin subsequently deposits. A vegetation is created that is initially sterile; however, vegetations may become infected during transient bacteremias that occur with trauma to any colonized mucosal surface. The adherence characteristics of the cell surface of gram-positive organisms explain the prevalence of staphylococci and streptococci in endocarditis. Other organisms, such as gram-negative rods, lack this type of surface. The organisms in a vegetation are protected from the host's immunologic system by the platelet and fibrin meshwork of the vegetation and by the avascular nature of the valve leaflet or chordae tendineae. The inability of polymorphonuclear leukocytes, antibody, and complement to reach the organisms in an effective manner explains why untreated bacterial endocarditis is almost uniformly fatal.

Acute bacterial endocarditis occurs on both normal and previously damaged heart valves. It is caused by organisms of higher virulence such as *S. aureus* and the pneumococci. Subacute bacterial endocarditis occurs on previously damaged heart valves and is caused by organisms with lower virulence such as viridans streptococci and *S. epidermidis*. The initial valvular damage may be secondary to intravenous drug abuse, congenital heart disease, degenerative heart disease such as calcific aortic stenosis and calcified mitral annulus, abnormal chordae tendineae as in mitral valve prolapse, or rheumatic fever.

Although the mitral valve is affected most often in infective endocarditis, the incidence of aortic valve involvement is increasing. This probably reflects the declining incidence of rheumatic heart disease and the increasing incidence of acute endocarditis from intravenous drug abuse and nosocomial infection, which more frequently involve the aortic valve. The tricuspid valve is involved less often than either of the left-sided valves, but it is a common site of involvement in intravenous drug users. Involvement of the pulmonic valve is unusual. Multiple-valve infection is not uncommon in situations where the degree of bacteremia is higher.

Organisms are present in high density within a vegetation and are continually shed into the bloodstream to produce a constant bacteremia. This sustained antigenic stimulation results in high titers of antibodies that form antigen-antibody complexes with free bacterial antigens. A vasculitis may result at endothelial sites where antigen-antibody complexes are deposited and is manifested most commonly as glomerulonephritis. Portions of the growing vegetations may embolize to cause both metastatic infection and infarction. Metastatic suppurative infection is more common with the pyogenic cocci that cause acute endocarditis than those organisms involved in

Table 6–13. *Frequency of Clinical Manifestations in Endocarditis*

Symptom	Percent	Sign	Percent
Fever	80	Fever	90
Musculoskeletal:		Heart murmur	85
Arthralgias	40	Embolic phenomena	50
Arthritis	30	Skin lesions	18–50
Myalgias	20	Splenomegaly	20–57
Chills	40	Clubbing	12–52
Weakness	40	Retinal lesions	2–10
Dyspnea	40		
Diaphoresis	25		
Anorexia	25		
Weight loss	25		
Malaise	25		
Cough	20		
Skin lesions	20		
Stroke	20		
Nausea and vomiting	20		

Source: Adapted from Scheld, W., and Sande, M. A.   Endocarditis and Intravascular Infections. In G. L. Mandell, R. G. Douglas, and J. E. Bennett (Eds.), *Principles and Practice of Infectious Diseases,* 2d Ed. New York: Wiley, 1985. Pp. 504–530.

subacute endocarditis. Local tissue damage at the site of the infection causes progressive valvular damage and insufficiency.

Diagnosis

The diagnosis of bacterial endocarditis may be difficult because the presenting symptoms and signs are both varied and nonspecific. Any combination of local valvular damage, systemic emboli with metastatic infection or infarction, vasculitis, or sepsis may confront the physician. A history of previous heart disease, rheumatic fever, heart murmur, cutaneous infection, intravenous catheters or drug abuse, procedures known to induce bacteremia, or antibiotic use is important. Table 6-13 lists the common presenting symptoms in bacterial endocarditis. Although fever is the most frequent sign, uremic patients, the elderly, and those previously treated with antibiotics may be afebrile.

In acute endocarditis the history is that of sudden onset of fever, chills, and malaise. Intravenous drug abuse is a frequent cause of acute endocarditis, and pulmonary complaints may occur because of septic pulmonary emboli and pneumonia. Symptoms of congestive heart failure may be seen early in acute endocarditis because of the invasive nature of the organisms. Subacute endocarditis has a more insidious onset with an estimated 2 weeks elapsing between the event likely to have caused the inciting bacteremia and the onset of symptoms. Another 5 weeks usually pass before the correct diagnosis is made. Patients may be symptomatic for months prior to diagnosis.

Physical Examination

The physical examination may reveal subtle clues that will lead to the correct diagnosis (see Table 6-13). Roth spots are pale, oval fundus lesions with a surrounding hemorrhage. Petechiae may be seen on the conjunctiva, oral mucosa, or extremities. Splinter hemorrhages are most commonly secondary to trauma, but multiple new splinters located proximally in the nail bed suggest endocarditis. Osler's nodes are small, 2- to 15-mm, red-blue, painful, nodular lesions. Janeway lesions are hemorrhagic, purple-red, painless macules with a predilection for the palms and soles. Both Osler's nodes and Janeway lesions are transient findings and may be present only for a few hours. Heart murmurs usually are present but may be absent in acute endocarditis, right-sided infection, or mural infection. A new or changing murmur is unusual and usually denotes acute staphylococcal endocarditis. Peripheral emboli can affect the circulation in the distal extremities. Abdominal findings may be secondary to visceral emboli.

Neurologic manifestations are common, and a sudden neurologic event in a young person, especially with fever or a murmur, suggests endocarditis. Focal central findings are usually secondary to emboli; seizures, toxic encephalopathy, visual changes, mononeuritis multiplex, and cranial nerve palsies also may be seen.

Laboratory Tests

Laboratory abnormalities are frequent but are not specific (Table 6-14). A normochromic normocytic anemia is secondary to chronic disease and worsens with duration of illness. Leukocytosis is common in acute endocarditis but unusual in subacute endocarditis. The sedimentation rate is elevated. An elevated rheumatoid factor and hypergammaglobulinemia are more common with increasing duration of illness. Low complement levels, an elevated creatinine level, and an active urinary sediment with proteinuria, red blood cells, and red blood cell casts can occur due to renal vasculitis and/or glomerulonephritis. With right-sided endocarditis the chest x-ray may show nodular embolic lesions or infiltrates. An electrocardiogram may reveal conduction defects or arrhythmias if myocardial abscesses, myocarditis, or coronary artery emboli exist.

Blood cultures are the most useful diagnostic test, since the hallmark of bacterial endocarditis is

Table 6–14. *Frequency of Laboratory Abnormalities in Endocarditis*

Laboratory finding	Percent
Positive blood culture*	
One culture	85–95
Two cultures	98–100
Elevated sedimentation rate	90–100
Anemia	70–90
Proteinuria	50–65
Rheumatoid factor	40–50
Microscopic hematuria	30–50
Leukocytosis	20–30
Thrombocytopenia	5–15
Leukopenia	5–15
Hypocomplementemia	5–15
Elevated serum creatinine	5–15
Urinary red cell casts	5–12

*In patients with a cultivable organism
Source: Compiled from Scheld, W., and Sande, M. A. Endocarditis and Intravascular Infections. In G. L. Mandell, R. G. Douglas, and J. E. Bennett (Eds.), *Principles and Practice of Infectious Diseases,* 2d Ed. New York: Wiley, 1985. Pp. 504–530.

a continuous low-grade bacteremia. A single blood culture has an 85 to 95 percent yield; a second increases this to 98 to 100 percent. Prior antibiotic therapy causes the culture-positive rate to decline to 64 to 91 percent for up to 2 weeks [71]. Antibiotics will lengthen the time required for cultures to become positive more often than they will completely sterilize them. Three blood cultures are recommended from different sites over a 1-hour period prior to instituting therapy in acute endocarditis and over 24 hours in subacute endocarditis. Repeated cultures over the next few days are necessary only if previous antibiotic therapy has been given or initial cultures were negative and endocarditis is likely. Some fastidious organisms and some common organisms inhibited by antibiotics may require up to 21 days to grow. Table 6-15 lists the organisms that most commonly cause endocarditis.

Echocardiography has been used for the diagnosis of endocarditis since 1973. The sensitivity of

Table 6–15. *Bacterial Causes of Endocarditis*

Organism	NVE (%)	PVE, early (%)	PVE, late (%)	IVDA (%)
Streptococci:	60–80	11	40	17
Viridans	30–40	5	29	6
Enterococci	5–18	4	10	8
Other	15–25	2	0	3
Staphylococcus aureus	10–27	19	10	38
Staphylococcus epidermidis	1–3	30	23	2
Aerobic gram-negative rods	1.5–13	18	11	15
Fungi	2–4	12	5	14
Culture negative	5–24	0	4	13
Miscellaneous	5	10	7*	2

*A high percentage of these may be diphtheroids.
Note: NVE = natural valve endocarditis; PVE = prosthetic valve endocarditis; IVDA = intravenous drug abusers
Source: Compiled from Scheld, W., and Sande, M. A. Endocarditis and Intravascular Infections. In G. L. Mandell, R. G. Douglas, J. E. Bennett (Eds.), *Principles and Practice of Infectious Diseases,* 2d Ed. New York: Wiley 1985. Pp. 504–530.

this technique has varied from 15 to 90 percent [42, 71]. A negative study never eliminates endocarditis. Vegetations may be too small to be seen or be too acoustically similar to surrounding structures to be defined. False-positive studies are unusual. Local complications such as valvular insufficiency, paravalvular leak, paravalvular abscess, and fistula may be defined by echocardiography.

Medical Therapy

Optimal therapy in endocarditis requires identification of the causative organism and a prolonged course of bactericidal parenteral antibiotics. Acute endocarditis should be treated empirically with antistaphylococcal therapy after blood cultures are drawn. Gentamicin may be synergistic with beta-lactam agents or vancomycin against staphylococci. When added to these agents, it may shorten the time required for defervescence and for blood cultures to become sterile [37]. The addition of gentamicin does not increase the overall cure rate, and it does increase the incidence of nephrotoxicity. Close observation is necessary in

acute endocarditis for signs of cardiac decompensation that may require emergent valve replacement.

In subacute endocarditis, antibiotic choice may be guided by culture results. Empiric therapy is indicated if significant valvular insufficiency exists. Either a semisynthetic penicillin or vancomycin plus an aminoglycoside is a reasonable choice.

An appropriate response to initial therapy is indicated by defervescence, a stable cardiac examination, a decreasing sedimentation rate and rheumatoid factor titer, and sterile blood cultures. Persistent fever suggests paravalvular, myocardial, or visceral abscess, ineffective antimicrobial therapy, or drug allergy. A deteriorating cardiac examination may occur with progressive infection or despite microbiologic cure if sufficient valvular damage has already occurred. Serum bactericidal titers have previously been poorly standardized and yielded inconsistent results. A recent study with large numbers of patients has correlated a peak bactericidal titer of 1 : 64 and a trough of 1 : 32 with 100 percent *microbiological* cure [90]. Table 6-16 lists the therapies of choice for common causes of bacterial endocarditis.

Table 6–16. *Therapy for Common Causes of Endocarditis*

Organism	Situation	Therapy	Duration
S. aureus	IVDA (uncomplicated)	Antistaphylococcal β-lactam 1.5–2 gm IV q4h or vancomycin 2 gm IV qd	4 weeks
	IVDA (complicated) or non-IVDA	Antistaphylococcal β-lactam 1.5–2 gm IV q4h or vancomycin 2 gm IV qd Aminoglycoside optional	4–6 weeks
	PVE	Antistaphylococcal β-lactam 1.5–2 gm IV q4h or vancomycin 2 gm IV qd Aminoglycoside or rifampin optional	4–6 weeks
S. epidermidis	PVE	Antistaphylococcal β-lactam 1.5–2 gm IV q4h or vancomycin 2 gm IV qd Plus aminoglycoside and/or rifampin	4–6 weeks
viridans strep.	Penicillin MIC ≤ 0.1 μg/ml and uncomplicated	APG 10–20 million units IV qd Plus streptomycin 500 mg IM q12h or gentamicin 3–5 mg/kg per day IV	4 weeks of penicillin alone or 2 weeks of the combination
	Penicillin MIC ≤ 0.1 μg/ml and complicated or penicillin MIC ≥ 0.1 μg/ml	APG 10–20 million units IV qd Plus streptomycin 500 mg IM q12h or gentamicin 3–5 mg/kg per day IV	Penicillin: 4 weeks; aminoglycoside: 2 weeks
Enterococci		PPG 20 million units IV qd or ampicillin 2 gm IV q4h or vancomycin 2 gm/IV qd Plus gentamicin 3 mg/kg per day IV (streptomycin 500 mg IM q12h acceptable if MIC ≤ 2000)	NVE: 4–6 weeks PVE: 6–8 weeks
Aerobic gram-negative rods		Aminoglycoside plus β-lactam	NVE: 4–8 weeks PVE: 4–8 weeks

Note: PPG = procaine penicillin G; APG = aqueous penicillin G; NVE = native valve endocarditis; PVE = prosthetic valve endocarditis; and IVDA = intravenous drug abuse.

Surgical Therapy

Indications for surgical therapy include refractory congestive heart failure, recurrent emboli, persistently positive blood cultures, valvular dysfunction on fluoroscopy, fungal etiology, valve ring or myocardial abscess, and purulent pericarditis [17]. If indicated, surgery should never be delayed in order to administer further antibiotic therapy. Antibiotics should be continued 4 to 6 weeks after surgery.

Prognosis depends on many factors. Poor prognostic factors include infection with organisms such as gram-negative rods, yeast, and *S. aureus*; involvement of the aortic valve; infection on a prosthetic valve; valvular damage with congestive heart failure; myocardial infection; and major embolic events, especially to the central nervous system. The mortality rate in endocarditis is 25 to 40 percent and rarely is due to resistant organisms [29]. The primary factor responsible for increased mortality is a delay in diagnosis and therapy.

Special Situations in Drug Abuse

Endocarditis due to intravenous drug abuse has a variable presentation. The tricuspid valve is involved more often, and pulmonary symptoms and signs are common. Owing to the invasive nature of the causative organisms, congestive heart failure may occur early. The white blood cell count tends to be elevated, and signs associated with left-sided endocarditis are generally absent. A heart murmur may be absent. Table 6-15 lists the most common organisms causing infective endocarditis in drug abusers, but there is some geographic variation. Empiric therapy for *S. aureus* should be started immediately after cultures are obtained. Close observation for signs of hemodynamic deterioration is essential. Empiric use of vancomycin is advised [42] when methicillin-resistant *S. aureus* is known to be prevalent or in patients with a history of prior oral cephalosporin use. Persons using intravenous amphetamines are at increased risk of *Pseudomonas aeruginosa* endocarditis and should receive empiric coverage for this organism also [42].

Prosthetic Valve Endocarditis

Prosthetic valve endocarditis is a serious complication of cardiac valve replacement [15]. The responsible organisms vary with the length of time the prosthetic valve has been in place (see Table 6-15). Infection of mechanical valves occurs on the valve ring, unlike infection on natural valves and to a lesser extent on porcine heterograft valves, where vegetations form on the valve leaflets. This paravalvular location of prosthetic valve endocarditis permits early spread of infection to the myocardium. Myocardial invasion is a poor prognostic sign and usually requires valve replacement. Echocardiography is less useful in this setting because the intense signals from the prosthesis interfere with the resolution of images around the valve.

Antibiotic therapy alone may be successful in uncomplicated cases of prosthetic valve endocarditis. However, complications are frequent, and surgery is a very common adjunct to medical therapy because the valve acts as an infected foreign body. Relapse with the initially infecting organism after replacement of an infected prosthetic valve occurs up to 15 percent of the time after surgery, and overall mortality is 29 to 54 percent [23].

Table 6–17. Prophylaxis for Endocarditis

Situation	Regimen
Dental procedures:	Penicillin 2 gm PO 1 hour before and 1.0 gm 6 hours after
Penicillin allergy	Erythromycin 1 gm PO 1 hour before and 500 mg 6 hours after
Unable to take oral	APG 2 million units IV or IM 30 to 60 minutes before and 1 million units 6 hours after
Unable to take oral, penicillin allergy	Vancomycin 1 gm IV over the hour before
Dental procedures in high-risk patients or genitourinary/ gastrointestinal procedures in moderate- to high-risk patients	Ampicillin 2 gm IM or IV plus gentamicin 1.5 mg/kg IM or IV ½ hour before and 8 hours after
Genitourinary/gastrointestinal procedures:	
Low-risk patient	Amoxicillin 3 gm PO 1 hour before and 1.5 gm 6 hours after
Penicillin allergy	Vancomycin 1 gm IV over the hour before with gentamicin 1.5 mg/kg IM or IV; repeat 8 to 12 hours after

Source: Adapted from Shulman, S. T., Amren, D. P., Bisno, A. L., et al. Prevention of bacterial endocarditis. *Circulation* 70: 1123A, 1984.

Gastrointestinal Infections

Infectious Diarrhea

Gastrointestinal (GI) infections as manifested by diarrhea are second only to the common cold in causing illness in the United States. Infectious diarrhea usually is the result of ingestion of food or water contaminated with infected feces. Direct person-to-person spread of infection via the fecal-oral route also occurs between sexual partners, in day-care centers, and is implicated in nosocomial infections. Symptoms frequently associated with diarrhea include nausea, vomiting, abdominal cramping, and systemic complaints of fever, myalgias, malaise, and headache. In evaluating the patient with diarrhea, a careful history should be taken with special attention to contact with other ill persons, travel, exposure to animals (including pets), food, water source, previous antibiotic use, sexual preference, underlying medical illnesses, recent surgery, and use of cancer chemotherapeutic agents.

DIAGNOSIS

Diagnosis is dependent on stool examination and culture. A stool examination must include appearance (watery, bloody), test for occult blood, and microscopic examination for fecal leukocytes (methylene blue or other stain). Depending on the patient's history, further tests may be appropriate, including dark-field examination for darting motility (Campylobacter jejuni), ova and parasite examination (Giardia lamblia, Entamoeba histolytica, helminths), and bacterial culture (Salmonella, Shigella). If Campylobacter, Yersinia, Clostridium difficile, or Vibrio species are suspected, the laboratory should be alerted, since these organisms require specialized selective media for isolation and identification. ELISA as well as other assays and culture are now available for detecting rotavirus in the stool. Rectal swabs for gonorrhea and herpes simplex may be required if symptoms suggest proctitis. Occasionally, sigmoidoscopy is used as an adjunct to stool examination when evaluating the patient with diarrhea. The rectal and colonic mucosa can be examined for ulcerations and the presence of pseudomembranes (C. difficile colitis). Biopsies and further stool samples can be obtained during this procedure. Rarely, small bowel biopsy (Giardia) and sampling of duodenal fluid (Strongyloides stercoralis) may be required.

Diarrheal illnesses can be grouped into four syndromes: (1) acute food poisoning, (2) watery diarrhea, (3) bloody diarrhea, and (4) chronic diarrhea.

Acute Food Poisoning

Symptoms, notably vomiting or diarrhea without fever, develop within 24 hours. Blood and fecal leukocytes are not found in stool specimens. Preformed toxins present in the food are produced by S. aureus, C. perfringens, B. cereus, and C. botulinum (onset of symptoms in botulism may be delayed and gastrointestinal symptoms may be minimal).

Watery Diarrhea

Watery diarrhea without fecal leukocytes or blood is caused by organisms that produce enterotoxins. These include V. cholerae, enterotoxigenic E. coli (traveler's diarrhea), rotavirus, and Norwalk-related viruses. Giardia and Cryptosporidium are usually included in this group, although the pathogenic mechanisms of these organisms are poorly understood.

Bloody Diarrhea

Bloody diarrhea with fecal leukocytes often accompanied by fever is caused by organisms that invade the intestinal mucosa. Some of these pathogens also may elaborate enterotoxins or cytotoxins. Invasive organisms include Shigella, Salmonella, C. jejuni, Y. enterocolitica, enteropathogenic E. coli, V. parahaemolyticus, non-01 V. cholerae, C. difficile, and E. histolytica. In the milder forms of these infections stools may not be grossly bloody, but fecal leukocytes are almost invariably present. Tests for occult blood are frequently positive.

Chronic Diarrhea

Chronic diarrhea (> 2 weeks) may be due to infectious organisms, although noninfectious causes predominate. Invasive diagnostic measures, which include endoscopy and small bowel biopsy, are often needed to determine the etiology. Organisms that must be considered in the differential diagnosis include *Giardia* and *E. histolytica*. In the immunocompromised patient, *Strongyloides* and *Cryptosporidium* should be considered.

TREATMENT

Fluid and electrolyte replacement is the mainstay of treatment for diarrhea. This can be achieved intravenously or orally. Most infections are self-limited and require no additional therapy. Antimicrobial therapy is reserved for patients with relatively severe illness with fever and bloody diarrhea. It also may be indicated when infection is prolonged and when there is a risk of person-to-person transmission, as in day-care centers. Use of symptomatic medications such as Pepto-Bismol and Lomotil is discouraged except in mild cases of nonbloody diarrhea. Antibiotic prophylaxis for traveler's diarrhea is not recommended because it may predispose the patient to more serious illness with invasive organisms and may encourage the growth of resistant organisms. Empiric therapy with tetracycline or trimethoprim-sulfamethoxazole may be used to shorten the course of traveler's diarrhea.

Mortality due to infectious diarrhea is rare in the United States, but diarrhea accounts for millions of deaths each year in the third world. Death results not from infection per se, but from circulatory collapse resulting from dehydration and electrolyte imbalance. Children and the elderly are most susceptible.

Antibiotic-Associated Diarrhea

Diarrhea associated with antibiotics (AAD) is common in hospitalized patients receiving antibiotic therapy; it also may occur after the cessation of such treatment. Almost all antibiotics have been associated, although ampicillin, clindamycin, and the cephalosporins are implicated most frequently [20]. This illness has a wide spectrum of symptoms from occasional loose stools to life-threatening systemic illness with fever, bloody diarrhea, pseudomembrane formation, leukocytosis, and severe abdominal pain. Late complications include dehydration, hypotension, and toxic megacolon.

DIAGNOSIS

Historically, *S. aureus* was believed to cause antibiotic-associated diarrhea; today, most investigators believe that this association was coincidental. Frequently no pathogen can be isolated. *Clostridium difficile* is the etiologic agent in almost all cases of antibiotic-associated diarrhea associated with pseudomembrane formation and it also may cause diarrhea without pseudomembrane formation. *Clostridium difficile* colitis also is seen in patients who are not receiving antibiotics. Cancer chemotherapeutic agents and mechanical manipulation of the bowel are thought to be predisposing factors. Laboratory diagnosis is based on culture of a strain of *C. difficile* that produces cytotoxin or demonstration of toxin in the stool. The clinical diagnosis can be made if pseudomembranes are seen with sigmoidoscopy.

TREATMENT

Treatment of mild to moderate cases of antibiotic-associated diarrhea includes replacement of fluids and discontinuation of antibiotic therapy; the latter is not essential if specific treatment is initiated. Severely ill patients usually are treated with oral vancomycin. Metronidazole is a less expensive alternative that can be used in milder cases. Relapse is not uncommon, and a second course of therapy may be required. Prognosis is good if the diagnosis is made early and treatment is adequate.

Enteric Fever

Enteric fever is a systemic illness acquired through the gastrointestinal tract. Gastrointestinal symptoms are often mild, but they may include nausea, vomiting, and diarrhea or constipation. Fever, headache, abdominal pain, and cough are common. Classically, "rose spots" are described, but they are found infrequently; other physical findings may include splenomegaly, relative bradycardia, rales or rhonchi, and occasionally, hepatomegaly and meningismus [35]. Bacteria are usually isolated from blood and may be found in stool and urine. Marrow culture is frequently positive and may be useful if blood cultures are negative. Leukopenia is often noted. *Salmonella* *typhi* is the usual etiologic agent, but other bacterial pathogens, including *Yersinia* spp., *C. fetus* spp. *fetus,* and *Salmonella* spp. other than *typhi* may cause similar syndromes. Chloramphenicol has been the drug of choice for seriously ill patients with *S. typhi,* but resistant organisms are now frequently reported. Alternative drugs include amoxicillin, ampicillin, and trimethoprim-sulfamethoxazole. Sensitivity testing is important in guiding therapy. Prognosis is good in otherwise healthy patients who receive appropriate therapy.

Intraabdominal Infections

Peritonitis

Inflammation of the peritoneum due to microorganisms can be either primary (spontaneous or idiopathic) or secondary. Primary peritonitis in adults occurs in patients with alcoholic cirrhosis and ascites. Rarely, patients with other causes of cirrhosis and ascites develop the illness, as do patients with no underlying disease. Secondary peritonitis from spillage of bowel contents results from many intraabdominal pathologic processes, which include surgery, trauma, bowel obstruction, vascular insufficiency, tumor, and abscess. It is also commonly associated with peritoneal dialysis [47].

DIAGNOSIS

Abdominal tenderness with rebound, ascites, and decreased or absent bowel sounds are common clinical findings. Diagnosis is based on clinical presentation, examination of peritoneal fluid, and culture of both fluid and blood. The white blood cell count of ascitic fluid is greater than 300/mm³ and usually greater than 1000/mm³ with leukocyte predominance. Gram's stain of the fluid is often helpful.

In primary peritonitis, enteric organisms, especially *E. coli,* are the most common isolates followed by *S. pneumoniae* and group A streptococci. Anaerobes are found less frequently. In secondary peritonitis, the predominant pathogen(s) is related to the endogenous flora of the segment of the bowel involved in the primary pathologic process. Mixed infections involving anaerobes are common. *Candida* spp. are also observed. Vaginal flora are isolated when the underlying disease is gynecologic in origin.

THERAPY

Empiric therapy directed against the most likely organisms should be initiated until culture results are available. Prognosis depends on the severity of the underlying illness.

Intraperitoneal Abscesses

Underlying diseases that may lead to abscess formation in the peritoneal cavity include abdominal surgery, appendicitis, diverticulitis, other ruptured viscus, biliary tract disease, and pancreatitis. Such abscesses are associated with spiking fevers, chills, and abdominal pain in the area of the abscess. Occasionally, the presentation may be subacute. Infections are mixed and include anaerobes and enteric gram-negative organisms. Radiologic examinations, including computed tomography, ultrasound, and radionuclide studies, are useful in confirming the diagnosis. Surgical or percutaneous drainage is the mainstay of treatment. Initial combination antibiotic therapy is modified as blood and abscess culture results become available.

Liver Abscesses
Liver abscesses may be caused either by bacteria or by *E. histolytica.* Classically, there is a single abscess in the right lobe. Bacterial abscesses may arise from direct extension from the biliary system or by arterial or venous routes. Usual pathogens include enteric gram-negative organisms and anaerobes. Amebic abscesses result from intestinal infection with subsequent invasion. This dissemination occurs in 3 to 9 percent of cases of amebic colitis [2]. They are more frequent in males.

DIAGNOSIS
Symptoms include fever, chills, right upper quadrant pain, and occasionally, cough and pleuritic chest pain. The liver is enlarged and tender. Jaundice is rare. Presentation may be that of an acute or subacute illness. Diagnosis, as with other intraabdominal abscesses, is based on radiologic imaging. The serum alkaline phosphatase level is usually elevated, but other liver function tests may be normal. Serologic tests are positive in 90 percent of cases of amebic abscess, but they may be misleading, since patients from endemic areas generally have positive titers even without current infection.

TREATMENT
Treatment includes antibiotics and drainage surgically or percutaneously. Multiple small abscesses have been cured with prolonged antibiotic therapy alone. Empiric antimicrobial therapy should be initiated pending culture results. Treatment is usually for a minimum of 4 weeks. Amebic abscesses are best treated with metronidazole; drainage is also recommended in order to establish the diagnosis and to prevent rupture. Rupture carries a mortality rate of 18 to 30 percent, whereas uncomplicated abscesses have less than a 1 percent mortality rate [48].

Cholecystitis/Cholangitis
Infection is not a cause of acute cholecystitis, but it develops in over half the patients with this disease. A major predisposing factor is previous biliary tract surgery. Jaundice in this setting indicates a high likelihood of bactobilia. Infectious complications of cholecystitis include cholangitis, abscess formation, empyema of the gallbladder, peritonitis, bacteremia, and liver abscess. Patients who develop these complications are acutely ill with fever, chills, right upper quadrant pain, leukocytosis, and jaundice. Other symptoms of sepsis may develop. Radiologic studies such as radionuclide scans and ultrasound are often useful in confirming the diagnosis of biliary tract disease. Organisms commonly cultured from the biliary tree include enteric gram-negative rods, enterococci, and anaerobes. Treatment includes surgical drainage and broad-spectrum antibiotics. Culture results should be used to guide antimicrobial therapy. Antibiotic therapy for uncomplicated cholecystitis is not routinely recommended; it is usually indicated, however, when the probability of bactobilia is high. Prognosis depends on the age of the patient and early treatment.

Helminths
Helminths may be the most prevalent of infections worldwide; in the United States alone it is estimated that there are 54 million persons with helminth infections [49]. The most common helminthic pathogens found in the United States are summarized in Table 6-18. Diagnosis is usually based on stool examination for eggs or passage of worms. Symptoms depend on the worm burden. This, in turn, determines whether patients should be treated.

Table 6–18. *Common Helminthic Pathogens Found in the United States*

Organism	Means of infection	Epidemiology	Symptoms	Treatment
Roundworms:				
Pin worm (*Enterobius vermicularis*)	Oral	Nationwide Families, children	Perianal pruritus	Mebendazole
Round worm (*Ascaris lumbricoides*)	Oral	Southeastern United States Families, children	Asymptomatic; occ. intestinal, biliary tract obstruction, pulmonary symptoms	Mebendazole
Hook worm (*Ancylostoma duodenale, Necator americanus*)	Skin	Southeastern United States Bare feet	Iron-deficiency anemia	Mebendazole Iron
Strongyloidiasis (*Strongyloides stercoralis*)	Skin	Southern United States Institutions, immunocompromised hosts	Autoinfection Abdominal pain, diarrhea, eosinophilia	Thiabendazole
Tapeworms:				
Beef tapeworm (*Taenia saginata*)	Oral	Undercooked beef	None	Niclosamide
Pork tapeworm (*Taenia solium*)	Oral	Undercooked pork	Seizures from cystircircosis	Niclosamide Praziquantel for cystircircosis
Fish tapeworm (*Diphyllobothrium latum*)	Oral	Raw fish	Anemia (vitamin B_{12})	Niclosamide Vitamin B_{12}, folate
Dwarf tapeworm (*Hymenolepis nana*)	Oral	Children	Abdominal cramps, diarrhea	Niclosamide
Echinococcosis (hydatid disease) (*Echinococcus granulosus*)	Oral	Sheep. cattle-raising areas	Liver cyst, eosinophilia	Surgery Mebendazole for disseminated disease

Central Nervous System Infections

Meningitis

The major infectious processes involving the central nervous system (CNS) include meningitis, encephalitis, brain abscess, and very rarely, subdural and epidural empyemas. Meningitis refers to inflammation of the subarachnoid space, and it has been defined by cerebrospinal fluid (CSF) pleocytosis, characteristically considered to be more than 5 white blood cells/mm³ [14]. Signs and symptoms vary with the etiology of the process. Although there is some overlap, meningitis can be divided into two clinically relevant categories on the basis of the cerebrospinal fluid examination. A positive Gram's stain of the cerebrospinal fluid or a polymorphonuclear cerebrospinal fluid pleocytosis is indicative of purulent meningitis, whereas a negative Gram's stain of the cerebrospinal fluid and mononuclear cerebrospinal fluid pleocytosis suggests an aseptic meningitis. Purulent meningitis is often an overwhelming infection and is a true medical emergency which requires rapid initiation of antibiotic treatment to avoid a tragic outcome.

Etiology

Hemophilus influenzae, Neisseria meningitidis, and *S. pneumoniae* together account for 80 percent of all cases of purulent meningitis. *Neisseria meningitidis* is the most frequent cause of meningitis in patients 5 to 30 years of age, and *S. pneumoniae* is the primary causal agent in patients over 30 years of age. In about 10 percent of patients with classic clinical and cerebrospinal fluid findings, no pathogen will be isolated, often because of prior inadequate antimicrobial therapy. *Listeria monocytogenes* is an uncommon pathogen that produces meningitis in the elderly, in immunocompromised hosts, and in neonates. *Staphylococcus aureus* is another infrequent meningeal pathogen causing meningitis secondary to contiguous infected foci or to hematogenous seeding during staphylococcal sepsis. Enteric gram-negative bacilli are very rare causes of meningitis.

Aseptic meningitis is most frequently due to viral infection. It is also produced by a variety of infectious and noninfectious causes, and several of the infectious causes may respond to antimicrobial therapy. The critical concern in managing patients with this syndrome is the prompt recognition of those who require such therapy. An etiology is determined in approximately 25 percent of the 3000 to 4000 cases of aseptic meningitis reported each year. The most frequently defined pathogens are the enteroviruses, which cause infections predominantly in the summer or early fall. Other agents include mumps, herpes simplex types 1 and 2, varicella zoster, cytomegalovirus, adenovirus, measles, Epstein-Barr virus, hepatitis A virus, poliomyelitis, and the encephalitis viruses. More important, meningeal irritation with mononuclear pleocytosis may be present in partially treated bacterial meningitis, parameningeal bacterial infections, tuberculosis, fungal meningitis, amebiasis, leptospirosis, syphilis, and Lyme disease. These treatable infections should not be overlooked. Noninfectious causes include systemic lupus erythematosus, sarcoidosis, carcinomatosis, drug reactions, chemical injury from intrathecal medication, Behçet's syndrome, and Mollaret's syndrome.

Diagnosis

Purulent bacterial meningitis primarily presents with fever, severe headache, and nuchal rigidity. Other symptoms that commonly develop include nausea, vomiting, photophobia, and mental aberration. Clinically, the meningeal irritation is reflected in nuchal rigidity, a positive Kernig's sign (pain in the hamstring and paraspinal muscles when the knee is extended with the hip flexed), and a positive Brudzinski's sign (flexion of the knees and hips when the neck is flexed). An abnormal state of consciousness is common; only 15 to 20 percent of patients appear totally alert on presentation. Papilledema is unusual; if present, a brain abscess or encephalitis should be considered. Occasionally, it is possible to identify an anatomic source for meningitis, and the initial examination should include a thorough evaluation of the sinuses and the middle ears and a search for a midline dermal sinus or occult skull fracture.

Viral aseptic meningitis presents with fever and signs of meningeal irritation (nuchal rigidity, severe headache, Kernig's and Brudzinski's signs) after a short prodromal illness. Unlike purulent meningitis, viral meningitis alone does not produce a change in mental status, and the presence of lethargy or confusion indicates either a purulent meningitis or concurrent encephalitis. Tuberculous and fungal meningitis have a more subacute presentation than is seen with bacterial or viral disease. Tuberculous infection evolves over a few days to weeks and fungal infections over a few weeks to months.

The major diagnostic test for meningitis is an examination of the cerebrospinal fluid. This should be performed in all patients in whom meningitis is a serious diagnostic consideration. Lumbar puncture lowers pressure in the spinal canal; individuals with localized increased intracranial pressure who undergo this procedure are at risk of uncal herniation from the pressure change. Individuals with papilledema or focal neurologic deficits (excluding ophthalmoplegias) should not have a lumbar puncture performed until a computerized axial tomographic (CT) scan has excluded a mass lesion. In a patient with a focal deficit in whom purulent meningitis is a possibility and a CT scan cannot be performed immediately, empiric antibiotic therapy should be started.

Examination of the cerebrospinal fluid includes cell count and differential count, determination of glucose and protein concentrations, a Gram-stained smear of the sediment, and culture. In the appropriate clinical settings, additional cerebrospinal fluid studies could include mycobacterial and fungal cultures, cryptococcal antigen, coccidioides antibody titer, VDRL, and cytocentrifugation for cytology. When purulent meningitis is present, the diagnosis is confirmed in 75 to 85 percent of patients by a Gram's stain of the cerebrospinal fluid demonstrating bacteria [21]. Purulent meningitis has several other characteristic cerebrospinal fluid findings: two-thirds of patients have a cerebrospinal fluid white blood cell count greater than 1000/mm^3 with a polymorphonuclear leukocytosis, approximately 75 percent have a cerebrospinal fluid glucose concentration less than 50 mg/dl, and 85 percent have an elevated protein concentration [33]. In patients with a negative cerebrospinal fluid Gram's stain, a cerebrospinal fluid white blood cell count over 1200/mm^3 with either a protein concentration greater than 150 mg/dl or a glucose concentration less than 30 mg/dl strongly suggests purulent meningitis. Patients with early bacterial meningitis may have normal cerebrospinal fluid examinations; if the clinical suspicion is high, the lumbar puncture should be repeated in several hours.

In most patients with viral meningitis, the cerebrospinal fluid examination reveals a normal glucose concentration, a protein concentration ranging from 50 to 200 mg/dl, and a white blood cell count of 50 to 1000/mm^3 [33]. Very early in the course of the illness neutrophils often predominate, but as the course progresses, a shift to more lymphocytic cells occurs within the first 24 hours. A low cerebrospinal fluid glucose concentration with a lymphocytic pleocytosis is seen in mumps and lymphocytic choriomeningitis infections. More commonly, this cerebrospinal fluid profile is associated with tuberculosis or fungal meningitis, partially treated bacterial meningitis, parameningeal infections, or carcinomatous or sarcoid meningitis. A lymphocytic pleocytosis and a high cerebrospinal fluid protein concentration should increase the concern about a parameningeal pyogenic process.

TREATMENT

The period of highest mortality with bacterial meningitis is the first 24 hours after onset and presentation [21]. Diagnostic evaluation must be performed immediately, and antibiotic therapy must be started as quickly as possible. In patients with possible meningitis who are acutely ill, a brief examination should be performed to exclude focal neurologic deficits or papilledema, and blood cultures and a lumbar puncture should be performed. If the cerebrospinal fluid is turbid, empiric antibiotic therapy should be instituted immediately. Since the predominant pathogens in adolescents and adults are *S. pneumoniae* and *N. meningitidis,* therapy with penicillin G (50,000 units/kg IV every 4 hours, approximately 20 to 24 million units per day in adults) should be started in the emergency department for these patients. Chloramphenicol (25 mg/kg IV every 6 hours) should be used in penicillin-allergic patients.

In patients whose symptoms are subacute, antibiotic therapy can be withheld until the initial results of lumbar puncture are known. If the studies are consistent with purulent meningitis, antibiotic therapy should be promptly initiated based either on the Gram's stain results or the age of the patient when the Gram's stain is negative. Crystalline penicillin G remains the agent of choice for pneumococcal and meningococcal meningitis. When the Gram's stain is suggestive of *H. influenzae,* treatment with ampicillin and chloramphenicol should be begun until the results of susceptibility testing are known. Ampicillin is the drug of choice for susceptible *H. influenzae* isolates; chloramphenicol or a third-generation cephalosporin is appropriate for ampicillin-resistant strains. Staphylococcal meningitis requires high-dose therapy with a penicillinase-resistant penicillin (nafcillin or oxacillin, 2 gm IV every 4 hours); vancomycin (500 mg IV every 4 hours) should be used for infections due to methicillin-resistant *S. aureus.* Either ampicillin or penicillin can be utilized for *L. monocytogenes* meningitis, with an aminoglycoside added in severe disease.

In patients who are immunocompromised, who have experienced trauma or cranial surgery, or who develop meningitis in the hospital, there is an increased risk that the infection is due to *L. monocytogenes, S. aureus,* or gram-negative enteric bacilli. Antibiotic therapy should provide coverage for these pathogens. If the lumbar puncture does not provide evidence for an etiologic agent, treatment with ampicillin (50 mg/kg IV every 4 hours, 2 gm IV every 4 hours in adults), vanco-

mycin (500 mg IV every 6 hours), and a third-generation cephalosporin (e.g., cefotaxime, 50 mg/kg every 6 hours) should be started in these patients and continued until there are culture results.

Supportive therapy for purulent meningitis includes maintenance of respiration (with mechanical ventilation if necessary), control of seizures, and careful control of fluids to minimize cerebral edema. Corticosteroids should be considered only if severe cerebral edema develops.

The appropriate treatment of aseptic meningitis is determined by the clinical setting. For example, during a summer epidemic of viral meningitis, mildly ill, alert patients who have a typical cerebrospinal fluid examination for an enteroviral meningitis do not necessarily require hospitalization if close follow-up can be arranged. However, if the patient presents during a nonepidemic period for enteroviral or arboviral infections, if there are any unusual features on physical examination or cerebrospinal fluid examination, or if the patient is not alert, then immediate hospitalization is indicated for close observation and additional diagnostic studies.

Patients who clinically have aseptic viral meningitis but whose cerebrospinal fluid examinations reveal a polymorphonuclear pleocytosis do not require immediate antimicrobial therapy. These patients can be watched without specific therapy and undergo a repeat cerebrospinal fluid examination in 12 to 24 hours to demonstrate the conversion of the polymorphonuclear pleocytosis to a lymphocytic pleocytosis [86]. This is appropriate only if repeat cerebrospinal fluid examination can be performed immediately if any change in the patient's condition occurs during observation. Otherwise, empiric antimicrobial therapy is indicated.

PREVENTION

There is an increased incidence of meningococcal disease in household contacts of patients with meningococcal infection. Rifampin can eradicate nasal carriage of meningococci and thus prevent systemic disease [56]. Rifampin (600 mg in adults, 5 mg/kg in children under 1 year, and 10 mg/kg for older children, given orally every 12 hours for four doses) is the best initial prophylaxis for close contacts of patients with meningococcal meningitis. Casual contacts such as with fellow workers, schoolmates, or health care workers do not require prophylaxis.

Encephalitis and Brain Abscess

Encephalitis is an infrequent complication of common infections and is caused primarily by viral agents, although bacterial, rickettsial, or parasitic pathogens are occasionally implicated. In the United States, epidemic encephalitis is produced by arthropod-borne viruses, which include eastern equine encephalitis, western equine encephalitis, St. Louis encephalitis, and California encephalitis. Herpes simplex virus (HSV) is the major cause of sporadic encephalitis. Rabies virus and slow viruses are rare causes of encephalitis. Rocky Mountain spotted fever and typhus are the major rickettsial diseases associated with encephalitis. The spirochetes of syphilis and Lyme disease also may produce encephalitis. Immunocompromised individuals are both at risk of encephalitis due to a wider spectrum of agents and have a higher incidence of encephalitis (see the section Immunodeficiency and AIDS).

DIAGNOSIS

In the normal host, viral encephalitis presents with fever, severe headache, nausea, vomiting, and alterations in state of consciousness ranging from mild lethargy to coma. With more severe disease there are focal signs, including seizures, motor weakness, abnormal deep tendon reflexes, tremors, aphasia, and paralysis. Concurrent signs of meningeal irritation may be present. While none of these findings is diagnostic of a specific pathogen, signs of temporal lobe involvement such as bizarre behavior, speech difficulties, olfactory hallucinations, or visual-field deficits suggest herpes simplex viral encephalitis. Encephalitis in the summer or early fall and a history of mosquito

exposure suggest disease due to an arthropod-borne agent.

Findings on cerebrospinal fluid examination are similar to those in aseptic meningitis. Red blood cells in the cerebrospinal fluid are seen commonly with herpes simplex viral encephalitis, and approximately 40 percent of these patients have more than 50 red blood cells/mm³ [96]. CT scans, electroencephalography, and brain scans also may demonstrate focal deficits in herpes simplex viral encephalitis.

TREATMENT

There is no current therapy for viral encephalitis, except for herpes simplex viral infection. Acyclovir (30 mg/kg per day for 10 days) has been demonstrated to be effective for herpes simplex viral encephalitis [94] and should be instituted empirically in patients with presumed viral encephalitis and focal neurologic findings. Other illnesses may mimic herpes simplex viral encephalitis. In patients who have undergone brain biopsy for presumed herpes simplex viral encephalitis, only 50 to 60 percent have had the diagnosis confirmed and about 24 percent have had another potentially treatable illness identified [95]. The small risk of brain biopsy is dependent on the experience of the surgeon, and the decision to perform a biopsy must be individualized. It should be considered in all patients with possible herpes simplex viral encephalitis and in patients with AIDS or other immunocompromising illnesses who develop encephalitis with focal lesions because of the wide diversity of potential etiologies.

Localized bacterial encephalitis, or brain abscess, is caused predominantly by mixed oral anaerobic bacteria and streptococcal species. *Staphylococcus aureus* and enteric gram-negative bacilli are implicated less frequently. Fifty percent of patients with a brain abscess have an apparent extracranial focus of infection. Brain abscesses present as an expanding intracranial mass lesion with generalized headache, nausea, vomiting, and the development of focal neurologic findings such as seizures and an abnormal state of consciousness [55]. Fever is not universally present and may be seen in only 30 to 40 percent of these patients [28]. Papilledema is observed occasionally. The CT scan demonstrates focal enhancing lesions in most patients, but with an early brain abscess it may be normal and a brain scan abnormal. Therefore, the latter should be considered in patients in whom an intracranial lesion is strongly suspected and the CT scan has no abnormalities.

Brain abscess and systemic bacterial and rickettsial disease associated with encephalitis will respond to appropriate antibiotic therapy. Patients with presumed brain abscess should be initiated on empiric antimicrobial therapy directed against the predominant pathogens. Penicillin G (20 million units per day IV in adults) and chloramphenicol (4 gm per day in adults) are effective. When the bacteriology is defined, intravenous metronidazole or a third-generation cephalosporin may be alternative agents. Neurosurgical consultation should be arranged for all patients with increased intracranial pressure or focal intracranial lesions.

Urinary Tract Infections

Urinary tract infection (UTI), a condition in which there is bacterial colonization of the usually sterile urine, can involve either the lower or upper urinary tracts or both. It may present with bacterially infected urine in an asymptomatic individual (asymptomatic bacteriuria) or as a symptomatic inflammatory process of the lower tract (cystitis or prostatitis) or kidneys (pyelonephritis). Asymptomatic bacteriuria is common, occurring in 1 to 3 percent of nonpregnant women, 4 to 7 percent of pregnant women, and 10 to 20 percent of elderly men and women. Bacteria found in the colon, such as *E. coli,* are the most common causes of community-acquired urinary tract infection. These organisms colonize the bladder by ascending the urethra from the periurethral area, a mechanism that explains the higher rates of urinary tract infection in females, in whom the urethra is shorter, and after sexual intercourse and instrumentation of the urethra and bladder [22, 84]. Patients with urinary tract infections acquired in the hospital after catheterization or who have structural abnormalities of the urinary tract are more likely to be infected with other gram-negative rods, such as *Proteus, Pseudomonas, Serratia, Klebsiella,* and *Enterobacter* species. Infection also can arise hematogenously, as with *S. aureus* bacteremia. Once colonization occurs, impairment of normal urinary flow with resulting stasis is the most important factor predisposing to the persistence and progression of infection. Obstructed flow enhances bacterial overgrowth and also facilitates retrograde infection of more proximal sites. Obstruction is caused by functional disorders (e.g., neurogenic bladder) or structural abnormalities (e.g., valves and stenoses of the urethra and ureters, prostatic enlargement, and renal calculi) [63].

Symptoms of lower tract infection arise from inflammation of the mucosa of the urethra and bladder and are characterized by dysuria, increased frequency and urgency of urination, and occasionally, suprapubic pain and the passage of cloudy or blood-tinged urine. Physical examination may reveal suprapubic tenderness, but fever and leukocytosis are uncommon without upper tract involvement. Similar symptoms can be caused by urethritis (usually due to a sexually transmitted disease) or vaginitis. Acute pyelonephritis is characterized by a sudden onset, fever and chills, and flank pain and tenderness; only 50 percent of patients have preceding symptoms of cystitis. On some occasions, symptoms of nausea, vomiting, and diarrhea are prominent, and the pain may radiate to the epigastrium or lower abdomen, suggesting the possibility of gallbladder disease, appendicitis, pelvic inflammatory disease, or a perforated viscus. Pain that is colicky or radiates to the groin suggests the presence of renal stone with or without infection. Infection of the kidney also may be subclinical and occurs in up to 20 percent of women with symptoms of cystitis and 40 percent of those with asymptomatic bacteriuria [79].

Diagnosis

Confirmation of the diagnosis of urinary tract infection requires evaluation of the urine by microscopy and culture. Pyuria, defined as greater than 10 white blood cells per high-power field in the sediment from a centrifuged urine, is present in 95 percent of patients with bacteriuria and less than 1 percent without infection. It is a sensitive indicator of urinary tract inflammation, although it is also present in 90 percent of patients with urethritis. The detection of a single bacterium on Gram's stain of urine also is a predictor of bacteriuria and correlates with $\geq 10^4$ organisms per milliliter in centrifuged urine and $\geq 10^5$ organisms per milliliter in uncentrifuged samples [78].

Proper handling of urine for culture requires that it be obtained by a method likely to avoid contamination (midstream specimen, single catheterization, sterile aspiration from the tube of a closed indwelling catheter, or suprapubic needle aspiration of the bladder) and processed or refrigerated within 30 minutes of sampling. While urine is normally sterile, some bacterial contamination from the urethra and periurethral skin is common, especially in voided specimens, making quantitation of culture results necessary in order to separate bacteriuria from contamination. Based on observations in women with asymptomatic bacteriuria and with pyelonephritis, a level of $\geq 10^5$ organisms per milliliter in midstream urine has been termed "significant bacteriuria" and accepted as a cutoff for true infection; patients without infection rarely have counts of $>10^4$/ml. While the level of $\geq 10^5$/ml is probably valid in patients with pyelonephritis or to define asymptomatic bacteriuria, a less stringent cutoff may be necessary for women with bacterial cystitis, 25 percent of whom will have counts of $<10^5$/ml. A lower cutoff, of 10^4/ml, is also appropriate in men, in whom contamination is less likely, and for

gram-positive organisms and fungi, which may be significant with counts between 10^4 and 10^5/ml. Blood cultures, if positive, are helpful in confirming the diagnosis of pyelonephritis and in determining the responsible organism in situations where urine cultures may be misleading, such as in patients with ureteral obstruction or in those with chronic polymicrobial lower urinary tract infection [32].

Although rarely necessary for the diagnosis of urinary tract infection, radiographic evaluation by intravenous pyelogram (IVP) to exclude structural abnormalities of the urinary tract is recommended for all children and men with bacteriuria. Among women, in whom urinary tract infections occur commonly despite a normal urinary tract, an intravenous pyelogram is usually reserved for the patient with complications, such as bacteremia, relapse after appropriate therapy, or frequent reinfection. Radiographic evaluation by intravenous pyelogram or ultrasound also may be useful in patients with pyelonephritis responding poorly to therapy in order to exclude renal calculi or renal or perinephric abscess.

Therapy

The successful treatment of urinary tract infection requires selection of appropriate antimicrobial agents, relief of obstruction if present, and follow-up cultures to detect relapse or recurrence. Many individuals with suspected pyelonephritis can be treated as outpatients with oral antibiotics; however, patients who are severely ill, unable to take oral medication, or infected with an organism not susceptible to oral agents should be hospitalized for parenteral therapy. The initial choice of therapy should be guided by the probability of likely organisms for the given clinical situation and the urine Gram's stain. Persistence of high bacterial counts in urine culture after 3 to 4 days of treatment indicates inadequate antimicrobial therapy, and continuing fever suggests the possibility of urinary tract obstruction or abscess. Therapy for symptomatic lower tract infection has traditionally included 7 to 10 days of an appropriate oral antibiotic; however, recent studies in women have demonstrated cure rates of 80 to 100 percent with regimens of single-dose oral antibiotics (trimethoprim-sufamethoxasole, 2 gm PO; amoxicillin, 3 gm PO; or sulfisoxazole, 2 gm PO). Single-dose regimens are not effective in upper tract infection and should not be used when symptoms of pyelonephritis or urologic abnormalities are present; they have not been evaluated in men. The approach to therapy of asymptomatic bacteriuria in children and pregnant women is the same as that for symptomatic lower urinary tract infection; other asymptomatic individuals with normal urinary tracts do not appear to benefit from treatment.

Approximately 50 percent of patients will experience recurrences of urinary tract infections within a year of treatment. Recurrence with the same organism is known as *relapse* and usually occurs within 2 weeks. It indicates persistent infection in renal or prostatic tissue and is common in patients with structural abnormalities. A recurrence caused by a new organism of the same or different species is termed a *reinfection* and usually occurs within 6 months; it is not commonly associated with anatomic abnormalities. All patients treated for urinary tract infections should be recultured within 1 to 2 weeks after finishing therapy to detect relapses, since these may be asymptomatic. Patients who relapse will often respond to longer courses of antibiotics: 10 to 14 days for those initially treated with single-dose regimens and 6 weeks for those relapsing after 10 to 14 days of treatment. If a relapse occurs after 6 weeks of therapy and no surgically correctable abnormality is present, long-term *suppressive* oral antiseptic or antibiotic therapy should be considered, especially for children or patients with structural abnormalities (which increase the risk of progressive renal damage) or symptoms. Patients with frequent reinfections also may benefit from *prophylactic* oral antibiotics after sterilization of the urine. Single-dose prophylactic antibiotics taken after each episode of sexual intercourse are useful in women whose recurrent urinary tract infections are associated with sexual activity. In patients without such clearly identifiable risk factors for reinfection, chronic administration of low doses of once-daily nitrofurantoin, trimethoprim, or trimethoprim-sulfamethoxasole will prevent 90 percent of reinfections. Infections that do occur during prophylactic therapy are usually caused by resistant organisms. Long-term suppressive or prophylactic therapy is ineffective in patients with indwelling catheters [67].

Prostatitis

Most bacterial infections of the prostate are due to enteric gram-negative organisms that ascend through the urethra. *Acute* prostatitis is characterized by fever and chills, symptoms of lower urinary tract infection, perineal or back pain, and a diffusely tender prostate on rectal examination. Pyuria is usually present, and urine cultures are positive. Prostatic massage should be avoided, since it may induce bacteremia. Most antibiotics penetrate the acutely inflamed prostate well, and therapy is usually successful. Complications include prostatic abscess or infarction, seminal vesiculitis, and epididymitis. *Chronic* bacterial prostatitis, probably the leading cause of relapsing urinary tract infections in men, is usually not preceded by acute infection. Many patients are asymptomatic; others experience intermittent or continuous perineal or low-back pain. Rectal examination and intravenous pyelography are usually normal unless chronic infection occurs in an otherwise enlarged or abnormal prostate. Diagnosis depends on the demonstration of higher bacterial counts in prostatic secretions expressed by digital massage and in postmassage voided urine than in first-voided (the first 5 to 10 ml) or midstream urine. Bacterial counts in chronic prostatitis are often low and may not exceed 10^3/ml, but microbiologic confirmation of infection is important, since chronic bacterial prostatitis can be mimicked by noninfectious conditions (e.g., nonbacterial prostatitis, prostatodynia) and since treatment requires prolonged antibiotic therapy. Oral trimethoprim-sulfamethoxasole penetrates the noninflamed prostate well, and administration for 1 to 4 months is currently the treatment of choice. Patients who relapse may benefit from chronic suppressive therapy [40].

Epididymitis and Orchitis

Epididymitis is an acute inflammatory condition of the epididymis usually caused by ascending infection from the urethra or prostate. In young, sexually active men, the most common preceding condition is urethral infection with *N. gonorrhea* or *C. trachomatis;* up to 20 percent of men with untreated gonorrhea may develop epididymitis. In children and older men, especially those with structural abnormalities or recent genitourinary procedures, epididymitis is usually associated with urinary tract infection by enteric organisms or *P. aeruginosa.* Epididymitis can be gradual or sudden in onset with predominant symptoms of scrotal pain and swelling. Examination usually reveals tenderness in the posterior scrotum over the epididymis and often erythema and edema of the scrotal wall. Patients with sexually acquired infection often have a urethral discharge. Inflammation also may progress to involve the testis and produce epididymo-orchitis. The diagnosis of epididymitis is based on the history and physical examination; laboratory studies may help determine the likely organism. A Gram-stained urethral swab specimen with white blood cells indicates urethritis and suggests *Chlamydia* or gonorrhea; Gram's stain and culture of midstream urine are useful in patients with a possible underlying urinary tract infection. The leading differential diagnosis of the acutely painful scrotum is testicular torsion, which is more common in adolescents than older men and which requires immediate surgery. White blood cells on urethral or urine Gram's stain make this diagnosis unlikely. Epididymitis generally responds well to medical therapy with appropriate antibiotics; complications such as testicular infarction and abscess require surgery. Bilateral epididymitis occasionally results in sterility.

Bacterial infection of the testes is rare except as a complication of epididymitis. Systemic viral infection by mumps or Coxsackie B can cause isolated testicular involvement. Mumps orchitis is most common in postpubertal men, occurring in 20 percent of cases. Testicular pain follows the onset of parotid symptoms by 4 to 6 days, is unilateral in 70 percent of patients, and usually resolves within a week. No specific therapy is available, and sterility seems to be a rare complication.

Sexually Transmitted Diseases

The intimate contact of skin and mucous membranes that occurs during sexual activity provides an excellent opportunity for transmission of a variety of generally fastidious bacteria, viruses, and protozoa. While these pathogens produce a wide spectrum of acute and chronic disease syndromes, most agents of sexually transmitted disease (STD) are asymptomatic in a large proportion of infected patients. This reduces the chances of their detection and increases the opportunity for transmission. Because of similarities in modes of transmission, infection with multiple pathogens is common in patients with sexually transmitted diseases. The important sexually transmitted viruses are discussed in other chapters (hepatitis A and B viruses in Chapter 5, human immunodeficiency virus in Chapter 7, and herpes simplex virus and human papilloma virus in Chapter 12); this discussion will focus on the important bacterial causes of sexually transmitted diseases: syphilis, gonorrhea, and infection with *Chlamydia trachomatis.*

Syphilis

Syphilis is a systemic illness with a wide variety of manifestations caused by the spirochete *Treponema pallidum.* The rates of new cases of syphilis in the United States have fallen by 95 percent since their peak during World War II, although approximately 25,000 cases are still reported per year, a third of which occur in homosexual men. While syphilis can be transmitted by direct inoculation, blood transfusion, and passage in utero, the vast majority of cases are sexually transmitted. Approximately one-third to one-half of the sexual contacts of patients with syphilis will become infected. This underscores the need for tracing and treatment of contacts.

DIAGNOSIS

Syphilis usually presents with a primary skin lesion, or chancre, at the site of inoculation after a mean incubation period of 21 days (range 3 to 90 days). The chancre begins as a papule, evolves into a painless, indurated ulcer, and heals over 3 to 6 weeks; multiple lesions may occur. Nontender regional lymphadenopathy is common. Primary syphilis may be asymptomatic in patients with a low inoculation titer of treponemes, prior syphilis, or a chancre at an inapparent site such as the oropharynx, anal canal, vagina, or cervix. Since *T. pallidum* cannot be grown by conventional culture, the diagnosis of primary syphilis is confirmed by demonstration under dark-field microscopy of motile spirochetes in exudate from the base of the chancre or by a positive serologic test for syphilis (STS). Primary syphilis must be distinguished from ulcers induced by genital herpes, infection with *Hemophilus ducreyi* (chancroid), or genital trauma, all of which are usually tender.

Without treatment, primary syphilis is followed within weeks or months by secondary syphilis, a systemic illness characterized by low-grade fever, malaise, generalized lymphadenopathy, and symmetrical mucocutaneous lesions. The syndrome is caused by hematogenous dissemination of treponemes and can be complicated by involvement of the central nervous system, eyes, liver, kidney, bones, and joints. The most typical feature is the maculopapular rash that often involves the palms and soles. Moist plaques in intertriginous areas, condyloma lata, and silvery mucous patches on genital or oral mucosa occur in 20 percent of patients. Secondary syphilis has a broad differential

diagnosis, but it can be easily confirmed by dark-field microscopy of moist skin lesions or serologic testing, which is invariably positive [13].

If untreated, syphilis progresses to a latent phase, defined as a positive serologic test in the absence of clinical disease. During "early latency," variably considered to be within 1 to 4 years of onset of infection, patients are infectious, and 25 percent will experience relapses of mucocutaneous lesions. "Late latent" syphilis is thought not to be infectious except through contact with a patient's blood (in utero or by transfusion), and individuals in this state are resistant to reinfection. More than 25 percent of persons with untreated latent syphilis may develop later complications, known as tertiary, or late, syphilis. These include gummas (granulomatous lesions of soft tissue or bones), cardiovascular syphilis (aortitis), and neurosyphilis (with meningovascular or parenchymal involvement) [13, 74].

There are two categories of serologic tests for syphilis: those which measure nonspecific, nontreponemal "reaginic" antibody (RPR, VDRL) and those which measure antibody directed against specific treponemal antigen (FTA-abs, TPHA-TP). The nonspecific tests are useful in screening and, because they tend to decline in titer after treatment, as indicators of the success of therapy or of reinfection. False-positive reactions can occur in a variety of situations: during acute and chronic infections, in pregnant women, in intravenous drug users, after immunization, and in autoimmune disease. A positive specific test is always necessary to confirm a diagnosis of syphilis. Once positive, treponemal-specific antibody persists for life, limiting its use in diagnosing reinfection.

TREATMENT

Since it became available, penicillin has been the drug of choice for syphilis. Although still exquisitely penicillin-sensitive, the slow rate of replication of *T. pallidum* makes prolonged drug exposure necessary. Syphilis of less than a year's duration is treated with a single 2.4 million unit intramuscular (IM) injection of long-acting benzathine penicillin G (LAB). Penicillin-allergic patients can be treated with tetracycline or erythromycin (2 gm per day orally for 15 days). For syphilis of unknown or greater than a year's duration, prolonged therapy with four weekly injections of long-acting benzathine penicillin G or 30 days of oral erythromycin or tetracycline is recommended. For neurosyphilis, high doses of parenteral penicillin G should be used in addition to long-acting benzathine penicillin G; chloramphenicol can be used in penicillin-allergic patients. Posttreatment testing by VDRL to ensure eradication of infection should be performed at 3, 6, and 12 months and, for secondary and late latent syphilis, at 24 months. Patients with neurosyphilis should be followed with serologic testing and cerebrospinal fluid evaluation for at least 3 years. Patients should be warned about the possibility of the Jarisch-Herxheimer reaction, a transient syndrome of fever, chills, malaise, arthralgia, and myalgia which begins within 2 to 6 hours of treatment and resolves within 24 hours. It occurs in 25 to 90 percent of patients treated for latent syphilis.

Gonorrhea

Gonorrhea is an infection of nonsquamous epithelium caused by *Neisseria gonorrhoea*. Although involvement is usually limited to mucosal surfaces of the genitalia, anus, and oropharynx, complications may arise from local extension of disease in up to 20 percent of patients and from blood-borne dissemination in 1 to 3 percent. In contrast to syphilis, gonorrhea has not been well-controlled, in part because of evolving antimicrobial resistance patterns, and it is currently the most common reportable communicable disease in the United States. Incidence rates rose to unprecedented levels in the 1970s and have since remained at approximately 1 million reported cases per year. While gonorrhea is occasionally transmitted by nonsexual contact, the vast majority of infections in adults are sexually transmitted. The risk of acquiring gonorrhea after a single exposure to an infected partner is 20 percent for men and up to 50 percent for women. Although

50 to 95 percent of newly infected persons develop symptoms, most cases are transmitted by asymptomatic individuals who do not come to medical attention and thus have prolonged infection. Identification and treatment of such contact should be carried out in every case of gonorrhea [31].

In men, gonococcal infection is most common in the urethra, where it produces symptoms of dysuria and purulent discharge in up to 95 percent of patients within 1 to 14 days of exposure. Local complications include epididymitis, lymphadenitis, and penile edema. Without treatment, symptoms resolve within several weeks, although patients occasionally remain culture-positive for months. In women, the endocervix is the most common site of involvement; the vagina, urethra, and anus may also be culture-positive. The rate of asymptomatic infection in women is unclear, although probably greater than that in men. Symptoms include vaginal discharge, abnormal menses, and dysuria, and many patients have a friable cervix and mucopurulent endocervical discharge on examination [10]. The most important local complication is ascending infection to the fallopian tubes, which produces pelvic inflammatory disease (PID). Pelvic inflammatory disease occurs in 10 to 20 percent of women with gonorrhea and is characterized by lower abdominal pain, adnexal tenderness, and occasionally, systemic toxicity with fever, chills, nausea, and vomiting. Pelvic inflammatory disease may be complicated acutely by tubo-ovarian abscess or pelvic peritonitis and chronically by fallopian tube scarring, which predisposes to ectopic pregnancy and infertility. A less common complication of ascending infection through the fallopian tubes is infection of the capsule of the liver, or perihepatitis.

Gonorrhea also can infect other sites in both men and women. Pharyngeal infection is usually asymptomatic and occurs in 3 to 25 percent of patients with genital infection. Anorectal infection occurs frequently in homosexual men and occasionally in women; less than 10 percent of infected persons develop symptoms of proctitis [27]. Ocular infection is the most common site of involvement in neonates and occurs occasionally in adults as conjunctivitis. Disseminated gonococcal infection (DGI) usually arises from asymptomatic mucosal sites and presents with fever, tenosynovitis, and characteristic petechial and pustular skin lesions on the extremities. Frank mono- or oligoarticular septic arthritis may subsequently develop either with or without preceding rash. The differential diagnosis of disseminated gonococcal infection includes other bacterial infections and seronegative arthritis such as Reiter's syndrome [30].

DIAGNOSIS

The diagnosis of gonorrhea requires detection of the organism in specimens from infected sites by Gram's stain or culture. A Gram's stain of purulent exudate from a mucosal surface which contains gram-negative intracellular diplococci is diagnostic and has a sensitivity of 95 percent in urethritis and 50 to 60 percent in cervicitis. Sensitivity is less for specimens obtained in the absence of purulent exudate or from heavily contaminated sites such as the rectum and pharynx. Cultures of mucosal sites on selective media have a sensitivity of 80 to 95 percent, and in screening for gonorrhea, they should be obtained from the sites of greatest risk: the urethra in heterosexual men, the endocervix in women, and the urethra, pharynx, and rectum in homosexual men. In disseminated gonococcal infection, neither Gram's stain or culture of skin lesions, joint fluid, or blood has a sensitivity of greater than 30 percent, and diagnosis depends on isolation of the organism from a mucosal site during a compatible clinical illness.

TREATMENT

Although sensitivity patterns have changed over the last 40 years, gonorrhea is susceptible to a variety of antimicrobials, and the choice of regimen depends on the site of involvement, local resistance patterns, patient compliance, and the likelihood of concomitant infection with *C. trachomatis*. The standard treatment for genital infection includes a single dose of a beta-lactam antibiotic (amoxicillin, 3.0 gm PO, or procaine penicillin G, 4.8 million units IM, plus 1 gm oral probenecid; ceftriaxone, 125 mg IM, is an alternative) followed by a week of oral tetracycline (2 gm per day) or doxycycline (200 mg per day) to eradicate *C. trachomatis*. The treatment of pelvic inflammatory disease requires 10 to 14 days of tetracycline or doxycycline and may require hospitalization and intravenous antibiotics. Patients infected with penicillinase-producing strains should receive intramuscular spectinomycin or ceftriaxone rather than a penicillin. Disseminated gonococcal infection responds quickly to the preceding regimens. Hospitalization and intravenous antibiotics are recommended for initial therapy of frank septic arthritis [66].

Chlamydia trachomatis *Infection*

Chlamydia trachomatis, an obligatory intracellular bacterium, produces a variety of clinical syndromes which include trachoma, perinatal conjunctivitis and pneumonia, and genital tract infections resembling those caused by gonorrhea. Because of the absence of widely available and sensitive diagnostic tests and a national reporting system, the extent of genital *C. trachomatis* infection in the United States is difficult to determine. The estimated 3 to 5 million cases per year, however, make *C. trachomatis* the most common cause of sexually transmitted diseases and a major public health problem. The prevalence of genital *C. trachomatis* infection in adults ranges from 3 percent in the general population to up to 20 percent in patients attending sexually transmitted disease clinics. Although less easily transmitted than *N. gonorrhoeae, C. trachomatis* is frequently a copathogen occurring in 25 to 50 percent of cases of gonorrhea. Infection is asymptomatic in up to 50 percent of patients and may persist for months, making tracing and treatment of sexual contacts an important element of control, analogous to the situation with syphilis and gonorrhea.

Like *N. gonorrhoeae, C. trachomatis* infects nonsquamous epithelium and causes mucosal inflammation, complicated occasionally by local extension into other anatomic sites. *Chlamydia trachomatis* has a longer incubation period than gonorrhea, 7 to 21 days, and generally produces a less brisk inflammatory response. In men, *C. trachomatis* is the etiologic agent in 30 to 50 percent of cases of nongonococcal urethritis (NGU) and also causes epididymitis and proctitis. In women, mucopurulent cervicitis, an often asymptomatic inflammation characterized by mucopurulent endocervical discharge and cervical friability, is as common as nongonococcal urethritis in men. It is present in 25 percent of women attending sexually transmitted disease clinics, and *C. trachomatis* is isolated in 60 percent of those patients. *Chlamydia trachomatis* also causes the urethral syndrome (dysuria and pyuria in the absence of significant bacteriuria), endometritis, perihepatitis, and most important, pelvic inflammatory disease which may occur in 10 percent of infected women. Genital *Chlamydia* infection has been also associated with Reiter's syndrome, most commonly in men. Lymphogranuloma venereum, a systemic disease produced by certain serotypes of *C. trachomatis,* is characterized by fluctuant regional lymphadenopathy and progressive fibrosis; it is rare in the United States.

While the clinical diagnosis of nongonococcal urethritis can be made by finding ≥ 4 polymorphonuclear leukocytes per oil-immersion field on a Gram's stain of urethral exudate, confirmation of *C. trachomatis* infection, especially in asymptomatic individuals or in those with other genital syndromes, relies on antigen detection or culture techniques [81, 82]. The former is more rapid and widely available but is only 80 to 90 percent as sensitive as the more expensive cell culture. *Chlamydia trachomatis* is sensitive to a variety of antimicrobials, including sulfonamides, the tetracyclines, and erythromycin, but its slow replication cycle makes prolonged therapy necessary. Thus far, the emergence of resistant organisms has not been a problem. Recommended therapy for lower genital tract infection includes tetracycline (2 gm daily), doxycycline (200 mg daily), or erythromycin (2 gm daily) for 7 days; treatment should be extended to 10 to 14 days for epididymitis and pelvic inflammatory disease. The use of these regimens for the treatment of gonorrhea will eradicate coexisting *C. trachomatis* infection and may enhance public health control of the *Chlamydia* problem.

Immunodeficiency and the Acquired Immunodeficiency Syndrome (AIDS)

Opportunistic infections are produced by organisms that are nonpathogenic and often part of routine colonizing microbial flora in the normal host but which cause disease when presented with the "opportunity" of a host with compromised defenses. The first lines of host defense are the intact anatomic barriers of skin and mucous membranes, which can be disrupted by trauma and iatrogenic procedures. Once these have been breached, the major mechanisms of protection against infection are humoral immunity, polymorphonuclear leukocytes (PMN), and cell-mediated immunity (CMI). Table 6-19 summarizes the disease states most commonly associated with defects in these three branches of host defense and a sampling of the most important pathogens

seen with each. Although more than one mechanism is usually involved in the control of infection with each of the listed organisms, several generalizations about specific defects are possible. First, patients with abnormal immunoglobulin levels or splenic dysfunction are at greatest risk for infection with pyogenic bacteria, whose protective capsule makes phagocytosis difficult without the presence of specific opsonizing antibody. Second, patients with abnormal function or number of polymorphonuclear leukocytes are predisposed to infection with skin and mucous membrane flora (e.g., staphylococci, enteric gram-negative bacteria, and *P. aeruginosa*) and fungi (e.g., *Candida* spp. and *Aspergillus* spp.). Third, patients with defective cell-mediated immunity are

Table 6–19. *Occurrence of Infections in Patients with Defects of Host Defense*

Humoral immunity	Hypogammaglobulinemia, splenectomy, multiple myeloma, chronic lymphocytic leukemia, nephrotic syndrome, cytotoxic therapy, AIDS	*Streptococcus pneumonia, Hemophilus influenza,* streptococci, *Pneumocystis carinii, Giardia lamblia*
Polymorphonuclear leukocytes	Cytotoxic therapy, nonlymphocytic leukemia, drug-induced granulocytopenia, aplastic anemia, chronic granulomatous disease	Staphylococci, gram-negative enteric bacteria, *Pseudomonas aeruginosa, Candida* spp., *Aspergillus* spp.
Cell-mediated immunity	AIDS, cytotoxic therapy, cortiocosteroid therapy, Hodgkin's disease, non-Hodgkin's lymphoma	*Mycobacterium* spp., *Listeria monocytogenes, Nocardia asteroides,* Herpes group viruses, *Candida* spp., *Pneumocystis carinii, Toxoplasma gondii*

susceptible to a variety of bacterial, fungal, protozoal, and latent DNA viral pathogens, many of which have the capacity to establish latent or quiescent intracellular infection (e.g., *M. tuberculosis, P. carinii, T. gondii,* and herpes group viruses). Most of the infectious processes manifested in these deficiency states develop from endogenous sources, which means that preventing infection is difficult [65, 68].

Neutropenia

Although there are a variety of disease- and drug-related causes of neutropenia, therapy of cancer with cytotoxic agents is the most common and probably the one associated with the most severe infections. The risk of infection during neutropenia is directly related to the depth of the decline, increasing significantly at <500 PMN/mm^3 and even more at <100 PMN/mm^3. The rapidity of onset and duration of neutropenia also increase the rate and severity of infection and are directly related to the intensity of therapy. Patients undergoing therapy for leukemia may be neutropenic for 3 to 6 weeks, during which time most will become febrile; therapy of solid tumors usually induces neutropenia of shorter duration. The site of infection is often related to chemotherapy-induced disruptions of skin and mucous membranes, which most frequently involve the lungs, oropharynx, skin and perianal area, and esophagus. Infections are generally caused by col-

onizing bacteria, and these are often hospital-acquired and resistant to multiple antibiotics [87]. Fungal infections by *Candida* spp. and *Aspergillus* spp. and mucormycosis are also common, probably in part because of the liberal use of broad-spectrum antibiotics for bacterial infection [75].

Although standard microbiologic and radiographic evaluation of neutropenic patients permits the diagnosis of most infections, their tempo and clinical presentation may be different than in normal hosts due to mobilization of inadequate numbers of polymorphonuclear leukocytes to sites of infection. Pulmonary infections are special problems in neutropenic patients [68]. They are common and have a mortality rate of over 50 percent due in part to delayed diagnosis and identification of the etiologic agent(s). Clinical findings and chest x-ray changes may take several days to develop, and purulent sputum for Gram's stain and culture is frequently not produced. Empiric antimicrobial therapy for likely pathogens is routine in the febrile neutropenic patient without localizing findings and has been advocated as an initial response to pneumonia of uncertain etiology [64, 83]. More invasive diagnostic procedures (e.g., transtracheal aspiration, bronchoscopy, and open lung biopsy) should be aggressively pursued in more complicated hosts, such as those with prolonged neutropenia, associated defects of cell-mediated immunity, or a poor clinical response to empiric therapy. Undue delay can result in clinical deterioration of the patient and increase the risk of invasive procedures and the likelihood of toxicity from broad-spectrum antimicrobials.

Acquired Immunodeficiency Syndrome

The acquired immunodeficiency syndrome (AIDS), first recognized in 1981, is caused by the human immunodeficiency virus (HIV), a lymphotropic retrovirus that infects T4 (helper) cells, B cells, and monocytes. There is a variable but usually progressive destruction of T4 cells which, because of their central role in immunoregulation, leads to a spectrum of immunologic disorders. These include decreases in lymphocyte proliferation response to antigens, delayed hypersensitivity, lymphokine production, natural-killer and cytotoxic T-cell activity, macrophage chemotaxis and killing, and B-cell response to new antigens. AIDS itself is a clinical syndrome, defined as the development of neoplasms or opportunistic infections which are predictive of a defect in cell-mediated immunity in the absence of known underlying causes of cellular immunodeficiency. While AIDS represents the most severe manifestation of progressive lymphocyte infection and depletion, it has occurred in only 20 to 30 percent of HIV-infected individuals over the 5 to 8 years of follow-up observation available so far. Once HIV infection occurs, however, it persists indefinitely and probably for the lifetime of the host. As of March 30, 1987, 33,482 cases of AIDS had been reported in the United States; the estimated number of individuals with subclinical HIV infection is greater than 1 million [19, 73].

Human immunodeficiency virus (HIV) is transmitted by intimate sexual contact, both homosexual and heterosexual, and by exposure to blood and blood products. Persons at risk of HIV infection include homosexual and bisexual men, intravenous drug users, hemophiliacs, blood transfusion recipients, heterosexual contacts of individuals within these groups, and infants born to infected women. Although heterosexual transmission of HIV has accounted for a minimal and constant proportion of AIDS cases in the United States and Europe, there is evidence that it is the primary mode of spread in Central Africa. Studies among household contacts and health care providers of AIDS patients indicate that HIV is very unlikely to be transmitted by casual contact. The requirement for intimate contact or exchange of blood is attributable to the fact that although HIV can be isolated from a variety of body fluids (e.g., blood, semen, urine, vaginal secretions, saliva, tears, and cerebrospinal fluid), only those containing T cells, such as blood and semen, are likely to be efficient vectors of infection.

The spectrum of manifestations of HIV infection is broad and not completely understood (Table 6-20). The largest group of patients with HIV infection are asymptomatic, chronically infected individuals (group II). Although some may experience a transient mononucleosis-like syndrome during the acute stage of their infection (group I), most acquire infection asymptomatically. The duration of the asymptomatic phase is variable, and the factors causing progression to more symptomatic stages are unknown. Most individuals who progress will develop persistent generalized lymphadenopathy (group III), which also may have a chronic, stable course or may accelerate into a further stage of disease. Development of frank AIDS occurs in up to 10 percent of these patients per year and may be heralded by regression of the lymphadenopathy. It has recently been appreciated that a spectrum of primary neurologic changes (group IVB) is common in HIV infection [40, 43]. Signs of neurologic deterioration precede frank immunodeficiency in 10 percent of AIDS patients, and it is possible that a large percentage of patients with HIV-induced dementia will never develop full-blown AIDS. The AIDS-related complex (ARC) has been variably defined but generally refers to individuals with constitutional symptoms (e.g., persistent fever and night sweats, sustained weight loss, persistent unexplained diarrhea, and profound fatigue; group IVA), some of whom develop "minor" opportunistic infections, i.e., those thought to be less predictive of impaired cell-mediated immunity (group IV, C1). The symptoms of AIDS-related complex are debilitating and may represent un-

Table 6–20. *CDC Classification of HIV Infection*

Group I: Acute infection: Mononucleosis-like syndrome, with seroconversion

Group II: Asymptomatic infection: Positive HIV antibody or viral culture, without symptoms

Group III: Persistent generalized lymphadenopathy: Lymphadenopathy (>1 cm) at two or more extrainguinal sites for more than 3 months in the absence of concurrent illness

Group IV: Other HIV disease:

  Subgroup A: Constitutional disease: One or more of the following: fever or diarrhea for more than 1 month or involuntary weight loss with no other explanation

  Subgroup B: Neurologic disease: One or more of the following: dementia, myelopathy, or peripheral neuropathy with no other explanation

  Subgroup C: Secondary infectious diseases: Infectious disease that is associated with HIV infection and/or at least moderately indicative of a defect in cell-mediated immunity:

    Category C1: Symptomatic or invasive disease due to 1 of 12 specified diseases listed in the surveillance definition of AIDS: *Pneumocystis carinii* pneumonia, chronic cryptosporidiosis, toxoplasmosis, extraintestinal strongyloidiasis, isosporiasis, candidiasis (esophageal, bronchial, or pulmonary), cryptococcosis, histoplasmosis, mycobacterial infection (*Mycobacterium avium* complex or *M. kansasii*), cytomegalovirus infection, chronic mucocutaneous or disseminated herpes simplex virus infection, and progressive multifocal leukoencephalopathy

    Category C2: Symptomatic or invasive disease due to 1 of 6 other specified diseases: oral hairy leukoplakia, multidermatomal herpes zoster, recurrent *Salmonella* bacteremia, nocardiosis, tuberculosis, and oral candidiasis

  Subgroup D: Secondary cancers: One or more of the following: Kaposi's sarcoma, non-Hodgkin's lymphoma, or primary lymphoma of the brain

  Subgroup E: Other conditions in HIV infection: Other diseases that may be attributable to HIV infection and are indicative of a defect in cell-mediated immunity (e.g., chronic lymphoid, interstitial pneumonitis, secondary infectious diseases, and neoplasms not listed above).

Source: *Morbid. Mortal. Weekly Rep.* 35: 334, 1986.

diagnosed opportunistic infection in some cases. The majority of patients with AIDS-related complex progress to AIDS.

The severe disorders that serve as the criteria for AIDS are included in categories C1 and C2 of group IV. The opportunistic infections are those which are seen rarely or only in localized form in normal hosts. The most common is *P. carinii* pneumonia (PCP), which occurs in 60 percent of patients with AIDS. The disease can be sudden in onset, but more commonly it progresses gradually over several weeks with symptoms of dry cough, fever, and shortness of breath. Physical examination is often unremarkable except for fever. The chest x-ray characteristically reveals bilateral interstitial infiltrates, but it is normal in 10 percent of patients, in which case hypoxemia or a gallium scan with diffuse pulmonary abnormalities may suggest the disease. Identification of *P. carinii* by staining of pulmonary specimens is required for a definitive diagnosis; obtaining such specimens usually requires bronchoscopy. The majority of pulmonary disorders in patients with suspected AIDS are due to *P. carinii* pneumonia with or without other pathogens; other processes include Kaposi's sarcoma and infection with *Mycobacterium avium-intracellulare* (MAI), cytomegalovirus (CMV), and a variety of bacteria and fungi. Treatment of *P. carinii* pneumonia with trimethoprim-sulfamethoxasole or pentamidine is effective in approximately 70 percent of patients, although up to 25 percent may have recurrences [91]. After the lungs, the gastrointestinal tract is the organ system most commonly involved with opportunistic infections in AIDS. Frequent problems include esophagitis caused by *Candida* spp., herpes simplex virus, and cytomegalovirus; gastroenteritis due to *M. avium-intracellulare*, intestinal protozoa, and enteric bacterial pathogens; and a chronic malabsorption syndrome. Central nervous system disease occurs in 35 to 40 percent of patients with AIDS. Although most commonly due to direct HIV-related neuropathy, opportunistic infections such as cryptococcal meningitis, central nervous system toxoplasmosis, and cytomegalovirus retinitis are also common.

The most important "opportunistic neoplasm" of the AIDS epidemic has been Kaposi's sarcoma (KS), a tumor of endothelial origin possibly related to cytomegalovirus infection. It occurs in 25 percent of AIDS patients, more frequently in homosexual men (36 percent) than intravenous drug users (4 percent). The disease presents with gradually progressive brown or purple nodules found on the trunk, extremities, and head and neck and often involves internal organs. Therapy with radiation, combined chemotherapy, and interferon has been of limited success, although the survival rate is almost three times as long for AIDS patients with Kaposi's sarcoma alone as for those with opportunistic infection.

Nosocomial Infections

A nosocomial infection is one acquired while the patient is in the hospital. It generally will appear at least 3 days after admission, but it may not present until after discharge. About 5 percent of hospitalized patients will develop a nosocomial infection; each leads to 5 to 10 additional hospital days per patient. Urinary tract infections are the most common (40 percent), followed by postoperative wound infections (20 percent) and pulmonary (15 percent) and blood (10 to 15 percent) infections [50]. Miscellaneous sites of infections, including the skin, peritoneum, and central nervous system, comprise the remaining 15 to 25 percent. Intensive care unit patients are at greatest risk. Common pathogens include enteric gram-negative rods, S. aureus, S. epidermidis, and enterococci. Many of these are resistant to commonly used antibiotics.

Most nosocomial urinary tract infections result from instrumentation; usually, this is placement of an indwelling urethral catheter. *Escherichia coli* is the most common pathogen; other frequent isolates include group D enterococcus, *P. aeruginosa,* and *Proteus/Providencia* spp. To prevent such infections, catheters should be used judiciously and removed as soon as possible. Aseptic insertion techniques, handwashing, and maintenance of closed sterile drainage are essential to reduce the incidence of infection.

Postoperative wound infections are a significant source of morbidity and occasional mortality. Rates of infection depend on the hospital, the surgeon, and the specific operation. Most of these infections are superficial and easily treated, but they can involve deep tissue spaces. In clean operations, S. aureus is the usual pathogen; in clean-contaminated operations, the endogenous flora of the organs involved in the resection are frequently isolated. Prevention is based on strict adherence to sterile surgical technique, short preoperative hospital stay, minimizing the duration of surgery, preoperative shower with antiseptic soap, shaving of body hair immediately before surgery, and judicious use of prophylactic antibiotics [51]. Because of the inherent risks involved (side effects, emergence of resistant organisms), intraoperative antibiotics should be used when there is a strong likelihood of infection or when the consequence of infection could be catastrophic, such as clean-contaminated or contaminated surgery or surgery in a person with a prosthetic heart valve. Antibiotic selection is based on knowledge of the endogenous flora found at the site of surgery; occasionally, preoperative cultures can guide the choice of drugs (e.g., urine culture prior to urologic surgery). Generally, antibiotics are given intravenously 1 hour before surgery and should be continued for 24 hours only.

Pneumonia

Pneumonia is the most common fatal nosocomial infection. Mortality is estimated at between 20 and 50 percent [52]. Gram-negative pneumonias are associated with the highest mortality rates. Organisms commonly isolated include *S. pneumoniae, Klebsiella* spp., *S. aureus, P. aeruginosa, E. coli,* and *Enterobacter* spp. Although less well documented, influenza viruses and respiratory syncytial virus (RSV) (pediatric wards) also cause nosocomial pneumonia.

Factors that predispose to development of nosocomial pneumonia include intubation, need for intensive care unit, antibiotics, surgery, chronic lung disease, advanced age, and immunosuppression [53]. Most of these pneumonias result from aspiration of mouth flora. Bacteremia from a distant primary source with subsequent seeding of the lungs is an important but less common cause. Diagnosis can be difficult. Important clues include worsening infiltrates on chest x-ray, increased purulent sputum production, and a decrease in P_{O_2}. Fever and leukocytosis may be present but are nonspecific. Sputum cultures frequently are difficult to interpret because of contamination with mouth flora; Gram's stain is sometimes useful in identifying a predominant organism in association with leukocytes. Blood or pleural fluid cultures are occasionally positive and may provide a definitive bacteriologic diagnosis.

Prevention includes close attention to handwashing and proper care of respiratory equipment and solutions. Yearly influenza vaccines for patient care providers can decrease the spread of this disease. Prophylactic antibiotics have not proven useful because they encourage colonization and subsequent infection with resistant organisms. Unfortunately, little progress has been made toward effective treatment or prevention of this very serious nosocomial infection.

Bacteremia

Nosocomial bacteremia is a very serious problem with mortality rates of 20 to 40 percent. It usually begins as a localized infection, but approximately one-fourth of cases are primary and are usually due to intravascular catheters. Bacteria gain access to the blood at the site where the catheter enters the skin. Any in-line site that provides access to or monitoring of the bloodstream is a potential site for introduction of bacteria.

Risk factors that predispose to catheter-associated bacteremia include extremes of age, immunosuppression, severe underlying illness, and the presence of infection elsewhere in the body [54]. The organisms most commonly isolated are endogenous skin flora (possibly altered by previous antibiotic therapy). *Staphylococcus aureus* and *S. epidermidis* are the most frequent pathogens; gram-negative organisms, especially *Klebsiella, Enterobacter, Serratia,* and *E. coli,* are also commonplace [46]. Very unusual isolates should alert the clinician to the possibility of contamination from a source other than the skin (e.g., contaminated intravenous solutions). Total parenteral nutrition (TPN) lines are a frequent source of *Candida.*

Catheters may be infected without obvious external signs; consequently, intravascular devices should be considered a very likely source of bacteremia when no other site can be found. Cultures of catheter tips are sometimes useful in confirming the diagnosis of device-related sepsis. In most cases of bacteremia due to intravascular catheters, the device must be removed in order to eradicate the infection. Occasionally, surgically implanted Broviac or Hickman catheters are left in place and the patient is treated with antibiotics.

Intravascular catheters should be placed with careful sterile or aseptic technique. Intravenous lines should be removed every 3 days and intraarterial lines should be removed every 4 days if possible [46]. Manipulation of the system should be minimized, and handwashing should be emphasized.

Nosocomial infection can be a serious, life-threatening complication of a routine hospitalization. Preventive measures must be incorporated into routine patient care. These include handwashing, assessment of need for all invasive procedures no matter how benign or commonplace, minimizing duration of invasion, and adherence to appropriate isolation measures. Empiric treatment of these infections is based on a knowledge of the microbial flora and antibiotic resistance patterns of the institution in which the patient is hospitalized, as well as an understanding of the pathogenic process.

Mycotic Infections

Although more than 100,000 species of fungi are recognized, only 100 species produce disease in humans. The term *fungus* is a general one encompassing a ubiquitous group of microorganisms which vary from spherical yeasts to filamentous molds. These are eukaryotic, have cell walls composed of chitin, cellulose, or other glucans, and are much larger than bacteria. The simplest form with which the physician is familiar is the yeast, which is oval or spherical and reproduces by budding. The vegetative structure of a mold is more complex and forms a threadlike, multicellular, tubular filament—a hypha—that may branch and be divided by septa into segments. The morphologic characteristics of these are helpful in diagnosis. Some fungi are dimorphic. They are molds when present in nature and convert into yeasts when they enter the tissues of humans or are grown at 37°C.

Mycotic diseases can be conveniently divided according to the portions of the body where the organisms commonly invade to produce disease. Some fungi grow in the presence of keratin and cause *superficial* mycoses on hair or skin (dermatophycoses). Others produce *subcutaneous* disease (e.g., sporotrichosis, chromomycosis). Some produce infection within the body and can disseminate throughout most tissues; examples of these *deep* mycoses include histoplasmosis, blastomycosis, coccidioidomycosis, and cryptococcosis. Although the distinction is somewhat arbitrary, it is useful to consider other fungi as *opportunistic*, since they are commonly present on the skin or in the environment and invade locally when the skin or mucosal defenses are altered or systemically when an individual is immunocompromised. The best known examples are candidiasis and aspergillosis. The preceding is a convenient clinical classification and is sufficient for most situations, but these patterns can be altered in any patient whose host defenses are compromised by immunosuppression, diabetes mellitus, or chronic pulmonary disease.

Superficial Mycoses

The dermatophytoses are caused by a group of fungi related by their predilection for invading skin, hair, and nails. The resulting infections are termed *tinea* (ringworm). Dermatophytic infections are caused by organisms which are indigenous to most countries and are found in the soil or are primary pathogens of animals. They may be spread from both these sources or from human to human by fomite contamination. Organisms of the genera *Epidermophyton, Microsporum,* or *Trichophyton* are responsible for most of these chronic infections. The infection is designated according to its anatomic location: tinea capitis, tinea corporis, tinea cruris (the intertriginous areas), and tinea pedis.

The diagnosis can be confirmed by laboratory examination of scrapings from the affected areas. These are treated with 10 percent potassium hydroxide to destroy the keratin and are stained with lactophenol blue. In these preparations, branching hyphal elements, arthrospores, and yeasts can be observed in tissue fragments, and spores can be seen within or on the surface of hair.

Subcutaneous Mycoses

Subcutaneous mycoses are chronic nonfatal diseases that usually remain localized to the subcutaneous tissues, although they may spread extensively therein. Infection is a result of the inoculation of spores, indigenous to the soil and vegetation, into the skin. The most common examples are sporotrichosis, chromomycosis, and mycetoma. Only the first occurs with any frequency in this country.

Sporothrix schenckii is a saprophytic fungus found throughout the world. In the United States, such infection is most common in the north-central areas. The organism is found in the soil and on rose bushes, sphagnum moss, tree bark, and other vegetation. As a result, this is primarily an occupational disease of gardeners, farmers, and horticulturists. The fungus enters through breaks in the skin, usually caused by the vegetation on which the organism resides, and produces a papule within 1 to 6 weeks. Thereafter, the lesion enlarges to become nodular and then spreads proximally through regional lymphatics to produce subcutaneous nodules and regional adenopathy. The nodules are not painful, but they may ulcerate and drain a thin, serous material. The histopathology is a combination of suppuration and granulomata. A characteristic finding is pseudoepitheliomatous hyperplasia, which can be confused with a malignancy. The organism is not easily seen in tissue, but it can be demonstrated by methenamine silver or periodic acid–Schiff stains. It usually is grown easily on Sabouraud's agar; the plates should be held for at least 4 weeks.

The disease rarely disseminates beyond the skin. A few cases of primary pulmonary sporotrichosis have been reported, and these are due to inhalation of the organism. The infection is usually limited to the lung and generally presents as a chronic pneumonia, often with thin-walled cavities. It mimics tuberculosis in many respects, as do most pulmonary fungal infections. When sporotrichosis disseminates, it involves the large joints and adjacent long bones about 80 percent of the time [97].

Subcutaneous disease is treated with oral potassium iodide. A saturated solution (SSKI) is given in doses of 3 to 4 ml (maximum) every 8 hours. The usual method is to begin with a low dose (1 ml) and increase to the maximum; an alternate but similar method is to treat by weight of drug, beginning with 50 mg per drop and increasing daily until 3 to 4 gm are given per day. The major side effects are gastrointestinal upset, rash, lacrimation, and parotid swelling [85]. Pulmonary or disseminated infections are usually treated with amphotericin B (see below). Ketoconazole has recently been shown to have efficacy in pulmonary disease and may replace am-

photericin B when more clinical experience has been gained.

Deep (Systemic) Mycoses

The systemic mycoses are generally acquired by inhalation of spores. In order for a fungus to survive under these conditions, it must be able to grow at 37°C, and this usually requires a shift in morphology from a mycelial to a yeast phase. As a rule, these infections are asymptomatic unless the exposure has been to a large inoculum. This is corroborated by the fact that millions of people have positive skin tests to these organisms but have never had manifestations of disease. In contrast to bacterial infections, humoral immunity plays little or no role in the defense against mycoses, although antibody titers may be useful for diagnostic purposes. Cell-mediated immunity (CMI) is primarily responsible for eliminating or containing disease. Conversely, suppression of cell-mediated immunity renders the host susceptible to acquisition or reactivation of a mycosis; the best current example is the incidence of cryptococcal meningitis in persons with the acquired immunodeficiency syndrome. The major infections which produce deep mycoses are acquired from a restricted geographic area, and this fact is very useful in limiting the diagnostic considerations when taking a medical history.

HISTOPLASMOSIS

The highly infectious fungus *Histoplasma capsulatum* usually causes acute, benign pulmonary disease in the normal host. Approximately one-half million persons acquire histoplasmosis annually in this country [92]. The infection is worldwide, but in the United States it is confined to persons who live or have lived in the great river valleys of the central part of the country. In Kentucky, southern Ohio, Missouri, and Tennessee about 90 percent of the population have positive skin tests for this organism. Its natural habitat is the soil, especially if it has been contaminated with the excreta of fowl, birds (starlings are the best described), or bats. The disease occurs in persons not directly exposed to these animals when construction or demolition is carried out and the spores are aerosolized from the soil.

The spores are inhaled into the alveoli, and after they germinate, they disseminate through the lymphatics to regional nodes and via hematogenous spread to the entire body. Many are removed by the reticuloendothelial system in the liver and spleen, and as a result, the manifestations of disease usually occur in these organs. In the normal host, a granulomatous reaction develops within the first 1 or 2 weeks; this contains the disease, and these caseating and noncaseating granulomata calcify over many years to produce the characteristic pulmonary and splenic calcifications. This sequence of events is similar to the pathophysiology of tuberculosis.

Heavy exposure to the organism, as in spelunkers or persons who work in chicken coops, may cause acute pulmonary histoplasmosis. This is an influenza-like syndrome which begins about 2 weeks postexposure. Fever, chills, and nonproductive cough dominate the clinical picture, and the chest x-ray reveals small, patchy, soft infiltrates that ultimately calcify. There is prominent hilar adenopathy which resolves after several weeks or months [24]. Progressive disseminated disease [24, 25, 76, 93] is uncommon, but it occurs in infants, older persons, and those with depressed cell-mediated immunity from any cause. The clinical illness can vary from a severe disease, more often seen in infants, to a chronic progressive disease which can extend from months to years. The systemic symptoms are hepatosplenomegaly, anemia, fever, chills, malaise, anorexia, and weight loss. This may be complicated by gastrointestinal ulcerations, cutaneous lesions, adrenal insufficiency, lytic bone lesions, lymphadenopathy, meningitis, and focal cerebritis.

Chronic pulmonary histoplasmosis usually occurs in the setting of chronic obstructive pulmonary disease [24] and begins as an interstitial pneumonitis that develops into a cavitary disease. It manifests itself, as do many chronic pulmonary infections, with malaise, weight loss, cough, night sweats, and an interstitial infiltrate that usually is in the apical and posterior areas of the lungs. Diagnosis of this cavitary or fibrotic pneumonitis requires demonstration of the organism in sputum (about a third to half of patients) or in biopsy material. Serial radiographs provide the best index of disease activity.

Diagnosis requires cultivation of the organism from sputum or marrow, biopsy of a lesion, or an appropriate body fluid. Tissue for histopathology is very useful, since the organisms are often demonstrated by the methenamine silver stain. Skin tests are not useful, since most individuals in endemic areas will react. Complement-fixation tests use two types of antigens: the yeast phase and the mycelial phase. The former becomes reactive within 1 to 2 weeks after exposure, the latter somewhat later. Since most persons with acute disease will be positive to both tests, the quantitative result is important; titers below 1 : 16 are suspect. At higher dilutions, a positive result is more likely to reflect acute disease, but it must be accepted with caution. A negative test is useful to eliminate the disease from diagnostic consideration. The titers may decline in disseminated histoplasmosis as the host becomes progressively debilitated.

COCCIDIOIDOMYCOSIS

Coccidioides immitis causes pulmonary infections in endemic areas of the United States. These infections, like histoplasmosis, are usually benign, but they can be chronic or disseminate. The endemic areas include the San Joaquin and adjacent valleys of California, southern Texas, Arizona and northern Mexico. Infection occurs relatively quickly in persons who move into these areas, since the arthrospores are inhaled whenever there are fresh diggings or dust storms. The clinical syndrome is an acute self-limited infection in 95 percent of persons [5]. About two-thirds of these will be asymptomatic, will develop a permanent immunity, and will be skin-test-positive. The remaining one-third develop an influenza-like syndrome after an incubation period of 1 to 3 weeks. In this group, a rash that is fine and macular also can appear, as can other manifestations of hypersensitivity—erythema nodosum or erythema multiforme are the best described. These are frequently accompanied by arthralgias and carry a good prognosis. This syndrome is known as "valley fever." The radiographic picture is a segmental pneumonia (about 50 percent), hilar adenopathy, and pleural infiltrates (about 20 percent); minimal reaction occurs in others. The organism can be recovered from the sputum in about half of primary infections. A positive culture is diagnostic, since the organism is not a commensal [5]. The laboratory should be notified of the probable diagnosis, since this organism is highly infectious and can cause laboratory outbreaks unless appropriate precautions are taken. Most patients who have acute disease do not require treatment, since the prognosis is excellent. Systemic antifungal therapy should be considered in persons who are at risk of developing chronic pulmonary or disseminated disease.

Chronic pulmonary disease can take the form of a progressive pneumonia, a miliary or cavitary disease, or a coccidioidoma [6]. Fewer than 1 percent of persons will have disseminated disease, but this generally is found in the following groups: infants, elderly, immunosuppressed persons, Filipinos, blacks, Mexicans, and pregnant women. Dissemination occurs within a few weeks of primary infection, but it can develop by reactivation of a latent focus. It can appear in any organ and is conceptually and clinically similar to disseminated histoplasmosis, which is described above.

Diagnosis is usually by cultivation of the organism, histopathology of affected tissues, and skin tests or serology. The skin test becomes positive within 4 weeks of the primary infection in 90 to 95 percent of patients. Conversion from negative to positive is useful, but a positive test in a prolonged illness is of much less value. Since the serology is affected by the skin test, it should be drawn before the coccidioidin is placed. The combination of precipitins, which appear within 4 weeks, and the complement-fixing antibodies, which develop between 4 and 12 weeks, are use-

ful. Since precipitins disappear in 4 to 6 weeks, their presence is important in the diagnosis of acute disease; the titer is not important. The complement-fixing antibodies persist, and a rising titer (greater than 1 : 16 to 1 : 32) suggests chronic or disseminated disease. Antibodies in the cerebrospinal fluid are considered pathognomonic of active coccidioidal meningitis.

Systemic antifungal therapy is indicated in all disseminated disease, and amphotericin B is the drug of choice. The role of ketoconazole or the other imidazoles is not completely clear, but the evidence indicates that these are inferior to amphotericin B [12].

BLASTOMYCOSIS

Blastomyces dermatitidis causes infections in normal hosts that are very similar to histoplasmosis. It is a dimorphic fungus which generally occurs in the central great river valleys and the mid-Atlantic and south-central states. Like *H. capsulatum*, it is a primary pathogen that produces asymptomatic infection about 60 percent of the time. Symptomatic patients can have an influenza-like illness which lasts for a few weeks. During this illness, the organism can be recovered from the sputum. Neither skin tests or serology are helpful for diagnosis because of the high incidence of false-negative and false-positive results. Chest x-rays are abnormal and may have multiple nodules, an interstitial infiltrate, or consolidation [70]. Since the natural history of this primary infection is not completely clear, there is debate as to whether it should be treated with antifungal agents. Infectious disease consultation is advised in the management of this process.

Chronic blastomycosis is quite variable [11]. The most common manifestations are in the lungs or skin. The complaints are of anorexia, malaise, weight loss, and fever if symptoms are present. The pulmonary findings are of cough, sputum production, and dyspnea. The chest x-ray is not specific. Skin lesions are a common presenting symptom [98]. They begin as small papules which enlarge and become verrucous, elevated, and crusted over several weeks. Bone lesions, when present, are lytic, as in histoplasmosis. The organism can infect the prostate, epididymis, or testes.

Amphotericin B has replaced the diamidines as therapy of choice; a total dose of 1.5 to 2 gm usually is necessary.

CRYPTOCOCCOSIS

Cryptococcus neoformans is usually found in association with bird droppings, especially those of pigeons. It is a saprophyte that infects normal and abnormal hosts. The portal of entry is usually the respiratory tract, and pulmonary infection is most common, but often without symptoms. As a result, this infection is infrequently diagnosed, and meningitis is the more common clinical presentation. Pulmonary infection is asymptomatic in about a third of patients; clinically significant disease has few constitutional signs or symptoms and is a subacute process. The organism provokes only a mild inflammatory process, and the usual indices of infection may be absent. Diagnosis requires evidence of tissue invasion by biopsy. The serologic test for cryptococcal antigen is positive in about half the cases. The prognosis of localized pulmonary disease is excellent. Observation is usually all that is necessary in pulmonary disease unless there is evidence of dissemination such as a positive culture of marrow or cerebrospinal fluid, the presence of antigen in the cerebrospinal fluid, or skin lesions. If the patient is an immunocompromised host, therapy is indicated irrespective of the severity of the clinical picture. Combined treatment with amphotericin B and 5-fluorocytosine is the treatment of choice [69].

The most common manifestation of disseminated disease is meningitis, and about half these patients have altered immunologic defense mechanisms. The most common symptoms are headache and altered mental status. Signs of meningeal irritation may not be noticed, but the cerebrospinal fluid will have a mononuclear cell infiltrate with a decreased glucose concentration. The organism can be demonstrated with an india ink preparation because of its large capsule in approximately half the patients. A positive crypto-coccal antigen in the cerebrospinal fluid is diagnostic, and is present in about 70 percent of patients.

Therapy is with both amphotericin B and 5-fluorocytosine [69]. The cerebrospinal fluid should be monitored weekly with culture, glucose, and cell count. The antigen should be checked monthly, and the cerebrospinal fluid reexamined every 3 to 4 months for a year after treatment, especially in an immunocompromised host. In patients with the acquired immunodeficiency syndrome, treatment may have to be continued for life.

Opportunistic Mycoses

Normal fungal flora, ubiquitously distributed in nature, are encountered with increasing frequency as opportunistic pathogens in humans with defects in host defense mechanisms. Disease generally occurs in those with depression of cell-mediated immunity but also occurs in diabetics and those with myeloperoxidase deficiency or chronic granulomatous disease of childhood. Pathologically produced air spaces, such as sinus tracts, ectatic bronchi, or emphysematous areas, can become colonized. Destruction of normal microbial flora by antibiotics allows the normal fungal flora to overgrow and predisposes to opportunistic mycoses. The most prevalent of these are candidiasis and aspergillosis.

Candida spp. are normal inhabitants of mucocutaneous body surfaces. The most common manifestations of overgrowth of these organisms are superficial skin infections and vaginitis. The specific alterations in the host which predispose to these infections are diabetes mellitus, treatment with corticosteroids or antibiotics, skin or mucosal damage (trauma, tumors, ulcerations, indwelling catheters, or similar devices), and immunosuppression, especially of cell-mediated immunity.

Oropharyngeal disease appears as white patches that are raised and may bleed slightly from a hyperemic base when scraped from the mucosa. Budding yeasts with pseudohyphae are seen microscopically. These lesions usually are treated with topical nystatin as a mouth rinse, 4 to 6 ml (100,000 units/ml) four times a day, or clotrimazole, as a 10-mg troche given four to five times a day. Vaginal disease is treated similarly with topical preparations of these agents or of micronazole as a cream or lotion. Amphotericin B also may be used in a topical form for vaginitis.

Oropharyngeal disease may prove to be a forme fruste of more widespread gastrointestinal candidiasis. Esophagitis is the most common manifestation [18, 36]. Gastritis may occur, as can invasion of the small and large intestines. The symptoms of retrosternal pain, dysphagia, nausea, and occasionally, gastrointestinal bleeding are more often found in patients with underlying cell-mediated immunity deficiencies from any cause or following treatment with broad-spectrum antibiotics. Many patients will have no symptoms. The diagnosis is made by esophagoscopy and demonstration of tissue invasion. Treatment is with nystatin suspension, 40 to 50 ml every 2 to 4 hours, or low-dose amphotericin B (see below).

Disseminated candidiasis is an important nosocomial infection in persons with lymphoma or leukemia and occasionally in persons with indwelling catheters or hyperalimentation lines. It presents similarly to bacteremias with fever, chills, and sometimes hypotension. The source is usually the gastrointestinal tract if the skin is not compromised. The hematogenous dissemination has some predilection for the kidneys, but, as with bacteremias, dissemination is in accordance with the cardiac output to a particular organ. Examination of the skin and eyes can provide evidence of the disease process. The former are small papular or pustular lesions in which the organisms can be demonstrated. Endophthalmitis occurs in persons with widespread candidiasis and may be asymptomatic or present with blurred vision or scotomata. Funduscopic examination reveals cotton wool exudates extending into the vitreous, although any portion of the eye may be involved. Diagnosis is by demonstration of the organism in blood cultures and skin biopsies or,

presumptively, from the eye findings in the appropriate clinical setting. In a setting of disseminated candidiasis, the possibility of endocarditis must be raised. This diagnosis and management of this complication are difficult and require infectious disease consultation. Treatment is with amphotericin B; the dose and duration vary with the clinical situation (see below). Fluorocytosine is not generally used in combination with this agent for candidiasis. Ketoconazole is not used in this disease.

Transient candidemia is associated with growth of the organism on indwelling catheters and hyperalimentation lines. If a blood culture is positive in such a patient, then all lines should be removed, if possible. A clinical determination should be made as to whether the person has disseminated disease (see above [34]). The patient can be observed for 48 hours without treatment if clinical conditions warrant it or treated with low-dose amphotericin B. Some authors prefer a full course of the drug in this situation [57].

Antifungal Therapy

These toxic agents are generally used in a seriously infected person, and an infectious disease consult should be required. There are many variations in dose and duration of treatment, and experts often do not agree on some specifics [7, 69, 85].

AMPHOTERICIN B

This agent acts by destruction of fungal cell membranes because of their content of ergosterol. Its differential toxicity is due to the fact that mammalian cell membranes contain cholesterol rather than ergosterol. The administration generally requires a test dose of 1 mg IV over several hours to determine if an individual will have a hypotensive reaction. The dose is incremented by 5 to 10 mg per day until a daily dose of 0.35 to 0.75 mg/kg per day is reached. In general, a dose of 50 mg per day is considered maximal in a normal adult male. In severely ill patients, the dose may be increased more quickly, but this is often accompanied by febrile reactions, chills, and hypotension. The major toxicity is renal, and the serum creatinine level should be checked every 3 days. If it rises above 2.5 to 3 mg/dl, then the drug should be discontinued or the dose decreased until it returns to normal. One method of accomplishing this is to change to an alternate-day regimen without decreasing the daily dose. Efficacy is determined clinically and by total dose of the drug rather than by daily dose or plasma concentration. Most systemic mycoses require 1.5 to 2.5 gm. Occasionally, *Candida* esophagitis or transient candidemia can be treated with a low-dose regimen. This consists of a test dose of 1 mg and then 5, 10, 20, 20, 20, 20 mg on consecutive days. When this is used, one should follow the patient carefully to be certain that disseminated disease is not masked by low doses of the drug. The major toxicity is renal, but most patients also experience fevers, chills, nausea, or vomiting. Anemia is common with prolonged therapy. Hypokalemia occurs in about one-fourth of patients due to the development of a renal tubular defect.

5-FLUOROCYTOSINE

This is an effective agent [7], but it is not used alone. Its major role is in combination with amphotericin B in the management of cryptococcal meningitis. It is converted to 5-fluorouracil by bacterial flora of the intestine, and this may produce an anemia. It is distributed into the total body water and enters the cerebrospinal fluid. It is well absorbed from the intestine and is given at a dosage of 50 to 150 mg/kg per day.

KETOCONAZOLE

This imidazole is useful against *Candida, Histoplasma, Coccidioides,* and *Blastomyces;* it is less active against *Sporotrix, Aspergillus,* and *Cryptococcus.* It interferes with sterol biosynthesis in fungi and in humans to a lesser extent; for this reason, it can produce some suppression of testosterone and corticosteroids in patients. It is given orally and is excreted by the liver; there is no alteration of dose in renal failure. The spectrum of use of this agent is still being developed. It has efficacy in chronic mucocutaneous candidiasis, dermatophyte infections, and thrush. It also has efficacy in blastomycosis, coccidioidomycosis, and histoplasmosis, but it should be used in these settings with an infectious disease consultant. The agent is promising because it can be given orally and is well tolerated, but at present it is recommended only for the two superficial fungal infections mentioned above.

References

1. Aduan, R. P., Fauci, A. S., and Dale, D. C. Prolonged fever of unknown origin. *Clin. Res.* 26: 558A, 1978.
2. Barbour, G. L., and Juniper, K., Jr. A clinical comparison of amebic and pyogenic abscesses of the liver in 66 patients. *Am. J. Med.* 53: 312, 1972.
3. Bartlett, J. G., and Gorbach, S. L. The triple threat of aspiration pneumonia. *Chest* 68: 560, 1975.
4. Bartlett, J. G., O'Keefe, P., Tally, F. P., Louie, T. J., and Gorbach, S. L. Bacteriology of hospital-acquired pneumonia. *Arch. Intern. Med.* 146: 868, 1986.
5. Bayer, A. S. Fungal pneumonias: Pulmonary coccidioidal syndromes: I. Primary and progressive primary coccidioidal pneumonias—Diagnostic, therapeutic, and prognostic considerations. *Chest* 79: 575, 1981.
6. Bayer, A. S. Fungal pneumonias: Pulmonary coccidioidal syndromes: II. Miliary, nodular, and cavitary pulmonary coccidioidomycosis—Chemotherapeutic and surgical considerations. *Chest* 79: 686, 1981.
7. Bennett, J. E. Antifungal Agents. In G. L. Mandell, R. G. Douglas, and J. E. Bennett (Eds.), *Principles and Practice of Infectious Diseases,* 2d Ed.

New York: Wiley, 1985. Pp. 263–270.

8. Bodey, G. P. Fungal infection and fever of unknown origin in neutropenic patients. *Am. J. Med.* 80(Suppl. 5C): 112, 1986.

9. Bolan, G., Broome, C. V., Facklam, R. R., Plikaytis, B. D., Fraser, D. W., and Schlech, W. F., III. Pneumococcal vaccine efficacy in selected populations in the United States. *Ann. Intern. Med.* 104: 1, 1986.

10. Brunham, R. C., Paavonen, J., Stevens, C. E., et al. Mucopurulent cervicitis: The ignored counterpart in women of urethritis in men. *N. Engl. J. Med.* 311: 1, 1984.

11. Busey, F., Baker, R., Birch, L., et al. Blastomycosis: A review of 198 collected cases in Veterans Administration hospitals (Blastomycosis Cooperative Study of the Veterans Administration). *Am. Rev. Respir. Dis.* 89: 659, 1964.

12. Catanzaro, A., Einstein, H., Levine, B., et al. Ketoconazole for treatment of disseminated coccidioidomycosis. *Ann. Intern. Med.* 96: 436, 1982.

13. Clark, E. G., and Danbolt, N. The Oslo study of the natural history of untreated syphilis. *J. Chron. Dis.* 2: 311, 1955.

14. Conly, J. M., and Ronald, A. R. Cerebrospinal fluid as a diagnostic body fluid. *Am. J. Med.* (Infectious Disease Supplement) July 28: 102, 1983.

15. Dinarello, C. A., and Wolff, S. M. Fever of Unknown Origin. In G. L. Mandell, R. G. Douglas, and J. E. Bennett (Eds.), *Principles and Practice of Infectious Diseases,* 2d Ed. New York: Wiley, 1985. Pp. 339–347.

16. Dinarello, C. A., and Wolff, S. M. Molecular basis of fever in humans. *Am. J. Med.* 72: 799, 1982.

17. Dinubile, M. J. Surgery in active endocarditis. *Ann. Intern. Med.* 96: 650, 1980.

18. Eras, P., Goldstein, M. J., and Sherlock, P. *Candida* infection of the gastrointestinal tract. *Medicine* 51: 367, 1972.

19. Fauci, A. S., Masur, H., Gelmann, E. P., et al. The acquired immunodeficiency syndrome: An update. *Ann. Intern. Med.* 102: 800, 1985.

20. Fekety, R. Recent advances in management of bacterial diarrhea. *Rev. Infect. Dis.* 5: 246, 1983.

21. Geisler, P. J., Nelson, K. E., Levin, S., Reddi, K. T., and Mose, V. K. Community-acquired purulent meningitis: A review of 1316 cases during the antibiotic era, 1954–1976. *Rev. Infect. Dis.* 1: 725, 1980.

22. Gillenwater, J. Y., Harrison, R. B., and Kunin, C. M. Natural history of bacteriuria in schoolgirls. *N. Engl. J. Med.* 301: 396, 1979.

23. Gnann, J. W., and Cobbs, C. G. Infections of Prosthetic Valves and Intravascular Devices. In G. L. Mandell, R. G. Douglas, and J. E. Bennett (Eds.), *Principles and Practice of Infectious Diseases,* 2d Ed. New York: Wiley, 1985. Pp. 531–539.

24. Goodwin, R. A., Jr., and Des Prez, R. M. State of the art in histoplasmosis. *Am. Rev. Respir. Dis.* 117: 929, 1978.

25. Goodwin, R. A., Shapiro, J. L., Thurman, J. H., et al. Disseminated histoplasmosis: Clinical and pathologic correlation. *Medicine* 59: 1, 1980.

26. Grayston, J. T., Kuo, C.-C., Wang, S.-P., and Altman, J. A new *Chlamydia psittaci* strain, TWAR, isolated in acute respiratory tract infections. *N. Engl. J. Med.* 315: 161, 1986.

27. Handsfield, H. H., Lipman, T. O., Harnisch, J. P., et al. Asymptomatic gonorrhea in men. *N. Engl. J. Med.* 290: 117, 1974.

28. Harrison, M. J. G. The clinical presentation of intracranial abscesses. *Q. J. Med.* 204: 461, 1982.

29. Hoeprich, P. D. Infective Endocarditis. In P. D. Hoeprich (Ed.), *Infectious Diseases,* 2d Ed. New York: Harper and Row, 1977. Pp. 979–1011.

30. Holmes, K. K., Counts, G. W., and Beaty, H. N. Disseminated gonococcal infection. *Ann. Intern. Med.* 74: 979, 1971.

31. Hook, E. W., and Holmes, K. K. Gonococcal infections. *Ann. Intern. Med.* 102: 229, 1985.

32. Jenkins, R. D., Fenn, J. P., and Matsen, J. M. Review of urine microscopy for bacteriuria. *J.A.M.A.* 255: 3397, 1986.

33. Katandanis, D., and Shulman, J. A. Recent survey of infectious meningitis in adults: Review of laboratory findings in bacterial, tuberculosis and aseptic meningitis. *South. Med. J.* 69: 449, 1976.

34. Klein, J. J., and Watanakunakorn, C. Hospital-acquired fungemia: Its natural course and clinical significance. *Am. J. Med.* 67: 51, 1979.

35. Klotz, S. A., Jorgensen, J. H., Buckwold, F. J., and Craven, P. C. Typhoid fever: An epidemic with remarkably few clinical signs and symptoms. *Arch. Intern. Med.* 144: 533, 1984.

36. Kodsi, B. E., Wickremesinghe, P. L., Kozinn, P. J., et al. *Candida* esophagitis: A prospective study of 27 cases. *Gastroenterology* 71: 715, 1976.

37. Korzeniowski, O., Sande, M. A., and The National

Collaborative Endocarditis Study Group. Combination antimicrobial therapy for *Staphylococcus aureus* endocarditis in patients addicted to parenteral drugs and in nonaddicts. *Ann. Intern. Med.* 97: 496, 1982.

38. Kreger, B. E., Craven, D. E., Carling, P. C., and McCabe, W. R. Gram-negative bacteremia: III. Reassessment of etiology, epidemiology, and ecology in 612 patients. *Am. J. Med.* 68: 332, 1980.

39. Kreger, B. E., Craven, D. E., and McCabe, W. R. Gram-negative bacteremia: IV. Reevaluation of clinical features and treatment of 612 patients. *Am. J. Med.* 68: 344, 1980.

40. Krieger, J. N. Prostatitis syndromes: Pathophysiology, differential diagnosis, and treatment. *Sex. Transm. Dis.* 11: 100, 1984.

41. Larson, E. B., Featherstone, H. J., and Petersdorf, R. G. Fever of undetermined origin: Diagnosis and follow-up of 105 cases, 1970–1980. *Medicine* 61: 269, 1980.

42. Levine, D. P., Crane, L. R., and Zervos, M. J. Bacteremia in narcotic addicts at the Detroit Medical Center: II. Infectious endocarditis: A prospective comparative study. *Rev. Infect. Dis.* 8: 374, 1986.

43. Levy, R. M., Bredesen, D. E., and Rosenblum, M. L. Neurological manifestations of AIDS: Experience at UCSF and review of the literature. *J. Neurosurg.* 62: 475, 1985.

44. Light, R. W., Girard, W. M., Jenkinson, S. G., and George, R. B. Parapneumonic effusions. *Am. J. Med.* 69: 507, 1980.

45. Lipsky, B. A., and Hirschmann, J. V. Drug fever. *J.A.M.A.* 245: 851, 1981.

46. Maki, D. G. Nosocomial bacteremia: An epidemiologic overview. *Am. J. Med.* 70: 719, 1981.

47. Mandell, G. L., Douglas, R. G., and Bennett, J. E. (Eds.). *Principles and Practice of Infectious Diseases.* New York: Wiley, 1985. P. 480.

48. Mandell, G. L., Douglas, R. G., and Bennett, J. E. (Eds.). *Principles and Practice of Infectious Diseases.* New York: Wiley, 1985. P. 493.

49. Mandell, G. L., Douglas, R. G., and Bennett, J. E. (Eds.). *Principles and Practice of Infectious Diseases.* New York: Wiley, 1985. P. 1562.

50. Mandell, G. L., Douglas, R. G., Jr., and Bennett, J. E. (Eds.). *Principles and Practice of Infectious Disease.* New York: Wiley, 1985. Pp. 1604–1605.

51. Mandell, G. L., Douglas, R. G., Jr., and Bennett, J. E. (Eds.). *Principles and Practice of Infectious Disease.* New York: Wiley, 1985. P. 1638.

52. Mandell, G. L., Douglas, R. G., Jr., and Bennett, J. E. (Eds.). *Principles and Practice of Infectious Disease.* New York: Wiley, 1985. P. 1620.

53. Mandell, G. L., Douglas, R. G., Jr., and Bennett, J. E. (Eds.). *Principles and Practice of Infectious Disease.* New York: Wiley, 1985. P. 1621.

54. Mandell, G. L., Douglas, R. G., Jr., and Bennett, J. E. (Eds.). *Principles and Practice of Infectious Disease.* New York: Wiley, 1985. P. 1613.

55. Mathisen, G. E., Meyer, R. D., George, W. L., et al. Brain abscess and cerebritis. *Rev. Infect. Dis.* 6: S101, 1984.

56. McCormick, J. B., and Bennett, J. V. Public health considerations in the management of meningococcal disease. *Ann. Intern. Med.* 83: 883, 1975.

57. Medoff, G. Controversial areas in antifungal chemotherapy: Short-course and combination therapy with amphotericin B. *Rev. Infect. Dis.* 9: 403, 1987.

58. Mitchell, D. P., Hanes, T. E., Hovampa, A. M., and Schenker, S. Fever of unknown origin: Assessment of the value of percutaneous liver biopsy. *Arch. Intern. Med.* 137: 1001, 1977.

59. Murray, H. W., Masur, H., Senterfit, L. B., and Roberts, R. B. The protean manifestations of *Mycoplasma pneumoniae* infections in adults. *Am. J. Med.* 58: 229, 1975.

60. Murray, P. R., and Washington, J. A., II. Microscopic and bacteriologic analysis of expectorated sputum. *Mayo Clin. Proc.* 50: 339, 1975.

61. Nicotra, M. B., Rivera, M., and Awe, R. J. Antibiotic therapy of acute exacerbations of chronic bronchitis: A controlled study using tetracycline. *Ann. Intern. Med.* 97: 18, 1982.

62. Peters, W. P., Friedman, P. A., Johnson, M. W., and Mitch, W. E. Pressor effect of naloxone in septic shock. *Lancet* 1: 529, 1981.

63. Petersdorf, R. G., and Beeson, P. B. Fever of unexplained origin: Report on 100 cases. *Medicine* 40: 1, 1961.

64. Pizzo, P. A., Robichaud, K. J., Gill, F. A., et al. Empiric antibiotic and antifungal therapy for cancer patients with prolonged fever and granulocytopenia. *Am. J. Med.* 72: 101, 1982.

65. Ramsey, P. G., Rubin, R. H., Tolkoff-Rubin, N. E., et al. The renal transplant patient with fever and

pulmonary infiltrates: Etiology, clinical manifestations, and management. *Medicine* 59: 206, 1980.

66. Rice, R. J., and Thompson, S. E. Treatment of uncomplicated infections due to *Neisseria gonorrhoeae*. *J.A.M.A.* 255: 1739, 1986.

67. Ronald, A. R. Current concepts in the management of urinary tract infections in adults. *Med. Clin. North Am.* 68: 335, 1984.

68. Rosenow, E. C., Wilson, W. R., and Cockerill, F. R. Pulmonary disease in the immunocompromised host. *Mayo Clin. Proc.* 60: 473, 1985.

69. Sarosi, G. A., Armstrong, D., Barber, R. A., et al. Treatment of fungal diseases. *Am. Rev. Respir. Dis.* 120: 1393, 1979.

70. Sarosi, G. A., Hammerman, K. J., Tosh, F. E., et al. Clinical features of acute pulmonary blastomycosis. *N. Engl. J. Med.* 290: 540, 1974.

71. Scheld, W., and Sande, M. A. Endocarditis and Intravascular Infections. In G. L. Mandell, R. G. Douglas, and J. E. Bennett (Eds.), *Principles and Practice of Infectious Diseases*, 2d Ed. New York: Wiley, 1985. Pp. 504–530.

72. Schimpff, S. C. Empiric antibiotic therapy for granulocytopenic cancer patients. *Am. J. Med.* 80(Suppl. 5C): 13, 1986.

73. Selwyn, P. A. AIDS: What is now known: III. Clinical aspects. *Hosp. Pract.* 21: 119, 1986.

74. Simon, R. P. Neurosyphilis. *Arch. Neurol.* 42: 606, 1985.

75. Singer, C., Kaplan, M. H., and Armstrong, D. Bacteremia and fungemia complicating neoplastic disease. *Am. J. Med.* 62: 731, 1977.

76. Smith, J. W., and Utz, J. P. Progressive disseminated histoplasmosis: A prospective study of 26 patients. *Ann. Intern. Med.* 75: 557, 1972.

77. Sprung, C. L., Caralis, P. V., Marcial, E. H., Pierce, M., Gelbard, M. A., Long, W. M., Duncan, R. C., Fendler, M. D., and Karpf, M. The effects of high dose corticosteroids in patients with septic shock. *New Engl. J. Med.* 311: 1138, 1984.

78. Stamm, W. E., Counts, G. W., and Running, K. R. Diagnosis of coliform infection in acutely dysuric women. *N. Engl. J. Med.* 307: 463, 1982.

79. Stamm, W. E., Wagner, K. E., Amsel, R., et al. Cause of the acute urethral syndrome in women. *N. Engl. J. Med.* 303: 409, 1980.

80. Stover, D. E., Zaman, M. B., Hadju, S. I., Lange, M., Gold, J., and Armstrong, D. Bronchoalveolar lavage in the diagnosis of diffuse pulmonary infiltrates in the immunosuppressed host. *Ann. Intern. Med.* 101: 1, 1984.

81. Swartz, S. L., Kraus, S. J., Hermann, K. L., et al. Diagnosis and etiology of nongonococcal urethritis. *J. Infect. Dis.* 138: 445, 1978.

82. Tam, M. R., Stamm, W. E., Handsfield, H. H., et al. Culture-independent diagnosis of *Chlamydia trachomatis* using monoclonal antibodies. *N. Engl. J. Med.* 310: 1146, 1984.

83. The EORTC International Antimicrobial Therapy Project Group. Three antibiotic regimens in the treatment of infection in febrile granulocytopenic patients with cancer. *J. Infect. Dis.* 137: 14, 1978.

84. Turck, M., Ronald, A. R., and Petersdorf, R. G. Relapse and reinfection in chronic bacteriuria: II. The correlation between site of infection and pattern of recurrence in chronic bacteriuria. *N. Engl. J. Med.* 278: 422, 1968.

85. Utz, J. P. Chemotherapy for the systemic mycoses: The prelude to ketoconazole. *Rev. Infect. Dis.* 2: 625, 1980.

86. Varki, A. P., and Puthuran, P. Value of second lumbar puncture in confirming a diagnosis of aseptic meningitis: A prospective study. *Arch. Neurol.* 36: 581, 1979.

87. Wade, J. C., Schimpff, S. C., Newman, K. A., et al. *Staphylococcus epidermidis*: An increasing cause of infection in patients with granulocytopenia. *Ann. Intern. Med.* 97: 503, 1982.

88. Weinstein, L. Clinically benign fever of unknown origin: A personal retrospective. *J. Infect. Dis.* 7: 692, 1985.

89. Weinstein, L., and Schlesinger, J. J. Pathoanatomic, pathophysiologic, and clinical correlations in endocarditis. Part I. *N. Engl. J. Med.* 291: 832, 1974.

90. Weinstein, M. P., Stratton, C. W., Ackley, A., Hawley, H. B., Robinson, P. A., Fisher, B. D., Alcid, D. V., Stephens, D. S., and Reller, L. B. Multicenter collaborative evaluation of a standardized serum bactericidal test as a prognostic indicator in infective endocarditis. *Am. J. Med.* 78: 262, 1985.

91. Wharton, J. M., Coleman, D. L., Wofsy, C. B., et al. Trimethoprim-sulfamethoxazole or pentamidine for *Pneumocystis carinii* pneumonia in the acquired immunodeficiency syndrome. *Ann. Intern. Med.* 105: 37, 1986.

92. Wheat, L. J., Slama, T. G., Eitzen, H. E., et al.

A large urban outbreak of histoplasmosis: Clinical features. *Ann. Intern. Med.* 94: 331, 1981.

93. Wheat, L. J., Slama, T. G., Norton, J. A., et al. Risk factors for disseminated or fatal histoplasmosis. *Ann. Intern. Med.* 96: 159, 1982.

94. Whitley, R. J., Alford, C. A., Hirsch, M. S., et al. Vidarabine versus acyclovir therapy in herpes simplex encephalitis. *N. Engl. J. Med.* 314: 144, 1986.

95. Whitley, R. J., Soong, S., Hirsch, M. S., et al. Herpes simplex encephalitis: Vidarabine therapy and diagnostic problems. *N. Engl. J. Med.* 304: 313, 1981.

96. Whitley, R. J., Soong, S., Linneman, C., Jr., et al. Herpes simplex encephalitis: Clinical assessment. *J.A.M.A.* 247: 317, 1982.

97. Wilson, D. E., Mann, J. J., Bennett, J. E., and Utz, J. P. Clinical features of extracutaneous sporotrichosis. *Medicine* 46: 265, 1967.

98. Witorsch, P., and Utz, J. P. North American blastomycosis: A study of 40 patients. *Medicine* 47: 169, 1968.

99. Young, L. S. Gram-Negative Sepsis. In G. L. Mandell, R. G. Douglas, and J. E. Bennett (Eds.), *Principles and Practice of Infectious Diseases,* 2d Ed. New York: Wiley, 1985.

100. Yu, V. L., Kroboth, F. J., Shonnard, J., Brown, A., McDearman, S., and Magnussen, M. Legionnaire's disease: New clinical perspective from a prospective pneumonia study. *Am. J. Med.* 73: 357, 1982.

101. Ziegler, E. J., McCutchen, A. J., Fierer, J., Glauser, M. P., Sadoff, J. C., Douglas, H., and Braude, A. I. Treatment of gram-negative bacteremia and shock with human antiserum to a mutant *Escherichia coli. New Engl. J. Med.* 307: 1225, 1982.

Metabolism and Endocrinology

7

Fred D. Hofeldt and
E. Chester Ridgway

Metabolism

Isolated free-living organisms or discrete functioning cells of a mammalian organ each survive in a complex environment. Their life processes involve homeostatic metabolic control mechanisms of cellular physiochemical changes in matter and energy. The hydrophobic properties of the phospholipids and certain proteins lead to the development of cellular and subcellular membranes that constitute the living cell and permit its subcellular organization. Genetically determined and metabolically regulated cell function within this environment is dependent on the presence of the proper concentrations of electrolytes, minerals, and nutrients, with hormones and local paracrine substances playing a regulatory role in more complex species. Metabolic processes maintain and protect the intracellular and extracellular environments against internal and external stresses. Intricate intracellular control mechanisms of intermediary metabolism of nucleic acid, proteins, lipids, and carbohydrates allow continued cellular function and survival in a complex environment. Unique cellular changes seen in some disease processes are dependent on the genome. In these diseases, abnormal gene regulation or gene products account for the molecular basis of the metabolic disorders. In other circumstances, alterations in the metabolic cellular milieu or homeostatic control mechanism underlie the disease process.

Diabetes Mellitus

Diabetes mellitus [26, 68] is a common clinical disorder having a prevalence of 3 to 5 percent and an incidence of approximately 100,000 new cases per year. At this time, it is estimated that approximately 4 million diabetics remain undiagnosed. Diabetes is a chronic catabolic disease that affects carbohydrate, protein, fat, water, and electrolyte metabolism. It is characterized by absolute or relative insulin deficiency and is associated with degenerative complications in the eyes, kidneys, nerves, and vasculature. Diabetes mellitus usually occurs as a primary condition (idiopathic), but secondary conditions need to be considered (Table 7-1). Diabetes may appear at any age, but it is more common in middle-aged and elderly persons who are obese (type II, non-insulin-dependent diabetes) (Table 7-2). Insulin-dependent diabetic patients (type I) usually are thin or of ideal body weight, usually have a more acute onset of their diabetes, and frequently have earlier complications. Type I diabetes is HLA-associated (HLA-B8, HLA-B18, HLA-DW3, HLA-DW4) with islet-cell antibodies present as a

Table 7–1. *Classification of Diabetes*
(Recommended by the National Diabetes Data Group)

I. Idiopathic diabetes mellitus (fasting plasma glucose >
140 mg/dl or OGTT*—peak glucose > 200 mg/dl; and
2-hour value > 200 mg/dl):
   A. Insulin-dependent (IDDM, type I)
   B. Non-insulin-dependent (NIDDM, type II):
      1. Nonobese
      2. Obese
II. Gestational diabetes (100-gm glucose load; fasting >
105 mg/dl, 1-hour > 190 mg/dl, 2-hour > 165, 3-hour
> 145 mg/dl; two abnormal values for diagnosis)
III. Other carbohydrate abnormalities:
   A. Impaired glucose tolerance (OGTT—a plasma
   glucose 1-hour value > 200 mg/dl and 2-hour
   value between 140 and 199 mg/ml)
   B. Previous abnormality of glucose tolerance
   C. Potential abnormality of glucose tolerance
   (identical twin with diabetes, family history of type
   II diabetes, pregnancy with live or stillborn child >
   4.5 kg, obesity, or islet-cell antibodies)
IV. Secondary diabetes (Cushing's syndrome, acromegaly,
glucagonoma, pheochromocytoma,
hyperaldosteronism, drugs, cystic fibrosis,
hemochromatosis, chronic pancreatitis, congenital
lipodystrophy, associated acanthosis nigricans,
autoimmune antibody to insulin or insulin receptor,
hypocalcemia)

---

*OGTT (oral glucose tolerance test): 75 gm oral glucose so-
lution is ingested following an overnight fast after ingesting
a 200- to 300-gm carbohydrate diet for 3 days with plasma
glucose samples at 0, 60, and 120 minutes.

manifestation of altered immune function. The islet-cell antibodies may precede the onset of clinically significant diabetes. Altered insulin secretory
reserve in these patients may be evaluated by periodic intravenous glucose tolerance tests, noting
a diminishing magnitude of readily releasable insulin which parallels clinical progression of the
diabetes. Some children have mild diabetes of an
autosomal-dominant inheritance (maternity-on-
set diabetes of young, MODY). Type II diabetes is
a familial disorder with high concordance rates in
identical twins.

DIAGNOSIS
History
Diabetes mellitus usually presents with clinical
features due either to acute metabolic alterations
or to chronic complications. The acute complica-

tions are a consequence of the hyperglycemia, dehydration, electrolyte and acid-base imbalance,
inability to combat infections (particularly skin
and vulvar), and poor wound healing. Clinically
significant diabetes exists when the patient has
polyuria, polydipsia, nocturia, weight loss, and
increased thirst. Nonspecific symptoms such as
tiredness, weakness, malaise, blurring of vision,
headaches, and drowsiness are common. With severe acute metabolic deterioration, the patient
may present with diabetic ketoacidosis or hyperosmolar coma. Many times the acute manifestations of diabetes are precipitated by infection or
other stresses that increase the need for insulin,
cause insulin resistance, and diminish insulin secretion. Some patients, especially the elderly,
present for the first time with chronic complications of diabetes related to deteriorating renal
function with hypertension, edema, or azotemia;
blindness or cataracts; neurologic complications
of a distal symmetrical polyneuropathy; or as isolated focal or multifocal neuropathies of cranial or
spinal nerve syndromes. Autonomic neuropathy
with impotence, urinary retention, gastroparesis
with early satiety, nausea, diarrhea, and orthostatic hypotension may be present. Accelerated
peripheral vascular disease, cerebrovascular disease, and coronary artery disease are more common in diabetics.

Physical Findings
Type I patients with diabetes frequently are thin
and may be undernourished, whereas type II diabetics may have insulin resistance with obesity.
Blood pressure and pulse should be taken supine
and upright for orthostatic changes. When cardiac
autonomic neuropathy is present, there will be no
pulse deceleration with a single deep breath.
Careful ophthalmologic examination for cataracts, venous dilation, exudates, hemorrhages,
microaneurysm, neovascularization, or retinal
scarring or detachment is important. Neurologic
examination should detail sensory losses (light
touch, pinprick, vibratory, position, temperature),
motor changes (weakness, atrophy, gait), and loss
of deep tendon reflexes. In the diabetic patient

Table 7–2. *General Characteristics of Type I and Type II Diabetes*

	Type I	Type II
Clinical:		
Occurrence:	6–10 percent diabetes population	80%
Onset:	Rapid	Usually gradual
Body habitus:	Thin	Obese
Acute complication:	Diabetic ketoacidosis	Dehydration, hyperosmolar coma
Chronic	Retinopathy	—
complications:	Neuropathy	Less frequent
	Nephropathy	—
	Atherosclerosis	Common
Medication:	Intensified insulin therapy is best	Diet with weight loss or oral hypoglycemic drugs; insulin when symptomatic
Pathophysiology:		
Metabolic state:	Insulin-deficient catabolic starvation state with abnormal lipid, protein, and carbohydrate metabolism	Insulin-resistant state with enhanced hepatic glucose production and insulin secretion adequate to prevent ketosis
Susceptibility:	In Caucasians linked to HLA B8, B18, Dr3, Dr4	Not HLA linked; genetic inheritance (multifactorial) (maturity-onset diabetes of youth is autosomal-dominant)
Pancreatic:		
Beta cell:	Destruction; autoimmune state with islet-cell surface and cytoplasmic antibodies; ? viral etiology; occasionally insulin antibodies	Normal with increased alpha cells and relative hyperglucagonemia

over age 40, a careful examination of the feet includes inspection for changes of skin color, ulcerations, venous stasis, palpation of peripheral pulses, sensory assessment, and assessment of hygiene and bony deformities.

In patients with acute decompensation, careful attention is given to the degree of dehydration, hypovolemia, breathing (Kussmaul), level of consciousness, temperature, and gastric distension. In these patients, a careful search is conducted for the precipitating stress of ketoacidosis or the hyperosmolar state.

Laboratory Tests

As a rule, fasting hyperglycemia (fasting plasma glucose level > 140 mg/dl on two occasions) establishes the diagnosis of diabetes mellitus, and an oral glucose tolerance test (OGTT) is not required. In elderly patients, the fasting plasma glucose level changes little with age, whereas there are significant postprandial glucose elevations of 10 mg/dl per decade after age 40. Hence a fasting

plasma glucose level greater than 140 mg/dl establishes the diagnosis of diabetes in all ages. During pregnancy, a diabetic oral glucose tolerance test after 100 gm oral glucose solution is seen when two or more of the following glucose values are exceeded: fasting > 105 mg/dl, 1 hour > 190 mg/dl, 2 hours > 165 mg/dl, and 3 hours > 145 mg/dl. Hemoglobin A1C is useful in following the course of therapy in diabetic patients, but is not useful in establishing the diagnosis. Each diabetic patient needs an initial and yearly assessment of renal function (serum creatinine and, if abnormal, a creatinine clearance and 24-hour urine protein excretion) and serum lipids (triglycerides, cholesterol, and high-density lipoproteins). Early in the disease, microalbuminuria (15 to 150 μg per minute) may be detected.

Special Tests

On the rare occasions, a 75-gm oral glucose tolerance test may be needed to establish the diagnosis in the nutrient-prepared patient (ingestion of 200 to 300 gm carbohydrates on 3 days prior to testing). In nonpregnant women less than 40 years old, the diagnosis of diabetes mellitus can be made when a fasting plasma glucose level is less than 140 mg/dl but a 2-hour glucose level exceeds 200 mg/dl plus any plasma glucose level at 30, 60, or 90 minutes that exceeds 200 mg/dl.

Impaired glucose tolerance in men and nonpregnant women is diagnosed by the oral glucose tolerance test when a fasting plasma glucose value is less than 140 mg/dl, a pre-2-hour plasma glucose value is greater than 200 mg/dl, and the 2-hour level is between 140 and 200 mg/dl. Those patients with impaired glucose tolerance should not be diagnosed as diabetics, since perhaps only 20 percent will ever advance to frank diabetes.

TREATMENT AND PROGNOSIS
Acute Management
DIABETIC KETOACIDOSIS. Diabetic ketoacidosis (DKA) occurs in type I diabetes and presents as a life-threatening medical emergency with profound metabolic derangements that result from a relative or absolute insulin deficiency leading to hyperglycemia, ketonemia, metabolic acidosis, dehydration, shock, and death (mortality 6 to 8 percent) [22, 32]. Diabetic ketoacidosis usually occurs when the diabetic patient fails to increase insulin dosage during the stress of an intercurrent illness or fails to continue insulin during periods of decreased food intake owing to nausea or loss of appetite. It also may be the presenting illness of a new diabetic patient.

Although the onset of diabetic ketoacidosis may develop acutely over 36 hours, the symptoms and signs can generally be recognized early enough to institute appropriate therapy. When diabetic ketoacidosis is precipitated by infection, the features of that infection (e.g., pneumonia, pyelonephritis, or gastroenteritis) may predominate.

The clinical suspicion should be confirmed immediately by demonstrating hyperglycemia (glucose level > 300 mg/dl by Dextrostix test on whole blood) and ketonemia (positive nitroprusside test). The ketone titer is determined by progressive dilutions (1 : 1, 1 : 2, . . ., 1 : 32) which continue to show a deep purple endpoint. Occa-

sionally, because of the predominance of beta-hydroxybutyric acid, the serum or urine ketone reaction, as measured by the Acetest tablet, may be falsely low. Precise laboratory measurements should corroborate the hyperglycemia, ketonemia, and acidemia with glucose, electrolyte, and arterial blood gas measurements.

The immediate goal of therapy in diabetic ketoacidosis is to correct the following seven abnormalities: (1) volume depletion, (2) hyperosmolality, (3) hyperglycemia, (4) ketonemia, (5) acidemia, (6) potassium depletion, and (7) precipitation event. Any underlying illness, such as an infection, myocardial infarction, cerebrovascular accident, or pulmonary embolism, must be evaluated and treated promptly. The best way to follow the rapid changes in clinical and metabolic status is with a well-maintained flow sheet.

To correct volume depletion and hyperosmolality, normal (0.9 percent) saline is infused at a rate of 500 to 1000 ml per hour in an adult. The rate of infusion must be individualized and decreased as evidence of volume depletion subsides, as noted by orthostatic blood pressures, pulse changes, and increasing urine output. Common total deficits are 5 to 10 liters of water, 300 to 700 mEq sodium, and 200 to 700 mEq potassium. After volume stabilization, half-normal (0.45 percent) saline may be used.

The low-dose continuous insulin infusion technique [4] allows fine adjustment of insulin delivery. After regular insulin (0.1 unit/kg) is injected rapidly intravenously (loading dose), then 50 units of regular insulin in 500 ml 0.9 percent saline (e.g., 1 unit per each 10 cc) is infused at a rate of 0.1 unit/kg per hour until the plasma glucose level has fallen to 250 mg/dl. Thus a 70-kg man would receive 7 units per hour or 70 cc per hour. Dextrose solutions are administered when the blood sugar level falls to 250 mg/dl or less to maintain the blood glucose level at about 250 mg/dl. The insulin infusion is continued until the acidosis is corrected.

Correction of acidemia usually is accomplished readily by the administration of adequate fluids and insulin. In profound acidemia, when a serum pH below 7.0 is present, the pH should be increased to, but not above, 7.2 with intravenous sodium bicarbonate. To avoid complications, complete restoration to a pH of 7.40 should be accomplished slowly within the first 24 hours with adequate insulin and saline.

Most patients with diabetic ketoacidosis have a profound deficit in total-body potassium (200 to 700 mEq), even though the serum potassium level may be high, low, or normal on admission. As a rule, potassium can be safely administered at a rate of 10 to 20 mEq per hour in concentrations of 20 to 40 mEq/liter. If hypokalemia is severe, potassium may be given cautiously with electrocardiographic monitoring at up to 40 mEq per hour in solutions that contain up to 40 mEq/liter. Such concentrated solutions are painful and may require administration through a central venous line.

Phosphate stores are commonly depleted in diabetic ketoacidosis, and with the administration of glucose-insulin solutions, serum phosphate levels fall because of the movement of phosphate into cells. If the serum phosphate level falls below 1 mg/dl, there is risk of hemolytic anemia, rhabdomyolysis, impaired white blood cell and platelet function, and central nervous system (CNS) and muscular dysfunction. With serum phosphate deficits of this magnitude, intravenous phosphate therapy is warranted. Most phosphate solutions contain very little potassium. Intravenous phosphate solutions can cause hypocalcemia due to extravascular precipitation of calcium phosphate crystals; therefore, these phosphate solutions must be given slowly; 1000 mg elemental phosphate or 0.16 m*M*/kg given parenterally as an 8-hour infusion is recommended. Oral phosphate replacement will correct most hypophosphatemic states of less severity.

After diabetic ketoacidosis has been reversed successfully, it is imperative for both the physician and the patient to review the initiating events to prevent further episodes.

NONKETOTIC HYPEROSMOLAR COMA. Nonketotic hyperosmolar coma (NKHC) is seen most commonly in elderly patients with mild type II diabetes and symptomatic polyuria when they lose their ability to ingest or to retain fluids as a result of illness, drugs, or central nervous system depression [40]. Enough insulin production persists to prevent ketoacidosis. During the osmotic (glucose) diuresis, water and solute loss continue, depleting extracellular volume. The glomerular filtration rate subsequently falls, and the protective effect of renal glucose excretion is lost, with a resultant rapid rise in the blood glucose level that produces and exacerbates the hyperosmolar state. Blood glucose concentrations in excess of 500 mg/dl usually are associated with azotemia; with concentrations of 800 mg/dl or higher oliguria usually is present.

Patients with the hyperosmolar syndrome may have altered serum sodium levels (range 120 to 188 mEq/liter). Total serum osmolarity may be 350 mOsmol/liter or higher (normal is 290 to 295 mOsmol/liter). Serum osmolarity can be estimated from the following formula:

Calculated serum$_{OSM}$

$$= 2 \times [Na^+] + \frac{[glucose]}{18} + \frac{BUN}{2.8}$$

Coma in this syndrome is due to the hyperosmolar state and intracellular dehydration. Focal or generalized seizure activity also may be present.

The therapy for this type of coma centers on replacement of fluid losses with hypotonic intravenous solutions. Relatively more water than saline has been lost. However, because of the hyperosmolar state, normal saline is hypotonic and is initially used to restore circulating volume and treat shock. This is followed by hypotonic saline solutions (0.45 percent saline). In the absence of ketoacidosis, these patients are often quite sensitive to insulin and respond to insulin infusion rates of 0.05 unit/kg per hour of regular insulin. Losses of phosphate and potassium occur with the osmotic diuresis and must be replaced. Extremely rapid correction of the hyperosmolarity is not desirable because the resulting sudden shift of water into the brain may delay recovery from coma or make coma worse. A reasonable goal is 50 percent correction of the calculated water deficit over the first 24 hours, with gradual completion of the deficit correction over the succeeding 24 hours. Because thrombotic events may occur in severe cases, prophylactic anticoagulation with low-dose heparin (5000 units every 12 hours deep SC) should be considered. The mortality rate is high in this condition (40 to 60 percent) usually because the severity of the precipitating event, which is frequently present for days prior to admission and is obscured by the metabolic derangement of the hyperosmolar state.

Long-Term Management

For diabetes mellitus, the fundamental treatment goals are to enable the patient to remain symptom-free, to achieve a near-normal metabolic state, and to escape the chronic complications. This is accomplished by achieving and maintaining ideal body weight, by appropriate diet, by an exercise program, and when necessary, by providing therapy with oral agents or insulin. The success of therapy depends largely on motivating and educating the diabetic patient to achieve self-care, which is best done by the diabetic nurse-practitioner, educators, dietitian, physician team. Unfortunately, despite strict control, vascular disease progresses because of its multifactorial etiology (i.e., hereditary, lipids, smoking, hypertension, obesity, coagulopathy). Since most type II diabetics are overweight, weight reduction is the cornerstone of their management. Calorie restriction to 1200 calories per day taken in three equal meals with behavior modification, food diaries, addition of fiber food, and membership in weight-loss support groups will help to achieve this goal. Complex carbohydrate should be provided with attention to the glycemic index of foods. Refined carbohydrates should be restricted to 8 to 10 percent total carbohydrate intake. The sulfonylureas are listed in Table 7-3. They are effective only in the type II diabetic and are given along with strict attention to diet and weight loss. The type I diabetic, particularly the juvenile-onset diabetic, requires additional nutritional calories (35 calories/kg body weight) for adequate growth, physical activity, and development. In the insulin-requiring patient, food must be distributed throughout the day in three meals with daytime snacking in the midmorning, midafternoon, and at bedtime to avoid hypoglycemia. Based on changes in physical activity, there is day-to-day regulation of this

Table 7–3. *Comparison of Oral Hypoglycemic Agents*

Drug	Daily Dose Range (mg)	Tablet size (mg)	Administration	Metabolism
First Generation:				
Tolbutamide	500–3000	250,500	bid, qid	Liver to inactive metabolites; short half-life (4 h)
Tolazamide	100–1000	100,250,500	qd, bid	Liver to inactivate and active metabolites; medium half-life (7 h)
Acetohexamide	500–1500	250,500	qd, bid	Short half-life (2 h), but liver metabolites have 6-hour hypoglycemic half-life
Chloropropamide	100–750	100,250	qd	Renal excretion of unmetabolized drug; long half-life (36 h)
Second Generation:				
Glyburide	1.25–20	1.25,2.5,5	qd, bid	Liver to inactivate and weakly active metabolites; medium half-life (10 h)
Glipizide	2.5–40	5,10	qd, bid	Liver to inactive metabolites; short half-life (4 h)

program. In order to control hyperglycemia, some type II patients may require insulin therapy. The second-generation oral agents have less drug-drug interaction because of nonionic protein binding. Their metabolites are inactive or weakly active, they promote free-water diuresis, and they are not associated with alcohol flushing. Sulfonylureas should be prescribed cautiously in elderly patients or those with significant renal or hepatic failure. They should not be given to pregnant women or nursing mothers. The greatest potential side effect is hypoglycemia. Chlorpropamide has been associated with an antabuse syndrome characterized by flushing following alcohol ingestion and inappropriate antidiuretic hormone syndrome.

INSULIN THERAPY. Frequently, insulin therapy is required to meet the criteria of controlling the metabolic alterations of the diabetic state, relieving symptoms, and promoting an adequate control of plasma glucose values. All type I diabetic patients are insulin-requiring and are prone to ketoacidosis when insulin-deficient. Insulin therapy should be intensified in these patients to establish good control. Intensified insulin therapy requires combinations of short-acting insulins (regular, semilente) in combination with intermediate-acting insulins (NPH, lente) or long-acting insulins (ultralente). Intensified insulin programs simulate the use of an insulin pump. The intermediate-acting insulins are given twice a day or long-acting insulin is given once a day to provide basal insulin requirements (i.e., bioavailable steady-state insulin similar to a pump's continuous basal insulin infusion). Since eating places additional anabolic demands on insulin requirements, diabetics require preprandial short-acting insulin given as two injections, one before breakfast and one before supper, or as three injections, one before each of the three meals. Occasionally, the evening NPH dose is not given a half hour before supper, but instead at bedtime to treat fasting hyperglycemia of the dawn phenomenon. The various insulin combinations can be premixed in the syringe prior to injection (i.e., NPH plus regular or ultralente plus a short-acting insulin). Insulin preparations available are the beef/pork combination, pure pork, pure beef, and human insulin. Human insulin is preferred in most diabetics. Commonly, the morning dose of insulin is two-thirds of the total daily amount, and usually 5 to 20 units of regular insulin will be required to cover each meal. Individual needs as determined by home glucose monitoring will modify this basic program.

In patients with type II diabetes who require insulin, some respond to a single injection of NPH given in the morning that is additive to the patient's insulin secretory capacity. If the daily NPH insulin dose is more than 30 to 40 units, it is advisable to split the NPH dose with before-supper NPH insulin. More complicated programs involve using split-mix combinations where regular insulin is added preprandially. In some poorly controlled type II patients, oral agents are added to the insulin program with variable degrees of effectiveness. In the difficult to manage type II patient, one must reinforce the importance of nutrition, diet, fiber food, restricted use of refined carbohydrate, and most important, weight loss. In some type I diabetics or patients with secondary diabetes due to pancreatic insufficiency, poor gastric emptying or nutrient absorption will complicate management. The appearance of insulin antibodies may prolong insulin action for both NPH and regular insulin. Severe insulin resistance where several hundreds of units of insulin are being prescribed may improve with use of human insulin or 40 to 60 mg prednisone daily. Insulin absorption is retarded in cigarette smokers and is enhanced when the injection site is an exercising extremity. Overinsulinization may lead to the rebound hyperglycemia (Smoygi effect) seen in patients with the erratic control. Insulin pumps, although initially more popular, are especially useful for pregnant diabetics and can be used in intelligent patients willing to adhere to strict home glucose monitoring, both preprandially and postprandially. A complication of insulin therapy is hypoglycemia. A decrease in caloric intake, exercise, alcohol ingestion, advancing renal failure, and hormone-deficiency states (hypopituitarism, adrenal insufficiency, or hypothyroidism) may additionally decrease insulin requirements. Illness or stress causes insulin resistance, in which additional preprandial regular insulin will be required. Insulin therapy is regulated by a home glucose monitoring program that assesses the plasma glucose profile in the fasting state before lunch, at 4:00 P.M., and at bedtime. Occasionally, a 2:00 A.M. blood sugar level is determined to evaluate the cause of fasting hyperglycemia (i.e., Smoygi versus dawn phenomenon). The rebound hyperglycemia of the Smoygi phenomenon is caused by excessive insulin administration, whereas the hyperglycemia of the dawn phenomenon represents early morning insulin deficiency from insulin undermedication with subsequent enhanced hepatic glucose production. A hemoglobin A1C level at 4- to 6-month intervals assesses long-term management of the hyperglycemia. During periods of illness, the patient is instructed in "sick-day rules," which include the more judicious use of home glucose monitoring, institution of short-acting insulin prior to each meal, continued caloric and electrolyte intake, and seeking of medical attention if nausea, vomiting, or ketonuria occurs. Every diabetic patient should have a bracelet or medical-alert card. With rapidly deteriorating metabolic control, the acute complication in a type I diabetic is diabetic ketoacidosis and in the type II diabetic is severe dehydration or hyperosmolar coma.

Chronic Complications

Diabetes mellitus is a chronic disease associated with long-term complications of retinopathy, nephropathy, neuropathy, and accelerated atherosclerosis. The duration of diabetes and degree of poor control are in many patients associated with more severe microvascular complications, especially in diabetic patients with HLA-DW4 tissue antigens. Remarkably, some patients are spared these complications despite poor control.

RETINOPATHY. Diabetes mellitus more often than any other systemic disease causes blindness. Features of diabetic retinopathy include microaneu-

rysms, irregular and tortuous veins, hemorrhages, exudates, neovascularization, and retinal detachment. Photocoagulation (argon laser) is beneficial in preventing severe visual loss in patients with proliferative retinopathy with or without hemorrhage. Focal photocoagulation may benefit some patients with macular edema. Vitrectomy may restore vision in selected patients with complicating retinal bleeds. As a minimum, diabetic patients should have a formal eye examination yearly, and examinations should be more frequent in those with established retinopathy.

NEPHROPATHY. Diabetic glomerulosclerosis (diffuse or nodular) is a specific type of renal lesion that occurs as a result of changes in the basement membrane and mesangium of the glomerular capillaries. Microalbuminuria is seen early in the course of diabetes and may respond to improved glucose control. Late-onset proteinuria heralds the onset of chronic renal disease, which many times progresses to end-stage, but blood pressure control may lessen the rate of progression of chronic renal insufficiency. Hence strict attention to blood pressure control to normal levels in those diabetic patients with and without renal insufficiency is important. Angiotensin-converting enzyme inhibitors have been shown to reduce proteinuria in some patients. Potentially treatable urinary tract infections as a cause of deteriorating renal function should be identified. Iodinated contrast radiologic studies should be done with caution and only in the well-hydrated patient. The management of renal failure in diabetes is the same as in other forms of chronic renal disease.

NEUROPATHY. Peripheral neuropathy often is a complication of long-standing diabetes. Motor, sensory, and autonomic nerves may be involved; the pattern is usually, but not always, symmetrical. The neuropathies may improve with better glucose control, but unfortunately, most often they do not. Chronic lower extremity peripheral neuropathy is most common in elderly patients and those whose duration of disease is greater than 10 years. Diminution or loss of vibration sense and absence of tendon reflexes are characteristic. Worsening symptoms (pain and paresthesias) may occur with poor glucose control. Ulcers on the feet and ankles secondary to trivial or unrecognized trauma are frequent. Because of diminished sensory perception secondary to peripheral neuropathy, such lesions often progress to deep infection resulting in osteomyelitis that may require amputation. Hence the diabetic foot should be examined at each visit. Involvement of the autonomic nervous system may cause overflow incontinence of urine, enteropathies, postural hypotension, disturbances of sweating and temperature regulation, and cardiac denervation.

Hypoglycemia

Hypoglycemia [21, 25, 30, 51, 65] is defined as a plasma glucose level less than 50 mg/dl (2.8 mmol/liter); it is a medical emergency and requires intravenous glucose as therapy. The usual causes of hypoglycemia are listed in Table 7-4. Fasting hypoglycemia presents with neuroglycopenic symptoms and is generally caused by serious underlying medical conditions. Reactive hypoglycemia occurs postprandially with adrenergic-mediated symptoms and is classified (see Table 7-4) as alimentary, diabetic, hormonal, or idiopathic. Although it is a popularly acclaimed disease, it is a relatively infrequently encountered eating disorder easily managed by dietary intervention with restriction of refined carbohydrates.

DIAGNOSIS
History
Determining the nature of the hypoglycemic disorder depends on age of presentation, underlying cause (see Table 7-4), family history, and whether the disorder occurs in the fasting or the postprandial state. The symptoms of fasting hypoglycemia are neuroglycopenic, including mental confusion, irritability, amnesia, stupor, and coma. Adrenergic symptoms include restlessness, shakiness, anxiety, hunger, palpations, nausea, and headache. The nonspecific symptoms may be caused

by a number of the conditions [31] listed in the differential diagnosis of adrenergic-mediated states ("spells") (Table 7-5). When considering hypoglycemia as the cause of a patient's symptoms, one should carefully exclude hypoglycemia due to the ingestion of drugs or alcohol, the use of insulin or oral sulfonylureas, or factitious drug use. Is the disorder made worse by exercise or fasting? Is there relief of symptoms with food ingestion? Whipple's triad includes the timely occurrence of symptoms and documented hypoglycemia which is relieved by glucose ingestion.

Physical Findings
Physical findings are related to the underlying cause of the hypoglycemia. Frequently, no physical findings are present except the observation of adrenergic-mediated symptoms during an attack (tremor, sweating, tachycardia, pallor, flushing). In neuroglycopenic states, the level of consciousness is depressed (lethargy, stupor, coma). Abdominal scars may suggest surgically altered gastrointestinal function. Tumors most frequently encountered are islet-cell, mesodermal, or adrenocorticocarcinoma and are frequently clinically inapparent unless there is extensive organ involvement or metastasis. Hormone-deficiency states are suggested by history and physical findings that indicate specific hormone deficiencies (see the section entitled Endocrinology). Hypoglycemia due to hepatic failure requires that approximately 80 percent of liver function be compromised, resulting in jaundice and other signs of liver decompensation. Inherited defects in hepatic intermediary metabolism are suspected in pediatric patients. The obtunded or agitated alcoholic may be hypoglycemic.

Laboratory Tests
A blood sample for glucose determination should be obtained at the time of hypoglycemia to confirm the diagnosis. If a pancreatic insulinoma or factitious hypoglycemia is suspected, a simultaneous insulin and C-peptide should be drawn (C-peptide levels are elevated in insulinoma and are

Table 7–4. *Classification of Hypoglycemic States*

I. Exogenous causes:
  A. Iatrogenic (related to treatment with insulin or oral hypoglycemic agents)
  B. Factitious (especially seen in paramedical personnel)
  C. Pharmacologic (Ackee nut, salicylates, antihistamines, monoamine-oxidase inhibitors, propranolol, phenylbutazone, pentamidine isethionate, phentolamine, alcohol)
II. Spontaneous hypoglycemia (endogenous metabolic processes):
  A. Fasting state hypoglycemia:
    1. Pancreatic disorders:
      a. Islet beta-cell hyperfunction (adenoma, carcinoma, hyperplasia)
      b. Islet alpha-cell hypofunction or deficiency
    2. Hepatic disorders:
      a. Severe liver disease (cirrhosis, hepatitis, carcinomatosis, circulatory failure, ascending infectious cholangeitis)
      b. Enzyme defects (glycogen-storage disease, galactosemia, hereditary fructose intolerance, familial galactose and fructose intolerance, fructose 1,6-diphosphatase deficiency)
    3. Pituitary-adrenal disorders (hypopituitarism, Addison's disease, adrenogenital syndrome, hypothyroidism)
    4. Central nervous system disease (hypothalamus or brainstem)
    5. Muscle (hypoalaninemia)
    6. Nonpancreatic neoplasms:
      a. Mesodermal (spindle-cell fibrosarcoma, leiomyosarcoma, mesothelioma, rhabdomyosarcoma, liposarcoma, neurofibroma, reticulum-cell sarcoma)
      b. Adenocarcinoma (hepatoma, cholangiocarcinoma, gastric carcinoma, adrenocorticocarcinoma, cecal carcinoma)
    7. Unclassified:
      a. Excessive loss or utilization of glucose and/or deficient substrate (prolonged or strenuous exercise, fever, lactation, pregnancy, renal glycosuria, diarrheal states, chronic starvation)
      b. Ketotic hypoglycemia of childhood (idiopathic hypoglycemia of childhood)
  B. Postprandial hypoglycemia (reactive to fed state):
    1. Reactive to glucose:
      a. Alimentary hypoglycemia (includes patients with previous gastrointestinal surgery, peptic-ulcer disease, disordered gastrointestinal motility syndromes, and asymptomatic gastrointestinal disease)
      b. Diabetes mellitus
      c. Hormonal (includes hyperthyroidism and deficient reserve syndromes of cortisol, epinephrine, glucagen, thyroid hormone, and growth hormone)
      d. Idiopathic
    2. Reactive to ingestion of other substrate (fructose, sugar, alcohol, leucine, galactose)
    3. Insulin or insulin receptor autoantibodies
III. Transitional low blood glucose state (asymptomatic biochemical hypoglycemia seen during oral glucose tolerance tests)
IV. Pseudohypoglycemia (chronic leukemia with white blood cell count generally in excess of 300,000)

Source: Adapted from Hofeldt, F. D. Reactive hypoglycemia. *Metabolism* 24: 1193, 1975. Used with permission of the publisher.

suppressed with factitious insulin administration). Proinsulin measurements are elevated in insulinoma. Stimulation tests (tolbutamide, leucine, glucagon, calcium) for diagnosing insulinomas are infrequently performed. The diagnosis of insulinoma is established by a prolonged fast with plasma glucose and insulin measurements at 6-hour intervals. Actually, most patients with an insulinoma will become hypoglycemic within 24 hours of fasting. A C-peptide suppression test, where elevated C-peptide levels (>1.2 ng/ml) are measured during controlled hypoglycemia using an insulin infusion (0.1 unit/kg), may be helpful in the difficult to diagnose insulinoma patient. Hormone-insufficiency states are assessed with routine laboratory measurements (see the section entitled Endocrinology). Toxicologic or alcohol determinations are done in cases of drug ingestion. Reactive hypoglycemia is diagnosed only after excluding other causes of adrenergic-mediated

Table 7–5. *Differential Diagnosis of Adrenergic-Mediated Symptoms ("Spells")*

I. Cardiovascular disease:
   A. Arrhythmias (sinus arrest, asystole, tachycardias, atrial fibrillation-flutter, tachybradycardia syndromes, to include sick-sinus syndrome, atrioventricular (AV) dissociation, and Stokes-Adams attacks)
   B. Pulmonary emboli and/or microemboli
   C. Orthostatic hypotension syndromes
   D. DaCosta syndrome (beta-adrenergic hyperresponsive state)
   E. Mitral valve or apparatus dysfunction
II. Psychoneurologic disease:
   A. Seizure disorders
   B. Autonomic insufficiency
   C. Diencephalic epilepsy
   D. Hyperventilation syndrome
   E. Cataplexy
   F. Anxiety neurosis
   G. Hysteria
   H. Migraine
   I. Syncope
   J. Psychophysiologic reaction
III. Gastrointestinal disorders:
   A. Dumping syndrome after gastrointestinal surgery
   B. Postprandial physiological dumping without prior gastrointestinal surgery
   C. Chinese-restaurant syndrome
   D. Irritable colon syndrome
   E. Food intolerance
IV. Endocrine-metabolic disorders:
   A. Hyperthyroidism
   B. Hypothyroidism
   C. Reactive hypoglycemia
   D. Fasting hypoglycemia
   E. Pheochromocytoma
   F. Carcinoid syndrome
   G. Hereditary angioneurotic edema
   H. Urticaria pigmentosa
   I. Hyperbradykinism
   J. Addison's disease
   K. Hypopituitarism
   L. Hypothalamic-pituitary dysfunction
   M. Menopause
   N. Diabetes mellitus
V. Miscellaneous disease:
   A. Sepsis
   B. Anemia
   C. Cachexia
   D. Hypovolemia (dehydration)
   E. Clonidine withdrawal
   F. Monoamine-oxidase inhibitors plus tyramine
   G. Idiopathic postprandial syndrome
VI. Stress

Source: Adapted from Hofeldt, F. D. Transitional low blood glucose. *Rocky Mt. Med. J.* 76: 30, 1979. Used with permission of the publisher.

symptoms (see Table 7-5). Oral glucose tolerance testing is rarely needed to establish this diagnosis. The diagnosis is best confirmed by timely home capillary glucose determinations during symptoms that demonstrate a blood glucose level below 50 mg/dl (2.8 mmol/liter). The 5-hour oral glucose tolerance test is nonphysiologic and should be used only as a research tool.

X-Ray and Special Tests
Localization of an insulinoma with an abdominal CT scan is helpful in 50 to 60 percent of the patients. Other localization procedures include pancreatic ultrasound, celiac arteriogram, and interoperative measurements in the portal-splenic circulation of insulin values. Pancreatic and nonpancreatic tumors causing hypoglycemia may require exploratory laparotomy if localization studies fail.

TREATMENT AND PROGNOSIS
Acute Management
Hypoglycemia should be suspected in all stuporous or comatose patients. Any delay in treatment and diagnosis may cause permanent brain damage. Treatment is always with glucose solutions, preferably intravenous (50 cc bolus of 50 percent dextrose solution or 5 to 10 percent dextrose infusion). Parenteral glucagon administration is unreliable and should not be used because it requires adequate hepatic glycogen stores, which may or may not be present.

Chronic Management
Reactive hypoglycemia is managed by elimination of refined carbohydrates and ingestion of well-balanced, mixed meals. Selected patients may require an oral antidiabetic agent, Probanthine, Phenytoin, calcium-channel blockers, or fructose.

For insulinoma patients, surgical removal of the tumor is imperative. Medical management of insulinomas includes frequent feedings (every 2 to

3 hours), diazoxide, streptozotocin, somatostatin or its analogues, and chemotherapy.

Hormone-deficiency states respond to replacement therapy (see the section entitled Endocrinology).

The prognosis depends on the etiology of the hypoglycemia (see Table 7-4). The drug-related causes are remedial once they are identified. In the diabetic with too much insulin or oral agents, home glucose monitoring is extremely helpful in discovering episodes of hypoglycemia and allowing dosage reductions. Reactive hypoglycemia is a benign disease readily treated by diet; it can be episodic, occurring when periods of dieting are combined with ingestion of convenient foods high in refined carbohydrates. When pancreatic insulinomas are identified, approximately 70 to 80 percent of these are benign adenomas and surgical removal of the lesion ameliorates the hypoglycemia. If the condition is due to islet-cell hyperplasia or carcinoma, then surgery, diet, and medical management are combined.

Disorders of Lipid Metabolism

Disorders of lipid metabolism [20, 24, 29, 58, 61, 73] are related to alterations in chylomicron and very-low-density lipoprotein (VLDL), triglyceride, cholesterol (low-density lipoprotein, LDL), and high-density lipoprotein (HDL) metabolism. They may occur on a genetic basis, may be induced by diet, may be secondary to other diseases, or may result from any combination of inheritance, disease, and diet. The clinical significance of these diseases is through their association with the early or accelerated development of atherosclerosis as manifested by cerebrovascular accidents, myocardial infarction, or peripheral vascular disease.

DIAGNOSIS

History

Since heredity plays a major role in these disorders, a very careful family history of lipid disorders, diabetes mellitus, hypothyroidism, or ath-

erosclerosis is important. The clinical significance of any abnormal laboratory test requires interpretation depending on personal or family history of the vascular complications. The chylomicronemia syndrome includes individuals whose postprandial triglyceride levels exceed 1000 mg/dl and may be associated with hepatosplenomegaly, recurrent bouts of pancreatitis, or eruptive xanthomas. Combined familial hyperlipidemia is characterized by the family members being heterogeneous as to elevated type(s) of lipid particle(s). In this disorder there is the frequent occurrence of vascular disease in family members. Since secondary conditions may cause hyperlipidemia, these should be assessed (diabetes mellitus, hypothyroidism, use of birth control pills, renal failure, liver disease, dysproteinemic states, use of diuretics and beta blockers, alcohol, and pregnancy). Dietary history may provide diagnostic and therapeutic insight. History of hypertension, gout, smoking, obesity, and exercise should be noted.

Physical Findings

The physical findings depend on which lipid particle is elevated. In the chylomicronemia syndrome one may see lipemia retinalis, eruptive xanthoma, hepatosplenomegaly, or acute pancreatitis. If the triglyceride elevation is due solely to very-low-density lipoproteins, the associated conditions include obesity, gout, and diabetes; the characteristic findings are eruptive, tuberoeruptive, and tuberous xanthomas. In familial dysbetalipoproteinemia (broad-beta disease, type III), patients may present with eruptive, tuberoeruptive, tuberous, and a peculiar palmar xanthoma. Palmer xanthomas also may be seen in biliary cirrhosis, where an abnormal lipoprotein particle exists. Patients with hypercholesterolemia have tendon xanthomas (hands, achilles), nonspecific xanthelasma, and arcus corneae juvenilis.

Laboratory Tests

Serum lipids should be drawn in the basal nonstressed, nondieting state after a 12-hour overnight fast. After acute stress, lipid levels are not considered basal for approximately 2 to 3 months. In the office or at bedside, serum can be separated, refrigerated, and noted for the presence of turbidity and particle layering. The very-low-density lipoprotein and remnant particles form a cloudy and turbid serum depending on their concentration. Chylomicrons are very large, aggregate particles that float, appear creamlike, and layer on the top of the serum. Cholesterol elevations do not contribute to turbidity. Patients with triglyceride disorders can be followed during therapy for plasma clearing. As part of the lipid assessment, the measurement of high-density lipoprotein levels are prognostic, since high-density lipoproteins, especially apolipoprotein A-I (apo A-I) and HDL$_2$, are associated with a reduced risk of occlusive vascular disease. A higher ratio of apolipoprotein B to apolipoprotein A-I is strongly related to increased risk of cardiovascular disease. Age- and sex-adjusted values must be used to interpret serum lipid values [61]. A rough guideline that defines the upper limits of normal values includes:

$$\text{Triglyceride} = 100 + \text{age}$$
$$\text{Cholesterol} = 175 + \text{age}$$
$$\text{Low-density lipoprotein} = 100 + \text{age}$$

If the triglyceride level is equal to or less than 400

mg/dl, low-density lipoprotein cholesterol can be accurately estimated by the following equation:

$$\text{LDL cholesterol} = \text{total cholesterol} - (\text{triglycerides}/5 + \text{HDL cholesterol})$$

Typical lipid values seen in the various hyperlipoproteinemias are shown in Table 7-6. According to this scheme, type I disease represents the chylomicronemia syndrome, type II represents hypercholesterolemic disorders, type III represents dysbetalipoproteinemia (broad-beta or remnant-removal disease), type IV represents the endogenous hypertriglyceridemic disorders, and type V represents a combined endogenous-absorptive hypertriglyceridemia.

THERAPY
General Guidelines
Maintenance of the ideal body weight with a balanced diet is the cornerstone of therapy. The diet should be the prudent cardiac diet, consisting of 35 percent fat, 300 mg cholesterol, and alteration of polyunsaturated-saturated fat ratio to >1. If further fat restriction is required, dietary fat is reduced from 35 to 20 gm and cholesterol is reduced to 300 to 100 mg per day. Alcohol should be eliminated in triglyceride disorders. Fiber food and fish oils may be helpful in hypertriglyceridemia. Exercise will raise high-density lipoprotein

Table 7–6. *Plasma Lipid and Lipoprotein-Cholesterol Concentrations in Dyslipidemic Subjects*

Hyperlipoproteinemic subjects	Plasma*		Cholesterol*		
	Cholesterol	Triglyceride	VLDL	LDL	HDL
Type I (n = 12)	324 ± 57	3316 ± 677	285 ± 57	22 ± 2	17 ± 2
Type II (n = 454)	354 ± 4	135 ± 4	24 ± 1	286 ± 9	44 ± 1
Type III (n = 66)	441 ± 54	694 ± 60	292 ± 19	111 ± 7	38 ± 2
Type IV (n = 299)	251 ± 4	438 ± 24	78 ± 4	132 ± 2	37 ± 1
Type V (n = 95)	373 ± 19	2071 ± 213	274 ± 22	72 ± 4	27 ± 1

*Values are means ± SEM (in mm/dl). VLDL represents the 1.006 gm/ml supernatant fraction and therefore includes chylomicrons when present and VLDL. To convert cholesterol and triglyceride values to millimoles per liter, multiply by 0.02586 and 0.01129, respectively.
Source: Reprinted from Schaefer, E. J., and Levy, R. I.   Pathogenesis and management of lipoprotein disorders. *N. Engl. J. Med.* 312: 1304, 1985. Used with permission.

levels. As triglyceride levels fall, high-density lipoprotein levels will rise.

Lipid-Lowering Agents

Hypertriglyceridemia is best treated with gemfibrozil (1200 to 1500 mg per day PO bid). Side effects include abdominal pain, nausea, vomiting, glucose intolerance, hyperuricemia, liver toxicity, hyperpigmentation, and rash. Clofibrate (1 gm PO bid) may have similar side effects, including myalgias, arthralgias, impotence, and cholelithiasis. The drug of choice for lowering cholesterol is the bile acid-binding resins (cholestyramine and colestipol). These agents may lead to constipation, rectal irritation, diarrhea, increased stool volume, and heartburn. Cholestyramine can interfere with the absorption of thyroxine, warfarin, and digoxin. Cholestyramine is given initially as 4 gm bid and should be increased to a maximum of 24 gm per day. Colestipol is given 5 gm PO bid, increased to qid if necessary. Compliance may be improved if these drugs are taken with juices, soft drinks, soups, or sauces. Nicotinic acid is used to treat both cholesterol and triglyceride disorders. The major side effects of flushing, gastrointestinal distress, and hepatotoxicity, which are minimized by starting at low doses of 100 mg PO tid and gradually increasing to 4 to 6 gm per day as required. Aspirin (300 mg PO) a half hour before each dose may reduce the vasomotor side effects. Specific competitive inhibition of the rate-limiting enzyme in cholesterol biosynthesis (HMG CoA reductase) with Levastatin provides new therapy for patients with hypercholesterolemia. The dose of Levastatin is 10 mg bid to 40 mg bid. Probucol is a well-tolerated cholesterol-lowering agent starting at a dose of 500 mg PO bid. Probucal will lower high-density lipoprotein cholesterol, but this effect is counteracted by the simultaneous use of both colestipol and probucal. Neomycin, a nonabsorbable antibiotic in a dose up to 2 gm per day PO, may be used. Side effects include ototoxicity and renal damage. D-Thyroxine lowers the low-density lipoprotein cholesterol, but the major side effect is hyperthyroidism, which can be harmful to patients with coronary artery disease.

PROGNOSIS

Triglyceride elevations are harmful in familial combined hyperlipidemia, diabetes mellitus, and peripheral vascular disease. Triglyceride levels over 700 mg/dl should be treated to avoid complications of pancreatitis. Elevated cholesterol levels (particularly low-density lipoprotein cholesterol) and reduced high-density lipoprotein levels are associated with advanced atherosclerosis, especially in familial hypercholesteremia. Normalizing these values is beneficial.

Eating Disorders

The eating disorders, i.e., anorexia nervosa, bulimia, and obesity, are common [2, 9, 27, 28, 38, 63, 69]. It is estimated that anorexia nervosa and bulimia affect 10 to 15 percent of adolescent girls and young women. The prevalence of bulimia among college women ranges as high as 20 percent. Anorexia nervosa is a syndrome characterized by extreme weight loss, body-image disturbances, and an intense fear of becoming obese. This pathologic fear of weight gain associated with faulty eating patterns, malnutrition, and unusual weight loss produces clinical illness. Bulimia is a syndrome distinct from anorexia nervosa and is characterized by secretive eating binges followed by self-induced vomiting, fasting, or abuse of laxatives or diuretics. Bulimic symptoms can be a part of the anorexia nervosa syndrome. The frequency of obesity increases with age in both sexes to about 35 percent in men and 50 percent in women. Black women are more frequently affected than white women. After age 65, obesity declines in the population. When body weight exceeds ideal standards, varying degrees of overnutrition are present. As a rule, when individuals are 10 to 19 percent over ideal body weight, they are considered overweight. Obesity occurs when ideal body weight exceeds 120 percent. Morbid obesity is defined as exceeding ideal body weight by 100 lbs or twice predicted ideal body weight.

DIAGNOSIS
History
A detailed history is obtained of the progression of weight changes, eating habits, family history of obesity, and family eating habits. Attempts at weight control are noted, particularly various compulsive acts or rituals used to control weight, which may include exercise, restrictive diets, starvation, vomiting, and diuretic or cathartic usage. Particular groups of individuals vulnerable to excessive weight loss include jockeys, wrestlers, gymnasts, models, ballet dancers, actors, and actresses. Eating behavior with regard to external stress and emotional changes such as anxiety, depression, or mood swings should be noted. Many weight disorders are associated with a distorted body image, and frequently, there may be underlying emotional disorders such as anxiety, depression, anger, resentment, or hostility. Antisocial behavior may exist, such as drug abuse, kleptomania, and sexual promiscuity. A 25 percent weight loss from original body weight defines anorexia nervosa. In cases of bulimia, a history of recurring episodes of binge eating associated with consumption of high-caloric food, inconspicuous eating behavior, and termination of eating episodes by abdominal pain, sleep, social activities, or self-induced vomiting may be noted. Weight fluctuations of 8 to 10 lbs may be associated with binging and fasting. These eating disorders may be associated with amenorrhea, oligomenorrhea, and decreased libido. The following questions may help ascertain information regarding this disorder. Do you feel helpless in the presence of food? Are you a binge eater? Do you try every new diet and always end up gaining back the weight you lose? Do you try to control your weight by vomiting, use of laxatives or diuretics, overexercise, or episodes of starvation? Do you eat when you are not hungry? Do you eat when you are anxious? Do you eat when you are depressed? Do you feel guilty after an eating

binge? Do you eat sensibly around other people, then "pig out" when you are alone?

When obesity exists, is there evidence of coexisting hypertension, diabetes, osteoarthritis, gallbladder disease, cardiovascular disease, or peripheral vascular disease? Both excessive obesity and anorexia nervosa syndromes may be associated with reproductive and menstrual disorders. The inadequate nutrition of anorexia nervosa may contribute to osteoporosis, whereas obesity contributes to degenerative joint disease.

Physical Examination
The physical examination should note the patient's general body habitus and distribution of nutrient stores, particularly in the face, neck, and skin fold areas, including the subscapular, abdominal, and tricep skin areas. Other clues include parotid swelling, gingival disease, or tarnished teeth. Patients with anorexia nervosa may manifest bradycardia, hypotension, unusual body leanness, hypercarotenemia, and the inability to maintain body temperature in the presence of heat or cold stress. Obesity can be defined by the percent over ideal body weight as projected from height and weight measurements (Fig. 7-1). Excessive obesity may be associated with pseudogynecomastia, pseudoacanthosis nigricans, dyshidrotic skin, and stasis dermatitis. The endocrine causes of obesity should be considered on physical examination to exclude Cushing's syndrome, hypothyroidism, and diabetes.

Laboratory Tests
Patients with anorexia nervosa and bulimia may manifest anemia, leukopenia, thrombocytopenia, and hypokalemia from diuretic or laxative abuse. A high urine pH in the absence of *Proteus mirabilis* infection suggests self-induced vomiting and metabolic alkalosis. Obesity may be associated with carbohydrate intolerance, diabetes mellitus, hyperuricemia, and altered hepatic enzymes. Elevated hepatic enzymes also might be seen in anorexia nervosa. Triglyceride levels are elevated in

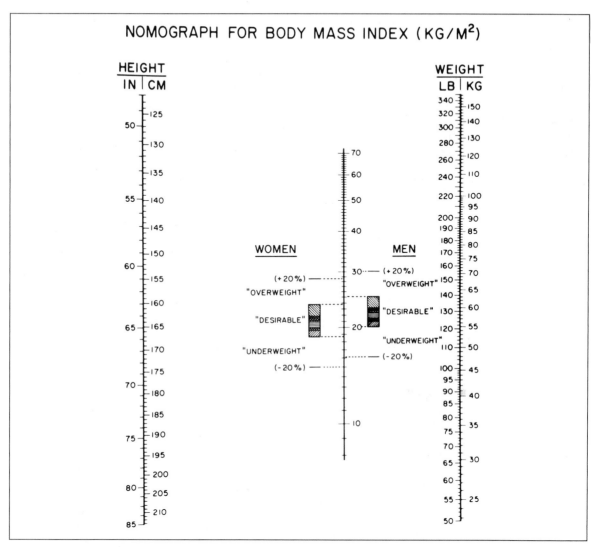

NOMOGRAPH FOR BODY MASS INDEX (KG/M²)

Figure 7–1. *The ratio of weight to height is read from the central scale. The ranges suggested as "desirable" from life insurance data must be interpreted with clinical judgment regarding relative skeletal muscle mass. (From A. E. Thomas, D. A. Kekay, and M. D. Cutlip, A normograph method for assessing body weight, Am. J. Clin. Nutr. 29: 302, 1976. Reprinted by permission.)*

obesity, and high-density lipoprotein levels are reduced.

Special Tests

In anorexia nervosa there may be a loss of the normal pulsatile secretion of gonadotropins and a blunted response to gonadotropin-releasing hormone (GnRH) testing, resulting in low sex steroid levels. Fasting inhibits the peripheral conversion of thyroxine (T_4) to triiodothyronine (T_3), resulting in a low T_3 state. Low basal growth hormone levels with depressed somatomedin C levels and hypercortisolism with blunted adrenocorticotropic hormone (ACTH) response to corticotropin-releasing hormone may be seen. The patient may not be able to concentrate urine normally in response to water deprivation and may manifest significant dehydration.

TREATMENT AND PROGNOSIS
Patients with obesity are best managed by a hypocaloric (1200-calorie) diet divided into three equal meals with the use of fiber food as a preprandial appetite suppressant that provides early satiety. Behavior modification programs include food diaries, caloric counting, exercise programs, and attention to mood alterations. The exercise program reinforces dietary compliance. The use of fad or ritualistic diets, anorectic agents, or thyroid hormone should be discouraged. Gastric bypass surgery in morbidly obese individuals who have failed medical management may be considered, but this is associated with a poor success rate. Use of gastric space-occupying balloons is experimental and associated with complications of gastric rupture or obstruction.

Treating patients with eating disorders should include attention to the patient's emotional insecurities and coexisting medical disorders, especially malnutrition and vitamin-deficiency states. In patients with anorexia nervosa or bulimia, a combined medical, psychiatric, and nutritional approach is needed. Insight-oriented therapy is more successful when the patient is made aware of their psychological defenses and underlying conflicts with adaptation of more realistic beliefs, goals, and behaviors. Behavior modification has been helpful in increasing weight gain, along with family interaction to encourage communication and cooperation, which is best accomplished through individual group and family therapy. Long-range drug therapy has not been effective. The goal of therapy is to help the patient regain physical health, reduce symptoms, increase self-esteem, and proceed with personal and social development. Patients with severe malnutrition, electrolyte abnormalities, or suicide risk may require hospitalization with nutritional support therapy and psychiatric therapy. The treatment of these eating disorders is notoriously difficult, and responses to therapy are seen in only a small number of patients.

Metabolic Bone Disease

When a disease process affects all parts of the skeleton, influencing all metabolic bone units, the disease is termed *metabolic bone disease*. This excludes localized bone disease, such as Sudeck's atrophy, bone cysts, Paget's disease, polyostotic osteodystrophy, and fractures. The metabolic diseases [11, 23, 34, 55, 56, 71] include osteitis fibrosa cystica of hyperparathyroidism, osteoporosis, osteomalacia, osteogenesis imperfecta, and renal osteodystrophy. The differential diagnosis of osteopenic bone conditions is presented in Table 7-7. Table 7-8 shows the differential diagnosis of osteomalacia.

DIAGNOSIS
History
The patient's sex, race, age of onset, and family history of the bone disease help to define the etiology. Idiopathic osteoporosis is divided into onset in youth, middle age, postmenopausal, or old age (senile). Osteogenesis imperfecta is manifested by fragile bones, blue sclera, deafness due to otosclerosis, fractures, and kyphoscoliosis. It has varying genetic expressions depending on its autosomal dominant or recessive forms. In evaluating osteomalacia, the history should include an extensive review of systems to determine if there is coexisting gastrointestinal disease, nutritional disorders, drug usage, or renal disease. Renal osteodystrophy occurs in the setting of advanced renal failure, phosphate retention, secondary hyperparathyroidism, metabolic acidosis, malnutrition, inactivity, and aluminum toxicity in hemodialysis patients. History of bone fracture(s), skeletal deformity, and loss of height should be noted. Contributing factors for osteoporosis include history of cigarette smoking, excessive alcohol and coffee drinking, early menopause, nulliparity, steroid usage, lactose intolerance, physical inactivity, and lack of sunlight exposure.

Table 7–7. *Osteopenia*

I. Age-related idiopathic osteoporosis:
   A. Juvenile osteoporosis
   B. Idiopathic osteoporosis of young adults
   C. Postmenopausal osteoporosis
   D. Senile osteoporosis
II. Osteopenic endocrine-metabolic disease:
   A. Hypogonadism
   B. Cushing's syndrome
   C. Hyperthyroidism
   D. Hyperprolactinemia
   E. Diabetes
   F. Calcium deficiency
   G. Malnutrition
III. Osteopenic medical disease:
   A. Rheumatoid arthritis
   B. Alcoholism
   C. Scurvy
   D. Immobilization
   E. Chronic obstructive pulmonary disease
   F. Chronic heparin administration
IV. Osteopenia of neoplastic disease:
   A. Multiple myeloma
   B. Systemic mastocystis
   C. Leukemia
   D. Lymphoma
V. Osteopenic connective-tissue disease:
   A. Osteogenesis imperfecta
   B. Homocystinuria
   C. Ehlers-Danlos syndrome
VI. Osteitis fibrosa cystica:
   A. Hyperparathyroidism, primary and secondary types
   B. Renal osteodystrophy (mixed metabolic bone disease)
VII. Osteomalacia (see Table 7-8) (frequently associated with secondary hyperparathyroidism)

Table 7–8. *Osteomalacia*

I. Vitamin D deficiency:
   A. Dietary
   B. Dietary plus low sunlight exposure
   C. Malabsorption state
II. Disorders of vitamin D metabolism:
   A. Decreased formation of 25-hydroxyvitamin D_3 in hepatic disease
   B. Decreased formation of 1,25-dihydroxyvitamin D_3:
     1. Renal failure
     2. Hyperphosphatemic disorders
     3. Vitamin D-dependent rickets, type I
     4. Aging
     5. Hypoparathyroidism
   C. Altered vitamin D metabolism by drugs:
     1. Anticonvulsants (barbiturates, phenytoin)
     2. Rifampin, isoniazid
   D. 1,25-dihydroxyvitamin D_3-resistant states:
     1. Renal failure
     2. Anticonvulsants
     3. Vitamin D-dependent rickets, type II
III. Disorders of phosphate metabolism (hypophosphatemic disorders with increased urinary phosphate loss):
   A. Vitamin D-resistant rickets (X-linked, sporadic, autosomal-recessive variants)
   B. Vitamin D-dependent rickets, type I
   C. Fanconi syndrome
   D. Oncogenic osteomalacia
IV. Abnormal mineralization disorders:
   A. Fibrogenesis imperfecta
   B. Hypophosphatasia
   C. Drugs (fluorides, diphosphonates)

Physical Findings

Patients' height, weight, and nutritional status should be assessed, with loss of height documented and deformities or fractures noted. Abdominal scars are clues to previous abdominal surgery or gastrectomy. Dorsal kyphosis (dowager's hump) with shortening and downward angulation of the ribs coming to rest on the iliac crest indicate long-standing osteoporosis. Blue sclera and disordered growth are seen in osteogenesis imperfecta. Senile osteoporosis may be associated with muscular atrophy and loss of subcutaneous tissue, giving the skin a transparent appearance.

Laboratory Tests

The evaluation of bones should include routine chest (posteroanterior and lateral) x-rays and lumbosacral spine and hip views in 15 degrees of internal rotation for the Singh index, which quantitatively rates bone loss by noting the presence or absence of trabecular stress lines of the femoral neck. Hand and skull films should be done in suspected hyperparathyroidism. Approximately 30 to 40 percent of bone mass must be lost before roentgenographic changes are noted. Basal laboratory tests include serum calcium, phosphate, electrolytes, blood urea nitrogen, and creatinine determinations, fasting urine pH, and 24-hour urine tests for calcium, phosphate, and creatinine. A urinary calcium level less than 50 mg per 24-hour sample characterizes osteomalacia, and values less than 100 mg are suspicious. Elevated urinary calcium levels greater than 250 mg per 24-hour sample may reflect a state of high bone turnover. Elevated serum bone alkaline phosphatase levels may be seen in high-turnover osteoporosis states, hyperparathyroidism, osteomalacia, healing fracture(s), and Paget's disease. Activity of bone breakdown can be assessed in Paget's disease with a urinary hydroxyproline measurement. Increased urinary osteocalcin (gamma-carboxyglutamic acid) reflects a high bone turnover state. When malabsorption is suspected, a quantitative 72-hour stool fat collection and a D-xylose absorption test is useful. A simple screening test may include qualitative stool examination for undigested food or Sudan III staining for fat. Specific endocrine causes are ruled out by appropriate laboratory tests (see the section entitled Endocrinology).

Special Tests

When hypercalcemia is present, hyperparathyroidism is suspected, especially if hyperchloremic metabolic acidosis exists. An elevated parathyroid hormone (PTH) level establishes the diagnosis. Low vitamin D levels, particularly 25-hydroxyvitamin D_3 occurs in osteomalacia. Low levels of 1,25-dihydroxyvitamin D_3 are seen in elderly patients, in renal disease, in type I vitamin D-dependent rickets, and in oncogenic osteomalacia. Radionuclide bone scanning will be positive in areas of bone fractures, metastatic carcinoma to bone, inflammation, or Paget's disease.

Bone densitometry will define osteopenia better than the conventional roentgenograms. Single-photon densitometry of the midradius and distal wrist are limited and do not accurately predict trabecular bone loss of the axial skeleton, but it is a useful technique to establish initial bone density and to follow changes that occur with disease progression or therapeutic intervention. The bone density of the spine is assessed by dual-photon densitometry or spinal computed axial tomographic (CAT) scanning, and both are sensitive for detecting early spinal osteoporosis. Bone biopsy with tetracycline labeling and histomorphologic assessment of bone mass, percent osteoid, percent resorption and formation surfaces, and osteoclast count may be needed in difficult cases.

TREATMENT AND PROGNOSIS

The prognosis for osteogenesis imperfecta as a genetic disease is poor, with impaired skeletal development and susceptibility to fractures early in life. Osteomalacia, when identified, is very remedial to therapy by supplying the necessary substrate for bone mineralization, such as calcium, vitamin D, or phosphate. Paget's disease may be incidentally noted, and if the location of the Paget's bone is in an asymptomatic area, little need be done. However, if critical weight-bearing bones are involved or associated with fracture, therapy is warranted with human or salmon calcitonin or the diphosphonates (etidronate). Calcitonin can be given as 100 I.U. subcutaneous daily to establish control of the disease, as assessed by symptoms and by following urinary hydroxyproline and serum alkaline phosphatase levels. When the disease is showing metabolic or clinical stability, maintenance therapy is decreased to 50 I.U. every other day. Alternatively, patients may be treated with the diphosphonate etidronate (5 to 10 mg/kg per day) not to exceed 6 months. The treatment with calcitonin and etidronate is intermittent and determined by the clinical and metabolic activity of the bone disease. In some instances, mithramycin, a chemotherapeutic agent, is useful, but there are frequent toxic side effects.

Renal osteodystrophy is an unrelenting condition unless recognized and treated early with control of hyperphosphatemia with aluminum hydroxide-containing antacids, adequate nutrition, vitamin D, calcium (1 to 1.5 gm per day), dialysis with calcium-containing dialysate, renal transplantation, and in selected patients parathyroidectomy. Deferoxamine may be helpful in treating aluminum-induced osteomalacia.

The prognosis in postmenopausal or senile osteoporosis is best with early detection and preventative treatment. Patients with senile osteoporosis are particularly prone to fractures because of the psychophysiologic deterioration of aging, falling secondary to household hazards, and polymedication, which renders the elderly patient drowsy, light-headed, and weak. Promoting physical activity with ambulation and exercise, ensuring adequate calcium intake (1 to 1.5 gm elemental calcium PO), and recognizing risk factors such as poor nutrition, alcoholism, and smoking are helpful. Preventive treatment of the high-risk postmenopausal patient before the onset of clinically significant bone disease with cyclic estrogen replacement therapy [0.625 mg conjugated estrogens (Premarin) or 30 to 45 μg ethinyl estradiol] daily for 21 days will best stabilize bone mass. Estrogens should be used with 10 mg medroxyprogesterone acetate (Provera) for the last 10 to 14 days of each menstrual cycle. The transdermal estrogens are reported useful in relieving the symptoms of menopause, but their efficacy in the long-term management of osteoporosis needs to be established. Side effects of estrogen therapy may include hypertension, fluid retention, breast tenderness, and gallbladder stones. Endometrial carcinoma is prevented if the patient is simultaneously treated with a progestin, as recommended above. Replacement doses of estrogens are not associated with the same increased hypercoagulable states seen with oral contraceptive medications. However, they should be used cautiously in patients known to have preexisting thromboembolic or peripheral vascular disease. In male patients and those females in whom estrogen therapy is contraindicated, stanozolol (2 mg qd to tid) may be equally effective. It is contraindicated in patients with carcinoma of the breast or prostate. In elderly patients in whom intestinal calcium absorption is poor, 1,25-dihydroxyvitamin D_3 (0.25 μg per day) promotes positive calcium balance. The use of sodium fluoride with informed consent (40 to 60 mg per day, keeping plasma concentrations at 10 to 20 μg/dl) with 1 to 1.5 gm calcium and vitamin D (50,000 units once to twice weekly) also may increase bone mass. Side effects of sodium fluoride include gastrointestinal irritability, arthralgias, and rheumatoid syndromes. Serum fluoride levels are followed to establish therapeutic range. Newer programs of activation and depression of the metabolic bone units (ADFR) are using oral phosphate as an activator followed by suppression with calcitonin or diphosphonate with a 3-month rest period and then a repeat cycle. This hopefully will establish an increased bone mass, but long-term studies are in progress to document the efficacy of this approach. Acute management of patients with fractures requires bed rest, analgesics, and support of the fracture site. Immobilization should be limited, and the patient should be ambulated as soon as possible.

Endocrinology

Inherent in the evaluation of endocrine disorders is an understanding of positive- and negative-feedback regulation of hormone biosynthesis and secretion. Hormones are secreted from a specific glandular tissue under servocontrol mechanisms that regulate the level of the hormone to best meet cellular and metabolic demands. Peptide hormones such as hypothalamic-releasing factors, pituitary hormones, parathyroid hormone, thyrocalcitonin, insulin, and glucagon are examples of hormones that act on target tissue by binding to specific membrane receptors on the cell, which, in turn, initiate hormone action through a complex process of generating intracellular mediators. Thyroid hormone, vitamin D metabolites, and the steroid hormones, which include the glucocorticoids, mineralocorticoids, androgens, and estrogens, readily permeate target-cell membranes. They act intracellularly to control metabolic function, particularly through regulation of DNA/RNA-protein synthesis. Hence cells are regulated by hormones that directly influence critical intracellular functions. The reserve secretory capacity of each endocrine gland is able to adapt to meet our changing metabolic needs through a system that rapidly responds to the various internal and external stressors.

Diseases of these endocrine glands result in either hormonal deficiency or hormonal overproduction. Hormonal-deficiency states may be due to destructive diseases, drugs, altered biosynthetic pathways, or end-organ resistance to hormone action. Deficiency states can be characterized as primary when the secretory gland is involved (thyroid, adrenal, gonad), as secondary if pituitary dysfunction occurs, and as tertiary with hypothalamic dysfunction. If the gland produces multiple hormones, such as, for example, the pituitary gland, deficiencies may be monotrophic, involve two or more hormones, or involve all hormones, resulting in a panhypopituitary state. Deficiencies of hormones are assessed by measuring plasma or urinary levels and noting their decreased secretion and production rates or through stimulation tests to assess the reserve capacity of a particular gland.

Endocrine conditions with excessive hormone production may be due to glandular hyperplasia, adenoma, or carcinoma. In these conditions, the measured levels of the hormone in the blood or urine exceed the usual normal secretory state. Hormone-excess states usually manifest themselves as specific endocrine syndromes easily recognized by history and physical examination and diagnosed by selective laboratory tests. Most overproduction states are characterized by autonomous hormone secretion that displays varying degrees of abnormal regulation.

Neuroendocrinology

The central nervous system regulates anterior and posterior pituitary function through the hypothalamus. Specific hypothalamic factors, such as thyroid-releasing hormone (TRH), gonadotrophin-releasing hormone (GnRH), growth hormone-releasing hormone (GRH), somatostatin (SRIF), corticotropin-releasing hormone (CRH), and prolactin-inhibitory factor (PIF, dopamine) have been isolated and shown to regulate pituitary gland function. Hypothalamic disease can, therefore, present as abnormal pituitary function. Hence the signs and symptoms of hypothalamic disease may present as a monotrophic or total anterior or posterior pituitary hormone-deficiency state. Since the hypothalamus also regulates other important functions, disease of this structure also may present as psychiatric disturbances, obesity or hyperphagia, thirst or compulsive drinking, essential hypernatremia, hypersomnolence, anorexia, or emaciation. In general, a destructive hypothalamic process causes all anterior pituitary hormone secretion to decrease except for prolactin, which increases. Thus the net effect of the hypothalamus on thyroid-stimulating hormone (TSH), luteinizing hormone (LH), follicle-stimulating hormone (FSH), adrenocorticotropic hormone (ACTH), or growth hormone (GH) is stimulatory, whereas the net effect on prolactin is inhibitory. If a specific pituitary hormone deficiency exists but its secretion can be stimulated by the hypothalamic releasing hormones, then the defect lies not in the pituitary, but at the level of the hypothalamus. In contrast, failure of the pituitary to respond to adequate stimulation by hypothalamic releasing factors implies that the defect is at the level of the pituitary gland.

Hypopituitarism

Hypopituitarism [1, 44] has multiple causes, including the previously discussed hypothalamic or pituitary disorders. Potential etiologies include space-occupying lesions, skull fractures, surgical ablation, radiation, tumors, infections, chronic granulomatous processes, infiltrative disease, or infarctions, as seen in postpartum hemorrhage (Sheehan's syndrome). When pituitary deficiencies occur, gonadotropins and growth hormone decline first, whereas corticotropin, thyrotropin, and prolactin are relatively well-preserved until the disease process advances to such an extent that total panhypopituitarism occurs.

DIAGNOSIS
History
The clinical features of hypopituitarism vary depending on the degree of pituitary destruction. The onset of pituitary failure syndrome may be insidious and evolve slowly over a period of several months to years. The symptoms of hypopituitarism include amenorrhea or impotence, weakness, fatigue, light-headedness, nausea and vomiting, intolerance to cold, loss of axillary and pubic hair, growth failure, and weight loss. With space-occupying lesions, headache and visual-field loss (bitemperal hemiopia) are noted. Polyuria and polydipsia suggest central diabetes insipidous.

Physical Findings
Signs of hypopituitarism include wasting, loss of axillary and pubic hair, pallor, atrophy of the skin, fine wrinkling or premature aging around the eyes and mouth, hypotension, bradycardia, hypothermia, and small testicles.

Laboratory Tests
The diagnosis depends on demonstrating reduced basal plasma levels of the pituitary trophic hormones, which fail to rise normally with stimulation. Differentiation of hypopituitarism of hypothalamic origin from intrinsic pituitary disease is done by testing thyroid-stimulating hormone reserve with thyrotropin-releasing hormone, follicle-stimulating hormone and luteinizing hormone reserve with gonadotropin-releasing hormone, prolactin reserve with the chlorpromazine or thyrotropin-releasing hormone, and adrenocorticotropic hormone reserve with metyrapone, vasopressin, insulin-induced hypoglycemia, or corticotropin-releasing hormone and growth hormone by growth hormone-releasing hormone, clonidine, arginine infusion, or insulin-induced

hypoglycemia. Table 7-9 shows the classic responses of pituitary hormones to hypothalamic testing (growth hormone-releasing hormone and corticotropin-releasing hormone are not currently commercially available for pituitary testing).

X-Ray and Special Studies
Whenever possible, the cause of the underlying hypopituitarism should be determined. In all cases, a space-occupying lesion of the sella, suprasellar areas, or hypothalamus is excluded by a contrast CT scan or magnetic resonance imaging (MRI). Coronal views are more helpful than axial views for smaller intrasellar lesions and for determining the degree of suprasellar involvement. Arteriograms are used rarely, but they can be used to exclude a vascular etiology.

TREATMENT AND PROGNOSIS
Therapy is directed toward treating the primary cause of the hypopituitary state. In the case of pituitary tumors, surgery or radiotherapy may be required (see Pituitary Tumors). Adequate substitution therapy of target-organ hormones that are deficient (estrogen, testosterone, glucocorticoids, mineralocorticoids, thyroxine, and DDAVP) always must be given. The prognosis in hypopituitarism is good, since adequate replacement therapy allows the individual to lead a normal life. Growth hormone deficiency results in retardation of linear growth in children and adolescents. In these patients, growth hormone replacement therapy is required to complete skeletal growth and maturation.

Pituitary Tumors
Space-occupying lesions in the sellar, suprasellar, or hypothalamic areas can produce varying degrees of pituitary hormone deficiency or can present as an anatomic lesion with headaches and optic nerve compression. If the hypophyseal portal system is interrupted, the patient will present with varying degrees of hypopituitarism

Table 7–9. *Hypothalamic-Pituitary Testing*

I. Hypopituitarism:
    A. Growth hormone deficiency: Need impaired response to two provocative tests for diagnosis:
        1. Insulin-induced hypoglycemia (ITT): 0.1 unit/kg IV with samples at 0, 30, 60 minutes; normal response is increment increase of 5 ng/ml or peak value > 7.5 ng/ml.
        2. Clonidine stimulation: 150 μg/m^2 of body surface area with samples at 0, 30, 60, 90 minutes; results the same as for ITT.
        3. Arginine: 0.5 gm/kg to a maximal dose of 30 gm IV as 30-minute infusion and samples at 0 time and every 30 minutes for 2 hours; results the same as for ITT.
        4. Growth hormone-releasing hormone test: 1 μg/kg IV with samples at 0, 30, 60 minutes; normal response is increment increase of 10 to 40 ng/ml over baseline.
    B. Thyrotropin and prolactin deficiency: Thyrotropin-releasing hormone test: 500 μg IV with samples at 0, 30, 60 minutes. Thyroid-stimulating hormone should increase by 5 microunits/ml, peak values > 20 microunits/ml are seen in early forms of mild primary hypothyroidism. Prolactin should at least double the baseline value.
    C. Gonadotropin deficiency:
        1. Gonadotropin-releasing hormone test for pituitary insufficiency: 100 μg IV with samples at 0, 30, 60 minutes for luteinizing and follicle-stimulating hormones. Luteinizing hormone should increase at least threefold with follicle-stimulating hormone increases of 1½ to 2 times basal.
        2. Clomiphene citrate for hypothalamic testing: 100 mg daily for 5 days with luteinizing and follicle-stimulating hormones measured morning of sixth day. Luteinizing hormone should double and follicle-stimulating hormone should increase by 50 percent over basal. In males, testosterone increases 1½ to 2 times.
    D. Corticotropin deficiency:
        1. See ITT above.
        2. Cortrosyn: 0.25 mg IV with samples at 0, 30, and 60 minutes for plasma cortisol, which should increase by 5 μg/dl and reach a peak value of >20 μg/dl.
        3. Metyrapone for hypothalamic testing: 500 mg every 4 hours × 6 or overnight test with 30 mg/kg at midnight; must show decrease cortisol to confirm blockade; serum 11-deoxycortisol increase > 7.5 μg/dl.
        4. Corticotropin-releasing hormone testing: 1 μg/kg IV with samples at 0, 15, 30, and 60 minutes; normal response is an increment increase of 10 to 40 pg/ml over baseline.
II. Acromegaly:
    A. 100-gm oral glucose solution suppresses to <2 ng/dl at 60 minutes.
    B. Thyrotropin-releasing hormone testing shows paradoxical increase in growth hormone.
III. Prolactinoma: Thyrotropin-releasing hormone testing shows blunted prolactin response.
IV. Cushing's disease (see Fig. 7-2)

and hyperprolactinemia. Nonfunctioning pituitary chromophobe adenoma may present as a space-occupying lesion. However, very few are truly null-secreting-cell tumors, and frequently they secrete either the glycoprotein hormones or their subunits. Craniopharyngiomas occur in a younger age group and are characterized by cystic and calcified components. Pituitary tumors may be hyperfunctioning and produce syndromes of acromegaly or gigantism with growth hormone excess, amenorrhea-galactorrhea with prolactin excess, Cushing's syndrome with adrenocorticotropin excess, and hyperthyroidism with thyroid-stimulating hormone overproduction.

SPECIAL STUDIES

The tumors may impair anterior and posterior pituitary function, producing deficiency states (see Hypopituitarism for testing procedure and Table 7-9). Formal visual-field testing detects optic nerve compression. Localization procedures include contrast head CT scan, magnetic resonance imaging, and arteriograms.

Acromegaly

Hypersomatotropism [16, 50, 66, 76] may produce the clinical syndrome of gigantism in children or adolescents and acromegaly in adults.

Ectopic production of the growth hormone-releasing factor (GRF) is a rare cause of acromegaly. The hypersecretion of growth hormone (GH) is usually by an eosinophilic or chromophobe pituitary adenoma. If the excessive growth hormone secretion occurs before puberty, then linear growth is accelerated and gigantism results. When the disorder occurs after puberty and epiphyseal closure is complete, then acral enlargement of the bones is the prominent feature.

DIAGNOSIS

History

The symptoms associated with acromegaly occur insidiously and include headaches, changes in hand or shoe size, photophobia, loss of vision, muscular weakness, sweating, arthralgias, amenorrhea, hirsutism, polyuria and polydipsia, rhinorrhea, decreased libido, and galactorrhea. Comparison of old photographs to document changes in the facial features is very helpful. Hypersomatotropism rarely occurs as part of the familial multiple endocrine neoplasia syndrome (MEN I).

Physical Findings

Acral enlargement and coarsening facial features lead to the classic physical features of acromegaly. These include thickened, coarse skin, doughy and sweaty palms, prominent supraorbital ridges (frontal bossing), conspicuous enlargement of the mandible (prognathism), widely spaced teeth, enlargement of the hands and feet, expansion of the ribs, crippling osteoarthritis, prominent lips, tongue, and nose, acanthosis nigricans, fibromas and skin tags, entrapment peripheral neuropathies, hypertension, hepatomegaly, cardiomegaly, goiter, and visual-field abnormalities. If hypogonadism and delayed puberty are present, eunuchoid body proportions are seen (gigantism).

Laboratory Tests

The diagnosis is established by serum growth hormone measurements, which are elevated in the basal state and do not suppress after glucose ingestion. Fasting values normally should not exceed 5 ng/ml. If an elevated value persists 1 hour after administration of 100 gm oral glucose solution, then the growth hormone level is considered nonsuppressible. In addition, measurement of somatomedin C levels that are elevated above the normal range are useful in confirming the diagnosis of acromegaly and in verifying the potency of the elevated growth hormone level. Growth hormone measurements following administration of thyrotropin-releasing hormone may show a paradoxical increase in acromegalics, a finding not seen in normal subjects. The loss of this responsiveness following therapy may indicate control of the disease process. Elevated prolactin levels may be seen in 30 to 40 percent of acromegalic patients.

Special Studies

[See Pituitary Tumors.]

THERAPY AND PROGNOSIS

The best therapeutic results are obtained with transsphenoidal hypophysectomy even for extensive suprasellar tumors. Transfrontal hypophysectomy is rarely required. Depending on the availability of community resources, external radiation [either photon beam (10,000 rads) or conventional radiation (5000 rads)] may be used. This may be reserved for residual or recurring tumors. Bromocriptine may be a useful adjunct to primary therapy. The effectiveness of therapy can be assessed by repeated measurements of growth hormone or somatomedin C. If hormonal elevations are present, recurrent tumor can be suspected and detected by pituitary contrast CT scan. Prognosis depends on early diagnosis and response to neurosurgical or radiation therapy. Bromocriptine therapy can control excessive hormone secretion, but not tumor size. Approximately 80 percent of patients treated with transsphenoidal hypophysectomy show a satisfactory response. With invasive adenomas, only about half are cured by surgery, since infiltration into dura, bone, or brain structures carries a poor prognosis. Complications of transsphenoidal surgery include rhinorrhea, meningitis, postoperative hemorrhage, and hypopituitarism. Treatment with radiation therapy is slow, and reduction of growth hormone levels may take 1 to 4 years. Other complications include optic nerve damage, hypopituitarism, encephalomalacia, and sphenoid sarcomas. Patients with elevated levels of both prolactin and growth hormone may respond better to bromocriptine therapy.

Prolactinomas

Prolactin-producing pituitary adenomas [50, 53, 76] may produce a syndrome of amenorrhea-galactorrhea, hypogonadism, osteopenia, and hirsutism. The predominant hypothalamic influence (dopamine) over pituitary prolactin secretion is inhibitory. Following pituitary stalk transection, the secretion of all anterior pituitary hormones decreases, whereas prolactin secretion increases. Hyperprolactinemia may be due to a variety of other physiologic, pharmacologic, and pathologic causes (Table 7-10). Hyperprolactinemia inhibits the hypothalamic-pituitary-gonadal axis by inhibiting hypothalamic gonadotropin-releasing hormone secretion, which results in low gonad-

Table 7–10. *Causes of Hyperprolactinemia*

 I. Physiologic (sleep, stress, exercise, pregnancy, chest-wall stimulation, coitus)
 II. Hypothalamic destructive lesion
 III. Pituitary stalk section
 IV. Pituitary tumor:
   A. Prolactinoma (microadenoma or macroadenoma)
   B. Acromegaly
 V. Endocrine disorders (hypothyroidism, adrenal insufficiency, i.e., Addison's disease)
 VI. Medical disorders (chronic renal failure, liver disease)
 VII. Drugs (phenothiazide, tricyclic antidepressants, sulpiride, opiate alkaloids, metoclopramide, cimetidine, methyldopa, reserpine, estrogen, thyrotropin-releasing hormone, prostaglandins, amphetamines)
 VIII. Ectopic prolactin production (bronchogenic carcinoma, hypernephroma)

otropin secretion (luteinizing and follicle-stimulating hormones), thereby interfering with gonadal steroidogenesis.

DIAGNOSIS

History

Characteristic features of patients with prolactinomas are caused by the pituitary tumor mass and prolactin excess. Symptoms include headache, visual loss, infertility, oligomenorrhea, amenorrhea, galactorrhea, and hirsutism. The male with prolactinoma may have diminished libido, impotence, oligospermia, or azospermia. Nonpituitary tumor causes (see Table 7-10) of hyperprolactinemia should be rigorously excluded.

Physical Findings

The signs include mild hirsutism, spontaneous or expressible galactorrhea, estrogen deficiency in the female, and in some cases a visual-field defect. Galactorrhea associated with normal menses is usually not associated with significant hyperprolactinemia. Some female patients have an androgen-excess state manifested by acne, hirsutism, and oligomenorrhea.

Laboratory Tests

Prolactin levels in excess of 300 ng/ml most often indicate a pituitary tumor. When the value is 100 ng/ml, a pituitary tumor is seen in 50 percent of patients. The normal range for prolactin is 0 to 20 ng/ml in females and 0 to 10 ng/ml in males. Values in the range of 20 to 100 ng/ml are difficult diagnostic problems and may occur under a variety of conditions (see Table 7-10). The thyrotropin-releasing hormone test has been used to investigate the functional autonomy of the lactotrope in hyperprolactinemic syndromes. In situations where the prolactin level is physiologically elevated, the prolactin concentration increases greater than twofold on stimulation with thyrotropin-releasing hormone. In contrast, most patients with prolactin-secreting tumors or hypothalamic disease will have a blunted response. The pituitary CT scan may localize the hypodense microadenomas or contrast-enhancing macro-adenomas. In patients with hirsutism, the plasma dehydroepiandrosterone sulfate level (DHEA SO_4) may be elevated.

Special Tests
[See Pituitary Tumors.]

TREATMENT AND PROGNOSIS
The treatment of hyperprolactinemia is directly related to the cause of the disorder. If a prolactin-secreting tumor is present, dopamine receptor agonist drugs, transsphenoidal hypophysectomy, or pituitary irradiation are the treatments of choice. Because of the effectiveness of bromocriptine in reducing prolactin levels and tumor size, it has become the initial treatment of choice. It is effective particularly in macroadenomas. The recurrence rate of microadenomas after transsphenoidal surgery is 20 to 50 percent. Macroadenomas may respond to the combination of bromocriptine followed by surgery, although long-term bromocriptine therapy may reduce the tumor size sufficiently to obviate the need for surgery. Most microadenomas are anatomically nonaggressive, and if the hyperprolactinemia is of concern because of galactorrhea or amenorrhea, then therapy may be required, preferably with bromocriptine. Otherwise, such patients can be followed with serial prolactin measurements once or twice yearly and repeat anatomic studies as needed. In most cases, 5 to 15 mg bromocriptine daily will reduce serum prolactin levels to normal. The side effects are less if the drug is started as a 2.5-mg evening dose and taken with food. Side effects include nausea, vomiting, postural hypotension, sleepiness, and depression. Female patients treated with bromocriptine rapidly regain normal ovulatory menstrual cycles and are fully fertile. If the patient becomes pregnant while on bromocriptine therapy, therapy can be discontinued during the pregnancy and the patient can be followed carefully for signs of pituitary tumor growth. If tumor growth recurs, bromocriptine

can be reinstituted or transsphenoidal hypophysectomy performed after delivery.

Prognosis depends on the correctable nature of the cause of the hyperprolactinemia (see Table 7-10). Surgery can be curative, but dopaminergic agonists as a first-choice agent can control hyperprolactinemia and cause tumor growth to regress.

Cushing's Disease
Excessive pituitary secretion of adrenocorticotropic hormone produces Cushing's disease [76]. These small corticotropin-producing pituitary adenomas are difficult to detect because abnormal pituitary sellas by conventional roentgenogram are seen in only 10 percent of cases and an abnormal pituitary CT scan is seen in only 60 percent of cases. Hence these tumors are difficult to localize prior to transsphenoidal pituitary surgery. Selective venous inferior petrosal sinus adrenocorticotropic hormone sampling has the potential to localize the tumor prior to surgery. These tumors characteristically produce mild adrenocorticotropic hormone hypersecretion (100 to 200 pg/ml), which stimulates the adrenal gland to secrete excessive quantities of cortisol. Large pituitary adrenocorticotropic hormone-secreting tumors may occur after adrenalectomy (Nelson's syndrome). These tumors secrete large amounts of adrenocorticotropic hormone and plasma levels may range from 700 to 1000 pg/ml or greater. These tumors are usually quite large and anatomically aggressive, frequently producing visual-field defects, suprasellar extension, and hypothalamic or brain invasion. Adrenocorticotropic hormone levels in Nelson's syndrome may be autonomous and not stimulated by corticotropin-releasing factor or suppressed with exogenous glucocorticoids. The adrenocorticotropic hormone levels in Cushing's disease can be both stimulated by exogenous corticotropin-releasing factor administration and suppressed by very high, but not low, doses of dexamethasone, thus establishing the diagnosis of hypothalamic pituitary-dependent Cushing's disease (Fig. 7-2).

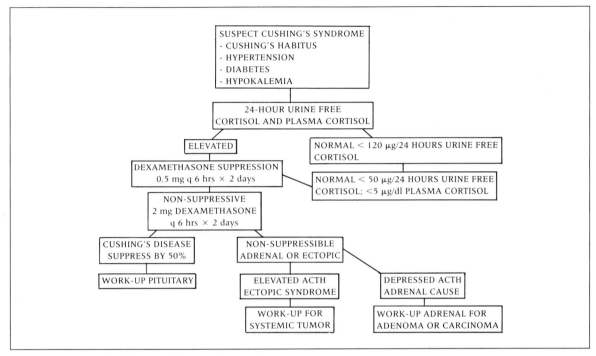

Figure 7–2. Algorithm for the evaluation of suspected Cushing's syndrome.

CLINICAL AND LABORATORY FEATURES
Since these features are largely the result of hypersecretion of cortisol, they will be discussed under the adrenal hypersecretory states of Cushing's syndrome (see Adrenal Disorders).

Central Diabetes Insipidus

The etiologies of diabetes insipidus [14, 52] include hypothalamic or pituitary tumors; infiltrative, granulomous or infectious disease; vascular accidents; skull fractures; and pituitary surgery. Some patients have an idiopathic form that may be familial. As a rule, the disease is due to neuronal damage to the neurohypophyseal centers of antidiuretic hormone (ADH) release, namely, the supraoptic and paraventricular nucleus. With antidiuretic hormone deficiency, polyuria occurs and only an intact thirst mechanism with increased water intake maintains normal plasma osmolality.

DIAGNOSIS
History
The symptoms consist of increased thirst, polydipsia (frequently with ice water ingestion), polyuria, and nocturia. Onset is usually abrupt. If stupor or coma develops, these patients are prone to severe dehydration, shock, and acute renal tubular necrosis. Severity of the polyuria depends on the location and completeness of the defects in antidiuretic hormone secretion. The volume of urine excreted may vary from a few to 20 liters per day.

Physical Findings
Physical signs are usually absent unless they are related to the underlying etiology. If fluid intake is decreased, severe dehydration results and central nervous system changes of agitation, stupor, and coma are seen.

Laboratory Tests

In complete diabetes insipidus a hyposthenuric urine with a specific gravity of 1.005 or less (urine osmolality 50 to 200 mOsmol/kg) is seen, whereas in partial diabetes insipidus concentrations of 400 to 450 mOsmol/kg can be reached with dehydration. With dehydration alone, serum osmolality is increased and serum sodium concentrations are elevated. The differential diagnosis of the polyuric state must include psychogenic water drinking, nephrogenic diabetes insipidus, and complete and partial diabetes insipidus. This is best evaluated by a carefully performed water dehydration test [52] followed by the administration of vasopressin. Responses of patients with complete diabetes insipidus show increased plasma osmolality with dehydration, while urine osmolality does not rise above that of plasma. Following vasopressin administration, urine osmolality increases by greater than 50 percent. Patients with partial diabetes insipidus show partial concentration of urine in response to dehydration and administration of vasopressin leads to further concentration (>10 percent increment), whereas patients with nephrogenic diabetes insipidus or psychogenic water drinking show very little response following maximal dehydration to the administration of vasopressin. Special studies to rule out an anatomic central nervous lesion include a head CT scan.

TREATMENT AND PROGNOSIS

Identifying the primary disorder and replacement therapy with vasopressin analogues afford long-term relief of the polyuric syndrome. Partial diabetes insipidus may respond to chlorpropamide, whereas complete diabetes insipidus requires intranasal use of deamino-8-D-arginine vasopressin (dDAVP) or parenteral aqueous vasopressin. For acute diabetes insipidus, aqueous vasopressin (2 to 6 units) usually is given IV or IM every 2 to 4 hours initially or dDAVP (1 to 2 μg IV or SC every 12 hours). For chronic diabetes insipidus, synthetic lysine vasopressin can be given frequently as a nasal spray or dDAVP can be given (0.1 to 0.2 cc qd to bid). The dose of vasopressin must be adjusted to keep the patient in water balance and prevent troublesome symptoms such as nocturia and sleep interruption; long-term management depends on the reversibility of the precipitating disorder.

Hypothyroidism

Hypothyroidism [5, 42, 57] is due mainly to failure of the thyroid gland (primary) and less commonly to failure of pituitary thyroid-stimulating hormone production (secondary) or hypothalamic thyrotropin-releasing hormone secretion (tertiary). Primary hypothyroidism occurs most frequently as a consequence of Hashimoto's thyroiditis, ^{131}I therapy, or thyroidectomy, but it may be seen as a familial or idiopathic disorder. Other causes include iodine deficiency, antithyroid drugs, congenital aplasia or dysplasia, neck irradiation for lymphoma, and infiltrative disease such as Riedel's chronic thyroiditis. In rare cases, the peripheral tissues are unable to respond to thyroid hormone (Refetoff syndrome).

DIAGNOSIS

History

The symptoms of hypothyroidism are due to the hypometabolic state induced by deficient thyroid hormone or thyroid hormone action. When the hypothyroidism is profound, it is termed *myxedema*. The symptoms of hypothyroidism include dry skin, coarse dry hair, weight gain, cold intolerance, constipation, lethargy, apathy, menorrhagia or oligomenorrhea, decreased libido, depression, deafness, hoarse voice, muscle cramps, paresthesias, sleep apnea, and memory impairment. A positive family history of autoimmune diseases is usually obtained in patients with Hashimoto's thyroiditis.

Physical Findings

Signs include round, puffy face, especially with periorbital edema; slow, hoarse speech with large tongue; hypokinesis; cold, dry carotenemic skin; dry, coarse hair with loss of lateral eyebrows; and delayed relaxation of the biceps or ankle reflexes.

The extremities are cool, and the patient may have hypothermia. The pulse is slow, and hypertension is commonly seen. Goiter is frequently palpable, and it may be diffused or nodular. A goiter is not seen in secondary and tertiary hypothyroidism or in primary hypothyroidism due to atrophic thyroiditis. Heart sounds may be distant; there may be cardiomegaly with and without pericardial or pleural effusions; a distended abdomen with ileus may be seen.

Laboratory Tests

The diagnosis is confirmed by a depressed serum thyroxine level (T_4) and T_3 resin uptake. Normal values for serum T_4 are 5.5 to 11.5 µg/dl, and for T_3 resin uptake they are 25 to 35 percent; however, these values for T_3 resin uptake may vary among laboratories. This gives a low thyroid index (multiplication product of serum $T_4 \times T_3$ resin uptake). The T_3 resin uptake test is an assessment of unbound thyroxine binding sites on thyroid-binding globulin (TBG). Multiplication of the measured serum T_4 by the T_3 resin uptake establishes a free thyroxine index and hence allows an interpretation of thyroid function tests when there are alterations in the serum binding proteins. A high T_3 resin uptake indicates that the levels of thyroid-binding globulin are low and that the low T_4 level is due to low binding proteins, not reduced thyroid function. A low T_3 resin uptake is seen in hypothyroidism or when there are increased levels of thyroid-binding globulin, as commonly seen in pregnancy or in patients on birth control pills. If both T_4 and T_3 resin uptakes are decreased, hypothyroidism is likely; if both T_4 and T_3 resin uptakes are increased, hyperthyroidism is likely. When T_4 and T_3 resin uptakes move in opposite directions, an excess or deficiency of thyroid-binding globulin is likely and the patient is usually euthyroid. An elevated serum thyroid-stimulating hormone level is the most important test to establish the diagnosis of primary hypothyroidism. Any reproducible elevation of thyroid-stimulating hormone in such patients indicates primary thyroid gland failure, even when serum thyroid hormone levels are normal (normal thyroid-stimulating hormone range 0.2 to 5.5 microunits/ml). Thus the serum thyroid-stimulating hormone measurement is the most valid and sensitive marker available for thyroid gland integrity.

Special Tests

In primary hypothyroidism, an exaggerated thyroid-stimulating hormone response to thyrotropin-releasing hormone testing occurs, and a diminished or flat response occurs in secondary hypothyroidism. A normal response of thyroid-stimulating hormone is noted in Table 7-8. The measurements of antimicrosomal and antithyroglobulin antibodies may establish the etiology as Hashimoto's thyroiditis when positive. Radioiodide uptake and scans are not required to evaluate the hypothyroid patient.

TREATMENT AND PROGNOSIS

Acute Management (Myxedema Coma)

Myxedema coma is a life-threatening complication of severe hypothyroidism. It is characterized by hypothermia, hypoventilation, hypotension, bradycardia, hyponatremia, and coma. It usually occurs after stress or trauma, a surgical procedure, or infection in a myxedematous patient. When myxedema coma is suspected clinically, it is critical that therapy be directed immediately at supporting vital functions and correcting the predisposing factors. Hypoventilation, CO_2 narcosis, and respiratory arrest are a constant threat and are best managed by assisted ventilation. Hypotension and hypovolemia are treated by replacing intravascular volume. A relative adrenal insufficiency is present, and hydrocortisone (200 to 300 mg daily) should be given intravenously until the patient improves. Drugs such as anesthetics, sedatives, and narcotics should be avoided or used in reduced dosage because their metabolic clearance rate is diminished. The thyroid hormone deficiency should be corrected by giving intravenous sodium levothyroxine, initially 300 to 500 µg as a bolus to immediately replace thyroxine total-body stores. This is followed by 50 to 100 µg daily to replace the normal daily production rate. Intravenous L-triiodothyronine will more rapidly reverse the hypothyroid state, but this is not commercially available in parenteral form. Vital signs should improve in 8 to 10 hours, and consciousness should return in 36 to 72 hours. Because of the profound nature of the hypothyroidism and the seriousness associated with the precipitating event, the mortality rate is high (40 to 60 percent). Possible complications of therapy include coronary ischemia, myocardial infarction, and electrolyte disorders (hypokalemia, hypophosphatemia). These patients, with their complicated predisposing factors, should be aggressively managed in intensive care units.

Long-Term Management
The object of long-term replacement therapy is to restore a normal metabolic state with L-thyroxine, usually 0.1 to 0.2 mg per day. Efficacy can be assessed clinically and by following serum thyroid-stimulating hormone levels. With adequate replacement therapy, the prognosis is excellent for a normal lifestyle.

Hyperthyroidism
Hyperthyroidism [15, 18, 46] is a clinical syndrome resulting from excessive tissue exposure to thyroxine (T_4) or triiodothyronine (T_3) or both. Thyrotoxicosis affects women much more frequently than men; it occurs at any age but is more common in young adults. The most common cause of hyperthyroidism is Graves' disease (diffused toxic goiter), toxic multinodular goiter, toxic adenoma (hot nodule), or subacute thyroiditis. Other causes include the factitious or iatrogenic use of exogenous thyroid hormone, silent thyroiditis (spontaneous resolving hyperthyroidism with lymphocytic thyroiditis), postpartum thyroiditis, struma ovarii, Jod Basedow hyperthyroidism (iodide-induced hyperthyroidism), thyroid-stimulating hormone-producing pituitary adenomas, functioning follicular metastatic thyroid carcinoma, or trophoblastic disease where human chorionic gonadotropin (HCG) is the thyroid stimulator.

DIAGNOSIS
History
Symptoms of hyperthyroidism include nervousness, irritability, emotional lability, tremor, anorexia or increased appetite, weight loss, heat intolerance, dyspnea, muscle weakness, palpitations, fatigue, insomnia, hyperdefecation, infertility, and oligomenorrhea. Eye complaints are noted if the patient has Graves' disease (photophobia, lacrimation, burning, sandy sensation, retrobulbar pain, and prominent eyes). The exophthalmus may precede or follow the thyrotoxicosis. Frequently, there is a family history of autoimmune thyroid disease. Many patients may relate the onset of Graves' disease to severe emotional stress.

Physical Findings
Signs of excessive thyroid hormone include a hypermetabolic state with rapid pulse, increased pulse pressure, increased respiratory rate, and increased body temperature. Warm, moist skin, palmar erythema ("liver palms"), fine-textured hair, Plummer's nails (onycholysis of nail bed), and pretibial myxedema may be seen in Graves' disease. Patients with Graves' disease may present with proptosis which is usually bilateral. There may be several eye signs of thyrotoxicosis (Graves' ophthalmopathy); these include infrequent blinking, tremor of the closed eyelids, lag of the upper lid on looking down, widened palpebral fissures with forward protrusion of the globe (exophthalmos), extraocular muscle palsy, corneal erosion and ulceration, or sight impairment (optic neuropathy). The neck should be visually examined and carefully palpated to determine whether the thyroid is enlarged diffusely or by single or multiple nodules. A thyroid bruit and palpable thrill may be present in Graves' disease. The thyroid examination is facilitated by having the patient swallow while observing the neck and during palpation of the thyroid gland. Cardiac examination will show a hyperdynamic precordium; atrial arrhythmias may be present.

Bowel sounds are active. Hepatomegaly rarely occurs, but splenomegaly and lymphadenopathy are common in Graves' disease. Muscle weakness, fine tremor, and increased deep tendon reflexes are noted. Ten percent of males may manifest gynecomastia.

Laboratory Tests
Hyperthyroidism is suspected on clinical presentation and the diagnosis is established on the basis of laboratory testing. Elevation in serum thyroxine (T_4) and/or serum triiodothyronine (T_3) levels must be demonstrated. Since abnormalities in thyroid-binding proteins (albumin, prealbumin) are common, both the serum T_4 and T_3 resin uptake must be interpreted together. The serum thyroid-stimulating hormone concentration is suppressed below limits of detection in all causes of hyperthyroidism except thyroid-stimulating hormone-producing pituitary adenomas, in which it is inappropriately elevated.

Special Tests
A flat thyroid-stimulating hormone response to thyrotropin-releasing hormone stimulation (500 μg given IV) with blood samples at 0, 30, and 60 minutes) characterizes hyperthyroidism and confirms a suppressed thyroid-stimulating hormone level. A thyroid radioiodide uptake test will help determine the type of hyperthyroidism. When the 24-hour thyroid radioiodide uptake is low or suppressed, the cause of hyperthyroidism is thyroiditis, iodide ingestion, the factitious use of thyroid hormone, or ectopic thyroid hormone production. In most states of hyperthyroidism, the uptake is elevated, indicating production of thyroid hormone by the thyroid gland. In these cases, a thyroid scan will determine the type of hypersecretory state (Graves' disease, toxic multinodular goiter, toxic adenoma, or Hashitoxicosis). Antimicrosomal or antithyroglobin antibodies will be elevated in Hashitoxicosis.

TREATMENT AND PROGNOSIS
Acute Treatment (Thyroid Storm)
Thyrotoxic crisis or storm [46] is a syndrome characterized by fever, dehydration, tachycardia or arrhythmias, agitation, and confusion. The disorder is characterized by high circulating levels of thyroid hormones similar to those found in hyperthyroidism. Usually the "thyroid storm" is triggered by another precipitating event, such as infection or another intercurrent illness. The diagnosis is usually suspected clinically.

Urgent treatment has four objectives: (1) to support vital functions, (2) to reverse the peripheral effects of excess thyroid hormone, (3) to reduce the production and release of thyroid hormone, and (4) to correct any precipitating factor. General supportive measures include vigorous support of intravascular volume, immediate treatment of cardiac dysfunction, and replacement of fluids, electrolytes, and glucose. A cooling blanket may be used to lower the temperature, but salicylates should be avoided because they may increase free thyroid hormones in serum. Since thyroid storm may result in relative adrenal insufficiency, hydrocortisone (100 to 300 mg IV daily) should be given. Steroids also decrease the peripheral conversion of T_4 to T_3. Peripheral adrenergic effects of thyrotoxicosis are controlled best with beta-adrenergic receptor antagonists such as propranolol. On occasion, intravenous propranolol is required; it should be used only in an intensive care unit with cardiac monitoring. Oral propranolol (40 to 80 mg every 4 to 8 hours) reduces the peripheral thyroid hormone effects and also inhibits conversion of T_4 to T_3. Methimazole (20 to 30 mg) or propylthiouracil (200 to 300 mg) should be given orally or by nasogastric tube every 4 to 8 hours to stop synthesis of thyroid hormone. Propylthiouracil, but not methimazole, also blocks conversion of T_4 to T_3. To prevent further release of thyroid hormones and block peripheral T_4 to T_3 conversion, iodine is given initially intravenously as sodium iodide (1 gm every 8 hours) and then orally as a saturated solution of potassium iodide (5 to 10 drops tid).

Long-Term Management

The treatment depends on the etiology. Graves' disease, multinodular goiter, and toxic nodular goiter can be treated with radioiodide, antithyroid drugs (propylthiouracil, 100 mg tid, or methimazole, 10 mg tid), or surgery. Subacute thyroiditis is a self-limited viral disease that spontaneously recovers. Postoperative or postradioiodide hypothyroidism occurs in 25 to 50 percent of patients. Elderly patients may have an apathetic or atypical presentation; they frequently require premedication with antithyroid drugs prior to radioiodide therapy. The ophthalmopathy of Graves' disease may be independent of the hyperfunctioning thyroid state but can be aggravated by hypothyroidism. It is treated with diuretics, elevation of the head of the bed, wearing sunglasses, artificial tears, Lacriserts, and, when severe, systemic steroids, orbital irradiation, or surgery.

Thyroid Neoplasms

Neoplasms of the thyroid gland [13, 17, 33, 47, 48, 74, 75] may be benign or malignant. Benign nodular disease of the thyroid is very common and increases with age. Autopsy studies suggest that 50 percent of the population has thyroid nodules, most of which are small and clinically insignificant. Malignant thyroid disease is actually an uncommon cancer accounting for only 20 to 25 cases per million population.

Cancers of the thyroid gland have been characterized as well-differentiated and undifferentiated tumors. The well-differentiated tumors include papillary, papillary-follicular, and follicular carcinomas. The undifferentiated tumors include medullary and anaplastic carcinomas. The occurrence of these tumors is such that papillary and mixed papillary variants account for approximately 65 percent; pure follicular carcinomas, approximately 20 percent, medullary carcinomas, 10 percent, and anaplastic carcinomas, 5 percent. The detection of thyroid carcinomas generally comes from evaluation of thyroid nodules. Anaplastic thyroid carcinoma may arise from preexisting well-differentiated thyroid carcinoma.

DIAGNOSIS

History

Thyroid carcinoma occurs more commonly in females than in males; it occurs particularly in males under age 40 and females under age 30. When papillary thyroid carcinoma occurs in patients over age 40, it has a more malignant course. Other determinants include a family history of thyroid cancer, particularly medullary carcinoma of the thyroid or multiple endocrine adenomatosis (MEA) type IIA or IIB. Malignant thyroid lesions are suggested by history of head and neck irradiation during childhood, recent growth or enlargement of the thyroid mass, change in voice, dysphagia, and weight loss. Any family history of pheochromocytoma or renal stones associated with hyperparathyroidism would indicate a workup for multiple endocrine adenomatosis syndrome. Familial medullary carcinoma of the thyroid gland may occur independent of the multiple endocrine adenomatosis syndromes.

Physical Examination

Examination of the neck may reveal a solitary nodule or a dominant nodule in a multinodular thyroid gland. Anterior and posterior cervical lymph nodes should be examined carefully. Most patients with thyroid cancer are euthyroid, having a normal physical examination (except for the thyroid nodule) and normal thyroid function tests. A careful systemic evaluation should be conducted for extrathyroid metastasis. A marfanoid habitus and mucosal neuromas would suggest multiple endocrine adenomatosis type IIB syndrome.

Laboratory Tests

Routine thyroid function tests (T_4, T_3 resin uptake, and thyroid-stimulating hormone are obtained to exclude coexisting abnormalities in thyroid function. Special x-rays of the neck may detect concentric calcification when associated with a hemorrhagic cyst, punctate calcification secondary to psammoma bodies (as seen in papillary carcinoma), or conglomerate calcification (as seen in medullary carcinoma). The thyroid scan will determine if the lesion is hypofunctioning (or "cold"), isofunctioning (or "warm"), or hyperfunctioning (or "hot"). Thyroid carcinoma is associated with solitary, cold, solid lesions. In lesions that are hyperfunctioning, the risk of thyroid cancer is negligible. Thyroid ultrasound will determine if the lesion is solid, mixed, or cystic. The thyroid fine-needle aspiration (FNA) biopsy should be performed in all thyroid nodules that are cold or hypofunctioning on thyroid scan. Cytologic examination of the fine-needle aspirate can be done using the stained-smear technique or fixed-cell block. The aspiration is performed using a 20-cc syringe with a 22-gauge needle. The chest film (posteroanterior and lateral) evaluates for possible metastatic disease and should always be performed prior to surgery. Human thyroglobulin measurements are of no value in preoperative assessment.

TREATMENT AND PROGNOSIS

The prognosis depends on the type of cancer found. Multinodular goiters are less commonly associated with thyroid cancer than are solitary, isolated, cold nodules. In the multinodular goiter, the dominant nodule can be initially biopsied; if it is benign, then L-thyroxine suppression therapy should be instituted. If the nodule enlarges while on suppression therapy, surgery or repeat biopsy of the lesion is warranted. All solitary, cold nodules should have aspiration biopsies; approximately 5 to 15 percent will be malignant and require surgical removal. If the nodule is benign, L-thyroxine suppression therapy should be instituted and monitored closely so that thyroid function tests are only minimally elevated and the serum thyroid-stimulating hormone level is undetectable. The long-term disadvantages of L-thyroxine suppression therapy are minimal, but accelerated osteoporosis has been reported. When thyroid cancer is detected in the thyroid nodule, total thyroidectomy is indicated for anaplastic and medullary carcinomas. Near-total thyroidectomy is the treatment of choice for follicular carcinoma. When papillary carcinoma is diagnosed, there is medical and surgical controversy as to the ideal type of treatment. Most often a subtotal thyroidectomy on the side of the lesion is performed and the patient is followed with long-term suppression therapy for recurrent disease. Another philosophy in papillary carcinoma is treatment with near-total thyroidectomy followed by radioiodide ablation of the residual thyroid bed and search for metastatic tissue. Recurrence rates have been shown to be less with this combined therapy. Postoperative hypoparathyroidism is diagnosed if persistent hypocalcemia is present. In both follicular and papillary carcinomas when metastatic disease is present, repeated large doses of 75 to 150 mCi ^{131}I will be required. In those patients who have been rendered disease-free by therapy, repeated thyroglobulin levels and diagnostic ^{131}I scanning procedures allow for detection of recurrent disease. Patients with known metastatic disease require a baseline technetium polyphosphate bone scan and yearly chest films. The prognosis is good for well-differentiated carcinoma of the thyroid gland with early surgery and long-term suppression with L-thyroxine. The dose of L-thyroxine for suppression is determined by a suppressed thyroid-stimulating hormone determination. Patients with anaplastic carcinoma have a poor outcome, with the mean survival being approximately 8 months. Similarly, the mean survival of medullary carcinoma of the thyroid gland is about 12 months. Metastatic disease in these two latter conditions is not remedial to radioiodide ablation therapy; hence anticancer chemotherapy agents or local radiation therapy is required.

Hypoparathyroidism

Hypoparathyroidism [3, 54, 62] occurs secondary to deficiency in parathyroid hormone production or its action (pseudohypoparathyroidism). Deficiencies in parathyroid hormone production are found in the following states: (1) after thyroid neck surgery when the parathyroid glands are inadvertently removed or suffer ischemic damage, (2) idiopathic, where an autoimmune process destroys parathyroid gland function (this may be part of a familial polyglandular failure syndrome when other endocrine glands such as the adrenal, thyroid, pancreas, and ovary undergo autoimmune endocrine failure), (3) rarely after radioiodide therapy, (4) as part of a rare DiGeorge's syndrome, which includes agenesis of the thymus and parathyroid glands, and (5) end-organ resistance to parathyroid hormone action, such as occurs in pseudohypoparathyroidism. This is a rare hereditary disorder associated with developmental defects such as shortened metacarpals and metatarsals, short stature, and dystrophic calcification. In pseudohypoparathyroidism, defects in hormone receptor activation of adenylate cyclase exist. These defects are characterized as type I or type II. In patients with the type I disorder, parathyroid hormone infusion is characterized by both deficient renal phosphaturia and urinary cAMP response, whereas in type II patients a normal urinary cAMP response is seen, but there is no renal phosphaturia. Patients with the type I disorder are classified as type Ia if there is deficient regulatory component of adenylate cyclase, as measured by a reduced erythrocyte N protein (G protein), whereas it is normal in type IIb. Some patients manifest the skeletal developmental defects of pseudohypoparathyroidism without the biochemical features and fulfill the criteria of pseudopseudohypoparathyroidism. Many of these patients may be seen in families with type Ia patients.

DIAGNOSIS

History

The etiology of hypoparathyroidism is suggested by history of previous neck surgery, familial occurrence of the disorder, or family history of multiple autoimmune endocrine disorders (hypothyroidism, adrenal insufficiency, hypogonadism, and diabetes). Most of the clinical symptoms are secondary to hypocalcemia with neuromuscular irritability, including peripheral and circumoral paresthesias, carpopedal spasm, muscle cramps, tetany, seizures, and bronchospasm or laryngeal stridor that can be provoked by anxiety attacks,

Table 7–11. Hypocalcemic Disorders

  I. Hypoparathyroidism: After thyroid or parathyroid surgery, idiopathic, after neck irradiation, pseudohypoparathyroidism, parathyroid agenesis (DiGeorge's syndrome)
 II. Altered vitamin D states (see Table 7-7)
III. Hyperphosphatemia: Rhabdomyolysis, tumor lysis with chemotherapy, renal failure, phosphate infusions or enemas
 IV. Hypomagnesemia
  V. Osteoblastic: "Hungry bones" after surgery for hyperparathyroidism or Graves' disease, osteoblastic prostate and breast metastasis
 VI. Medical illness: Hypoalbuminemia, pancreatitis, malabsorption, after blood transfusion
VII. Neonatal hypocalcemia

hyperventilation, exercise, or menstrual cycle. Mental changes include irritability, paranoia, depression, and frank psychosis. Occasionally, elevated cerebrospinal fluid pressure and papilledema may occur and mimic a cerebral tumor. Since hypocalcemia is the cardinal feature of this disorder, the differential diagnosis of other causes of hypocalcemia must be considered (Table 7-11).

Physical Findings

Physical findings are usually related to the hypocalcemia or the associated conditions causing the hypocalcemia. Patients with pseudohypoparathyroidism are characterized by shortened stature with shortening of the fourth metacarpal or metatarsal. Subcutaneous calcifications may be noted. In idiopathic hypoparathyroidism, one may see alopecia, moniliasis of nail beds, vitiligo, cataracts, or defective dental development, or other autoimmune deficiency syndromes may be present. Signs of hypocalcemia include Chvostek's and Trousseau's signs, but some normal subjects also may show a Chvostek's sign. The classic electrocardiographic finding is a prolongation of the QT interval. Electrocardiographic changes also may include the T-wave peaking or inversion. The hypocalcemia may be associated with congestive heart failure resistant to digitalis.

Laboratory and Special Tests

Hypocalcemia and hyperphosphatemia with normal renal function suggest hypoparathyroidism. The serum parathyroid hormone level is low in most forms of hypoparathyroidism, but it is normal or elevated in pseudohypoparathyroidism. In this latter case, a parathyroid hormone infusion shows changes in urinary phosphate and cAMP response, which, as discussed above, characterizes the various types of pseudohypoparathyroidism. Diminished erythrocyte G-unit activity occurs in patients with type Ia disorder.

TREATMENT AND PROGNOSIS

Acute Management

Acute medical management for hypocalcemia requires the intravenous administration of calcium salts, usually available as 10 percent solutions given as 5 to 10 mg/kg elemental calcium over 6 to 8 hours. Prognosis depends on the underlying condition.

Chronic Management

Long-term correction of the hypocalcemia requires the use of vitamin D and calcium supplements. These patients are moderately vitamin D-resistant and require 50,000 to 150,000 units of vitamin D per day with 1 to 2 gm elemental calcium to correct the hypocalcemia. Individual variations exist with regard to the correct therapeutic dosage. A short-acting but expensive vitamin D preparation, 1,25-dihydroxyvitamin D_3 (calcitriol), provides more rapid correction of the hypocalcemia at a dose of 0.5 to 1.25 μg per day. Serum calcium levels during therapy should vary from 8 to 9 mg/dl to avoid hypercalciuria and the complications of nephrolithiasis. Vitamin D correction of the hypocalcemia will improve the renal phosphate excretion and lower serum phosphate levels, but some patients may require phosphate-binding antacids to correct the hyperphosphatemia. Complexity of therapy depends on the underlying etiology. Once these patients are regulated, they tend to remain relatively stable, giving a good long-term prognosis. However, patients must be carefully observed during periods of intercurrent illness associated with dehydration or if glucocorticoids (which antagonize vitamin D action) are administered.

Hyperparathyroidism

Parathyroid hormone overproduction [43, 54] is seen in primary hyperparathyroidism or secondary hyperparathyroidism. In most cases, primary hyperparathyroidism is usually due to a single adenoma of the parathyroid gland, whereas hyperplasia of all four glands is seen in 10 percent of cases. Chronic renal failure with hyperphosphatemia and secondary hypocalcemia is commonly associated with parathyroid hyperplasia (secondary hyperparathyroidism), which may lead to autonomous function of the enlarged parathyroid gland (tertiary hyperparathyroidism). Hyperparathyroidism also occurs as part of familial multiple endocrine adenomatosis syndromes.

DIAGNOSIS

History

The symptoms of hyperparathyroidism are due to the hypercalcemia. The differential diagnosis of hypercalcemic disorders is listed in Table 7-12.

Table 7–12. *Causes of Hypercalcemia*

I. Hyperparathyroidism
II. Non-parathyroid hormone dependent:
  A. Malignancy:
    1. With osseous metastasis
    2. Humoral hypercalcemia of malignancy
  B. Benign (familial hypercalcemic hypocalciuria
  C. Endocrine disorders: Hyperthyroidism, adrenal insufficiency
  D. Immobilization: Especially with coexisting Paget's disease, rheumatoid arthritis, adolescent growth
  E. Granulomatous disease: Sarcoidosis, tuberculosis, berylliosis, histoplasmosis, fungal diseases
  F. Drugs: Thiazides, milk alkali syndrome, vitamin A and D intoxication
  G. Miscellaneous: Artifactual (hyperproteinemia), dialysis, after renal transplant surgery, diuretic phase of acute renal failure associated with rhabdomyolysis

Generally the symptoms of hypercalcemia are nonspecific and include weakness, fatigue, lethargy, renal colic, weight loss, headache, mental disturbances, depression, constipation, epigastric pain, nausea, vomiting, polyuria, polydipsia, anorexia, pruritus, arthralgias, bone pain, hypercoagulation state, and occasionally coma. Unexplained causes of urinary calculi, renal colic, peptic ulcer disease, pancreatitis, or altered mental status should alert the physician to the diagnosis. Fractures and bone cysts (brown tumors) may be present in advanced disease.

Physical Findings

Few physical findings are seen in hyperparathyroidism, and when present, such findings are related to the cause of the hypercalcemia (see Table 7-12). Signs of hypercalcemia include hypertension and soft-tissue calcification, especially band keratopathy. A slit-lamp ophthalmologic examination may show band (calcified) keratopathy. Parathyroid adenomas are rarely palpable, and when they are palpable on physical examination, one should suspect the very rare parathyroid carcinoma. When a familial syndrome is present, the associated endocrine tumors may provide leads to the diagnosis of hyperparathyroidism.

Laboratory Tests

The characteristic laboratory findings in primary hyperparathyroidism are hypercalcemia, hypophosphatemia, and a mild hyperchloremic metabolic acidosis. The two most common disorders causing hypercalcemia are primary hyperparathyroidism and hypercalcemia of malignant disease. Parathyroid hormone-mediated hypercalcemia is suggested by low fasting phosphate levels (<2.8 ml/dl), high chloride levels (>104 mEq/liter), and an elevated chloride-phosphate ratio (>33). An elevated serum parathyroid hormone level establishes the diagnosis. However, if renal failure is also present, then clearance of the parathyroid hormone is delayed and spuriously high values may be seen. Serum and urinary calcium with creatinine measurements are helpful in excluding familial benign hypercalcemic hypocalciuria by showing a calcium clearance/creatinine clearance of greater than 0.01. Elevations in serum alkaline phosphatase may indicate active bone changes, which may be associated with periosteal bone resorption on x-rays, particularly of the hands, skull, and clavicles. Bone biopsy shows osteitis fibrosa cystica with osteopenia, increased osteoclast count, and a high bone turnover state. Localization studies prior to surgery have been notoriously poor. Ultrasound of the neck or thallium-technetium scanning may detect large adenomas. Venous parathyroid hormone catheterization studies are indicated only after a negative neck exploration. In hypercalcemia of malignancy, clinical evidence of a cancer is usually obvious, the serum calcium level may be quite high, the serum phosphate level is usually normal or high, the chloride-phosphate ratio is below 30, and the parathyroid hormone level is suppressed.

TREATMENT AND PROGNOSIS

Acute Management

Hypercalcemia with levels >14 mg/dl is a medical emergency. First-line treatment should always be vigorous saline hydration, since these patients are always volume-depleted. Once volume is repleted, intravenous furosemide can initiate a further calciuria. Treatments of acute and chronic hypercalcemia are presented in Table 7-13. In many cases, the hypercalcemia is mild and does not require urgent therapy. In untreated patients, when intercurrent illnesses lead to dehydration, severe hypercalcemia may occur. The treatment of choice for hyperparathyroidism is surgery, even in early asymptomatic patients. Long-term medical management may be more expensive than surgery. It is imperative that an experienced neck surgeon perform the operation. Most patients will require removal of a single adenoma. Hyperplasia of all four glands is treated by removal of 3½ half glands. Prognosis for cure is good in primary hyperparathyroidism with surgery, particularly when only one gland is removed. Removal of multiple glands raises the risk of hypoparathy-

Table 7–13. *Therapy of Hypercalcemia*

I. Urgent therapy:
  A. Saline:
    1. Generally safe with 200 to 300 cc per hour, but may need 10 to 20 liters per day with careful monitoring. Use NS:D$_5$W alternately in a 4:1 ratio with 20 mEq KCl per bottle (can follow urinary K$^+$, Na$^+$, and volume to document Na$^+$, and volume to document losses)
    2. May need 15 mg magnesium per hour
  B. Saline plus furosemide:
    1. With aggressive management, 80 to 100 mg furosemide IV q1–2 h and replace urinary electrolytes
    2. Less urgent management, 40 mg furosemide q4–6 h
    3. Before using furosemide, be sure patient is adequately hydrated
  C. Calcitonin: 4 to 8 MRC units/kg SC q6–12 h
  D. Calcitonin plus glucocorticoids:
    1. 4 to 8 MRC units/kg q6–12 h
    2. Prednisone, 40 to 60 mg per day
  E. Intravenous phosphate: Given as 1000 mg elemental phosphate (0.16 mM/kg) over 8 to 12 hours during each 24-hour period (*caution:* Can cause hypotension)
  F. Intravenous EDTA: Avoid use, since forms insoluble calcium compounds that will damage kidney
  G. Dialysis
II. Chronic therapy (adjunct therapy in addition to treating primary cause):
  A. Mobilization
  B. Oral phosphates:
    1. 1000 to 2000 mg elemental phosphate (i.e., K-Phos, 3 tablets tid)
    2. Avoid use if elevated serum phosphate level
  C. Mithramycin: 25 μg/kg in 50 cc D$_5$W given as infusion over 3 hours
  D. Glucocorticoids: Prednisone, 4 to 60 mg per day
  E. Diphosphates: Didronel, 5 to 20 mg/kg per day PO or 7.5 mg/kg with 3 liters saline given over 24 hours daily for 3 days
  F. Indomethacin: 25 to 50 mg tid

roidism requiring permanent long-term vitamin D and calcium therapy. Postoperatively, patients may experience transient hypocalcemia due to suppressed parathyroid hormone function in normal glands or rapid uptake of calcium by depleted bones. This can usually be managed with a low-dose calcium infusion of 150 to 250 mg elemental calcium over 6 to 8 hours or with oral calcium supplementation. 1,25-Dihydroxyvitamin D$_3$ may be the more ideal form of vitamin D therapy for early postoperative hypocalcemia, since it allows a more rapid correction of the serum calcium level and can be discontinued at a later time to determine if permanent hypoparathyroidism is present.

Chronic Management
Treatment of chronic secondary hyperparathyroidism of osteomalacia or chronic renal failure may require calcium and vitamin D to elevate the serum calcium level and decrease parathyroid hormone levels. Patients with chronic renal failure require normalization of the serum phosphate level with phosphate-binding antacids prior to the administration of 1,25-dihydroxyvitamin D$_3$. Other methods of managing hypercalcemia are shown in Table 7-13. Prognosis depends on the underlying condition and is poor when the cause is neoplasia.

Adrenal Disorders
Adrenal disorders manifest as specific syndromes depending on whether hormone excess or deficiency exists. The hormones from the adrenal cortex include glucocorticoids, aldosterone, androgens, and some estrogens. Epinephrine and norepinephrine arise from the adrenal medulla. These hormones regulate metabolic requirements and are secreted in response to physiologic stress. In disease states, the excessive production of estrogens by an adrenal adenoma causes gynecomastia in the male, whereas the excessive production of androgens in the female causes hirsutism and varying degrees of virilization. Cortisol excess produces Cushing's syndrome. Excessive production of adrenal mineralocorticoids (11-deoxycorticosterone, corticosterone, and aldosterone) or catecholamines produces a moderate to severe hypertensive state. Adrenal glucocorticoid deficiency may result from primary glandular failure, may be secondary to pituitary failure, or may be tertiary to hypothalamic failure.

Adrenal Insufficiency

Adrenal insufficiency [10, 37, 41, 60, 70] results from inadequate secretion of adrenal glucocorticoids and is caused by conditions listed in Table 7-14. These patients manifest primarily the clinical features of deficient mineralocorticoids, glucocorticoids, or sex steroids depending on the nature of the primary lesion.

DIAGNOSIS

History

The major clinical manifestations include weakness, anorexia, nausea, vomiting, abdominal pain, constipation or diarrhea, salt craving, lightheadedness, weight loss, fatigue, lethargy, muscle and joint pains, apathy, confusion, and on occasion, psychosis. Increased skin pigmentation characterizes primary adrenal insufficiency, whereas skin depigmentation occurs in hypothalamic-pituitary causes of adrenal insufficiency. When infection, surgical procedures, trauma, prolonged fasting, or other stresses are superimposed, acute adrenal crisis may be precipitated. Less often, acute adrenal insufficiency may result from bilateral adrenal hemorrhage due to trauma, anticoagulants, or infection. Adrenal crisis is char-

Table 7–14. Causes of Adrenal Insufficiency

I. Primary adrenal insufficiency:
  A. Autoimmune atrophy (Addison's disease)
  B. Destructive processes such as tuberculosis, histoplasmosis, blastomycosis, sarcoidosis, infarction, carcinomatosis, acquired immunodeficiency syndrome (AIDS), irradiation
  C. Congenital adrenal hyperplasia (deficiency of 20-hydroxylase, 3β-hydroxysteroid dehydrogenase, 17α-hydroxylase, 21-hydroxylase, 11β-hydroxylase)
II. Hormone unresponsive syndromes:
  A. Adrenocorticotropic hormone unresponsiveness (congenital adrenocortical unresponsiveness)
  B. Cortisol resistance
III. Secondary adrenal insufficiency:
  A. Selective adrenocorticotropic hormone deficiency
  B. Panhypopituitarism
IV. Tertiary adrenal insufficiency (hypothalamic disease)
 V. Following discontinuation of suppressive doses of glucocorticoids

acterized by increased anorexia, nausea, abdominal distress, fever, hypotension, shock, and coma. If the adrenal insufficiency is secondary to congenital adrenal enzymatic defects, presentation may be as the adrenogenital syndrome, manifest in childhood with ambiguous genitalia and precocious puberty or in the adult as hirsutism. If secondary adrenal insufficiency is present, loss of other pituitary trophic hormones is likely to be present. Similarly, patients with primary adrenal insufficiency may have symptoms of other autoimmune endocrine disorders, such as hypothyroidism (Schmidt's syndrome), Graves' disease, hypoparathyroidism, pernicious anemia, premature ovarian failure, and insulin-dependent diabetes mellitus.

Physical Findings

Characteristically, the patient presents with lean body habitus, weight loss, buccal and skin hyperpigmentation (especially over sun-exposed or pressure-sensitive areas), hyperpigmentation in scars, hypotension, vitiligo, and calcified ear cartilage. Pituitary disease is suspected when deficiencies of the other pituitary hormones are manifest. In adrenal crisis, moderate to severe hypotension, hypovolemia, loose skin, shrunken eyeballs, dry tongue, mental confusion, fever, and shock occur.

Laboratory Tests

Laboratory abnormalities include hyponatremia, hyperkalemia, mild metabolic acidosis, hypercalcemia, hypoglycemia, anemia, eosinophilia, lymphocytosis, and elevation of the blood urea nitrogen (BUN) level with a normal serum creatinine level. The diagnosis of adrenal insufficiency is established by demonstrating low adrenal secretory products and failure of the glands to respond to stimulation. The blood cortisol level is less than 5 μg/dl, and urinary 17-hydroxycorticosteroids (17OHCS) are less than 2 mg per 24 hours. An adrenocorticotropic hormone test is performed with blood samples drawn at 0, 30, and 60 minutes following the administration of 0.25 mg Cortrosyn intravenously. In acutely ill patients this test can be performed after pretreatment with dexamethasone. A normal response is a plasma cortisol rise to greater than 20 μg/dl and an increase of more than 5 μg/dl over the baseline value. In differentiating primary from secondary adrenal insufficiency, a plasma adrenocorticotropic hormone level is elevated in the primary disorder and low in secondary and tertiary adrenal insufficiency. Adrenal autoantibodies are positive in Addison's disease. An adrenal CT scan will show small adrenal glands as a presumptive diagnosis of autoimmune Addison's disease, whereas enlarged adrenal glands represent infiltrative disease. Occasionally, a flat plate of the abdomen will demonstrate adrenal calcification.

TREATMENT AND PROGNOSIS
Acute Management

Therapy of acute adrenal insufficiency is directed toward replacing glucocorticoids, fluids, and electrolyte imbalances. Hydrocortisone phosphate or Solu-Cortef (100 mg) is given as a rapid intravenous injection. This is followed by 50 to 100 mg hydrocortisone or Solu-Cortef IM or IV every 6 hours or 100 mg hydrocortisone as an infusion given over 4 to 6 hours. A total of 300 to 400 mg of these short-acting steroids is given in the first 24 hours. The total deficit in extracellular fluid is often 20 percent of the extracellular fluid volume and should be replaced with isotonic saline. Steroids are rapidly tapered to replacement levels over 4 days unless complicating medical conditions are present. Attention should be given to the presence of hypoglycemia. The hyperkalemia and hyponatremia will correct with saline replacement, steroids, and glucose administration. If volume expansion is slow in correcting the hypotension, temporary use of sympathomimetic agents is warranted. Identifying the underlying precipitating condition is important. The adrenal crisis itself is remedial to therapy within 12 to 48 hours, and prognosis is good if the underlying provoking condition is successfully managed. Long-term maintenance therapy with glucocorticoids and mineralocorticoids is required in these patients.

Chronic Management

Maintenance therapy for chronic adrenal insufficiency should simulate the normal diurnal variation of cortisol secretion (i.e., 20 mg hydrocortisone or 25 mg cortisone acetate at 8:00 A.M. and 10 mg hydrocortisone or 12.5 mg cortisone acetate at 6:00 P.M.). Mineralocorticoid replacement (i.e., Florinef, 0.05 to 0.2 mg every morning) is required for patients with primary adrenal insufficiency, whereas patients with hypothalamic-pituitary adrenal insufficiency may maintain adequate electrolyte balance with glucocorticoid supplementation plus adequate salt intake. During times of medical, surgical, or psychiatric stress, supplemental corticosteroids must be given to avoid acute adrenal crisis; usually for minor illness the patient doubles or triples the daily dose. For surgical stress, hydrocortisone phosphate (50 mg) or its equivalent should be given intravenously 12 hours before surgery and 100 mg should be given intravenously immediately before the surgical procedure. In addition, 50 mg intramuscularly or intravenously is required for every 4 hours of surgery. Alternately, 100 mg hydrocortisone phosphate or Solu-Cortef can be given as an intravenous infusion over 4 to 6 hours of surgery. Hydrocortisone equivalents (300 mg) are given the first day with rapid tapering over the next 2 to 4 days. Patients with adrenal insufficiency must understand their dependence on supplemented stress steroids. They should carry identifying information on their person at all times, such as a Medic Alert bracelet or card. Prognosis in chronic primary adrenal insufficiency is good when the patient is educated as to the disease process, limitations, and illness precautions.

Cushing's Syndrome

Cushing's syndrome [6, 12, 35, 76] is a clinical state of glucocorticoid excess that results from adrenocortical hyperplasia due to excessive pituitary adrenocorticotropic hormone production (Cushing's disease), excessive production of cortisol by adrenal adenoma or adenocarcinoma, ectopic production of adrenocorticotropic hormone or corticotropin-releasing hormone by neoplasms, or iatrogenic secondary to the exogenous administration of adrenal steroids. Hence, Cushing's Syndrome represents all the causes of the clinical state of glucocorticoid excess while Cushing's Disease includes only those due to a hypothalamic pituitary ediology.

DIAGNOSIS
History
The common symptoms are weakness (especially proximal muscle), fatigue, weight gain, amenorrhea, oligomenorrhea, facial plethora, easy bruising, thromboembolic events, hirsutism, emotional difficulties, back pain, fractures, and susceptibility to infection. The onset may be insidious or sudden, with clinical manifestations developing over a 4- to 6-week period.

Physical Findings
Characteristically, the patient presents with a rounded, full-moon face with reddening of the cheeks. There is redistribution of fat into the central trunkal area with thinning of the extremities due to protein wasting and fullness of the supraclavicular fossa with a dorsal fat pad ("buffalo hump"). Skin changes include the thin, fine skin, acne, purple striae, hypertrichosis, ecchymosis, purpura, acanthosis nigricans, and peripheral edema. When adrenal hyperfunction occurs, excessive production of androgens will produce increasing baldness, increasing muscular habitus, hirsutism, and virilism. Excessive mineralocorticoid production may produce mild to moderate hypertension.

Laboratory Tests
Impaired glucose tolerance or diabetes with an insulin-resistant state is common with Cushing's syndrome. The complete blood count will show leukocytosis, lymphopenia, eosinopenia, and occasionally, polycythemia. A hypokalemic metabolic alkalosis occurs, especially in ectopic Cushing states. Diagnosis of Cushing's disease is dependent on showing high cortisol production rates which fail to suppress with varying doses of

exogenous glucocorticoids (dexamethasone), as shown in Fig. 7-2. Measuring a 24-hour urine free cortisol level is the most sensitive test for diagnosing cortisol overproduction. An overnight dexamethasone suppression test is performed to determine whether normal feedback regulation of the pituitary-adrenal axis is present. If the plasma cortisol level at 8:00 A.M. after 1 mg PO dexamethasone at 11:00 P.M. the night before is less than 5 μg/dl, the result is normal. When the plasma cortisol level is greater than 5 μg/dl, further workup is warranted. Formal evaluation consists of measuring adrenal steroid response (urinary 17-hydroxycorticosteroids, free cortisol, or plasma cortisol) to low-dose (0.5 mg q6h × 8) and high-dose dexamethasone (2 mg q6h × 8). About 70 percent of the endogenous cases of Cushing's syndrome are due to Cushing's disease which fails to suppress on low-dose but does suppress after a high-dose dexamethasone administration. Adrenocorticotropic hormone levels are high in ectopic states and low when an adrenal cortisol-producing tumor is present.

Special Tests: Cushing's Disease
Pituitary CT or magnetic resonance imaging scans are only positive in 50 to 60 percent of patients with pituitary microadenomas producing Cushing's disease. Adrenocorticotropic hormone venous sampling of inferior petrosal sinuses may establish a lateralizing pituitary gradient for adrenocorticotropic hormone that strongly suggests a pituitary source for the Cushing's disease. In addition, stimulation tests with corticotropin-releasing factor help distinguish Cushing's disease due to small pituitary microadenomas (positive response with increase in adrenocorticotropic hormone of 10 to 40 pg/ml above baseline) from adrenal adenomas or ectopic adrenocorticotropic hormone production (negative or flat response). Adrenal adenoma and carcinoma may be identified by abdominal CT scan, nephrotomograms, ultrasound, iodocholesterol scan, or adrenal venograms. Metabolic bone survey or bone-density measurements document the osteoporosis. In ectopic Cushing's syndrome, one must identify the

site of the tumor in the thymus, lung, kidney, or breast.

TREATMENT AND PROGNOSIS

Treatment and prognosis of Cushing's syndrome depend on the underlying cause. When caused by Cushing's disease, transsphenoidal hypophysectomy is recommended. If localization studies by CT scan have not been helpful, then information obtained from venous adrenocorticotropic hormone samplings of the inferior petrosal sinuses may localize the lesion to one side of the pituitary or the other. Depending on the extent of pituitary surgery, the patient may require replacement therapy of glucocorticoids or other pituitary hormones. Prognosis depends on extent of pituitary surgery and residual pituitary function. Adrenal tumors should be surgically removed; prognosis depends on early diagnosis and extent of malignancy. The suppressed normal adrenal gland will require 2 to 6 months to fully recover. Neoplasms producing ectopic adrenocorticotropic hormone should be resected if possible. Medical adrenalectomy for adrenal tumors or resistant ectopic cases can be achieved by the administration of the aminoglutethimide, metyrapone, or mitotane (O,P'-DDD). Prognosis is poor in these malignant conditions, with tumor progression and increasing metabolic deterioration due to the Cushing's syndrome.

Hyperaldosteronism

The states of mineralocorticoid excess are listed in Table 7-15, and they include hyperaldosteronism, which may be due to either primary or secondary disorders. Primary hyperaldosteronism [49, 72] is a sodium-retention, volume-expansion state with hypokalemic metabolic alkalosis and hypertension. Many of the causes of secondary hyperaldosteronism are associated with volume depletion and sodium retention.

DIAGNOSIS

History

The symptoms of primary hyperaldosteronism include hypertension, polyuria, polydipsia, nocturia, fatigue, weakness, muscle cramps, paresthesias, and occasionally paralysis.

Table 7–15. *Causes of Hypermineralocorticoid States*

I. Primary hyperaldosteronism (low renin activity):
   A. Primary aldosteronism (adrenal adenoma)
   B. Idiopathic aldosteronism (adrenal nodular hyperplasia)
   C. Dexamethasone remedial hyperaldosteronism
   D. Adrenal carcinoma
II. Secondary hyperaldosteronism (elevated renin activity):
   A. Renovascular hypertension
   B. Malignant hypertension
   C. Edematous disorders with arterial hypovolemia (cirrhosis, nephrotic syndrome, heart failure, idiopathic edema)
   D. Bartter's syndrome (normal to low blood pressure, elevated renin and aldosterone)
   E. Primary reninism (renin-secreting tumors)
   F. Estrogen therapy (increased renin substrate)
   G. Renal salt-wasting diseases
III. Elevation of other mineralocorticoids (low renin activity):
   A. Desoxycorticosterone-secreting adenomas
   B. Glucocorticoid synthesis defects (17-alpha- and 11-beta-hydroxylase deficiencies; elevated adrenocorticotropin levels stimulate desoxycorticosterone and corticosterone production)
   C. Ectopic adrenocorticotropic hormone production
   D. Cushing's disease
   E. Licorice ingestion

Source: From Reller, L. B., Schalch, D. S., and Rudolph, M. C. Endocrine and Metabolism. In L. B. Reller, S. A. Sahn, and R. W. Schrier (Eds.), *Clinical Internal Medicine.* Boston: Little, Brown, 1987. P. 397. Used with permission of the publisher.

Physical Findings

Hypertension may range from a mild benign type to, occasionally, a more severe form. In primary hyperaldosteronism edema is usually absent, whereas in secondary hyperaldosteronism edema may be present. Orthostatic hypotension may be noted. Depression of the deep tendon reflexes, tetany, and periodic paralysis may be seen secondary to hypokalemia.

Laboratory Tests

The laboratory findings of primary aldosteronism are an elevated plasma aldosterone level, a suppressed plasma renin level, hypokalemic metabolic alkalosis, hypomagnesemia, submaximal concentration of urine unresponsive to vasopressin, and carbohydrate intolerance. Electrocardiographic abnormalities may include depression of the ST segments and T-wave abnormalities with appearance of U waves, premature ventricular contractions, and ventricular fibrillation. A normal serum potassium value does not exclude primary hyperaldosteronism, particularly in the salt-depleted patient. Plasma aldosterone levels greater than 22 ng/dl and urinary aldosterone levels greater than 20 μg per 24 hours in the presence of suppressed renin activity indicate primary hyperaldosteronism. Demonstrating autonomy of aldosterone secretion is done by infusing 2 liters of saline intravenously over 4 hours or with the administration of 0.3 mg Florinef every 12 hours for 3 days and repeating the aldosterone measurements. The inability to demonstrate elevated plasma renin activity with volume depletion by furosemide (40 mg PO) and upright posture for 4 hours establishes the suppressed low renin state. In contrast, high plasma renin and aldosterone values are seen in secondary forms of hyperaldosteronism. Adenomas are characterized by decreasing plasma aldosterone levels following upright posture, whereas with adrenal hyperplasia plasma aldosterone levels rise on standing.

Special Studies

To search for adrenal tumors an adrenal CT scan or iodocholesterol scan is useful. Adrenal vein catheterizations studies hormonally define and localize the lesion, allowing a distinction between adenoma and bilateral adrenal hyperplasia.

Treatment and Prognosis

The treatment depends on the etiology of the hyperaldosteronism. In the case of an adenoma, surgery gives an 80 percent success rate. Spironolactone may be used in nonresponding patients. When bilateral hyperplasia is present, there is characteristically a poor response to surgery, which should be avoided; use of spironolactone, amiloride, or an angiotensin-converting enzyme inhibitor will normalize the potassium and improve the blood pressure.

Pheochromocytoma

Pheochromocytomas [8] (or functioning paraganglioma) occur in only a small percent of the hypertension population (<1 percent), but when identified, they represent a surgically curable form of hypertension. Pheochromocytoma is a great masquerader, often suggesting other diseases such as diabetes, hypercalcemia, thyrotoxicosis, anxiety, neurosis, severe infections, Cushing's syndrome, and even carcinoid syndrome. It is a potentially fatal disease unless diagnosed and treated. The disease may occur on a familial autosomal-dominant basis or as part of multiple endocrine neoplasia with autosomal-dominant inheritance. Such patients, once identified, require genetic counseling and surveillance.

DIAGNOSIS

History

The clinical manifestations of circulating catecholamine excess include headache, hypertension, palpitations, sweating, orthostatic hypotension, pallor, flushing, tremor, anorexia, nausea, weight loss, epigastric pain, constipation, chest pain, dizziness, weakness, nervousness, anxiety, paresthesias, and syncope. The classic triad includes hypertension, sweating, and palpitations and is seen in 90 percent of patients. A familial syndrome is suggested by other family members with the disorder or the familial occurrence of renal stones or medullary thyroid cancer.

Physical Findings

The most common sign is hypertension, which may be either sustained or paroxysmal and is associated with episodic symptoms of sweating, palpitations, or tachycardia. Hypertension is usually severe and may be malignant. Hypertensive retinal changes and sweaty, clammy skin may be seen, but otherwise, the physical examination is relatively nonspecific. The pheochromocytoma may be associated with neurocutaneous disorders, café-au-lait spots, hyperplastic corneal nerves, marfanoid habitus, neurofibroma, and mucosal neuromas. Palpation of the abdomen usually does not reveal a tumor, but abdominal or suprapubic palpation may induce a rise in blood pressure and symptoms.

Laboratory Tests

Diagnosis is established by demonstrating increased levels of catecholamines or their metabolites, e.g., normetanephrine, metanephrine, or vanillylmandelic acid (VMA) in the urine. Creatinine should be determined in the urinary samples so that the results can be expressed per unit of creatinine. In most assays, the upper limits for a normal urinary vanillylmandelic acid level is 7 to 10 mg per day, and the upper level for total metanephrines is 1.3 mg per day. Total urinary free catecholamines should be less than 100 to 150 μg per day and may be fractionated into epinephrine (normal < 20 μg per 24 hours) and norepinephrine (normal < 70 μg per 24 hours). When plasma catecholamines are measured, they must be obtained under basal conditions with the patient lying supine and sampling from an indwelling venous catheter that has been inserted approximately 30 minutes prior to sampling. Values below 500 pg/ml make the diagnosis unlikely, whereas values of above 2000 pg/ml characterize pheochromocytoma. Alternatively, increased plasma catecholamine levels which do not suppress after clonidine administration (0.3 mg) may assist in diagnosing the condition. The clonidine suppression test assists in interpreting borderline values. Other pharmacologic tests for pheochromocytoma are considered obsolete and dangerous.

Special Studies

Most pheochromocytomas can be localized readily because of their large size; hence they are frequently identified with the abdominal CT scan. In special circumstances, radionuclide scanning with *meta*-[¹³¹I]iodobenzylguanidine (MIBG) is useful. Since these tumors are quite vascular, they localize easily with arteriography; however, the patient should be studied only after adequate pharmacologic adrenergic blockade prior to this procedure to avoid hypertensive crisis. An occasional patient may require venous sampling for localization.

Acute Management

Phentolamine or nitroprusside infusion treats hypertensive emergencies. After a 0.5- to 1-mg intravenous phentolamine test dose, blood pressure is controlled by repeated doses (2 to 5 mg) or a 0.5 mg per minute intravenous infusion. Careful attention is paid to volume status, arrhythmias, and monitoring.

Chronic Management

The definitive treatment of pheochromocytoma is surgical excision. Hypertension is controlled preoperatively with alpha-adrenergic blockade with phenoxybenzamine (20 to 80 mg per day). Liberal salt intake and control of tachycardia or cardiac arrhythmias with beta-adrenergic blockade are necessary. An experienced anesthesiologist carefully selects premedications and anesthetic agents that do not sensitize the myocardium to catecholamines. Intraoperative management requires electrocardiographic, intraarterial pressure, and central venous pressure or Swan-Ganz monitoring. Intraoperative blood pressure and arrhythmias are controlled with volume replacement, phentolamine, propranolol, pressor agents, lidocaine, and nitroprusside. The chronic management of unresectable malignant pheochromocytoma requires phenoxybenzamine or prazosin for hypertension. Alpha-methyl-paratyrosine is used to decrease catecholamine synthesis. Prognosis in these patients is poor.

Male and Female Sexual Disorders

A clinical consideration of sexual disorders of the adult male and female include male and female hypogonadism and sex hormone overproduction states such as hormonally functioning endocrine tumors that cause estrogenized effects in the male and androgenized features in the female.

Amenorrhea

Amenorrhea [36] is an early manifestation of female hypogonadism that presents as a result of either primary or secondary causes. Primary amenorrhea consists of never having menstrual cycles; secondary amenorrhea is the absence of menstrual flow in female patients who have previously menstruated. As noted in Table 7-16, primary amenorrhea may be associated with abnormal chromosomal analysis, as seen in Turner's

Table 7–16. Amenorrhea

I. Primary amenorrhea:
   A. Gonadal abnormalities:
      1. Turner's syndrome
      2. Gonadal dysgenesis variants
      3. Gonadal agenesis
      4. Hypoplastic ovaries ("resistant ovary syndrome")
      5. Male pseudohermaphradite (testicular feminization and other androgen-resistant variants)
   B. Extragonadal abnormalities:
      1. Müllerian duct anomalies (maldevelopment of hymen, vagina, cervix, uterus)
      2. Müllerian agenesis (Mayer-Rokitansky-Kuster-Hauser syndrome)
II. Secondary amenorrhea:
   A. Endometrial destruction* (infection, surgery, after D&C, irradiation)
   B. Acquired ovarian failure (menopause, premature ovarian failure, surgical castration, radiation)
   C. Central nervous system (hypothalamic-pituitary disease)*
   D. Hormonal disorders* (congenital adrenal hyperplasia, hypothyroidism, acanthosis nigricans with insulin resistance, polycystic ovaries, Cushing's syndrome, adrenal insufficiency, hyperthyroidism, feminizing or masculinizing ovarian tumors)
   E. Metabolic (obesity, starvation, diabetic, alcoholism, weight loss-induced amenorrhea)
   F. Acute and chronic illness (hepatic, hematologic, renal, cardiac, pulmonary, infectious, oncologic)
   G. Prolactinoma*
   H. Stress (psychogenic, anorexia nervosa, bulimia, runners, pseudocyesis)
   I. Drugs (psychotrophic drugs, spironolactone, steroids, oral contraceptives, "postpill," drug addiction, progestins)
   J. Pregnancy
   K. Idiopathic

*If this occurs before puberty, it may cause primary amenorrhea.

syndrome, gonadal dysgenesis, and testicular feminization, or it may be associated with structural and developmental anomalies of the genital tract. In cases of secondary amenorrhea, lesions of the hypothalamic-pituitary-ovarian axis need be considered. One must always exclude oral contraceptive usage, pregnancy, and menopause.

Diagnosis

History

Important in evaluating amenorrhea is the nature of the onset of the menstrual disorder, whether of a primary or secondary type. The history of sexual development and progression of puberty should include the age of onset of menarche, the regularity of periods, degree of menstrual flow or spotting, menstrual pain, and premenstrual tension. Associated medical conditions, other endocrine conditions (including hypothyroidism, hirsutism, obesity, diabetes), headaches, extent of exercise, abnormal eating behavior, galactorrhea, infertility, pregnancy histories, psychic stress, and use of medications, especially hormones, should be noted. Absence of menstrual periods by age 14 associated with delayed growth and absence of secondary sexual characteristics or absence of menstruation with normal growth and secondary sexual characteristics by age 16 constitutes primary amenorrhea.

Physical Findings

Physical examination should include assessment of sexual development, the presence of axillary and pubic hair, and stage of breast development. Examination should assess vaginal estrogen effect, urogenital development, presence of inguinal hernia, ovarian-uterine size, and the presence of ovarian or abdominal masses. In the case of Turner's syndrome, the patient's short stature, shield chest with widely spaced nipples, webbed neck, and cubitus valgus are characteristic. Patients with other forms of gonadal dysgenesis may be tall and eunuchoid. Presence of an enlarged thyroid, galactorrhea, hirsutism, or virilization would suggest other endocrinopathies.

Laboratory Tests

Measurement of pituitary gonadotrophins (luteinizing and follicle-stimulating hormones) is best determined by pooling three separate samples taken at 10-minute intervals when gonadotrophins are low. When gonadotrophins are high, a karyotype is needed to evaluate gonadal dysgenesis and intersex disorders. In some cases, abdominal ultrasound or CT scans may be needed to evaluate the ovarian and uterine sizes. Special stimulation tests of pituitary-ovarian function may include the administration of clomiphene citrate (50 mg bid) for 5 days with the measurement of pituitary gonadotrophins on the morning of the sixth day or the use of 100 μg gonadotropin-releasing hormone with the measurement of luteinizing hormone and follicle-stimulating hormone levels at 0, 30, 60, and 90 minutes. A vaginal smear can be taken to assess estrogen effect. Basal body temperatures may determine the presence of ovulation.

TREATMENT AND PROGNOSIS

In all forms of female hypogonadism where estrogen deficiency is present, the institution of estrogen replacement is warranted. In patients with secondary amenorrhea due to ovarian failure, vasomotor symptoms of "hot flashes" and tissue estrogen deficiency with urogenital atrophy and dyspareunia are relieved by estrogen therapy. In younger patients, estrogen is especially indicated to avoid the long-term consequence of osteoporosis. Replacement therapy consists of 0.625 to 1.25 mg Premarin daily for 21 days each month with 10 days of a progestin (10 mg medroxyprogesterone acetate) during the last 10 days of the cycle. In the cases of amenorrhea due to hyperprolactinemia, treatment is with bromocriptine alone or in combination with pituitary surgery. In selected patients in whom fertility is desired, ovulation induction can be initiated with clomiphene citrate, and in patients with gonadotropin failure, ovulation can be initiated with human chorionic gonadotropin and Pergonal. The prognosis depends on the underlying condition (see Table 7-16).

Male Hypogonadism

The causes of male hypogonadism are listed in Table 7-17. They include disorders of diminished pituitary-gonadotropin reserve (hypogonadotrophic hypogonadism) or testicular failure (hypergonadotrophic hypogonadism) [45, 59].

Table 7–17. Male Hypogonadism

I. Hypogonadal hypogonadism:
  A. Hypothalamic-pituitary disease:
    1. Hypothalamic
    2. Panhypopituitarism
    3. Selective gonadotropin deficiency:
      a. Biologically inactive gonadotropins
      b. Acquired deficiency due to hypothalamic-pituitary disease
      c. Kallmann's syndrome (associated with diminished olfactory function)
      d. Rosewater's syndrome (X-linked recessive gonadotropin deficiency)
      e. Fertile eunuch (luteinizing hormone deficiency)
      f. Isolated follicle-stimulating hormone deficiency
      g. Laurence-Moon-Biedl syndrome (autosomal-recessive associated with mental retardation and retinitis pigmentosa)
      h. Prader-Willi syndrome (a syndrome of childhood obesity, neonatal hypotonia, short stature, cryptorchidism, and mental retardation associated with a defection in chromosome 15)
  B. Delayed puberty
  C. Feminizing adrenal tumors and congenital adrenal hyperplasia
  D. Systemic illness or stress
  E. Drugs (sex hormones, anabolic agents, alcohol)
II. Hypergonadotrophic hypogonadism:
  A. Sex chromatin-positive: Klinefelters and its variants
  B. Sex chromatin-negative:
    1. XYY hypogonadism
    2. Androgen resistance syndrome (5α-reductase disorders or androgen insensitive to include testicular feminization and Reifenstein syndrome)
    3. Functional prepubertal castrate, rudimentary testes, or bilateral anorchia
    4. Noonan's syndrome (male Turner's)
    5. Sertoli-cell only syndrome (Del Castillo syndrome)
    6. Myotonic dystrophy
    7. Gonadotropin-producing pituitary tumor
    8. Adult testicular failure (mumps, gonorrhea, leprosy, tumor, lymphoma, irradiation, chemotherapy, trauma, alcohol, starvation)

DIAGNOSIS

History

Specific features regarding the time and nature of onset of the hypogonadal state should be noted, particularly the relationship to normal growth and sexual development and regression of secondary sexual characteristics of axillary and pubic hair and genital growth. Diminished sexual function is noted with regard to potency, infertility, sexual drive (libido), aggressive behavior, and erectile function. Alterations in taste and smell would suggest Kallmann's syndrome (isolated gonadotropin deficiency). History of testicular trauma, mumps, or other orchitis should be obtained. Many drugs affect sexual performance, especially antihypertensive medication. Headache and loss of other endocrine function would suggest a hypothalamic or pituitary lesion. Vasomotor symptoms may occasionally be seen with testicular failure, especially if abrupt.

Physical Examination

Physical examination includes the patient's height, with floor to pubic and pubic to crown measurements and span-to-height ratio to determine if a eunuchoid body proportion is present. Eunuchoid features include a span that is 2 inches greater than height and a sole-to-symphysis measurement that is 2 inches greater than the symphysis-to-crown measurement. Body hair density and distribution should be noted. Other androgen-dependent tissues are the prostate, larynx, and muscle mass. The normal male testicle is at least 5 cm in diameter and firm in consistency. A testicular size less than 5 cm represents a prepubital size, and testicles 2.0 to 2.5 cm in size suggest Klinefelter's syndrome. Testicular masses, inguinal hernias, varicocele, and penile and scrotal development should be noted. Hypospadias would suggest a 5α-reductase deficiency. Gynecomastia may be seen with excessive estrogen production or decreased testosterone production and is caused by alterations in the circulating testosterone-estrogen ratio. Other estrogenized effects include soft skin, palmar erythema, and spider angiomas. A normal semen analysis requires a hormonally and structurally intact gonadal system.

Laboratory Tests

Initial evaluation consists of measurement of pituitary gonadotrophins (luteinizing hormone and follicle-stimulating hormone) and testosterone. The measurement of pituitary gonadotrophins allows one to approach the differential diagnosis of possible causes of the disorder (see Table 7-17). When pituitary gonadotrophins are elevated and testosterone is normal or low in patients with small testicles and gynecomastia, then the diagnosis of Klinefelter's syndrome is entertained and a karyotype is indicated. 5α-Reductase deficiency is characterized by end-organ insensitivity to testosterone with poor masculine development and varying manifestations of male pseudohermaphroditism. It is diagnosed by measuring androgen metabolites in culture fibroblasts. Male pseudohermaphroditism results from enzymatic defects in androgen biosynthesis, defects in androgen end-organ response, and defects in Müllerian regression. When pituitary gonadotrophins are low, a pituitary workup should be instituted to exclude other pituitary hormone-deficiency states (see Hypopituitarism). However, as with other pituitary hormones, low gonadotropin levels are difficult to distinguish from normal levels; therefore, a stimulation test is needed to establish if gonadotrophin secretion is deficient. The gonadotropin-releasing hormone test, which involves administering 100 µg gonadotropin-releasing hormone and measuring pituitary gonadotrophins (luteinizing hormone and follicle-stimulating hormone) at 0, 30, 60, and 90 minutes, will determine pituitary gonadotrophin reserve. Hypothalamic testing can be performed with clomiphene stimulation using 50 mg twice a day for 5 days and measuring pituitary gonadotrophins and testosterone on the sixth day. A basal prolactin value is indicated in acquired male hypogonadism to rule out pituitary prolactinoma. Specific tests for taste and smell are needed if one suspects Kallmann's syndrome.

TREATMENT AND PROGNOSIS

Androgen replacement therapy is best accomplished with 200 mg intramuscular testosterone every 2 weeks. Sublingual replacement with 30 to 50 mg methyltestosterone per day is less effective, and blood testosterone levels are not reliably maintained. An orally effective androgen is Halotestin (5 to 20 mg per day), but fluid retention and gastrointestinal side effects (nausea, cholestatic jaundice, abnormal liver function tests) may limit its use. Testosterone replacement will protect against osteoporosis and will return sexual potency, drive, and erectile function in most patients.

IMPOTENCE

Impotence [70] characterizes male sexual dysfunction. It must be distinguished from loss of libido (sex drive or impulse), which may be caused by psychological or organic factors. Impotence is the inability to obtain or sustain penile erection that is most frequently secondary to emotional or neurologic disorders. It is seen in about 50 percent of adult male diabetics as part of autonomic neuropathy. A history of early morning erections implies normal neurocirculatory function. Psychological sexual fears, phobias, guilt, or deteriorating marital relationships may be responsible. Endocrine causes are rare, but one should consider testicular failure, pituitary failure, hypothyroidism, and diabetes mellitus. Drugs are an increasingly important cause of impotence, particularly antihypertensive medications such as thiazide diuretics, beta-adrenergic blocking drugs, and alpha-methyldopa.

Androgen-Excess States

When an androgen-excess state occurs in the female, a characteristic syndrome of hirsutism and/or virilization is produced [64]. These disorders in the male may escape detection unless they occur at a young age, causing precocious puberty, increased growth, or short stature. Table 7-18 lists the various causes of androgenizing conditions in the female patient.

Table 7–18. Conditions Associated with Hirsutism

   I. Physiologic (puberty, pregnancy, menopause)
  II. Genetic (racial, familial)
 III. Pituitary (Cushing's disease, acromegaly, prolactinoma)
 IV. Adrenal:
    A. Adenoma, carcinoma
    B. Congenital adrenal hyperplasia (adrenogenital syndrome):
      1. 21-Hydroxylase deficiency
      2. 11-Hydroxylase deficiency
  V. Ovarian:
    A. Polycystic ovary disease (Stein-Leventhal syndrome)
    B. Hyperthecosis
    C. Tumors (adrenoblastoma, adrenal rests, hilus cell, pseudomucinous cystadenoma)
 VI. Intersex problems:
    A. Male pseudohermaphroditism
    B. Variants of gonadal dysgenesis
    C. Testicular feminization
 VII. Miscellaneous endocrine disorders:
    A. Achard-Thiers syndrome (hirsute patient with diabetes mellitus)
    B. Juvenile hypothyroidism
VIII. Drugs (Dilantin, androgens, anabolic agents, corticosteroids, progestins, diazoxide, minoxidil)
 IX. Idiopathic

DIAGNOSIS

History

Important historic features include the age of onset of the symptoms, growth and sexual development, and family history for similar disorders. A careful history of medications, particularly birth control pills, phenytoin, minoxidil, and anabolic steroids, should be obtained. Hirsutism is frequently the presenting complaint. Its onset may coincide with puberty, pregnancies, or the menopausal state. Fertility history, ethnic background, change of voice, obesity, associated acne, change in libido, regularity of menstrual cycle, and frequency and method of hair removal should be obtained.

Physical Examination

Distribution of hair is noted on the upper lip, chin, sideburn area, neck, postcervical area, shoulder, chest, breasts, abdomen, thighs, and legs. Significant abnormal hair (hirsutism) needs to be distinguished from ethnic hair (hypertrichosis). In the female, hair growing above the umbilicus or on the shoulders, the ear, the sternum, and the thighs usually indicates significant hirsutism. Virilizing signs include frontal balding, deep voice, and male body habitus and muscle mass. A careful pelvic examination should note clitoromegaly and ovarian or abdominal masses. Physical findings also may suggest Cushing's syndrome, acromegaly, or prolactinoma.

Laboratory Tests
Laboratory measurements include luteinizing hormone, follicle-stimulating hormone, testosterone, or free testosterone. An adrenal source of the androgens is indicated when there is an elevation in the plasma DHEA-sulfate level. Plasma testosterone levels in excess of 300 ng/ml usually indicate an ovarian or adrenal tumor.

Special Tests
Consideration of Cushing's syndrome may require a dexamethasone suppression test and urinary free cortisol measurements. If a congenital adrenal enzyme deficiency is suspected, plasma 11-deoxycortisol (compound S) or 17-hydroxyprogesterone for 11-hydroxylase and 21-hydroxylase deficiencies, respectively, is measured. Mild cases of congenital adrenal hyperplasia require an adrenocorticotropic hormone stimulation test with measurements of cortisol, compound S, and 17-hydroxyprogesterone and their ratios. To evaluate for ovarian pathology, ultrasound scans of the ovaries or abdominal CT scans are needed. In some cases, laparotomy or laparoscopy may be indicated.

TREATMENT AND PROGNOSIS
Treatment consists of electrolysis to remove the excess hair, particularly in the cosmetically apparent areas. Electrolysis is expensive and requires long treatment periods to remove small amounts of hair. When increased adrenal androgen production exists, dexamethasone (0.75 to 0.1 mg hs) is given for adrenal suppression. In cases of Stein-Leventhal syndrome (polycystic ovarian syndrome) wedge resection of the ovaries may result in fertility. However, a trial of clomiphene citrate may be equally effective. With an ovarian androgen source or in idiopathic hirsutism, low-dose birth control pills can be used. Antiandrogen therapy using spironolactone (100 to 400 mg per day), cimetidine (400 to 1200 mg per day), or medroxyprogesterone acetate have been effective in reducing the amount of hair regrowth. When an anatomic lesion in the ovary or adrenal is identified, exploratory surgery for tumor removal is necessary. Prognosis for complete reversal of the hirsutism in most cases is poor, and significant psychosexual stress and emotional disorders may coexist.

Endocrine Tumors
Endocrine tumors [4, 7, 19, 39, 67] may be hormonally functioning or nonfunctioning. When they occur as nonfunctioning tumors, they result in the destruction of endocrine tissue and may present as a metastatic carcinoma syndrome. When hormonally functioning, they may present as the distinct syndromes noted in Table 7-19. Some endocrine tumors produce a number of hormones, and some nonendocrine tumors produce an ectopic hormone(s) that stimulates an endocrine gland(s).

DIAGNOSIS
History
Symptoms of weight loss, cachexia, and a specific endocrine syndrome (see Table 7-19) raise the suspicion for these tumors. Each syndrome has been previously discussed. Astute clinical judgment allows early detection.

Physical Examination
The physical examination may show a large mass or evidence of metastasis. A distinct clinical presentation such as Cushing's syndrome, acromegaly, Zollinger-Ellison syndrome, hirsutism with virilization, or carcinoid syndrome suggests a neoplastic etiology. In the case of ectopic Cushing's syndrome, the patient may not manifest the

Table 7–19. Classification of Endocrine Tumors

I. Solitary glandular tumors (functional and nonfunctional): This category includes tumors originating in the hypothalamus, pineal body, pituitary, thyroid, parathyroid, adrenal cortex, adrenal medulla, pancreas, ovary, and testes.

II. Polyglandular syndromes (multiple endocrine adenopathy), syndromes (tumor or hyperplasia):
Type 1: Pituitary, pancreas, parathyroid.
Type 2a: Medullary thyroid carcinoma, pheochromocytoma, parathyroid.
Type 2b: Medullary thyroid carcinoma, pheochromocytoma, ganglioneuroma phenotype.
Type 3: Other polyglandular endocrine tumor associations.

III. Monoglandular syndromes (one APUD clone making multiple hormones): This category includes carcinoid, medullary thyroid carcinoma, and nesidioblastosis (pancreatic islet-cell hyperplasia)

IV. Ectopic syndromes (tumorous aberrant APUD clone making one or many peptides): This includes secretion of tumor markers and the clinical syndromes of antidiuretic hormone excess, Cushing's syndrome, hypoglycemia, hypercalcemia, precocious puberty, gynecomastia, erythrocytosis, hypophosphatemia, hyperpigmentation, acromegaly, and watery diarrhea

Source: from Eckel, R. H., and Hofeldt, F. D. Endocrinology and Metabolism in the Elderly. In R. W. Schrier (Ed.), *Clinical Internal Medicine in the Aged.* Philadelphia: Saunders, 1982. Used with permission of the publisher.

classic clinical stigmata of Cushing's, but instead may present with marked cachexia, wasting, electrolyte abnormalities, and increased pigmentation or freckling caused by the high adreno-corticotropic hormone–melanocyte-stimulating hormone–like peptides.

Special Tests

The diagnosis of nonfunctioning endocrine tumors is made with organ-imaging studies and a search for metastatic disease in lung, liver, bone, and brain. When hormonally functioning tumors are suspected, suppressive studies to determine autonomy of the endocrine-secreting tumor is warranted. In certain situations, such as thyroid medullary carcinoma or gastrinomas, stimulation tests are used. Some endocrine tumors secrete abnormal hormonal products such as the alpha subunits of the glycoprotein hormones in some apparently nonfunctioning pituitary tumors, unusual androgen metabolites in adrenal carcinoma, elevated beta-human chorionic gonadotropin in testicular carcinoma, and proinsulin in islet-cell carcinoma.

TREATMENT AND PROGNOSIS

The treatment and prognosis depend on early detection and surgical removal of the primary lesion with selective chemotherapy or radiation therapy for metastasis. When the tumor is an adenoma, surgical removal alleviates the condition. In certain hormonally functioning tumors, hormonal therapy that antagonizes the primary tumor is available. Prognosis depends on the extent and degree of control of the primary malignancy. Certain tumors, such as gastrinomas and thyroid medullary carcinomas, have long-term prognoses that are good with medical management.

References

1. Abboud, C. F. Laboratory diagnosis of hypopituitarism. *Mayo Clin. Proc.* 61: 35, 1986.
2. Albrink, M. J. Obesity. *Clin. Endocrinol. Metab.* 5: 297, 1976.
3. Akita, Y., Sajto, T., Yajima, Y., and Sukuma, S. Stimulatory and inhibitory guanine nucleotide-binding proteins of adenylate cyclase in erythrocytes from patients with pseudohypoparathyroidism type I. *J. Clin. Endocrinol. Metab.* 61: 1012, 1985.
4. Ballard, H. S., Frame, B., and Hartsock, R. J. Familial multiple endocrine adenoma–peptic ulcer complex. *Medicine* 43: 481, 1964.
5. Bastenie, P. A., Bonnyns, M., and Vanhaelst, L. Natural history of primary myxedema. *Am. J. Med.* 79: 91, 1985.
6. Besser, G. M., and Edwards, C. R. W. Cushing's syndrome. *Clin. Endocrinol. Metab.* 1: 451, 1972.
7. Block, M. B., Roberts, P., Kadair, R. G., Seyfer, A. E., Hull, S. F., and Hofeldt, F. D. Multiple en-

docrine adenomatosis type IIb. *J.A.M.A.* 234: 710, 1975.

8. Bravo, E. L., and Gifford, R. W. Pheochromocytoma: Diagnosis, localization and management. *N. Engl. J. Med.* 311: 1298, 1984.

9. Bray, G. A. Obesity in America. *Int. J. Obesity* 3: 363, 1979.

10. Burke, C. W. Adrenal insufficiency. *Clin. Endocrinol. Metab.* 14: 947, 1985.

11. Campbell, G. A., Kemm, J. R., Hosking, D. J., and Boyd, R. V. How common is osteomalacia in the elderly. *Lancet* 2: 386, 1984.

12. Carpenter, P. C. Cushing's syndrome: Update of diagnosis and management. *Mayo Clin. Proc.* 61: 49, 1986.

13. Charles, M. A., Dodson, L. E., Waldeck, N., Hofeldt, F. D., Ghaed, N., Telepak, R., Ownbey, J., and Burstein, P. Serum thyroglobulin levels predict total body iodine scan finding in patients with treated well-differentiated thyroid carcinoma. *Am. J. Med.* 69: 401, 1980.

14. Cobb, W. E., Spare, S., and Reichlin, S. Neurogenic diabetes insipidus: Management with DDAVP. *Ann. Intern. Med.* 88: 183, 1978.

15. Cooper, D. S., and Ridgway, E. C. Antithyroid drugs: Pharmacology and therapeutic guidelines. *Thyroid Today* 7: 1, 1984.

16. Davidoff, L. M. Studies in acromegaly: II. Historical note. *Endocrinology* 10: 453, 1926.

17. DeGroot, L. J., and Reilly, M. Comparison of 30 and 50 mCi doses of iodine-131 for thyroid ablation. *Ann. Intern. Med.* 96: 51, 1982.

18. DeGroot, L. J., Inbar, S. H., Mazzaferri, E. L., and Tzagournis, M. Look for these clues to thyrotoxicosis. *Patient Care* 17: 143, 1983.

19. Eckel, R. H., and Hofeldt, F. D. Endocrinology and Metabolism in the Elderly. In R. W. Schrier (Ed.), *Clinical Internal Medicine in the Aged.* Philadelphia: Saunders, 1982.

20. Eckel, R. H. Diabetes and Hyperlipidemia. In Sussman, Draznin, James (Eds.), *Clinical Guide to Diabetes Mellitus.* New York: Alan R. Liss, 1986.

21. Fischer, K. F., Lees, J. A., and Newman, J. H. Hypoglycemia in hospitalized patients. *N. Engl. J. Med.* 315: 1245, 1986.

22. Foster, D. W., and McGarry, J. D. The metabolic derangements and treatment of diabetic ketoacidosis. *N. Engl. J. Med.* 209: 159, 1983.

23. Frame, B., and Parfitt, A. M. Osteomalacia: Current concepts. *Ann. Intern. Med.* 89: 966, 1978.

24. Freedman, D. S., Srinivasan, S. R., Shear, C. L., Franklin, F. H., Webber, L. A., and Berenson, G. S. The relation of apolipoproteins A-I and B in children to parental myocardial infarction. *N. Engl. J. Med.* 315: 721, 1986.

25. Gale, E. Hypoglycemia. *Clin. Endocrinol. Metab.* 9: 461, 1980.

26. Harris, M., and Cahill, G. Classification of diabetes mellitus and other categories of glucose intolerance. *Diabetes* 28: 1039, 1979.

27. Health and Policy Committee, American College of Physicians. Eating disorders: Anorexia nervosa and bulimia. *Ann. Intern. Med.* 105: 790, 1986.

28. Herzog, D. B., and Copeland, P. M. Eating disorders. *N. Engl. J. Med.* 313: 295, 1985.

29. Hoeg, J. M., Gregg, R. E., and Brewer, B. An approach to the management of hyperlipoproteinemia. *J.A.M.A.* 255: 512, 1986.

30. Hofeldt, F. D. Reactive hypoglycemia. *Metabolism* 24: 1193, 1975.

31. Hofeldt, F. D. Transitional low blood glucose. *Rocky Mt. Med. J.* 76: 30, 1979.

32. Hofeldt, F. D., and Kelly, M. Low-dose insulin regimens in the management of diabetic ketoacidosis. *Minn. Med.* 66: 25, 1983.

33. Hofeldt, F. D., Bornemann, M., Treece, G. L., Sims, J., Kidd, G. S., McDermott, M. T., Clark, J., and Ghaed, N. Practical application of fine-needle thyroid aspiration biopsy in clinical medicine. *Milit. Med.* 149: 522, 1984.

34. Hofeldt, F. D. Proximal femoral fractures. *Clin. Orthop.* 218: 12, 1987.

35. Howlell, T. A., Rees, L. H., and Besser, G. M. Cushing's syndrome. *Clin. Endocrinol. Metab.* 14: 911, 1985.

36. Huffman, J. W. Delayed female sexual maturation. *Postgrad. Med.* 78: 239, 1985.

37. Irvine, W. J., and Barnes, E. W. Adrenal insufficiency. *Clin. Endocrinol. Metab.* 1: 549, 1972.

38. James, W. P. T. Obesity. *Clin. Endocrinol. Metab.* 13: 435, 1984.

39. Keiser, H. R. Sipples syndrome: Medullary thyroid carcinoma, pheochromocytoma and parathyroid disease. *Ann. Intern. Med.* 78: 561, 1973.

40. Khardori, R., and Soler, N. G. Hyperosmolar hyperglycemic nonketotic syndrome. *Am. J. Med.* 77: 899, 1984.

41. Kozak, G. P. Primary adrenocortical insufficiency. *Am. Fam. Physician* 15: 124, 1977.

42. Ladenson, P. W., Goldenheim, P. P., and Ridgway,

E. C. Rapid pituitary and peripheral tissue responses to intravenous L-triiodothyronine in hypothyroidism. *J. Clin. Endocrinol. Med.* 56: 1252, 1983.

43. Lafferty, F. Primary hyperparathyroidism. *Arch. Intern. Med.* 141: 1761, 1981.

44. Lamberton, R. P., and Jackson, I. M. D. Investigation of hypothalamic-pituitary disease. *Clin. Endocrinol. Metab.* 12: 509, 1983.

45. Lipsett, M. D. Physiology and pathophysiology of Leydig cell. *N. Engl. J. Med.* 277: 351, 1980.

46. Mackin, J. F., Canary, J. J., and Pittman, C. S. Thyroid storm and its management. *N. Engl. J. Med.* 291: 1396, 1974.

47. Mazzaferri, E. L., and Young, R. Papillary thyroid carcinoma. *Am. J. Med.* 70: 511, 1981.

48. McCowen, K. D., Adler, R. A., Ghaed, N., Verdon, T., and Hofeldt, F. D. Low dose radioiodide thyroid ablation in postsurgical patients with thyroid cancer. *Am. J. Med.* 61: 52, 1976.

49. Melby, J. C. Diagnosis and treatment of primary aldosteronism and isolated hypoaldosteronism. *Clin. Endocrinol. Metab.* 14: 977, 1985.

50. Melmed, S. Pituitary tumors secretory growth hormone and prolactin. *Ann. Intern. Med.* 105: 238, 1986.

51. Merimee, T. J. Spontaneous hypoglycemia in man. *Adv. Intern. Med.* 22: 301, 1977.

52. Miller, M., Moses, P. M., and Streeten, D. H. Recognition of partial defects in antidiuretic hormone secretion. *Ann. Intern. Med.* 73: 721, 1970.

53. Molitch, M. E. (Bromocriptine Study Group). Bromocriptine as primary therapy for prolactin-secreting macroadenomas. *J. Clin. Endocrinol. Metab.* 60: 698, 1985.

54. Purnell, D. C., and VanHeerden, J. A. Management of symptomatic hypercalcemia and hypocalcemia. *World J. Surg.* 6: 702, 1982.

55. Raisz, L. G., and Kream, B. E. Regulation of bone metabolism. *N. Engl. J. Med.* 309: 25, 1983.

56. Richelson, L. S., Wahner, H. W., Melton, L. J., III., and Riggs, B. L. Relative contributions of aging and estrogen deficiency to postmenopausal bone loss. *N. Engl. J. Med.* 311: 1273, 1984.

57. Ridgway, E. C., McCammon, J. A., Benotti, J., and Maloff, F. Acute metabolic responses in myxedema to large doses of intravenous L-thyroxine. *Ann. Intern. Med.* 77: 549, 1972.

58. Rifkind, B. M., and Degal, P. Lipid Research Clinics Program reference values for hyperlipidemia and hypolipidemia. *J.A.M.A.* 250: 1869, 1983.

59. Sacks, S. A. Evaluation of impotence. *Postgrad. Med.* 74: 182, 1983.

60. Savage, M. D. Congenital adrenal hyperplasia. *Clin. Endocrinol. Metab.* 14: 893, 1985.

61. Schaefer, E. J., and Levy, R. I. Pathogenesis and management of lipoprotein disorders. *N. Engl. J. Med.* 312: 1300, 1985.

62. Schneider, A. B., and Sherwood, L. M. Pathogenesis and management of hypoparathyroidism and other hypocalcemic disorders. *Metabolism* 24: 871, 1975.

63. Schwabe, A. D. Anorexia nervosa. *Ann. Intern. Med.* 94: 371, 1981.

64. Schwartz, F. L. Hirsutism: Pathophysiology, clinical evaluation, treatment. *Postgrad. Med.* 77: 81, 1985.

65. Seltzer, H. S. Drug-induced hypoglycemia. *Diabetes* 21: 955, 1972.

66. Serri, O., Somma, M., and Hardy, J. Acromegaly: Biomedical assessment of cure after long-term follow-up of transsphenoidal selective adenomectomy. *J. Clin. Endocrinol. Metab.* 61: 1185, 1985.

67. Steiner, A. L., Goodman, A. D., and Powers, S. R. Study of a kindred with pheochromocytoma, medullary thyroid carcinoma, hyperparathyroidism and Cushing's disease: Multiple endocrine neoplasia type 2. *Medicine* 47: 371, 1968.

68. Sussman, K. E., and Metz, R. J. S. *Diabetes Mellitus*, 4th ed. New York: American Diabetes Association, 1975.

69. Thomas, A. E., Kekay, D. A., and Cutlip, M. D. A normograph method for assessing body weight. *Am. J. Clin. Nutr.* 29: 302, 1976.

70. Tzagournis, N. Acute adrenal insufficiency. *Heart Lung* 7: 603, 1978.

71. Wahner, H. W. Assessment of metabolic bone disease. *Mayo Clin. Proc.* 60: 827, 1985.

72. Weinberger, M. H. Primary aldosteronism: Diagnosis and differentiation of subtypes. *Ann. Intern. Med.* 100: 300, 1984.

73. Witztum, J., and Schonfeld, G. High-density lipoproteins. *Diabetes* 28: 326, 1979.

74. Woolner, L. B. Thyroid carcinoma. *Semin. Nuclear Med.* 1: 481, 1971.

75. Young, R. L., Mazzaferri, E. L., Rahe, A. J., and Dorfman, S. G. Pure follicular thyroid carcinoma. *J. Nuclear Med.* 21: 733, 1980.

76. Zervas, N. T., and Martin, J. B. Management of hormone-secreting pituitary adenomas. *N. Engl. J. Med.* 302: 210, 1980.

Rheumatology and Immunology

8

David Collier and
James Steigerwald

Over 36 million people in the United States suffer from some sort of rheumatic disease, accounting for 20 percent of all visits to health care providers [54]. These diseases, which affect the musculoskeletal system and supporting structures, are unique in a number of ways. They are frequently chronic in nature and may be associated with pain and deformities. They vary widely in suspected etiologies from simple trauma to a joint eventually resulting in degenerative joint disease to widespread immune-complex deposition resulting in a disease such as systemic lupus erythematosus.

Because these diseases are so protean in their manifestations, it is difficult to outline one simple approach to the diagnosis and treatment of each patient. In a general sense, however, rheumatic diseases can be divided into three different categories depending on the patient's predominant clinical manifestation (Table 8-1). There will obviously be some overlap of diseases into other categories, and some diseases may progress from one category to another, especially when an acute arthritis (septic, for example) causes permanent and chronic joint changes. Nevertheless, we feel that this classification allows the clinician to focus on the most likely diagnosis in any one patient.

We will not attempt to cover all the more than 100 rheumatic disorders, but we will concentrate on those seen most commonly in clinical practice.

Evaluation of the Patient

There are some aspects of rheumatic disease that need to be understood before a patient can be classified as having one or another type of disease. Certain terms need to be defined because their use implies different etiologies to a patient's illness:

Arthritis: Joint inflammation frequently associated with swelling and aggravated by moving the joint.
Arthralgia: Pain in a joint without any signs of inflammation—common in viral illness.
Myalgia: Pain in a muscle without any signs of inflammation—common in viral illness.
Myositis: Tenderness and pain in a muscle with associated findings of inflammation.
Tendinitis: Inflammation of a tendon usually secondary to acute or chronic strain.
Tenosynovitis: Inflammation of a tendon and its synovial sheath, often seen in septic arthritis, rheumatic arthritis, or the axial arthropathies.
Synovitis: Inflammation of the synovial lining cells causing pain and swelling of a joint.
Enthesopathy: Inflammation where fibrous tissue (tendon) attaches to a bone—common in the axial arthropathies.

Certain laboratory examinations also may be useful in the evaluation of rheumatic diseases. The erythrocyte sedimentation rate (ESR), al-

Table 8–1. Classification of Rheumatic Diseases

I. Articular diseases:
  A. Monarticular:
    1. Acute (septic arthritis, crystalline arthritis)
    2. Chronic (traumatic arthritis)
  B. Polyarticular:
    1. Acute (viral arthritis)
    2. Chronic (rheumatoid arthritis, ankylosing spondylitis, Reiter's syndrome, psoriatic arthritis, enteropathic arthritis, osteoarthritis/degenerative joint disease)
II. Systemic disease: Systemic lupus erythematosus, Sjögren's syndrome, systemic sclerosis (scleroderma), polymyositis/dermatomyositis, mixed connective-tissue disease, vasculitis, polymyalgia rheumatica
III. Nonarticular: Fibrositis, back pain, shoulder pain, hip pain, elbow pain, sports-related injuries

Table 8–2. Causes of an Elevated Erythrocyte Sedimentation Rate

Inflammation
Infection
Malignancy
Increased plasma immunoglobulins
Pregnancy (third trimester)
Oral contraceptives
Anemia
Obesity (especially in women)
Elevated serum cholesterol
Low serum albumin
Hypothyroidism

Source: From Soy, H. C. and Liang, M. H. The erythrocyte sedimentation rate guidelines for rational use. *Ann. Intern. Med.* 104: 515, 1986.

though nonspecific, may be helpful diagnostically in differentiating systemic inflammatory diseases from functional, nonorganic complaints. Because it is influenced by acute-phase reactants, such as fibrinogen, which are produced during a variety of inflammatory, infectious, or other injurious stimulants, it also may be helpful in following the course of certain inflammatory diseases, especially rheumatoid arthritis and systemic lupus erythematosus.

The Westergren method for the erythrocyte sedimentation rate is much more accurate than the microtube method and should be used whenever available. Normal values for the Westergren method at the University of Colorado Health Sciences Center are 0 to 15 mm per hour in men and 0 to 25 mm per hour in women up to the age of 50 years. The rate does gradually rise with age, so that a useful rule of thumb is to consider the result normal if it is below half the age of the subject. Besides the rheumatic diseases, other common causes of an elevated sedimentation rate are shown in Table 8-2.

Synovial fluid analysis is the other laboratory examination pertinent in any rheumatic disease. The indication for aspiration and analysis of synovial fluid is the presence of *any* unexplained

active than the others, synovial fluid should be aspirated and analyzed because of the increased incidence of infection in an already damaged joint.

Once fluid is obtained, three routine examinations should be performed on it [38]:

1. White blood cell (WBC) count and differential, using saline as the diluent for the synovial fluid. When the usual white blood cell diluent is used, the hyaluronic-acid-protein complexes precipitate because of the acetic acid in the diluent. This may cause a falsely low white blood cell count in the fluid.
2. Examination of the fluid for crystals by polarized light microscopy.
3. Gram's stain and routine cultures for bacteria; fungal or mycobacterial cultures should be obtained if they are clinically indicated.

Other studies on synovial fluid, including total protein, glucose, and complement levels, are rarely helpful and should not be ordered routinely. Table 8-3 lists the typical synovial fluid findings in various disease states [38].

Table 8–3. *Characteristics of Synovial Fluid in Various Disease States*

Disease	Appearance	Leukocyte count* (per ml)	Crystals	Comments*	Class
Normal	Clear, straw-colored	<75 (15% PMN)	None		
Noninflammatory:					
Acute traumatic arthritis	Clear or bloody	<1000 (25% PMN)	None	Red blood cells may be present	1
Osteoarthritis	Clear, straw-colored	<1000 (15% PMN)	None	Occasional cartilage fragments	
Systemic lupus erythematosus	Clear or cloudy	1000 to 5000 (10–15% PMN)	None	Decreased SF complement	
Inflammatory:					
Rheumatoid arthritis	Cloudy, light yellow	10,000–20,000 (60–75% PMN)	None	Occasional cholesterol crystals; decreased SF complement	2
Gout	Cloudy, white or yellow	10,000–20,000 (60–70% PMN)	Sodium urate	Strongly negative birefringent crystals	
Pseudogout	Cloudy, white	10,000–40,000 (60–70% PMN)	Calcium pyrophosphate	Weakly positive birefringent crystals	
Reiter's syndrome	Cloudy, light yellow	10,000–30,000 (70% PMN)	None	Reiter's cells	
Infectious:					
Bacterial	Cloudy, gray or yellow	50,000–75,000 (90% PMN)	None	—	3
Tuberculosis	Cloudy, gray or yellow	25,000 (50% PMN)	None	Synovial biopsy often needed	
Viral	Clear	2000–20,000 (variable differential)	None	Decreased SF complement with prodrome of hepatitis B	
Hemorrhagic:	Cloudy, red	Variable		Red blood cells present	4
Trauma:					
Hemorrhagic					
Scurvy					
Anticoagulant therapy					
Pigmented villonodular synovitis					

*PMN = polymorphonuclear leukocytes; SF = synovial fluid.
Note: The complement level in synovial fluid is characteristically decreased in active rheumatoid arthritis and in the prodromal arthritis associated with some cases of hepatitis B; it usually is normal or increased in the other diseases listed.
Source: From Gatter, R. A. *A Practical Handbook of Joint Fluid Analysis.* Philadelphia: Lea and Febiger, 1984. P. 4–5.

Monarticular Disease

Virtually any form of arthritis may be monarticular at onset. There is, however, a group of diseases that characteristically begin and remain monarticular. These diseases include the following:

Infectious arthritis:
  Bacterial
  Tuberculous
  Fungal
Crystalline arthritis:
  Gout
  Calcium pyrophosphate deposition disease (pseudogout)
  Hydroxyapatite disease
Traumatic arthritis
Avascular necrosis
Pigmented villonodular synovitis
Malignant tumors
Osteoid osteoma

Acute Monarticular Disease

INFECTIOUS (SEPTIC) ARTHRITIS

A pyogenic infection in a joint is a medical emergency. Rapidity of diagnosis is important; the more quickly the treatment begins, the more likely the patient will recover and the less likely there will be chronic residual changes in the joint.

Infectious agents primarily are involved in arthropathies by direct invasion of the synovium or bone. These agents are comprised of bacteria, including spirochete and mycobacteria, fungi, protozoa, worms, and viruses. Viruses tend to cause polyarticular disease and are covered under Polyarticular Disease. Infections can indirectly cause a secondary arthritis with sterile synovium. The mechanism of this arthritis is incompletely understood, although it is widely believed to be due to immune complexes. Examples of this are subacute bacterial endocarditis, Whipple's disease, and hepatitis B virus. Arthritis can occur after the inciting infection has subsided. Examples of this are rheumatic fever, Reiter's syndrome, and Jaccoud's syndrome (after rheumatic fever) [119].

This section will be concerned primarily with direct invasion of a joint by bacteria or fungi.

The primary focus of an infection leading up to an infected joint is usually remote from that joint. The organism is generally spread hematogenously by eluding serum bactericidal activity and the reticuloendothelial system to reside in synovial tissue or juxta-articular bone. Thus a damaged joint or impaired host predisposes to joint infections. An infected joint is rarely due to a direct inoculation by a penetrating wound, steroid injection, or surgery. There can, however, be local invasion into a joint from a contiguous infection. Table 8-4 lists the organisms most commonly responsible for acute pyogenic arthritis, and Table 8-5 lists the organisms most commonly responsible for acute pyogenic arthritis by age.

Immunologic derangements can predispose to infectious arthropathies; these include hypogammaglobulinemia, chronic granulomatous disease, and treatment with immunosuppressive drugs

Table 8–4. Organisms Commonly Responsible for Acute Pyogenic Arthritis

Organism	Percent in adults	Percent in children
Gram-positive cocci:		
Staphylococcus aureus	35	45
Streptococcus pyogens	10	25
Gram-negative cocci:		
Neisseria gonorrhoeae	50	5
Mycobacteria/fungi	<1	<1

Table 8–5. Organisms Commonly Responsible for Acute Pyogenic Arthritis by Age

Age	Organism
<6 months old	*S. aureus*, gram-negative
<2 years	*S. aureus*, *H. influenzae*
2–15 years	*S. aureus*, *S. pyogens*, *S. pneumoniae*
16–50 years	*N. gonorrhoeae*, *S. aureus*
Over 50 years	*S. aureus*, Enterobacteriaceae

Table 8–6. *Chronic Diseases Commonly Associated with Specific Organisms*

Disease	Organism
Cancer	Gram-negative
Liver disease	Gram-negative bacilli, *S. pneumoniae*
Diabetes mellitus	Gram-positive and -negative
Chronic renal failure	*S. aureus*
Hemoglobinopathies	*S. pneumoniae, Salmonella*
Complement deficiency (especially C5–C9)	*N. gonorrheae*
Rheumatoid arthritis	*S. aureus*
IV drug use	*S. aureus, Pseudomonas, Serratia*

(i.e., corticosteroids or cytotoxic drugs). Certain chronic diseases are associated more commonly with specific organisms [40, 41, 119], as shown in Table 8-6.

Clinical Presentation

Pyogenic arthritis presents as a relatively sudden onset of pain, warmth, and swelling in a joint. Decreased range of motion and pain on movement can be the most sensitive signs of infection. It is monarticular in 85 percent of cases. The joints most often involved are knees, hips, ankles, and shoulders, although any joint can be involved. Intravenous (IV) drug abusers will commonly be afflicted with infections in their vertebrae, sternoclavicular joint, or sacroiliac joint [6, 41]. Gonococcal and meningococcal arthritis can begin with migratory polyarthritis [71]. The majority of patients have fever, usually low grade, and about 25 percent have rigors. If the infection begins or spreads to the bone (osteomyelitis), chronic systemic symptoms of fever and weight loss generally occur. Neonates and infants can present with signs of septicemia, such as lethargy, fever, tachycardia, and hypotension.

Diagnostic Studies

Whenever infection in a joint is considered, it is mandatory to aspirate and examine the joint fluid. The most important test is to culture the joint fluid on the appropriate medium. Joint fluid is usually cultured in chocolate agar, but it is also cultured on special media for a specific suspected organism. For example, fungi are mainly cultured on Sabouraud's agar, and mycobacteria are cultured commonly on egg-glycerol-potato medium. Cultures are positive in 80 percent of all infections [41].

The next step is to examine the synovial fluid for crystals and then to do a Gram's stain. The Gram's stain is positive 50 to 70 percent of the time in pyogenic infections [41]. The white blood cell count and differential in the synovial fluid usually demonstrate a white blood cell count of over 50,000 with over 90 percent polymorphonuclear leukocytes. Rarely is the white blood cell count less than 20,000. It would be very uncommon for any other disease process to give a synovial fluid white blood cell count greater than 100,000 [41].

Studies of peripheral blood demonstrate that the erythrocyte sedimentation rate is elevated and there is a leukocytosis in about 90 percent of patients. Blood cultures are positive 35 to 50 percent of the time [40, 41].

When the synovial fluid cultures yield no diagnosis and an infection is still considered, a synovial biopsy can be extremely helpful. The organisms may be seen concentrated in the synovium, especially in tuberculous or fungal infections. Culture of the synovium with Gram's stain rarely misses the organism.

X-Ray Studies

Radiographs during the first week of infection may show soft-tissue swelling or appear normal. It is nevertheless useful to obtain these radiographic studies as a baseline for following the progression of the infection. As early as 10 days, but usually after 3 weeks, localized osteoporosis and rarefaction of subchondral bone can be observed, followed by erosions of the juxta-articular bone and narrowing of the joint space due to destruction of the articular cartilage. If osteomyelitis is present, both bone destruction and new bone formation can be present, and radiolucent areas of lysis and increased bone density are seen [41].

Early in the course of an infection, radioisotope

scanning techniques may detect the site of infection even when radiographic studies are normal. Technetium (^{99m}Tc) diphosphonate and gallium (^{67}Ga) citrate radioisotope scans can be helpful, especially if the patient does not have an underlying inflammatory or degenerative process. Both studies are nonspecific but the gallium scan tends to be more specific for infection than the technetium diphosphonate scan. A three-phase radionucleotide study performed by scanning as the isotope is injected, immediately after injection, and then 2 to 3 hours later can help make the diagnosis of osteomyelitis.

Computerized axial tomographic (CT) scanning is most helpful with complex structures such as the spine or difficult to assess areas such as the sacroiliac joint or sternoclavicular joint. In osteomyelitis, an increased density in medullary bone tissue can be seen before bony destruction and cavitation can be documented. The CT scan is specially helpful in documenting soft-tissue abscess.

General Treatment Principles
A patient with a septic joint should be hospitalized and given intravenous antibiotics. The choice of antibiotic depends on the Gram's stain, age of the patient, and clinical situation. The duration of therapy depends on the organism, delay of therapy, host factors, and response to therapy. Usually 2 to 6 weeks of parenteral antibiotics are given, followed by 2 to 6 weeks of oral antibiotics. The infected joint should be needle aspirated daily until no fluid is obtained or the white blood cell count in the synovial fluid is normal. Surgical drainage is indicated in hip infections, sternoclavicular joint involvement, vertebral involvement with cold compression, prosthetic joints, and difficult to aspirate joints or in joints that respond poorly to needle aspiration [15]. Initially, over the first 2 to 3 days, the joint is immobilized, and then active and passive range of motion are increased as signs of inflammation are decreased.

Specific septic joint infections will now be discussed.

NEISSERIA GONORRHEAE. The most common infectious arthritis in the 15- to 45-year age group is *N. gonorrheae*. From 0.1 to 3 percent of patients with gonococcal urethritis develop disseminated gonococcal infection (DGI). Most gonococcal arthritis is seen in sexually active females, with symptoms most striking during menstruation, pregnancy, and postpartum. Other groups susceptible to disseminated gonococcal infection are homosexual males and those patients with C5–C9 complement deficiency [28].

Clinically, these patients have a slight fever with polyarthralgias; two-thirds of patients will develop a tenosynovitis, usually in the wrist, fingers, or ankles. There is a dermatitis seen in the majority of patients, which can be anything from an acromacule that blanches to papules to vesiculopustules [71]. In the evaluation of these patients it is important to culture the urethra or cervix, throat, rectum, and joint fluid. *Neisseria gonorrheae* pharyngitis predisposes to disseminated gonococcal infection. The skin lesions are rarely culture-positive [28, 71]. Table 8-7 indicates the usual treatment regimens.

Rarely are the organisms resistant to penicillin. A response to treatment should be seen in 1 to 3 days. Also, unlike most other pyogenic infections, after the first joint tap there is usually no need to do repeated needle aspirations of the infected joint.

STAPHYLOCOCCAL ARTHRITIS. This is the most frequent infectious agent when all age groups are considered. Usually, infection is spread hematogenously from a primary site. The most common joints affected are the knees and hips [41]. The synovial fluid is culture-positive 75 to 90 percent of the time [40]. The treatment is nafcillin, 8 to 12 gm IV per day, or alternatively, cephalothin, 6 to 8 gm IV per day, vancomycin, 2 gm IV per day, or clindamycin, 1 to 3 gm IV per day. Frequent needle aspirations of the joint are a vital part of therapy.

OTHER BACTERIAL ORGANISMS. Streptococcal infection is an uncommon cause of a septic joint and is seen more often in patients with liver disease or hemoglobinopathies [41]. The organism is usually cultured in the synovial fluid and blood.

Table 8–7. Treatment Regimens for N. gonorrheae *Arthritis*

Initial "loading"				Maintenance therapy			
Drug	Dose	Route	Duration	Dose	Route	Duration
Aqueous crystalline penicillin G*	10×10^4 U	IV	Until improved	0.5 gm qid*	PO	To complete 7 days treatment
Ampicillin	3.5 gm	PO	1 dose†	0.5 gm qid	PO	4 days
Amoxicillin	3.0 gm	PO	1 dose†	0.5 gm qid	PO	4 days
Tetracycline HCL‡	—	—	—	0.5 gm qid	PO	7 days
Erythromycin‡	—	—	—	0.5 gm qid	PO	7 days
Spectinomycin HCL‡	—	—	—	2.0 gm qid	IM	3 days

*Initially and then ampicillin, 0.5 gm PO qid for maintenance until 7 days of treatment completed.
†With 1.0 gm probenecid.
‡Same regimen initially and for maintenance therapy in penicillin sensitive patients.

Treatment is intravenous penicillin G, 10 million units per day, or intravenous erythromycin, 2 to 4 gm per day.

Gram-negative infections have been seen with increasing frequency. Usually, entry site is the genitourinary or gastrointestinal systems. The arthritis is commonly monarticular. Treatment is gentamicin, 4.5 to 6 mg/kg IV per day, plus carbenicillin, 30 gm IV per day [6].

Mycobacterial infections in the United States are generally seen in the urban nonwhite population, with a male predominance (2 : 1) [7]. Articular tuberculosis is frequently a combination of arthritis and osteomyelitis. Radiographic studies demonstrate that the infection proceeds slowly from the periphery of a joint, with joint-space narrowing occurring late. There is bony destruction without much reactive new bone formation. Involvement is most common in the knees, hips, ankles, wrist, and spine [7]. The purified protein derivative test is almost always positive, but active pulmonary disease is seen in only 10 to 50 percent of these patients [7]. Treatment is with two or three drugs, usually a combination of isoniazid, 300 mg per day PO, and rifampin, 600 mg per day PO, with ethambutol, 1.5 to 2.0 gm per day added if there is any suggestion of drug resistance [7].

LYME ARTHRITIS. Lyme disease was first recognized in 1975 because of clustering of arthritis in children in Lyme, Connecticut that was at first thought to be juvenile rheumatoid arthritis. Lyme arthritis is caused by a spirochete, *Borrelia burgdorferi*, transmitted by the tick *Ixodes damini* [110]. It is a seasonal disease (summer) that is most common in children and young adults [109]. Early in the disease the patient has circulating immune complexes, elevated IgM antibody, and cryoglobulins, which are probably responsible for the early clinical symptoms [110].

The early manifestations are a skin rash, erythema chronicum migrans, that begins as a red macule or papule [109]. The area of redness expands and leaves an area of central clearing. About half the patients at this time develop secondary annular lesions, malaise, fatigue, headache, fever, and chills [109]. Later manifestations include meningeal irritation, as manifested by headache and stiff neck [110]. Cardiac involvement is sometimes seen with fluctuating degrees of arterioventricular block to myopericarditis [110]. The arthritis may precede the rash, but usually it occurs a few weeks to as late as 2 years after onset of illness. Typically it begins as migratory joint tendon and bursae pain. Frank arthritis, most commonly in the knees, begins months after the illness [110]. Large and small joints may be affected.

Laboratory examination may reveal 500 to over 100,000 white blood cells in the synovial fluid with normal synovial glucose concentrations. The erythrocyte sedimentation rate is usually elevated, and liver function tests may be abnormal. There is a specific IgM antibody test to the spirochete that peaks the third to the sixth week after onset [110].

Treatment early in the illness is either oral tetracycline, 250 mg four times a day, for 10 to 20 days or phenoxymethyl penicillin, 500 mg orally four times a day, for the same duration. Erythromycin also has been used at 30 mg/kg per day in divided doses four times a day for 15 to 20 days, but it is less successful. Patients with meningitis or frank central nervous system abnormalities should be given intravenous penicillin G, 20 million units a day, in divided doses for 10 days. Established Lyme arthritis also can be treated with the same intravenous penicillin G regimen [111].

CRYSTALLINE ARTHRITIS

There are three types of crystalline arthritis, and each has an acute and chronic form:

Acute Crystalline Arthritis	Chronic Crystalline Arthritis
Acute gout	Tophaceous gout
Pseudogout	Calcium pyrophosphate deposition disease
Hydroxyapatite	Milwaukee shoulder/knee syndrome

Gout

Gout is a metabolic disease found exclusively in humans due to a lack of the enzyme uricase. It is caused by the deposition of monosodium urate monohydrate crystals in joints. The prevalence of gout is 2 to 3 per 1000, with an increase in prevalence due to age and serum urate concentration [63]. Gout affects males more than females, and in 20 percent of patients there is a strong family history. In males, the disease begins after puberty. In females, the disease usually begins after menopause, and in patients with enzyme defects leading to gout, the disease may begin at birth [63]. The manifestations of gout include not only arthritis and tophi, but also inflammation and stones in the kidney resulting from increased urate [11].

SERUM URATE AND GOUT. A serum uric acid level over 7.0 mg% by the uricase method is abnormal [63]. Females normally have 1 mg% less than males. Hyperuricemia is caused either by increased production or decreased excretion of monosodium urate. This can be determined by collecting a 24-hour urine sample for uric acid. Usually, the 24-hour urine uric acid level is less than 600 mg on a purine-free diet and less than 800 mg on a normal diet. Over 1000 mg per day of uric acid is clearly abnormal [11, 63]. Table 8-8 lists the causes of hyperuricemia.

Reduced renal elimination is the cause of gout in the majority of patients with gout.

CLINICAL PRESENTATION. There are four stages in gout: asymptomatic hyperuricemia, acute gouty arthritis, intercritical gout, and chronic tophaceous gout. The chance of a gout attack or renal stones increases with increasing amounts of serum uric acid. In males with a uric acid level above 9 mg%, the likelihood of a gout attack is 50 percent. With a serum uric acid level greater

Table 8–8. Causes of Hyperuricemia

  I. Increased production of urate: Genetic causes:
     A. Idiopathic hyperuricemia
     B. Genetic mutations of controlling enzymes in the production of urate activity:
        1. Increased phosphoribosylpyrophosphate synthetase activity.
        2. Glucose-6-phosphatase deficiency
        3. Hypoxanthine guanine phosphoribosyltransferase (HGPRT) abnormality.
 II. Acquired increased production:
     A. Myeloproliferative disorders
     B. After therapy with cytotoxic drugs
     C. High purine intake
     D. Alcohol consumption
     E. Obesity and hypertriglyceridemia
III. Reduced renal elimination of urate:
     A. Genetic, intrinsic underexcretion of urate
     B. Acquired:
        1. Intrinsic renal disease, acute or chronic
        2. Polycystic kidney disease
        3. Lead nephropathy
        4. Hypertension
        5. Lactic acidosis or ketosis
        6. Drugs: Diuretics, low-dose aspirin, pyrazinamide, ethambutol, nicotinic acid, fructose, levodopa, and methoxyflurane.

than 13 mg% or a urine uric acid level greater than 1100 mg per 24 hours, there is a 50 percent chance of getting renal stones [63]. It usually takes 20 to 30 years between onset of hyperuricemia and the first attack of gout. The first gouty attack peak age is around 50 years. If a patient comes in with a gouty attack and is less than 30 years old, he (or she) may have an enzyme defect [123]. The initial attack is usually monarticular and in 50 percent of patients affects the first metatarsophalangeal (MTP) joint. In 90 percent of patients the first metatarsophalangeal joint is involved at some time [105]. Other joints frequently involved in a relative order of greater to lesser frequency are the instep, ankle, knee, wrist, and fingers. The classic gouty attack occurs at night or early in the morning. The pain comes on quickly and reaches a maximum in hours. It can be so painful that the afflicted does not even want the bed sheets on the painful joint. Accompanying the pain can be swelling of the joint and redness in the surrounding skin (gouty cellulitis). The attack resolves within 1 day to a week, occasionally longer. If the gout goes untreated, the attack frequency may increase over time. Precipitating factors include trauma, surgery, alcohol, certain drugs, dietary excess, and dehydration.

The intercritical period is the asymptomatic period between gout attacks. In the first year, up to 62 percent of patients will have a second gouty attack [63]. As the attack rate increases, the attacks more often become polyarticular.

If the gout is left untreated, up to 70 percent of patients will develop tophi. Tophi are deposits of urate that can occur anywhere, but most commonly they are found on the helix of the ear, the fingers, hands, knees, and feet. If these are aspirated, a white chalky material is found. Tophi correlate with urate renal disease. The average time from first attack to tophi is 12 years, ranging from 3 to 42 years [63].

Two types of renal disease are related to gout: urate nephropathy and uric acid nephropathy. In urate nephropathy, deposits of urate crystals are found in the interstitium of the medulla and pyramids in the kidney with surrounding giant-cell

reaction [11]. On urinalysis, albuminuria, mild number of cells, and a concentrating defect can be found. Progressive renal failure may be seen in 15 to 25 percent of patients with untreated gout [11, 63]. This high incidence, however, has recently been challenged [21]. The renal failure is associated with hypertension and gouty attacks. Uric acid nephropathy can be of two types. The first is uric acid stones, which are seen in 10 to 25 percent of patients with primary gout. Chronic acidosis with acid urine predisposes to stone formation. The second type of uric acid nephropathy is the precipitation of uric acid crystals in collecting ducts and ureters causing an acute renal failure. Precipitating factors include excessive exercise, dehydration, and leukemias and lymphomas treated with chemotherapy.

LABORATORY EVALUATION. In evaluating a patient with gout, the standard laboratory tests of complete blood count and SMA-18 are obtained. It is important to know the serum uric acid level. Uric acid is the breakdown product of purine metabolism, being the final product produced by the enzyme xanthine oxidase. Serum uric acid level is measured by several different methods. It is important to know the normal ranges used in your laboratory. Other useful routine tests are a cholesterol and triglyceride level and a urinalysis. If the patient has some evidence of renal failure, urinary lead excretion after EATA stimulation is useful, since increased lead intake is associated with urate nephropathy. A 24-hour urine sample is obtained for uric acid. If the patient excretes over 600 mg per day while on a low-purine diet or over 800 mg per day on a normal diet, this person is considered a hypersecretor [11, 63]. Synovial fluid examination can make the diagnosis of gout. The synovial fluid is a class II or III fluid (see Table 8-3). The diagnosis is made when needle-shaped negatively birefringent crystals are seen intracellularly in a phagocytic white blood cell.

The classic roentgenographic changes are erosions that are sharply marginated and lucent with a "punched out" appearance. These are most often observed in subchondral bone in bases or heads of the phalanges. This marginated lucent pocket is continuous with adjacent bone contour and gives the appearance of an overhanging margin. Despite the erosion, there is relative preservation of joint space and osteoporosis is generally not prominent unless the disease is allowed to progress [55].

TREATMENT. There is some controversy about the treatment of asymptomatic hyperuricemia [69]. Most physicians would treat patients with serum uric acid levels greater than 12 mg% or with 24-hour urines showing greater than 1100 mg uric acid per 24 hours. The acute gouty attack can be treated with a nonsteroidal anti-inflammatory agent or colchicine [93]. The usual drug of choice is indomethacin, 50 mg qid for 2 days and then decrease the dosage. Other nonsteroidals are effective. For patients who cannot take medicine by mouth, colchicine can be given intravenously, 1 to 2 mg in 20 ml normal saline over 20 minutes. This can be repeated in 6 hours.

Chronic suppressive therapy usually involves either a uricosuric agent or an agent that prevents the production of urate. In general it is good to instruct the patient on weight loss, the importance of preventing dehydration, the use of high-purine foods, and the association with alcohol consumption [11, 104]. If the patient has had three or more gouty attacks and has tophi or renal failure, chronic suppressive therapy is started after the patient is over the acute attack. Allopurinol is a competitive inhibitor of xanthine oxidase and prevents urate formation. It is used when the 24-hour urine demonstrates a hypersecretor, the glomerular filtration rate (GFR) is less than 50 ml per minute, or the patient has tophi, renal stones, a lymphoproliferative disorder, or is given cytotoxic therapy [11, 104]. The initial dosage of allopurinol is 100 mg per day; then it is increased weekly by 100 mg per day up to 600 mg per day, until the uric acid level is below the upper limits of normal. Serious drug interactions may occur with azathioprine, thiazides, and ampicillin. Otherwise, if the patient is not a hypersecretor and does not have any of the other problems listed above, the uricosurics are used. Probenecid competitively inhibits uric acid resorption by tubules. Dosage starts at 250 mg bid and increases to 500 mg bid. Higher dosages are sometimes used by increasing by 500 mg every 2 weeks as the serum uric acid level is followed. Sulfinpyrazone is given at a beginning dosage of 50 mg bid and then is increased 100 mg each week to a maximum dosage of 800 mg per day. Usually a nonsteroidal anti-inflammatory agent or colchicine at 0.6 mg bid is given for 3 months or longer concomitantly with chronic suppressive therapy to prevent an acute attack of gout.

Calcium Pyrophosphate Deposition Disease (CPDD)
Calcium pyrophosphate dihydrate (CPPD) crystals in a joint are the cause of the disease. Symptomatic calcium pyrophosphate deposition disease is about half as common as gout. It generally is a disease of the elderly, with onset usually at age 50 years or over [96]. The prevalence is slightly greater in males than females.

This disease is a great mimic and can superficially resemble various other types of arthritis. There are six common types of presentations [96]:

1. *Type A: Pseudogout.* This is an acute or subacute self-limiting attacking rarely as severe as gout. Like gout, the patient is pain free between attacks. It can be provoked by surgery or severe medical illness. The predominant joint is the knee and other appendicular joints. The knee is to pseudogout what the first metatarsophalangeal joint is to gout. Inflammation may spread from the initial "mother" joint to "daughter" joints.

2. *Type B: Pseudo-rheumatoid arthritis* (5 percent). This presentation is similar to rheumatoid arthritis. Multiple joints are involved, including the wrists, elbows, metacarpophalangeals, knees, and shoulders. The patient may have systemic symptoms of morning stiffness, fatigue, and synovial thickening. The erythrocyte sedimentation rate may be elevated and 10 percent of patients have low-titer positive rheumatoid factors, confusing the picture even more. Attacks may last weeks to several months.

3–4. *Type C and D: Pseudo-osteoarthritis.* This type of presentation is one of progressive degeneration of multiple joints, especially the knees, wrists, metacarpophalangeals, hips, spine, shoulders, elbows, and ankles. Involvement is generally symmetrical. There can be stigmata of primary osteoarthritis, such as Heberden's nodes (nodules on the distal interphalangeal joint) or Bouchard's nodes (nodules on the proximal interphalangeal joint). This is probably the chance association of two common types of arthritis in the elderly. Women predominate in this type of disease. About a third of patients with pseudo-osteoarthritis have superimposed acute attacks and have been classified as type C. Type D seems not to have superimposed acute inflammation.

5. *Type E: Lanthanic* (asymptomatic calcium pyrophosphate deposition disease). This is the most common form. Calcium pyrophosphate dihydrate is seen on roentgenograms, but the patient has no symptoms.

6. *Type F: Pseudoneuropathic joint.* A patient with denervation of a joint, as is seen in tertiary syphilis, can develop a totally destroyed joint, termed a Charcot joint. This disease has been seen in association with a typical Charcot joint. Calcium pyrophosphate deposition disease has also been seen in joints that resemble Charcot joints but in which there is an absence of neurologic abnormality.

Secondary forms of calcium pyrophosphate deposition disease have been associated with the following diseases [96]:

Hemochromatosis
Hyperparathyroidism
Gout
Diabetes mellitus
Hypophosphatasia
Wilson's disease
Ochronosis
Hypothyroidism—especially at the beginning of thyroid replacement

Hereditary forms have been described in Czechoslovakia, Chile, Holland, and France.

LABORATORY TESTS. It is important to obtain cal-

cium, phosphorus, glucose, uric acid, and liver function tests in the initial screening. If a secondary form of this disease is suspected, iron studies, thyroid studies, and a parathyroid hormone level should be obtained. Synovial fluid analysis usually demonstrates an inflammatory fluid. The diagnosis can be made when the disease is suspected clinically and rhomboid crystals that are weakly positively birefringent are seen.

Roentgenograms can be very helpful in making the diagnosis, since the calcium pyrophosphate crystals can be deposited on fibrocartilage, on hyaline (articular) cartilage, in ligaments, and in joint capsules. Radiopaque lines of calcium pyrophosphate are classically seen in the fibrocartilage of the pubic symphysis, wrist, knee meniscus, and annulus fibrosis; the hyaline cartilage in the knee, hips, shoulders, and elbows; and the spinal disks along the outer margins [27]. Patients with hemochromatosis will commonly have involvement of the metacarpophalangeal joint, which is unusual for primary calcium pyrophosphate deposition disease.

TREATMENT. If there is a primary underlying condition associated with this disease, an attempt is made to try to correct the underlying condition. For acute attacks, nonsteroidal anti-inflammatory agents are the treatment of choice. Intra-articular steroids are used if one joint has prolonged involvement with pain and inflammation. For chronic synovitis, nonsteroidal anti-inflammatory agents are used.

Hydroxyapatite Crystal Deposition Disease (HCDD)
Hydroxyapatite crystal deposition disease is a group of diseases of basic calcium phosphate crystal deposition associated with calcific periarthritis, tendinitis, and bursitis. The study of this group of diseases has been hampered by a lack of a simple, reliable diagnostic test. Clinically, the patient presents with an acute calcific periarthritis that consists of localized warmth, redness, swelling, and pain over a single joint, most commonly the shoulder [72]. An acute gouty-like attack also can be seen with hydroxyapatite crystals. Roentgenograms may demonstrate periarticular calcifica-

tion. Round or fluffy calcifications that vary in size from a few millimeters to several centimeters are seen. Synovial fluid can reveal shiny, laminated, coin-like lesions, but more often the hydroxyapatite crystals are so small they are beyond the limits of resolution of optical microscopy. When the crystals are seen, they are tiny needle or platelike spots with rare birefringence.

The more chronic type of hydroxyapatite crystal deposition disease is termed Milwaukee shoulder/knee syndrome [73]. This is seen in the elderly, with a mean age in one study of 72 years. Females predominate, with a female-to-male ratio of 4 : 1 [73]. The dominant shoulder is the most affected, and the symptoms are variable [73]. Mild to moderate pain, especially after use, is common. Limitations of motion, stiffness, and pain also are described. Rotator cuff lysis can be demonstrated on arthrogram. Radiographs demonstrate joint degeneration, bony destruction of the humeral head, and small osteophytes. Soft-tissue calcifications are seen 40 percent of the time. Synovial fluid analysis surprisingly reveals a low leukocyte count [43]. Hydroxyapatite aggregates and particulate collagen are seen in nearly all these patients [43].

TREATMENT. Treatment for acute calcific periarthritis has been nonsteroidal anti-inflammatory agents and colchicine [73]. Surgical removal of large calcific deposits usually provides permanent symptomatic relief [73]. However, medical treatment of Milwaukee shoulder/knee syndrome is generally unsatisfactory. Nonsteroidal anti-inflammatory drugs, repeated shoulder aspirations, and decreased shoulder use moderately control the symptoms. Surgical approaches have been generally successful and include anterior acromioplasty, repair of the rotator cuff, and total shoulder replacement.

Polyarticular Disease

Acute Polyarticular Disease
VIRAL ARTHRITIS
Viral arthritis is always associated with viral infection.

Hepatitis B
Between 10 and 30 percent of patients infected with hepatitis B virus will develop a transient arthritis. The arthritis typically involves the small joints of the hands in a symmetrical fashion, but it also can affect the shoulders, elbows, wrist, knees, ankles, and feet. Occasionally, the arthritis will spare the small joints and involve larger joints in an asymmetrical fashion. The joints may be red, hot, and swollen, or there may be no objective signs of inflammation. In addition to arthritis, tendinitis has been reported. Skin manifestations frequently accompany the arthritis. The rash is most often urticarial, but it may be maculopapular or even petechial [59]. It can occur on the trunk or the extremities. Both the arthritis and the rash tend to occur during the anicteric phase of the hepatitis [59]. Both last from days to about 3 weeks or when jaundice develops. No instance of chronic arthritis resulting from hepatitis B virus has been reported.

The pathogenesis of the arthritis may relate to circulating immune complexes. During the early stages of the disease, when the arthritis occurs, the hepatitis B surface antigen (HBsAg) is in excess. It binds to antibody, and the complex, because it contains primarily IgG1 and IgG3, binds complement. Therefore, complement levels are depressed both in the serum and in the synovial fluid. The typical white blood cell count in the synovial fluid will vary widely, but the mean count is approximately 20,000 cells/mm^3 with greater than 50 percent polymorphonuclear cells [59]. Cultures of the synovial fluid or tissue have been negative, but immunofluorescence and electron microscopic examinations of synovium in some cases have demonstrated virus particles within the tissue.

The arthritis associated with hepatitis B infection is self-limited. When active, it can be treated in most patients with aspirin or other nonsteroidal anti-inflammatory drugs.

Rubella

Rubella arthritis is the most common example of arthritis in association with a viral disease. In most series, 15 to 30 percent of patients with rubella develop arthritis [112]. Although it can occur in children and men, it is predominantly a disease of women. The arthritis typically involves the small joints of the hands and wrist in a symmetrical fashion. It also may be associated with a carpal tunnel syndrome. Symptoms generally occur a few days after the rash is seen and last for 3 to 4 weeks.

The pathogenesis of the arthritis may involve a direct infection, since virus has been cultured from the synovial fluid of a few patients. However, immune complexes also have been isolated from involved joints. The virus may serve as an antigenic component and when combined with immunoglobulin initiates an acute inflammatory response in the joint. The disease is self-limited and responds well to treatment with salicylates or nonsteroidal anti-inflammatory drugs.

Arthritis following rubella vaccine immunization occurs in 35 to 40 percent of women receiving live attenuated rubella virus vaccine [112]. The incidence of arthritis in children is much lower, in the range of 1 to 4 percent. The arthritis is similar to that seen following natural infection, but it does tend to last longer and may be associated with recurrent attacks. It is, however, eventually self-limited and not associated with chronic arthritis. Treatment is the same as for the natural infection.

Other Viral Infection

Adenovirus may be associated with rheumatic complaints, and they generally follow an acute upper respiratory infection. The arthralgias and arthritis are polyarticular in presentation, last only a few days to weeks, and resolve without sequelae [112].

Mumps arthritis may occur in 0.5 to 1 percent of patients with the disease. It is seen from 1 to 15 days after the onset of parotitis, is found primarily in the larger joints, and is also a self-limited disease [112].

Chronic Polyarticular Disease

RHEUMATOID ARTHRITIS

Rheumatoid arthritis is a chronic systemic disease with the major manifestation being a symmetrical synovitis that may lead to erosion and destruction of the joint cartilage, the supporting structures, and eventually bone. This will give rise to the typical joint deformities that are seen clinically and on radiographs.

Rheumatoid arthritis is the most common of the inflammatory rheumatic diseases. It occurs worldwide, with up to 3 percent of women and 1 percent of men being affected [78]. The age of onset varies from infancy to old age, with the peak between the ages of 35 and 45 years [78]. There is no racial predominance nor personality type and no true hereditary pattern, although there is an HLA relationship. HLA-DR4 is found three times as often in adult rheumatoid arthritis as in a control population of patients, suggesting that there may be some hereditary predisposition to the disease [115]. Of particular interest is the fact that the disease does not appear to have been in existence prior to the last few hundred years [3]. The explanation for this awaits the discovery of the etiology(ies) of the disease.

The onset of the arthritis, characterized by inflammation of arthrodial (synovial) joints, is highly variable. It may develop as an acute polyarthritis over the span of a few days or may have a more insidious onset with stiffness and arthralgias at the onset eventually developing into frank synovitis. It is very difficult, if not impossible, however, to diagnose rheumatoid arthritis in the absence of painful and swollen joints [76]. It is our feeling that if swelling is not observed within the first 6 to 12 months of disease, it is unlikely that the patient has rheumatoid arthritis.

The pattern of joint involvement is typically

symmetrical, with both small and large joints affected. Occasionally, however, a monarticular or oligoarticular onset will be seen. These latter are more commonly seen in the juvenile form of rheumatoid arthritis. Because this is a disease of synovial lining cells, all diarthrodial joints may be eventually involved. Included in these are the temporomandibular, sternoclavicular, and acromioclavicular joints, the facet joints of the spine, and rarely, the sacroiliac joints.

Involvement of two areas may pose life-threatening problems to the patient. The first is synovitis at the C1–C2 vertebral level. Chronic synovitis at this level may eventually erode through the transverse ligament, the ligament that stabilizes the upper cervical spine. If this occurs, the spinal column is able to move anteriorly or posteriorly and even superiorly. Because of the close proximity of the spinal cord and the brain, serious neurologic problems can occur. Lateral radiographs of the cervical spine in flexion and extension can alert the physician to the presence of this problem, which, if severe, may require surgical stabilization. Less severe displacement may respond to the use of a firm cervical collar [76].

The second area of joint involvement that is potentially life-threatening is involvement of the cricoarytenoid joint. This joint sits in direct apposition to the vocal cords. If inflamed on a chronic basis, the synovium will eventually fix to the vocal cords and immobilize them. If the vocal cords are fixed in an abducted position, patients will report that they are chronically hoarse. They also may have sore throats during the acute inflammatory process. If the cords become fixed in an adducted position, the vocal chink becomes very narrow. In such patients, a superimposed upper respiratory infection may cause respiratory distress and precipitate a respiratory emergency requiring tracheostomy. If a patient reports episodes of stridor, the cords should be observed. If they are severely narrowed, thought should be given to a partial arytenoidectomy. Other synovial structures, such as tendon sheaths and bursae, can be involved with rheumatoid inflammation, particularly around the shoulder, elbow, wrist,

and knee. Tenosynovitis, especially of the extensor tendons of the hand and wrists, may lead to tendon rupture. Involvement of the volar side of the wrist frequently causes the carpal tunnel syndrome (median nerve compression). Rapid distention of a joint capsule or bursa may cause it to rupture. The typical example of this in rheumatoid arthritis is a ruptured popliteal (Baker's) cyst. The synovial fluid that leaks from the cyst dissects down the posterior leg causing swelling and pain. Clinically, it may resemble thrombophlebitis, but it can be clearly differentiated by an arthrogram or ultrasound of the calf [76]. The preferred treatment is injection of the knee with a corticosteroid preparation.

The clinical course of rheumatoid arthritis in the adult tends to follow one of three patterns. The first is a monocyclic course, in which the disease is active for 6 months to 2 years [86]. It then tends to go into remission and does not recur. About a third of patients follow this pattern. The second and most common pattern is the polycyclic course, occurring in 50 percent or more of patients [46]. In these patients, the disease exhibits remissions and exacerbations with slowly progressive changes in the joints. The third type, the progression pattern, occurs in 10 to 15 percent of patients, who never seem to experience a true remission of their disease [46]. These are the patients with the most significant joint deformities, and they are also the ones who seem to experience more of the extra-articular manifestations of the disease.

The extra-articular manifestations of rheumatoid arthritis tend to occur later in the course of the disease and correlate with a number of laboratory findings [42, 58], including the following:

1. High-titer rheumatoid factor
2. Serum immune complexes
3. Decreased serum complement
4. Eosinophilia

Specific extra-articular manifestations [42, 46, 58, 76] of rheumatoid arthritis include the following:

1. *Rheumatoid nodules.* These subcutaneous nodules are usually found over extensor surfaces or pressure points or along tendons or tendon sheaths. They occur in 25 to 35 percent of patients and are highly specific for the disease. Histologically, the nodule resembles an infectious or foreign-body granuloma.

2. *Lymphadenopathy.* Lymph node enlargement is common in rheumatoid arthritis, especially in those patients with active disease. There are two specific syndromes associated with rheumatoid arthritis and lymphocytic hyperplasia. Felty syndrome is characterized by diffuse lymphadenopathy, splenomegaly, neutropenia, an increased incidence of vasculitic skin ulcers, and recurrent infections. Sjögren's syndrome is also characterized by lymphadenopathy and the sicca syndrome: dry eyes and dry mouth because of infiltration of the lacrimal and salivary glands with lymphocytes. The lymphadenopathy in Sjögren's syndrome may even mimic malignant lymphoma. On rare occasions, especially in Sjögren's syndrome not associated with a connective-tissue disease, a malignant lymphoma may develop.

3. *Pleuropulmonary.* Pleuritis and/or pleural effusions are the most common pleural manifestations of rheumatoid arthritis. Pleuritis, when present, generally occurs during periods of activity of the arthritis. Pleural effusions are generally asymptomatic unless the effusion becomes so massive as to cause respiratory problems. The pleural effusions are characterized by a high protein content (serous exudates), mildly inflammatory white blood cells with either mononuclear or polymorphonuclear cells predominating, and a low glucose content, generally below 20 mg% and occasionally 0 mg% [42]. Complement levels in the pleural effusions are depressed, suggesting that immune complexes may play a role in the pathogenesis of the effusion.

Pulmonary involvement may be manifest either by the presence of rheumatoid nodules in the lung parenchyma or by pulmonary fibrosis. The pulmonary nodules may be single or multiple and may on occasion cavitate. Unfortunately, even though most nodules occur in rheumatoid patients who have peripheral nodulosis, there is no absolute way to differentiate them from a neoplasm, short of lung biopsy. Interstitial fibrosis, bibasilar in most cases, occurs in about 5 percent of patients with rheumatoid arthritis. It is generally only an incidental finding, but occasionally it will progress to respiratory insufficiency.

4. *Cardiac.* Involvement of the heart in rheumatoid arthritis is commonly reported at autopsy but rarely is a significant clinical problem. Pericarditis is the most frequent finding (35 to 50 percent) on autopsy, but it is detected in less than 10 percent of living rheumatoid arthritis patients and even in this latter group it is rarely symptomatic. An occasional patient is seen who requires surgical decortication secondary to chronic constrictive pericarditis.

5. *Ocular.* Eye involvement in rheumatoid arthritis stems from two distinct causes. Most common is the patient who complains of an irritating dryness in the eye, i.e., the patient with Sjögren's syndrome secondary to lymphocytic infiltration of the lacrimal glands and dry eyes. The second, less common, but potentially more serious eye involvement occurs in the patient who develops episcleritis, a diffuse hyperemia of the deeper vessels. This lesion is related to the presence of rheumatoid nodules. Occasionally, the granuloma will involve the sclera, causing widespread necrosis with thinning of the sclera and perforation of the eye (scleromalacia perforans).

6. *Vasculitis.* Vasculitis occurs in a small percentage of patients with long-standing, but frequently inactive arthritis. It may involve the small vessels of the digits, ranging from small skin infarctions to ulcers and frank gangrene of the digit. It also may involve larger vessels, i.e., the nutrient vessels of peripheral nerves, which can result in loss of sensory and motor functions of the nerve. Clinically, this manifests by such findings as wrist drop (radial nerve) or foot drop (posterior tibial nerve). Pulmonary hypertension secondary to vasculitis also has been described. These complications are most difficult to treat, frequently requiring cytotoxic therapy in an attempt to arrest the vasculitis.

Laboratory Findings

HEMATOLOGY. Anemia is present in most patients with long-standing rheumatoid arthritis [42]. It may be on the basis of iron deficiency secondary to the gastrointestinal blood loss associated with the medications used in the treatment of the disease. Most often, however, the anemia is the anemia of chronic disease with a low serum iron level and a low serum iron-binding capacity.

Leukopenia is seen in those patients with Felty's syndrome, and a leukocytosis may be seen in patients with very active disease. Typically, however, the white blood cell count is normal.

SEROLOGY. *Rheumatoid factor:* Rheumatoid factors are immunoglobulins of any class that possess antigenic specificity for the FC fragment of IgG. Although they have been found among all classes of immunoglobulins, only IgM rheumatoid factor is measured in clinical practice. The most common test for measuring rheumatoid factor uses IgG-coated latex beads. Serum is incubated with these beads, and aggregation is noted if rheumatoid factor is present in the serum. Quantitation is performed by serially diluting the serum, with the final result expressed as the highest dilution yielding detectable aggregation.

Rheumatoid factor is not specific for rheumatoid arthritis. About 80 percent of adult patients with rheumatoid arthritis will have rheumatoid factor in their sera—generally in a titer of over 1 : 160 dilution. Rheumatoid factor is also found, however, in other connective-tissue diseases, including systemic lupus erythematosus (30 percent), Sjögren's syndrome (79 percent), and scleroderma (20 percent) [46]. Rheumatoid factors also are found to various degrees in nonrheumatic illnesses, especially chronic infections, as well as in the "normal" healthy population. The incidence of rheumatoid factor in the population over 65 years of age will reach up to 20 percent. In almost all instances, however, the titer will be low.

Antinuclear antibodies (ANA): Autoantibodies directly against cell nuclei are characteristically seen in systemic lupus erythematosus and will be discussed in more detail under that heading. They are also seen in up to two-thirds of patients with rheumatoid arthritis, being most prevalent in those with active long-standing disease. They are generally found in lower titers than what is seen in systemic lupus erythematosus.

Complement: Complement levels are depressed in synovial fluid and in effusions (pleural or pericardial) in rheumatoid arthritis. Serum complement levels are normal except in those patients with widespread rheumatoid vasculitis [57].

Synovial fluid: Rheumatoid synovial fluid is characterized as an inflammatory fluid. The average white blood cell count varies from 10,000 to 15,000 cells/mm^3 with a predominance of polymorphonuclear cells. During very active disease, the white blood cell count may rise to more than 50,000 cells/mm^3. As noted earlier, synovial fluid complement levels are reduced.

Radiographic Findings

Early in the course of the disease the only findings on x-ray will be soft-tissue swelling and periarticular osteoporosis. As the disease progresses, however, there is loss of cartilage space and juxta-articular erosions. Later stages of disease show complete loss of the articular cartilage, bony destruction, and deformity of the joint [46]. Secondary degenerative changes may eventually be superimposed on the inflammatory changes of rheumatoid arthritis.

Treatment

Since there is no definitive cure for rheumatoid arthritis, the goals of treatment are to reduce the pain, prevent deformities, and maintain function. To this end, treatment should involve the patient and the patient's family as well as the physician. Additionally, there may be times during the illness when physical and occupational therapists, social workers, visiting nurses, and orthopedic or hand surgeons may need to participate in the care of the patient.

One accepted approach to the treatment of this disease is to follow the pyramidal plan shown in Table 8-9, beginning at the base and progressing to the apex of the pyramid as necessary [46, 98].

Table 8–9. *Pyramidal Treatment Plan for Rheumatoid Arthritis*

			Investigational therapy and procedures				
		Immunosuppressive	Reconstructive surgery	Rehabilitation center			
	Penicillamine	Sulphasalazine	Methotrexate	Oral steroids	Preventive surgery		
	Auranofin (oral gold)	Gold salts	Antimalarials	Nonnarcotic analgesics	Intra-articular steroids	Orthopedic devices	
Education: patient, family, society	Heat, cold	Therapeutic exercise	Occupational therapy	Emotional, joints, systemic rest	Nutrition	Salicylates to tolerance	Nonsteroidal anti-inflammatory drugs

Table 8–10. *Nonsteroidal Anti-Inflammatory Drugs*

Drug	Daily dosage	Frequency per day
Ibuprofen	1600–3200 mg	4
Indomethacin	75–150 mg	3
Naproxen	500–1500 mg	2
Tolmetin	800–2000 mg	3
Sulindac	200–400 mg	2
Meclofenamate sodium	300–400 mg	4
Piroxicam	10–20 mg	1

Salicylates are usually used as the first medication because of their cost and equal efficacy to the nonsteroidal anti-inflammatory drugs. Because of toxicity, however, most patients will require a trial with one or more of the newer nonsteroidal anti-inflammatory drugs [118]. There are numerous drugs of this class on the market with more to be approved in the near future. A partial list of nonsteroidal anti-inflammatory drugs and their dosages as used in rheumatoid arthritis is shown in Table 8-10.

If the patient fails to respond to nonsteroidal anti-inflammatory drugs within a few months, it is wise to progress to the slower-acting but generally more effective medications. The drugs, either auranofin or oral gold, the antimalarials, or the injectable gold salts, are used in addition to salicylates or nonsteroidal anti-inflammatory drugs. These drugs require 4 to 6 months to achieve maximal benefit, but 50 to 65 percent of rheumatoid patients will benefit from their use.

If the arthritis still remains active, the next level of medication should be considered. Penicillamine and sulphasalazine are also slow-acting agents that seem to have about the same efficacy as the three previous agents but may have more toxicity. Oral corticosteroids are effective, but their long-term use is significantly limited because of the multiple steroid side effects. Methotrexate, either by intramuscular injection or orally, is the newest drug in this category. Given in three divided doses at a total weekly dose of 15 mg or less, it appears to be very useful in alleviating persistent synovitis. At these lower dosages, side effects to date have been generally acceptable.

In patients with the most aggressive disease, especially those with vasculitis, the use of other immunosuppressive agents, especially cyclophosphamide, has been necessary.

Finally, reconstructive orthopedic surgery has allowed many patients to continue to be active despite severe joint disease.

Prognosis
The course of rheumatoid arthritis is variable, with periods of exacerbation and remission. Approximately 65 percent of patients, however, will

have some degree of disability from their disease [33]. Factors associated with a poorer prognosis include persistent disease for more than 1 year in a person less than 30 years of age, presence of subcutaneous nodules or other extra-articular manifestations, sustained disease despite adequate treatment, and high titers of rheumatoid factor.

AXIAL ARTHROPATHIES

The axial arthropathies can be placed into two categories due to similar physical findings in each category:

Category I:
  A. Ankylosing spondylitis
  B. Enteropathic arthropathies:
    1. Ulcerative colitis
    2. Crohn's disease (regional enteritis, granulomatous colitis)
Category II:
  A. Reiter's disease
  B. Psoriatic arthropathy

There are terms used repeatedly in discussing these diseases that should be clearly understood by the reader before proceeding to the rest of this chapter:

Axial arthropathy: An arthritis involving the spine.
Ankylosis: Fusion of a joint as a result of a disease process, with fibrous or bony union across the joint.
Sacroiliitis: Inflammation of the sacroiliac joint.
Spondylitis: Inflammation of one or more vertebrae of the spine.
Osteophytes: A bony outgrowth.
Syndesmophyte: A bony outgrowth from a ligament in the spine, usually linking one vertebral body to the next.
Entheses: A ligamentous or articular-capsular attachment to the bone such as where the Achilles tendon attaches to the calcaneus.
Synchondrosis: A union between two bones formed by cartilage; examples are articulations formed by

vertebral bodies and the cartilaginous disk or the manubriosternal joints.

In general, these diseases are grouped together because they share certain characteristics [82]:

1. They have radiographic evidence of sacroiliitis.
2. Many have spondylitis.
3. Peripheral joint involvement usually occurs in the lower extremity.
4. They have enthesopathies—inflammation in areas of entheses commonly manifested by heel pain or by swollen fingers or toes (sausage digits), called dactylitis.
5. They are different from rheumatoid arthritis in that they are rheumatoid factor-negative, have no subcutaneous nodules, and the arthritis is usually not symmetrical.
6. These diseases tend to run in families.

Ankylosing Spondylitis (AS)

Ankylosing spondylitis is not a rare disease. The clinical prevalence of overt disease is about 0.1 percent. However, populations screened by x-rays have demonstrated that 1 percent may have this disease. Ankylosing spondylitis is predominantly a male disease (10 to 7 : 1 male-to-female ratio). The onset is in young adults 16 to 40 years old, but there is a juvenile form that may begin as early as 8 years of age [19]. Ankylosing spondylitis is very common in certain Native American tribes and is rare in Central Africa, and the incidence in Caucasians is between these two extremes.

Clinical history is very helpful. With five bits of information the diagnosis can be made with a 95 percent sensitivity and 85 percent specificity [17]:

1. The onset of back pain is insidious.
2. The back pain began before the age of 40.
3. The back pain has lasted over 3 months.
4. The pain is worse in the morning.
5. The pain is better with exercise.

The back pain is the most prominent presenting symptom, but over the course of the disease, 35 percent of patients also will have a peripheral arthritis. The peripheral joints most commonly involved are the hips and shoulders. As described later, extra-articular problems also occur.

PHYSICAL EXAMINATION. The back should be inspected, and one should look for an unusually straight back or a humped back. The range of motion may be severely limited in all directions. A special test to measure this limitation of motion is the Schoeber test. The patient stands straight up and a mark is made at the sacral dimples; 10 cm up from this mark a second mark is made. The patient bends over and the distance between the two marks is measured again. This should measure 15 cm. Less is abnormal. It is not unusual for a patient with ankylosing spondylitis to measure less than 11 cm while bending over. As the disease progresses, the spine may fuse slowly from the lumbar spine up to the cervical spine. A crude way to measure this is the occiput-to-wall examination. The patient presses his or her back against a wall and then is asked to touch his or her head to the wall. Measure the distance of the occiput from the wall as an indication of spinal involvement [19].

Owing to the synchondrosis in ankylosing spondylitis, the ribs may not move where they are connected to the sternum. Chest expansion, therefore, may be less than 1 inch, whereas 2 inches is normal [121]. Sacroiliac involvement can be difficult to assess clinically. Pressing on the pelvic bones from the front or sides may elicit diffuse buttock pain representative of inflammation in the sacroiliac joint [19]. The Faber test, i.e., flexion, abduction, and extension with rotation of the leg, also elicits sacroiliac pain.

Many extra-articular manifestations can occur [19, 82]:

1. Constitutional symptoms such as fatigue, weight loss, and low-grade fever.
2. Conjunctivitis or iritis.
3. Apical pulmonary fibrosis, often confused with early tuberculosis, can be seen in patients with severe disease.
4. Cardiovascular disease is manifested by heart block or aortic valve disease.
5. Neurologic problems related to spinal inflammation and ankylosis include the cauda equina syndrome (buttock pain and/or sensory and motor impairment due to spinal entrapment of nerves), C1–C2 subluxation, and spinal fracture.

LABORATORY TESTS. The erythrocyte sedimentation rate is elevated in most patients with active disease. The alkaline phosphatase level is sometimes elevated. The rheumatoid factor and antinuclear antibodies are usually negative in all the groups with axial arthropathies. The HLA-B27, which is discussed below, is positive in about 90 percent of Caucasians.

The test that is most diagnostic is roentgenograms of the sacroiliac joint and the spine. Over time, all patients will have some evidence of sacroiliitis. In ankylosing spondylitis, the involvement is typically bilateral, affecting the lower two-thirds of the sacroiliac joint [19]. The evidence on radiographs can be subtle, with joint space widening, to juxta-articular sclerosis and joint space loss, to complete ankylosis of the joint. In the early phase of ankylosing spondylitis, the spine may show squaring of the vertebrae with "shiny corners." Later, syndesmophyte formation becomes prominent and will progress in a minority of patients such that the spine fuses into one solid bone (bamboo spine) [121]. The fusion process starts in the lumbar spine and progresses cranially such that 20 percent of patients have cervical spine fusion. Peripheral joint space loss and erosions can be seen, mainly in the hips. Very early in the disease the radiographs can appear normal, but bone scan or CT scan can detect abnormalities.

Colitic Arthropathies

Ulcerative colitis and Crohn's disease are both associated with an arthritis that appears identical to ankylosing spondylitis. Some patients present with a more peripheral arthritis instead of a predominantly central arthritis. The axial type of arthritis is seen in 5 to 8 percent of patients with ulcerative colitis and Crohn's disease [83]. The peripheral arthritis is more prevalent, being seen in 9 to 12 percent of patients with ulcerative colitis and up to 20 percent of patients with Crohn's disease [83]. There is a male predominance in the central arthritis presentation (2 : 1), but the peripheral arthritis favors no sex.

The axial arthritis associated with colitis appears in every way as ankylosing spondylitis. The arthritis can precede the bowel disease by years, and the arthritis does not parallel the course of the bowel disease.

In contrast, the peripheral arthritis is more common in ulcerative colitis patients with very active bowel disease. Peripheral arthritis precedes the disease in only 10 percent of patients [83]. The typical peripheral attack occurs as an asymmetrical lower extremity arthritis coming on very quickly, reaching a peak of pain in 24 hours, and lasting 2 months, although it may persist indefinitely [83]. This arthritis is usually evident within 5 years of the onset of bowel disease.

The extra-articular manifestations particularly associated with the colitic arthropathies include the following:

1. Clubbing of the fingers, where the finger becomes more bulbous and the angle of the nail is lost
2. Pyoderma gangrenosum, a necrotizing skin lesion
3. Stomatitis, ulcers in the mouth
4. Uveitis, inflammation of the eye
5. Erythema nodosum, skin lesion consisting of raised macules

LABORATORY TESTS. A complete blood count and erythrocyte sedimentation rate should be assessed, since these patients are usually anemic and the sedimentation rate is usually elevated. The synovial fluid is a class II fluid. The HLA-B27 is positive in over 70 percent of ulcerative colitis patients and over 55 percent of Crohn's disease patients who have the axial arthropathy type of presentation [83]. Patients with peripheral arthritis have no increased incidence of HLA-B27.

Radiographs of colitic arthritis patients can be indistinguishable from those of patients with ankylosing spondylitis. They can have symmetrical sacroiliitis and similar spinal involvement. The patients with peripheral joint disease have little erosive disease. Periostitis (new bone formation) may be seen.

Reiter's Syndrome
Reiter's syndrome is an asymmetrical, predominantly lower extremity arthropathy that is associated with one or more of the following:

1. Urethritis or cervicitis
2. Diarrhea
3. Eye disease manifested by conjunctivitis or anterior uveitis.
4. Mucocutaneous disease of balanitis (penile skin rash), oral ulcers, or a skin rash on the palms or soles called keratoderma blennorrhagicum

The patient may have all these signs (a third of patients) or some of these signs (a third of patients) or may just have a typical arthritis (a third of patients). The prevalence is similar to ankylosing spondylitis, about 0.1 percent of the adult population, but the male predominance is even greater in Reiter's syndrome: 10 to 50 : 1. The disease most commonly occurs in people 16 to 40 years of age [20].

CLINICAL HISTORY. The clinical history can be very helpful. About two-thirds of patients relate having an infectious diarrhea or infectious urethritis days to weeks prior to the onset of the arthritis. Organisms causing diarrhea and related to the induction of Reiter's syndrome include *Shigella flexneri, Salmonella typhimurium enteritidis, Yersinia enterocolitica, Campylobacter fetus,* and *Klebsiella pneumoniae* [2, 37, 62, 66]. The patient may have had an infectious urethritis associated with *Neisseria gonorrhoeae* or *Chlamydia trachomatis* [2, 62]. In a third of patients there is no known antecedent infectious cause.

The arthritis, in general, has an acute onset in a lower extremity joint, predominantly the knees and ankles [37, 62]. This arthritis may be short-lived or, as is more frequent, persistent or recurrent. Back pain is seen in about half the patients.

Enthesopathies are prominent in these patients. Especially frequent is heel pain related to a plantar fasciitis or Achilles tendinitis. Dactylitis is also common [20].

PHYSICAL EXAMINATION. A careful physical examination should search for evidence of arthritis, sacroiliitis, enthesopathies, and the extra-articular manifestations (see below). The joints involved tend to be asymmetrical lower extremities, predominantly the knees. The arthritis can be florid with a large effusion and much pain on movement. Evidence of sacroiliitis is seen in 50 to 70 percent of patients. The heel and Achilles tendon should be palpated for signs of inflammation and tenderness. The fingers and/or toes may be swollen. In the United States, 80 percent of patients have evidence of a urethritis some time in the course of their disease [20]. Conjunctivitis is seen in half these patients and may precede the arthritis. Mucocutaneous lesions include painless oral ulcers, balanitis (a penile skin rash), and bumps or hyperkeratotic lesions on the palms and soles called keratoderma blennorrhagicum [20]. This latter rash resembles pustular psoriasis. Nail changes, including pitting and onycholysis, are seen in 10 percent. If the disease progresses, cardiac involvement, including aortic insufficiency, heart block, pericarditis, and myocarditis, can occur. A chronic uveitis can develop that, if left untreated, can lead to blindness. Rarely, fusion of the spine is seen.

LABORATORY TESTS. If the patient is having symptoms of urethritis or diarrhea, an attempt should be made to culture one of the implicated organisms from a urethral or cervical swab or from the stool. A mild anemia, leukocytosis, and elevated erythrocyte sedimentation rate are often present. The synovial fluid is generally class II. Characteristically, the complement level is elevated in patients with Reiter's syndrome and is normal to low in most other types of synovitis. The antinuclear antibody and rheumatoid factors are negative. The HLA-B27 is positive in 50 to 80 percent of whites and in 45 to 50 percent of blacks [115].

Radiographs can show osteoporosis, joint space loss, and erosions. Periostitis at tendon insertions with subtle erosions can be seen. Radiographs of patients with central arthritis usually show an asymmetrical sacroiliitis, but it occasionally is symmetrical. There are distinct syndesmophytes of the spine; they are generally large, asymmetrical, and nonmarginal [20].

Psoriatic Arthritis

Psoriatic arthritis is a seronegative inflammatory arthritis associated with psoriasis. Psoriasis is seen in 2 percent of the population, and 7 percent of these patients have arthritis [60]. Skin lesions of psoriasis usually begin at ages 16 to 20 and 45 to 55. The arthritis associated with psoriasis begins at ages 35 to 50 [81].

CLINICAL HISTORY. The psoriatic skin lesions usually precede the arthritis, although in up to 15 percent of patients the arthritis can herald the skin lesions. The onset is acute in half the patients [81]. A family history of psoriasis is found in a third of patients.

PHYSICAL EXAMINATION. Psoriatic arthritis is divided into five subgroups of disease process. These can be seen in "pure" form, but it is more common that these subgroups overlap [60, 80, 81]:

1. Spondylitic type of involvement is seen similar to Reiter's syndrome (5 to 20 percent of patients). There is asymmetrical sacroiliac involvement. Syndesmophytes, although unusual, may occur and arise from the lateral and anterior surfaces of the vertebral bodies instead of the margins.
2. Distal interphalangeal joints are predominantly, although rarely (5 percent) exclusively, involved. This arthritis correlates best with abnormal nail changes.
3. The arthritis mutilans type is fortunately rare (5 percent). Widespread destruction and dissolution of bones in the hands and feet are seen.

4. A rheumatoid arthritis pattern of involvement with symmetrical polyarthritis is seen, except that the rheumatoid factor is negative and the patient has psoriasis.
5. A single or asymmetrical oligoarthritis is seen in the majority of patients.

Sausage digits are especially common in this axial arthropathy. The skin rash may be diffuse, guttate, or pustular. It also may be subtle and seen only in hidden areas such as behind the ear, under the arm, or on the buttocks. Nail changes are common. More than 20 nail pits on a hand is distinctly unusual in control subjects, but these are seen in 80 percent of patients with psoriatic arthritis. Onycholysis is also common where the nail leaves its nail bed. Rarely, the other extra-articular manifestations described above are seen.

LABORATORY TESTS. The laboratory blood tests and synovial fluid analysis are similar to the other axial arthropathies. The uric acid level is elevated 20 percent of the time [81]. The HLA studies correlate with the type of arthritis presentation [60]:

1. Sacroiliitis and spondylitis associated arthritis: HLA-B27 is positive 90 percent of the time.
2. Peripheral arthritis is associated with HLA-B38.
3. Symmetrical rheumatoid-type arthritis is associated with HLA-DR4.
4. Psoriasis alone is associated with HLA-B13 and B17.

Roentgenographic studies can be very helpful in making the diagnosis of psoriatic arthritis [80, 81]. Hand films may demonstrate distal interphalangeal joint involvement with erosions and expansion of the base of the terminal phalanx. The distal interphalangeal joint can have a virtually pathognomonic appearance of a pencil pointing into a cup. The distal tufts of the finger can be absorbed. Arthritis mutilans demonstrates severe joint destruction and bony absorption throughout the hand. The sacroiliitis and syndesmophytes were already described above.

The HLA-B27 Story

Human leukocyte antigens (HLA) are polymorphic cell surface glycoproteins with genetic determinants on the short arm of chromosome 6. Within this HLA region lie six currently well-defined HLA loci: HLA-A, HLA-B, HLA-C, HLA-DR, HLA-DQ, and HLA-DP. Antigens determined by the A, B, and C loci are found on the surface of virtually every human cell. HLA-DR is on the surface of selected cells involved in immune responses (macrophages, certain T cells, and B cells). Every person possesses two HLA regions, one paternally and one maternally derived. HLA antigens are autosomal-dominant.

It is now recognized that HLA-B27 is probably more than one molecule, but none of the more specific molecules is more associated with the axial arthropathies than any other. In 1973, a very strong association between HLA-B27 and ankylosing spondylitis was discovered. Since then, innumerable studies have demonstrated the following associations among Caucasians [60, 82, 115]:

Disease	Range of Percent Positive
Controls	4–14
Ankylosing spondylitis	81–100
Reiter's syndrome	57–96
Inflammatory bowel disease	50–100
Juvenile arthritis	39–42
Psoriasis and arthritis	7–43

There are, however, a few caveats to keep in mind. Not all patients with HLA-B27 develop disease. The association is less strong among blacks and Japanese. Finally, the HLA-B27 test is generally not helpful in making the clinical diagnosis of one of the axial arthropathies, and it is our opinion that this test should be ordered only in difficult or confusing cases where all the information that can be gathered is helpful or for genetic counseling [18].

Treatment of the Axial Arthropathies

In general, the goals in treating the axial arthropathies are to control pain and prevent deformities. Good posture is emphasized in work and in daily activities. Avoidance of occupations which necessitate frequent bending should be recommended, and the patient should be counseled on sleeping on a firm mattress. Active aerobic exercise is beneficial in these patients, especially exercise that promotes good posture and promotes hip and shoulder range of motion. Swimming is an ideal exercise for this type of arthritis.

The nonsteroidal anti-inflammatory drugs are used in all the axial arthropathies. Any of this group of drugs is useful, but typically, indomethacin is used first because it is the most consistently effective nonsteroidal anti-inflammatory drug. Intra-articular steroids are used for persistent peripheral joint arthritis. If over time a peripheral joint becomes destroyed, joint replacement can be very useful.

In Reiter's syndrome, antibiotics are used for infectious agents associated with this disease. For particularly severe, unresponsive peripheral arthritis, low-dose methotrexate in one weekly dose may control the disease. In psoriatic arthritis, the skin lesions should be treated. For patients who have a rheumatoid-like pattern of involvement, standard disease-modifying agents used to treat rheumatoid arthritis can be used with good success. Methotrexate and azathioprine have been used for severe disease.

Osteoarthritis

Osteoarthritis or degenerative joint disease in its primary form affects peripheral and central articulation and is characterized by degeneration of cartilage, subchondral bone thickening, eburnation or marbling of bone, marginal spur formation, and subarticular bone cysts. A *heritable primary form* involving Heberden's nodes and multiple joints and occurring around menopause has been reported [64]. Inflammatory erosive forms, primarily involving the hands, also have been seen.

The term *secondary osteoarthritis* is used if there are known direct causes of the arthritis. Included in this category are the osteoarthritic problems secondary to previous inflammatory joint disease, metabolic or endocrine diseases, previous trauma to the joint, and those joints with developmental abnormalities and subsequent biomechanical dysfunction [68].

Osteoarthritis affects primarily weight-bearing joints, the lumbar and cervical spines, and the distal interphalangeal and proximal interphalangeal joints of the hands. It is primarily a disease of cartilage, with early changes limited to the cartilage matrix. Eventually there is deterioration of the collagen fibers with loss of the cartilage. Subchondral bone is also affected, and as the body attempts to repair the damage with new bone formation, the characteristic marginal spurs or osteophytes are formed [88].

Clinical History

Symptoms, localized to the joints involved, are pain, particularly on motion and weight-bearing, mild stiffness after periods of rest, and aching at times of changes in the weather. Signs of inflammation are uncommon except in a severe form known as erosive osteoarthritis. Crepitation, limitation of motion, malalignment, and deformities are seen in later stages of the disease. Tenderness and effusions may occur, especially after trauma or vigorous overuse of the involved joint. Heberden's (distal interphalangeal) and Bouchard's (proximal interphalangeal) nodes in the hands are common, especially in females, and they tend to occur in families.

Laboratory Tests

Laboratory studies disclose no abnormalities; the erythrocyte sedimentation rate is normal, and the rheumatoid factor is usually negative. The synovial fluid characteristically is noninflammatory, except when hemorrhage or traumatic synovitis supervenes. Radiographic evaluation shows the absence of osteoporosis and marginal erosions, but subchondral sclerosis, cysts, marginal osteophyte formation, and, in time, irregular loss of cartilage space occur [13].

Treatment

The objectives of treatment are to relieve pain, minimize disability, and delay progression of the disease. Correction of factors producing excessive joint strain, i.e., obesity or differences in leg length, are essential. Physical measures, especially rest, heat, exercise, and supportive devices, are helpful in selected patients.

Mechanical causes of pain without much secondary inflammation may respond well to analgesics alone. There is good evidence, however, for mild inflammation in most patients, with up to 30 percent having calcium pyrophosphate dehydrate or hydroxyapatite crystals found in synovial fluid or in the surrounding tissues. Therefore, nonsteroidal anti-inflammatories may be quite beneficial (Table 8-11).

Because of the potential renal toxicity of these drugs, careful follow-up of renal function should be done, especially in the elderly.

Intra-articular corticosteroid injections may be used two to three times a year in any one joint if medication has not given substantial relief.

If severe pain or disability persists despite optimal medical therapy and roentgenograms show progression of disease, surgery should be considered. The three procedures most often utilized are arthroscopic debridement to remove loose bodies, realignment procedures, or total joint replacement.

Table 8–11. Nonsteroidal Anti-Inflammatory Drugs in Osteoarthritis

Drug	Daily dose	Frequency per day
Salicylates	1.8–3.6 gm	3–6
Indomethacin (Indocin)	50–100 mg	2–4
Ibuprofen	1200–3600 mg	3–4
Naproxen (Naprosyn)	250–1000 mg	2
Sulindac (Clinoril)	200–400 mg	2
Meclofenamate sodium (Meclomen)	300–400 mg	2
Piroxicam (Feldene)	10–20 mg	1

Systemic Disease

Systemic Lupus Erythematosus

Systemic lupus erythematosus (SLE) is a multisystem disease of unknown etiology characterized by the presence of multiple autoantibodies that participate in immunologically mediated tissue injury [25]. Of the connective-tissue diseases (CTD), it is second in occurrence only to rheumatoid arthritis, with an incidence of systemic lupus erythematosus in the United States of 7.6 cases per 100,000 population per year. This disease occurs more commonly in females (9 : 1 female-to-male preponderance), but this marked difference occurs only after puberty [91]. It is more prevalent in black females aged 15 to 64 years in the United States, in whom there is 1 case per 245; in comparison, the rate in all females aged 15 to 64 years is 1 case per 700 [91].

Estrogens appear to play a role in this increased prevalence in females because (1) there are reported cases in which monozygotic twins were discordant for systemic lupus erythematosus, with the nonaffected twin having undergone castration at an early age; (2) oral contraceptive therapy increases the risk of a flare in systemic lupus erythematosus patients; and (3) the disease is associated with Klinefelter's syndrome, in which there is evidence for persistent estrogenic stimulation [66].

There also appears to be some genetic predisposition to the disease. In one report of 16 pairs of monozygotic twins, 11 of the pairs were concordant for clinical systemic lupus erythematosus and only 5 pairs were discordant. Additionally, there appears to be an increased percentage of

Table 8–12. Criteria for the Classification
of Systemic Lupus Erythematosus (1982)

1. Malar rash
2. Discoid lupus
3. Photosensitivity
4. Oral ulcers
5. Arthritis
6. Proteinuria (>0.5 gm per day) or cellular casts
7. Seizures or psychosis
8. Pleuritis or pericarditis
9. Hemolytic anemia, leukopenia, lymphopenia, or thrombocytopenia
10. Antibody to DNA or antibody to Sm or false-positive STS
11. Positive fluorescent antinuclear antibody (FANA)

two of the histocompatibility locus antigens (HLA-DR2 and HLA-DR3) in patients with this disease [25].

In 1982, the American Rheumatism Association modified the preliminary criteria for the classification of systemic lupus erythematosus. The new classification is based on 11 criteria (Table 8-12). The diagnosis can be made if at least 4 of the 11 criteria are present serially or simultaneously during the period of observation.

The onset of systemic lupus erythematosus may mimic many other diseases, especially when only one organ system is initially involved. Thus thrombocytopenia may be present for months to years and diagnosed as idiopathic thrombocytopenic purpura (ITP) until involvement of other organ systems occurs and the correct diagnosis is made. Because of this and the fact that any organ system may be involved at the onset of the disease, we find it useful to consider each organ system individually.

CUTANEOUS MANIFESTATIONS

Up to 80 percent of patients will have skin involvement sometime in the course of their disease, with approximately 25 percent having cutaneous involvement as a presenting feature of the disease [91].

Skin lesions related to systemic lupus erythe-

matosus may be classified into three groups: chronic, subacute, and acute. Discoid lesions constitute the most common chronic form of skin disease, but a nodular panniculitis also may be seen. The subacute variety of skin disease occurs as a widespread erythematous superficial rash and, in contrast to the discoid lesion, does not scar. Acute forms of cutaneous lupus include the malar erythema (butterfly rash), a more widespread macular erythema, or a wide spectrum of cutaneous necrotizing vasculitis [91].

MUSCULOSKELETAL MANIFESTATIONS

Polyarticular joint pain is the most common feature of systemic lupus erythematosus, occurring in more than 90 percent of patients [91]. Characteristically, there is no evidence for inflammation, but it may be associated with swelling, tenderness, and limited range of motion, especially in the hands. Volar subluxation of the metacarpophalangeal joints resembling rheumatoid arthritis in lupus is termed Jaccoud's deformity. These anatomic derangements occur because of tendon laxity and intrinsic muscle tightness. Cartilage destruction, subchondral cysts, and erosions are not usual features of systemic lupus erythematosus.

LUNG INVOLVEMENT

Parenchymal and pleural involvement in lupus is common. Pleuritic chest pain, present at the time of diagnosis or at some time during the course of the disease, may occur in as many as 80 percent of patients. Pleural effusions occur in 15 to 40 percent. The pleural effusion is usually an exudate with an elevated white blood cell count (either lymphocytes or neutrophils). Glucose levels in the fluid are normal, but complement levels are frequently depressed.

Parenchymal lung involvement in systemic lupus erythematosus may take either an acute or chronic form. Acute lupus pneumonitis frequently presents a dramatic clinical picture. The patient typically appears toxic, with fever, dyspnea, and hypoxemia. A dry cough is usually present, and despite the fact that there may be widespread, diffuse alveolar infiltration, physical findings in the lung may be minimal. Even with aggressive therapy, the mortality rate is high [91].

Massive pulmonary hemorrhage is also an acute complication of systemic lupus erythematosus, but fortunately, it is rare. A sudden decrease in hematocrit at the onset of respiratory distress may provide a valuable differential clue.

Other more chronic problems include diffuse interstitial pneumonitis, pulmonary hypertension, diaphragmatic involvement, fibrosing alveolitis, and infection [91, 108].

CARDIAC MANIFESTATIONS

Pericarditis is the most common manifestation, occurring in as many as a third of patients, often in association with pleuritis. Symptomatic pericardial effusions may be associated with clinical symptoms, but asymptomatic effusions can be detected by echocardiograph in as many as two-thirds of patients [114].

Clinical myocarditis is present in about 10 percent of patients, usually in conjunction with skeletal muscle inflammation. Verrucous endocarditis (Libman-Sacks disease) is often present on pathologic examination. The vegetations are usually found under the mitral valve leaflets in autopsy studies, but they rarely cause significant clinical problems.

Chronic coronary artery disease may occur as a result of small-vessel vasculitis, but it is much more commonly related to accelerated coronary atherosclerosis. Hyperlipidemia is a common risk factor for coronary artery disease, as are corticosteroid use, hypertension, and the nephrotic syndrome, all of which may be seen in systemic lupus erythematosus.

Conduction-system disease is only occasionally seen in adults with systemic lupus erythematosus, but newborn infants of mothers with lupus having anti-SS-A antibodies are at risk for congenital heart block [35].

GASTROINTESTINAL MANIFESTATIONS

Although gastrointestinal symptoms occur in over half of systemic lupus erythematosus patients, most are nonspecific and frequently related to the drugs used in treatment. Specific manifestations of lupus include serositis of the peritoneum with or without ascites, visceral vasculitis with bloody diarrhea, usually in the setting of cutaneous vasculitis and active lupus, and pancreatitis [53].

Clinically significant liver disease is unusual in systemic lupus erythematosus, although some patients seem predisposed to hepatotoxicity from aspirin and the nonsteroidal anti-inflammatory drugs [91].

NEUROPSYCHIATRIC MANIFESTATIONS

Central nervous system (CNS) disorders appear as the initial symptom of systemic lupus erythematosus in about 10 percent of patients, most frequently in the form of generalized motor seizures or psychiatric illness [1, 34]. Significant neuropsychiatric dysfunction occurs sometime during the course of disease in 50 percent of patients and overall is second to nephritis as the most common organ-related cause of death. Strokes, cranial neuropathies, or transverse myelitis possibly may be related to focal vascular events. The cause of organic mental syndromes, encephalopathy, chorea, or psychosis is less clear, but since they are often transient or reversible, it is unlikely that brain-cell death is involved.

RENAL MANIFESTATIONS

Nephritis is the initial manifestation in systemic lupus erythematosus in roughly 5 percent of patients, although 50 to 75 percent will ultimately have clinical renal involvement [90]. Despite this high frequency, death from renal failure occurs in fewer than 10 percent of patients. Clinical signs of significant renal disease include hypertension, nephrotic syndrome (or lesser degrees of proteinuria), hematuria, pyuria, active urinary sediment, and renal failure, which may present in an acute or chronic form [90].

A widely accepted histologic classification of lupus nephritis subdivides this disease into four categories: focal proliferative, mesangial, diffuse proliferative, and membranous glomerulonephritis. Patients with focal proliferative and mesangial glomerulonephritis may have active sediment or significant proteinuria, but they very rarely develop renal failure. Diffuse proliferative glomeru-lonephritis connotes widespread glomerular scle-rosis and proliferative change, frequently with accompanying interstitial tubular atrophy. If un-treated, the majority of these patients develop some degree of azotemia and consequently have a poorer prognosis [4]. Membranous glomerulo-nephritis resembles idiopathic membranous ne-phritis without cellular infiltration or necrosis by light microscopy. Although hypertension and frank azotemia are less common, profuse protein-uria is characteristic. This subgroup also carries a less favorable prognosis for long-term survival [90].

LABORATORY MANIFESTATIONS

The hallmark of systemic lupus erythematosus is the wide variety of autoantibodies produced by virtually all patients. These antibodies are directed not only against nuclear and cytoplasmic com-ponents, but also against circulating proteins and cell membranes [44] (Table 8-13). The LE cell phenomenon is an example of an autoantibody (antinucleoprotein antibody) interaction with an-tigen (nuclear debris), which in turn is engulfed by a phagocytic cell (the polymorphonuclear cell).

Detection of Antibodies

The detection of these antibodies requires a num-ber of special techniques. The fluorescent anti-nuclear antibody test is the most commonly used screening method. The antinuclear antibody test gives a number of fluorescent patterns, commonly classified as diffuse (homogeneous), rim (periph-eral), speckled, or nucleolar. These patterns may appear mixed, reflecting the detection of more than one type of antibody. The rim pattern is the most specific for systemic lupus erythematosus, but the speckled and diffuse patterns are seen more commonly [44]. Antinuclear antibodies de-tected by this technique are by no means diag-nostic for systemic lupus erythematosus, because they are also seen in high titers in mixed connec-tive-tissue disease and in low titers in many other rheumatic and nonrheumatic diseases [44]. Sub-typing the antinuclear antibodies requires other techniques available at specialized laboratories. Detecting these antibodies is useful for a number of reasons. Antibodies to Sm antigen are consid-

Table 8–13. *Classification of Antinuclear Antibodies**

Antibodies to DNA:	
Single stranded (ss) DNA	Present in many diseases
Double stranded (ds) DNA	High titers in 70 percent of patients with SLE; lower titers in other rheumatic diseases
Antinucleoprotein:	
Requires DNA, protein complex	LE cell in SLE and other rheumatic diseases
Antibodies to histones	Drug-induced LE and idiopathic SLE (30 percent of patients)
Antibodies to nonhistone proteins:	
RNP	High titer in MCTD, other rheumatic diseases
Sm	Probably specific for SLE (25 percent of patients)
SS-A (Ro)	"ANA-negative" SLE, other rheumatic diseases
SS-B (La)	Sjögren's syndrome, other rheumatic diseases
Scl-70	High specificity for PSS
PCNA	SLE (7 percent of patients)
Anticentromere antibodies	PSS, CREST syndrome
Antinucleolar antibodies	PSS, other rheumatic disease, especially in association with Raynaud's phenomenon

*Abbreviations: ANA = antinuclear antibodies; MCTD = mixed connective-tissue disease; PSS = progressive systemic scle-rosis; SLE = systemic lupus erythematosus; RNP = ribonucleoprotein; CREST = calcinosis, Raynaud's phenomenon, esoph-ageal hypomotility, sclerodactyly, and telangiectasia; PCNA = proliferating cell nuclear antigen; Sm = Smith antigen, named after the first patient in whom the antibody was described; SS-A, SS-B = Sjögren's syndrome antibodies A and B.

ered to be markers for systemic lupus erythematosus, whereas high-titer antibody to native double-stranded DNA (n-dsDNA) is seen almost exclusively in systemic lupus erythematosus [44]. Antibodies to n-DNA can be further subdivided according to immunoglobulin subclasses and also according to whether or not they fix complement. This appears to be clinically useful, since most patients with active lupus nephritis have IgG complement-fixing antibody to n-DNA. Furthermore, many patients with lupus nephritis demonstrate increased levels of anti-n-DNA antibody during an exacerbation of their renal disease. This is frequently accompanied by a decrease in levels of either total hemolytic serum complement or complement components, such as C3 or C4. There also have been suggestions that those patients with low titers of antibodies to n-DNA and specificities limited to Sm or ribonucleoprotein (RNP) have less renal involvement. Clinicians are certainly more comfortable with the diagnosis of systemic lupus erythematosus if antinuclear antibodies are detected, but approximately 5 percent of patients remain repeatedly negative. In many of these an anticytoplasmic antibody (SS-A) is detected.

In addition to the role in diagnosing systemic lupus erythematosus, antinuclear antibodies have been shown to play a significant role in producing organ damage, particularly in renal, skin, and vascular tissues. Complexes of anti-DNA antibody and DNA have been detected in the dermal-epidermal junction of the skin, in the glomerulus, and as free circulating immune complexes. The activation of complement by these complexes induces an inflammatory response that results in tissue damage [102]. Furthermore, antibodies bound to circulating proteins or cell membranes have been shown to produce functional defects in the respective proteins or cells (e.g., antibodies to white blood cells may be related to the leukopenia frequently seen in lupus) [122].

In addition to the presence of antinuclear antibodies, patients with systemic lupus erythematosus may have a number of hematologic abnormalities. These include leukopenia, thrombo-cytopenia, or a hemolytic anemia. Circulating anticoagulants occur in as many as 10 percent of patients. They rarely cause problems with bleeding, and in the patients with anticardiolipin antibodies, there is an increased risk for thrombosis of vessels.

COURSE AND PROGNOSIS

The course of systemic lupus erythematosus is characterized by periods of remissions and exacerbations over many years. Patients with a poorer prognosis are those with serious central nervous system disease, renal or myocardial disease, and those requiring high-dose corticosteroids and/or immunosuppressive therapy for long periods of time. More than 90 percent of patients will survive over 10 years. The leading cause of death in most series is now infections or other complications relating to treatment.

TREATMENT

Treatment depends on the severity of the disease and the organ systems involved. For those with mild disease and no serious organ involvement, symptomatic treatment with nonsteroidal anti-inflammatory drugs is recommended [113]. Antimalarials such as hydroxychloroquine (200 to 400 mg per day) have been used successfully in treating the arthralgias and arthritis, as well as the milder forms of skin rash, pleuritis, or pericarditis [113]. More serious disease with renal, central nervous system, pulmonary, pericardial, or hematologic involvement requires corticosteroids for treatment. Immunosuppressive agents such as azathioprine and cyclophosphamide may be required for very aggressive disease or for their steroid-sparing effects [4, 113].

Sjögren's Syndrome

Sjögren's syndrome may be defined as a combination of two of the following: (1) keratoconjunctivitis sicca (dry eyes), (2) xerostomia (dry mouth), and (3) a connective-tissue disease, usually rheumatoid arthritis or less frequently systemic lupus erythematosus, scleroderma, or dermatomyositis [100]. When a connective-tissue disease is present, the patient is considered to have secondary Sjögren's syndrome. Primary Sjögren's syndrome is diagnosed in the absence of another connective-tissue disease.

Pathologically, Sjögren's syndrome is characterized as a chronic inflammatory disease secondary to glandular infiltration of lymphocytes and plasma cells [61]. This results in diminished lacrimal and salivary gland secretion, which is known as the sicca complex. In some patients, the lymphoid infiltrates are more invasive than in others, resulting in destruction of the lymph node architecture [24]. These patients are considered to have a pseudolymphoma, and some may actually terminate in a true malignant lymphoma.

CLINICAL FEATURES

Clinical features include symptoms related to the dry eyes, dry mouth, and associated connective-tissue disease. Other findings include lymph node and glandular enlargement in over 50 percent of patients, muscle weakness, or lower extremity purpura [100]. Renal tubular acidosis also may be seen in a number of patients [61].

LABORATORY FINDINGS

Hypergammaglobulinemia is present in most patients. Rheumatoid factor, often in high titer, is seen in essentially all patients, even those without rheumatoid arthritis. Antinuclear antibodies, including antibody to SS-A (Ro) or SS-B (La), are also detected in 80 percent of primary Sjögren's syndrome patients [61]. Antibodies to SS-A (Ro) and SS-B (La) are detected to a lesser extent in secondary Sjögren's syndrome, especially in patients with rheumatoid arthritis.

TREATMENT

Treatment is purely symptomatic, using methylcellulose eye drops (artificial tears) for the dry eyes and lozenges plus frequent ingestion of fluids to relieve the symptoms of a dry mouth.

Scleroderma

Systemic sclerosis (scleroderma) is a multisystem disease characterized by varying degrees of proliferative changes in small arteries and arterioles, obliterative microvascular lesions, and fibrosis in the skin and internal organs [48, 89, 103]. Raynaud's phenomenon is the classic example of the widespread vascular abnormalities seen in scleroderma [103]. Defined as the paroxysmal ischemic episodes in the fingers and toes brought on by exposure to cold or emotional upset, Raynaud's phenomenon is present in over 95 percent of patients with scleroderma and may predate any other manifestations of the disease by as little as a few months or as long as 40 years [92, 117]. Scleroderma may exist in a mild form with calcinosis, Raynaud's phenomenon, esophageal involvement, sclerodactyly, and telangiectasia (the CREST syndrome) or may be rapidly progressive until the patient dies from renal or cardiopulmonary disease within months to a few years [92, 103]. The cause of scleroderma is not known, but it may be primarily a disease of blood vessels [48, 89]. Immunologic aberrations also play a role, and most recently, an increased number of mast cells have been found in the skin during early active disease [47].

CLINICAL HISTORY

The most common initial complaint is Raynaud's phenomenon, which may antedate any of the other signs or symptoms by months or years. Skin involvement is the characteristic finding in scleroderma, and it occurs early in the course of the disease [117]. It is possible for scleroderma to exist without skin involvement, but this is extremely uncommon (less than 1 percent of scleroderma patients). The skin involvement may be localized to the extremities (sclerodactyly) or may involve the entire body. The skin becomes tight and thick; hyperpigmentation or hypopigmentation, telangiectasia, soft-tissue calcification, and skin ulcers also may occur [117].

Musculoskeletal involvement, manifested by arthralgias or arthritis, occurs in over 75 percent of patients with classic scleroderma [94]. The characteristic feature of the synovial involvement is the abundance of fibrin deposition, which may cause a friction rub to be heard over the joints when they are moved [94]. Myositis may develop in 30 to 40 percent of patients, although it is not as severe as the myositis seen in dermatomyositis or polymyositis.

Gastrointestinal involvement leads to hypoperistalsis or aperistalsis in the esophagus with secondary reflux; stricture formation occurs as a late complication. Replacement of smooth muscle by fibrous tissue in the small bowel may result in hypotonia and malabsorption secondary to bacterial overgrowth. Involvement of the large bowel occurs in 25 percent of patients and is characterized by wide-mouthed diverticulae seen on barium enema studies [77, 89, 103].

Pulmonary involvement, caused by replacement of lung parenchyma with fibrous tissue, is manifested by shortness of breath and cough. Chest radiographs may show fibrosis at the lung bases; there is a decreased diffusing capacity in over 50 percent of patients. Progressive pulmonary disease may cause right-sided heart failure and lead to a cardiopulmonary death. Pulmonary hypertension may occur in the absence of parenchymal lung disease [77, 103].

Cardiac disease may be secondary to pulmonary involvement or may be related to fibrosis of the myocardium. Acute and chronic pericarditis does occur and is a poor prognostic sign, especially when associated with pericardial effusions [77, 89, 103].

Renal disease first manifested by proteinuria and then by a rapidly increasing serum creatinine level is the most fulminant of the scleroderma variants. It is often, although not always, associated with hypertension. Control of blood pressure, although difficult, will frequently reverse the course of the fulminant renal failure [48, 89]. Two of the newer antihypertensive drugs, captopril or enalapril, have been particularly useful in controlling the blood pressure. If the hypertension or renal failure is not controlled, however, dialysis or even renal transplantation may be necessary.

LABORATORY TESTS

Antinuclear antibodies are present in the sera of over 95 percent of patients with scleroderma [48]. By immunofluorescence, seven different patterns of antinuclear antibodies can be differentiated in either the nucleus or the nucleolus. Three of these antibodies have shown some specificity for scleroderma. The least specific is an antibody to 4S and 6S RNA. The antigen is a low-molecular-weight RNA present in the nucleolus. The second antibody is an antibody directed against the kinetochore at the centromere region of a chromosome. This antibody is present in about 35 percent of all scleroderma patients, but it correlates very strongly with the clinical scleroderma variant CREST syndrome. The third antibody is a marker antibody—found in 10 to 20 percent of scleroderma patients and rarely in other diseases. It is referred to as antibody to Scl-70, a 70,000 molecular weight chromosome-associated basic protein [44].

TREATMENT

There is no cure for scleroderma. Treatment is purely symptomatic, but it should be aggressive to try to minimize deformity and disability. This is especially true for the gastrointestinal tract, where treatment of acid reflux into the esophagus may prevent stricture formation.

Polymyositis/Dermatomyositis

The inflammatory myopathies are a group of diseases in which the muscles are diffusely damaged by a perivascular and/or interstitial infiltration of inflammatory cells, predominantly lymphocytes.

DIAGNOSIS

The five criteria for diagnosis listed in Table 8-14 include proximal muscle weakness [8, 9], which is the initial manifestation in greater than two-thirds of patients and is present overall in 98 percent at some time during the disease course. Patients will have difficulty in rising from a sitting position or in climbing stairs. Similarly, raising the arms over the head becomes very difficult.

Table 8–14. *Criteria for Diagnosis of the Inflammatory Myopathies*

1. Symmetrical muscle weakness
2. Electromyographic changes characterized by myositis
3. Elevated serum muscle enzymes
4. Muscle biopsy abnormalities
5. Characteristic dermatologic features

Source: From Bohan, A. and Peter, J. B. Medical Progress: Polymyositis and dermatomyositis, Part I. *N. Engl. J. Med.* 292: 344, 1975.

Table 8–15. *Classification of the Inflammatory Myopathies*

1. Primary idiopathic adult polymyositis (34 percent)
2. Primary idiopathic adult dermatomyositis (29 percent)
3. Dermatomyositis/polymyositis associated with malignancy (8.5 percent)
4. Childhood dermatomyositis/polymyositis associated with vasculitis (7 percent)
5. Dermatomyositis/polymyositis associated with connective-tissue disease (21 percent)

Source: From Bohan, A. and Peter, J. B. Medical Progress: Polymyositis and dermatomyositis, Part I. *N. Engl. J. Med.* 292: 344, 1975.

Dysphagia is present in 20 to 50 percent of patients. Facial muscles are involved infrequently, and extraocular muscles are spared [8, 52]. The second criterion is the electromyographic (EMG) changes characteristic of myositis. These include small polyphasic potentials, increased insertional irritability and fibrillation, and bizarre high-frequency repetitive discharges [9]. The third criterion is elevated serum muscle enzymes (creatine phosphokinase, aldolase, SGOT, and lactate dehydrogenase) [9]. The fourth criterion is muscle biopsy abnormalities, including necrosis, degeneration and regeneration, phagocytosis, and an interstitial or perivascular inflammatory response. And finally, there are the characteristic dermatologic features, which include an erythematous, scaly rash of the face, neck, shawl area, and extensor surfaces of the knees, elbows, and medial malleoli and a heliotrope rash (periorbital violaceous discoloration) and Gottron's papules (scaly erythematous dermatitis over the dorsum of the metacarpophalangeal and proximal interphalangeal joints of the hands) [9].

There are five major classes of patients with the inflammatory myopathies [88], as shown in Table 8-15.

There are about five new cases per million people per year, which makes the inflammatory myopathies about a tenth as common as rheumatoid arthritis. The disease may involve other organ systems, including the gastrointestinal tract, where there may be difficulty swallowing along with abnormal motility of the esophagus and small bowel [52]. Ulceration of the bowel with bleeding is sometimes seen in childhood. Lung involvement includes aspiration pneumonia, hypoventilation, interstitial fibrosis, drug-related pneumonitis (methotrexate), or infection [52]. Raynaud's phenomenon occurs in 35 percent of patients, and arthralgias or arthritis occurs in about 50 percent [52]. Cardiac involvement, although common, is usually asymptomatic, with only electrocardiographic changes, mitral valve prolapse, or systolic clicks [52].

The association with malignancy is intriguing. The overall prevalence is 5 to 11 times the expected incidence, with 95 percent of the malignancies occurring in patients over the age of 40 years. Myositis precedes the diagnosis of malignancy in two-thirds of patients by an average of 1 to 2 years. The common tumors are breast, lung, ovary, and gastrointestinal malignancies [12].

No specific etiology has been determined for these myopathies, but definite abnormalities of both the humoral and cell-mediated immune systems are common.

TREATMENT

Treatment requires the initial use of high-dose corticosteroids (60 to 100 mg per day). The immunosuppressive agents methotrexate or azathioprine have been used with some success in those who are steroid failures or who have developed major steroid side effects [9, 52].

The overall survival in recent series of adult patients is 85 to 90 percent, with most of the deaths occurring in the group with the malignancies [10,

26]. The average duration of treatment required is 1 to 2 years [9, 52].

Mixed Connective-Tissue Disease

The features of several connective-tissue diseases can overlap in the same patient. Patients with combined manifestations of systemic lupus erythematosus, scleroderma, and polymyositis have high titers of antinuclear antibody to ribonuclear protein (RNP) [99]. Most patients are females. No racial or ethnic predominance has been recognized. The syndrome usually presents with arthralgias or arthritis, diffuse swelling of the hands leading to a tapering or sausage appearance of the fingers, Raynaud's phenomenon, myositis, and esophageal hypomotility [99]. Pulmonary involvement, serositis, lymphadenopathy, rashes, splenomegaly, and hepatomegaly also occur [99]. Renal and central nervous system involvement are distinctly less common than in systemic lupus erythematosus.

LABORATORY TESTS

Laboratory abnormalities include a high titer of antinuclear antibody with a speckled pattern (>1 : 1000), a high titer of antibody to ribonuclear protein, elevated creatine phosphokinase and aldolase levels, abnormal electromyograms, a muscle biopsy consistent with polymyositis, abnormal cineesophagrams and manometric studies (decreased motility in the lower two-thirds of the esophagus), and abnormal pulmonary functions tests in 50 percent of patients, with a restrictive pattern and decreased diffusion capacity [99]. Complete evaluation also should include urinalysis, a 24-hour urinary protein determination, and creatinine clearance, since 5 percent of patients develop glomerulonephritis.

TREATMENT

Most patients respond to low-to-moderate doses of steroids (40 mg per day or less), although those with far-advanced, widespread disease and those whose major manifestations are secondary to scleroderma may not respond as rapidly or com-

pletely [84]. Duration of treatment is often measured in months to years.

Acute Rheumatic Fever

Rheumatic fever is an inflammatory disease that occurs as a sequela to infection with group A streptococci. The most common clinical feature of this disease is arthritis, but there is heart involvement in a third to half of patients, and Sydenham's chorea occurs in 5 percent or less of cases as a late manifestation. The characteristic rash of rheumatic fever, erythema marginatum, is rare; it is an evanescent erythema of the trunk or proximal extremity that is nonpruritic and painless. Small subcutaneous nodules are characteristic but rare.

The arthritis is characterized by migratory involvement; large joints of the extremities are most often affected. The arthritis responds rapidly to salicylate therapy, and seldom are there any permanent sequelae. In rare instances, a nonprogressive arthropathy of the hands and feet, known as Jaccoud's arthritis, occurs. In these patients, ulnar deviation of the fingers is accompanied by flexion at the metacarpophalangeal joints and hyperextension at the distal interphalangeal joints. It is differentiated from rheumatoid arthritis by lack of pain, heat, and redness in the joints and absence of rheumatoid factor in the blood.

Vasculitis

Vasculitis is a pathologic process characterized by inflammation and necrosis of blood vessels. The clinical spectrum of disease is wide, since essentially any vessel in the body may be affected by the vasculitis, with dysfunction dependent on the organ system involved. There are numerous classifications of vasculitides [23], but one that we have found useful is shown in Table 8-16.

The remainder of this discussion will concentrate on the three major causes of vasculitis, the polyarteritis group, the small-vessel hypersensitivity vasculitides, and the large-artery or giant-cell arteritides.

Classic polyarteritis nodosa, a necrotizing vas-

Table 8–16. *Classification of the Vasculitides*

  I. Medium and small arteries (polyarteritis group):
    A. Polyarteritis nodosa
    B. Allergic granulomatosis
  II. Small vessels (hypersensitivity vasculitis group):
    A. Hypersensitivity vasculitis
    B. Serum sickness and serum sickness-like reactions
    C. Henoch-Schönlein purpura
    D. Essential mixed cryoglobulinemia
    E. Vasculitis associated with systemic lupus
       erythematosus and rheumatoid arthritis
    F. Vasculitis associated with malignancies
  III. Large arteries (giant-cell arteritis):
    A. Temporal arteritis (giant-cell arteritis)
    B. Takayasu's arteritis
  IV. Wegener's granulomatosis
  V. Lymphomatoid granulomatosis
  VI. Mucocutaneous lymph node syndrome (Kawasaki's
    disease)
  VII. Thromboangiitis obliterans (Buerger's disease)
  VIII. Central nervous system vasculitis
  IX. Behçet's disease
  X. Vasculopathy associated with atrial myxoma:
    Clinically resembles systemic vasculitis but is caused
    by embolization of myxomatous tissue and
    subsequent invasion of the arterial wall.

Source: From Cupps, T. R. and Fauci, A. S. The Vasculitides. Philadelphia: Saunders, 1981.

culitis of small and medium-sized arteries, was first described by von Rokitansky in the mid-1800s. The lesions in the vessels are frequently segmental, with nodules grossly visible along the course of involved vessels [95]. The disease is mediated by the deposition of immune complexes within the vessel wall [31]. Complement is activated with the subsequent attraction of polymorphonuclear white blood cells to the site of the immune-complex deposition [31]. These events result in the release of proteolytic enzyme with destruction of the vascular structure.

The disease is most common between the ages 30 and 50 years and occurs more commonly in men (2 : 1). Patients appear systemically ill, with hypertension and renal involvement common [29, 95]. Additionally, involvement of the gastrointestinal tract is common, as is hepatic involvement. An association has been noted between hepatitis, hepatitis B surface antigen, and the development of polyarteritis nodosa. Mononeuritis multiplex is seen in 50 percent of pa-

tients, with significant central nervous system disease present in 23 percent [23]. A skin rash is distinctly uncommon, although vasculitic nodules are present and palpable in 30 percent of patients.

Aggressive treatment of the disease with cyclophosphamide and prednisone is the initial approach, along with control of hypertension. With the early use of cyclophosphamide, the mortality from the disease has been substantially reduced [67].

The hypersensitivity vasculitides include not only hypersensitive vasculitis, but also serum sickness and Henoch-Schönlein purpura [39]. Pathologically, the skin lesions dominate the picture with inflammation of arterioles, capillaries, and venules. The most common lesion, palpable purpura, is seen in essentially all patients and occurs in the lower extremities [39]. Other organ systems that may be involved include the gastrointestinal tract with melena or hematemesis, renal involvement manifested by hematuria in a third of patients, and arthritis/arthralgias in about 40 percent. Most patients do well with this disease, and recovery occurs after months to 1 to 2 years [39]. No treatment is effective; therefore, management involves supportive care.

Giant-cell arteritis consists of two clinical syndromes, temporal arteritis and Takayasu's arteritis [70]. Temporal arteritis is a systemic disease affecting primarily elderly Caucasians. Ninety percent of the patients are over 60 years of age [30, 49]. Constitutional symptoms, including malaise and fever, are common, and other large arteries, both extra- and intracranial, may be involved. The major concern is functional visual impairment because of involvement of the ophthalmic vessels. Some reports suggest that visual impairment may occur in up to a third of patients [30, 50]. Polymyalgia rheumatica appears to coexist in 30 to 60 percent of patients [49]. Polymyalgia rheumatica is a clinical syndrome present in patients over the age of 50 years and characterized by proximal muscle pain and morning stiffness [22]. It does not involve the kidney.

The most useful diagnostic procedure is a temporal artery biopsy. Treatment with corticosteroids can be begun prior to the biopsy. Treatment of choice is prednisone (1 mg/kg per day for a week). Then a *very* slow taper can be begun. It often takes 2 years to completely suppress the disease.

To summarize, suspect vasculitis in the following situations:

1. Multisystem disease with prominent constitutional systems
2. Skin diseases characterized by
   a. Palpable purpura
   b. Chronic or recurrent urticaria
   c. Nonspecific erythematous macular or papular rash
   d. Subcutaneous nodules, livedo reticularis, ulcerations, or peripheral gangrene
3. Nonspecific glomerulonephritis
4. Unexplained progressive central nervous system disease, intellectual deterioration, confusion, headache, impaired consciousness, and seizures

A biopsy of an involved area is almost always required for diagnosis.

Polymyalgia Rheumatica

Polymyalgia rheumatica usually presents in elderly patients as an acute illness characterized by severe stiffness, aching muscular pain, fatigue, lethargy, anorexia, and weight loss. Often the patient first notices the symptoms upon getting out of bed after feeling well the night before, although symptoms may occur insidiously. The muscular symptoms usually are confined to the neck, shoulder, pelvic girdles, and back [22].

CLINICAL MANIFESTATIONS
One usually finds a distraught patient who appears acutely ill, with tender muscles and shoulder joints, but without true muscle weakness, even though getting out of bed or a chair may be difficult. A nonspecific synovitis may occur in hands, wrists, and shoulders and may be confused with rheumatoid arthritis. Symptoms and physical findings of giant-cell arteritis, particularly headache, visual symptoms, and tender temporal arteries, should be sought, since these two entities often coexist [49].

LABORATORY TESTS
Laboratory abnormalities include a markedly elevated erythrocyte sedimentation rate greater than 50 mm per hour, mild anemia, nonspecific elevation of alpha$_2$- and gamma-globulins, normal creatine phosphokinase and aldolase levels, and a normal electromyogram. Giant-cell arteritis is found in 20 to 40 percent of patients with polymyalgia rheumatica who have a temporal artery biopsy [22, 30, 49].

TREATMENT
Because visual disturbances, including blindness from ophthalmic artery involvement, may occur in up to 50 percent of patients with positive temporal artery involvement, treatment with moderate doses of steroids is advisable. Response characteristically is dramatic, with complete resolution of symptoms within several days. The sedimentation rate is helpful in following the course of the disease. There is a high incidence of relapse if steroids are withdrawn in the first 2 years of treatment. Because of the osteoporosis seen in many patients who require corticosteroids for this period of time, all patients also should be given calcium (1500 mg per day) and vitamin D (50,000 IU once or twice a week) when they are begun on corticosteroid treatment.

Nonarticular Rheumatic Disease

Fibrositis

Fibrositis is characterized by symptoms of diffuse musculoskeletal aching, accompanied by multiple sites of deep myofascial tenderness but few, if any, objective signs of inflammation. Although it can affect anyone, it is seen most commonly in women between the ages of 20 and 50 years [124]. It may exist as a primary fibrositis or in association with other connective-tissue diseases, including rheumatoid arthritis.

Although the etiology is unknown, most feel that fibrositis is the result of an interaction of several factors. They include a perfectionist-type personality, emotional stress, psychological disturbance, and a disturbed sleep pattern [79, 106]. Among the most common areas of pain and tenderness are the cervical spine and the paravertebral area [106, 124].

The pain of fibrositis is diffuse and poorly localized, but it tends to be away from joints. It is described as a deep aching pain that seems almost constant. Superimposed on this are areas of specific tenderness (trigger points) which cause excruciating pain if bumped or squeezed [106]. Associated with the pain is the constant feeling of extreme fatigue. Most patients admit that they sleep poorly at night, but even those who feel they sleep well are almost all "light" sleepers [79].

On physical examination nothing is found suggesting inflammation, but frequently there are multiple painful trigger points which, when touched, cause severe pain.

Laboratory studies are all within normal limits, as are roentgenograms.

TREATMENT

Treatment of fibrositis is difficult. The patient needs to understand that this is not a crippling disease but one that may cause significant discomfort at times. An attempt should be made to alter the sleep pattern so that the patient will awake more refreshed. Tricyclic antidepressants help reduce alpha sleep wave pattern intrusions into deep sleep and allow for improvement in the quality of sleep. Physical modalities such as heat, ice, or injection of trigger points may be of some benefit, while analgesics or anti-inflammatory medications also may prove useful. In some patients the knowledge that someone (their physician) believes they really do have a specific disorder is enough to allow them to carry on their daily lives.

Back Pain

Low-back pain is second only to respiratory infections as a cause of lost work in the United States. Although the differential diagnosis of back pain is quite broad and includes many serious and potentially remediable disorders, only a small percentage of patients have infectious, neoplastic, inflammatory, or metabolic disease as the cause of their pain (Table 8-17). Most patients have back pain as a result of either structural weakness of the back or direct spinal nerve compression.

The lumbar spine is a complex system comprised of several pain-sensitive structures, such as the anterior and posterior longitudinal ligaments and the periosteum. Paraspinal muscles also may account for pain, but probably the most important pain-causing structure is the facet joint, the posterior articulation of the inferior facet of one vertebral body with the superior facet of the next.

Pain arising from the structures just mentioned is usually dull and aching and, therefore, easily distinguished from the radicular pain of nerve root compression caused by a herniated nucleus pulposus. In interpreting nerve root compression syndromes it is necessary to recognize that although nerve roots exit from the spinal column below the correspondingly numbered vertebral body, they are most vulnerable to compression by disk herniation at the level above that vertebral body. This is shown in Table 8-18.

It should be possible to distinguish between low-back pain caused by weakness of supporting structures of the spine (lumbosacral sprain syndrome) and disk herniation with spinal nerve en-

Table 8–17. *Differential Diagnosis of Low-Back Pain*

Possible causes of pain	Diagnostic procedures
Lumbosacral sprain syndromes	See text
Nerve root compression (disk herniation)	See text
Infection (bacterial and tuberculous)	ESR, cultures, skin tests, bone scans
Fracture (traumatic and pathologic)	Radiographs
Axial arthropathies	Radiographs of sacroiliac joint and lumbosacral spine; ESR, HLA typing
Osteoporosis and osteomalacia	Serum calcium, phosphate, alkaline phosphatase
Paget's disease	Serum calcium, phosphate, alkaline phosphatase
Neoplasm (bone, spinal cord, and nerve root)	Tomography, scintiscan, serum protein electrophoresis, marrow examination
Scoliosis	Routine radiographs
Vascular causes (aneurysm and claudication)	Vascular studies
Referred visceral pain (e.g., pancreas or prostate)	Gastrointestinal or genitourinary evaluation

Table 8–18. *Disk Herniation, Symptoms and Signs*

Root	Disk	Pain radiation	Sensory deficit	Motor deficit	Deep tendon reflexes
L5	L4–5	Back, dorsum of foot, great toe	Lateral leg, mediodorsal foot	Foot, great toe extensors	Normal
S1	L5–S2	Back, sole and heel	Heel, lateral foot	Plantar flexors	Absent ankle jerk

Table 8–19. *Clinical Features of Lumbosacral Sprain and Nerve Root Compression*

Variable	Lumbosacral sprain syndrome	Nerve root compression syndrome
Age	Variable	Third to fourth decade (when disk is weakest)
Course	Acute or chronic	Acute or recurrent
Pain quality	Deep, aching, poorly localized	Sharp, lancinating
Valsalva maneuver	No change	Pain increased
Neurologic findings	None	Sensorimotor deficit, loss of deep tendon reflexes

trapment (nerve root compression syndrome). The cardinal points in the differential diagnosis are shown in Table 8-19.

Most disk herniations occur at one of the lowest two levels of the vertebral column, probably because of factors related to weight-bearing. Each of the two presents characteristic features (see Table 8-18).

DIAGNOSIS

The history and physical examination are the most important tools for diagnosing and distinguishing the lumbosacral sprain syndrome and the nerve root compression syndrome. Besides the findings already listed, patients with nerve root compression often will experience pain on straight leg raising, especially when the maneuver is augmented by great toe hyperextension or thumb pressure on the sciatic nerve in the popliteal fossa.

Routine laboratory studies are not helpful in most cases of low-back pain. Anteroposterior, lateral, and oblique radiographs of the spine should be obtained of most new patients; they may show such abnormalities as osteoarthritis, osteopenia, or spondylolisthesis. Computerized axial tomography (CT) and magnetic resonance imaging (MRI) are extremely helpful in the diagnosis, but they should be reserved for patients in whom the diagnosis is elusive or in whom a surgical procedure is contemplated. Other tests should be chosen sparingly according to the clinical situation. Table 8-17 lists the differential diagnosis of back pain along with various procedures that may be helpful in establishing each diagnosis.

TREATMENT

Most cases of low back pain, whether due to sprains or disk herniations, can be managed conservatively. Surgical procedures have a very limited role in the therapy of low-back pain. They are reserved for specific neurologic complications of the nerve root compression syndrome. Most proved disk herniations, however, improve within 3 to 6 weeks on medical management.

General measures include (1) bed rest (with firm mattress or bed board), (2) analgesics and anti-inflammatory agents, (3) local heat, (4) mild sedation (to relieve muscle spasm and facilitate bed rest), and (5) exercises aimed at strengthening the back and decreasing lumbar lordosis. Absolute indications for laminectomy in a documented disk herniation are (1) cauda equina syndrome (bowel and bladder dysfunction), (2) marked muscular weakness, and (3) progressive neurologic deficit despite adequate conservative management. Relative indications for laminectomy include (1) intolerable pain in an emotionally stable patient, (2) pain unrelieved by complete bed rest for 3 to 6 weeks, and (3) recurrent, incapacitating sciatica.

Shoulder Pain

Evaluation of the patient with shoulder pain often presents the physician with a difficult diagnostic challenge. Symptoms referable to the shoulder may arise from the shoulder joint itself (glenohumeral articulation) or the accessory joints of the shoulder (acromioclavicular, sternoclavicular, and scapulothoracic); the periarticular structures overlying the joint (tendons, bursae, muscle, and capsule); adjacent or distant musculoskeletal structures; vascular, neurologic, or visceral lesions (diaphragmatic irritation); or even psychogenic causes. This discussion focuses on intrinsic, nonarticular causes of shoulder pain, since these occur more commonly.

DIAGNOSIS

The most common causes of shoulder pain (excluding fractures, dislocations, and acromioclavicular separation) are calcific supraspinatus tendonitis, subacromial and subdeltoid bursitis, bicipital tenosynovitis, adhesive capsulitis, and tears of the musculotendinous (rotator) cuff. Symptoms may be acute, with sudden onset of pain, tenderness, and limitation of active and passive motion, or more commonly, subacute or chronic in nature. The precipitating factor is most often trauma caused either by direct injury, unaccustomed or prolonged repetitive activity, or sudden effort or exertion. Calcific tendonitis is thought to be caused by chronic trauma that results in minute fiber tears, fibrillation, and low-grade inflammation. The supraspinatus tendon is affected most commonly, with secondary involvement of the subacromial bursa often causing a bursitis. Clinically, this overstress condition of the shoulder is referred to as impingement syndrome, since, as you elevate the arm, the inflamed or damaged tissue impinges on the subacromial area and beneath the coracoacromial ligament. Adhesive capsulitis may follow as a sequela to arthritis or any periarticular inflammation. Limitation of motion is usually severe and quite limiting, with pain varying from very mild to severe. Rotator cuff tears most often involve the supraspinatus tendon; a partial rupture is most common. Acute trauma nearly always is responsible, although tears may occur in association with rheumatoid arthritis. Pain and tenderness over the greater tuberosity and limitation of motion are the common symptoms [101].

Examination and radiographs are usually helpful in differentiating the preceding problems. Acute subacromial bursitis and calcific supraspinatus tendonitis may be difficult to differentiate, since they often occur together. Most often a radiograph will show calcific deposits in the soft tissue above the humeral head and below and lateral to the acromion.

TREATMENT

Medical management includes local heat, range-of-motion exercises, nonsteroidal anti-inflammatory agents, and local injection with lidocaine and long-acting steroids. When the problem is recurrent or chronic, a surgical procedure may be required to remove extensive calcium deposits.

A rotator cuff tear may be suspected when a patient felt or heard a "snap" following an injury to the shoulder that resulted in acute pain and limitation of shoulder motion. Loss of the ability to initiate abduction suggests a complete tear. Evaluation should proceed immediately with an arthrogram of the involved shoulder. Complete ruptures require surgical intervention. Partial tears may be managed conservatively with heat, sling, rest, analgesics, and oral anti-inflammatory agents. After healing, a course of physical therapy is usually necessary to restore range of motion; otherwise adhesive capsulitis may ensue.

Acute bicipital tenosynovitis is relatively easy to diagnose, since the symptoms are usually localized to the anterior of the shoulder joint. The tendon is tender to palpation and is rolled easily under the thumb. Pain may be reproduced maximally with forced supination of the elbow at 45 degrees of flexion. Response to oral nonsteroidal, anti-inflammatory agents or local injection of lidocaine and steroids or both is usually satisfactory.

Hip Pain

Pain in the hip may arise from many structures in addition to the hip joint; these include bursae, tendons, muscles, and the sacroiliac joints, as well as periosteal, vascular, neurologic and visceral lesions. A careful history is mandatory, since it suggests the diagnosis as often as the physical examination and radiographs.

Pain in the hip joint itself is primarily felt in the groin and not the buttocks; it may radiate along the inner aspect of the thigh to the knee in the distribution of the obturator nerve. Sometimes hip-joint pain may present as knee pain with few symptoms referable to the hip. Pain often is aggravated by weight-bearing and activity such as climbing stairs. Other causes of groin pain simulating hip disease include acute trauma with muscle or ligament strain (groin pull), inguinal hernia, iliopsoas bursitis, phlebitis of the iliac veins, local lymphadenopathy, and inflammation and masses involving the external genitalia.

Pain over the lateral aspect of the hip often is due to greater trochanteric bursitis. It is aggravated by weight-bearing and lying on the involved side. Pain in the buttock area can be due to a variety of problems ranging from disease of the lower lumbar vertebrae, muscle spasm, sacroiliitis, vascular insufficiency, and ischial tuberosity bursitis to visceral disorders in the pelvis and abdomen. Root compression from herniation of the lower lumbar disk usually results in low-back pain with radiation to the buttocks and down the posterior aspect of the legs; it is aggravated by walking, sitting, coughing, or sneezing.

Physical examination is helpful in confirming the source of pain. Because the hip joint lies so deep to musculocutaneous structures, one rarely appreciates heat, redness, or effusions of the joint. Tenderness, pain on motion, and measurement of the limitation of motion and of leg length are the primary objective means by which the status of the hip joint is evaluated. Observations of gait, standing, and sitting in a chair are also helpful. The most common problem causing hip pain is degenerative joint disease. Other causes include trauma, axial arthropathies, rheumatoid arthritis, sepsis, gout, pseudogout, and aseptic necrosis of the femoral head.

Greater trochanteric bursitis is diagnosed by tenderness over the bursa, pain over the lateral aspect of the hip on weight-bearing, external rotation, and active abduction of the hip. Tenderness over the ischial tuberosity and pain in the same area when sitting denote ischial bursitis. Tenderness over the sacroiliac joints is an important sign in sacroiliitis.

TREATMENT

Treatment varies according to the disease process involved, but it includes bed rest, heat, exercises, analgesics and anti-inflammatory agents, local steroid injections, and antibiotics and open drainage when sepsis is involved.

Elbow Pain

Lateral epicondylitis, or tennis elbow, refers to a condition of chronic inflammation of the common extensor muscle origins at the lateral humeral epicondyle. It may occur in tennis players, usually beginning or less experienced individuals, and is caused most often by improper technique when using the backhand stroke. It also occurs as an occupational hazard among carpenters and gardeners or in anyone performing a task requiring frequent pronation and supination of the arm.

The injury is generally due to an acute inflammatory process with or without partial rupture of the tendon at the tendon-periosteal junction. Predisposing factors include inadequate forearm, wrist, or metacarpophalangeal extensor power and flexibility.

Diagnosis is made on historical grounds and the finding of tenderness at the lateral epicondyle of the humerus. Various treatments have been tried, including rest, exercises, massage, heat, fitting an elastic band around the proximal forearm, and anti-inflammatory agents. The best relief of symptoms is by avoiding the activity responsible for the symptoms and local injection of steroids. Even if

symptoms recur or persist, the condition is generally self-limiting, with a duration of not longer than 6 to 12 months.

Sports-Related Running Injuries

RUNNING INJURIES: THE KNEE

Tables 8-20, 8-21, and 8-22 present a classification of runners and the incidence and etiology of runner's injuries [14, 87]. The knee is extremely vulnerable to many stresses applied to the lower extremity. Because of its anatomic location, an abnormality proximally in the hip or distally in the ankle or foot or malalignment of all or part of the leg may be the source of the problem encountered at the knee. To fully evaluate a knee problem, the entire lower back, hip, and lower extremity must be examined.

Table 8–20. Classification of Runners

Level I:	Jogger	Novice or recreational runner averaging 2 to 18 miles per week (mpw) at 8 to 16 minutes per mile
Level II:	Sports runner	20 to 40 miles per week at 8 to 10 minutes per mile
Level III:	Long-distance runner	40 to 70 miles per week at 7 to 8 minutes per mile (most marathon runners)
Level IV:	Elite	70 to 170 miles per week at 5 to 7 minutes per mile (world class)

Table 8–21. Overuse Syndrome in Runners: Relationship Between Distances Run and Incidence of Injuries

Miles per week	Injured runners (%)
0–20	48
20–40	32
40–60	13
60–80	5
80 +	2

Source: From Pagliano, F., and Jackson, J. W. Overuse syndrome in runners. *Runners World* 8: 42, 1980.

Table 8–22. *Etiology of Running Injuries*

Training errors (60 percent):
  Excessive mileage
  Intensive workouts
  Rapid change in routine
  Terrain (hills, hard surfaces, sand, sloped or banked
    surfaces)
  Interval training (multiple runs of short duration with
    little rest between bursts)
Anatomic factors (20 percent):
  Pronated foot
  Caves foot
  Leg-length difference
Shoes (20 percent):
  Soft heels increase force on heel
  Wide heels allow hyperpronation
  Inflexible soles increase muscle stress
  Flat soles give poor traction in mud and snow, so should
    be studded
  Irregular wear of heel or sole causes increased muscle
    stress

To best determine the cause of the patient's knee problem, a thorough history must be elicited, followed by localization of the discomfort and identification of the structure involved. Basic understanding of the anatomy is obviously very important. A *differential diagnosis* can be developed by considering problems that arise from extra-articular structures and those which are related to intra-articular structures. This discussion will focus on some of the more common extra-articular injuries.

Iliotibial Band Syndrome

This is an inflammation of the tissue between the iliotibial band and the lateral femoral condyle caused by the repeated rubbing as the knee is flexed and extended. Characteristically, this is seen in long-distance runners who have dramatically increased their mileage.

TREATMENT. Treatment includes decreasing the running distance, ice for 20 minutes after exercise, stretching exercises, nonsteroidal anti-inflammatory drugs, steroid injection, and correction of footwear, if necessary.

Pes Anserinus Bursitis

This is seen most commonly in runners. The hamstrings act as knee flexors and internal rotators of the tibia. The bursa located between the tibial insertion of the medial collateral ligament and the three tendons as they cross to attach to the proximal medial tibia is locally tender with swelling.

TREATMENT. Treatment includes limitation of activity (running), ice after exercise, nonsteroidal anti-inflammatory drugs, steroid injection, and shoe orthotics to correct foot deformity, if present.

Patellar Tendinitis

Also known as jumper's knee, this is an inflammation to the lower pole of the patella. It is particularly common in basketball players, certain track athletes, and occasionally runners.

TREATMENT. Treatment includes decreased activity, ice after exercise, nonsteroidal anti-inflammatory drugs, neoprene patellar stabilizer, *no* steroid injection, and surgery (rarely indicated).

Joint Laxity

Joint laxity as an inherited trait or ligamentous laxity secondary to an old ligament tear may be a source of knee pain after running or jumping activity. Usually, there is a small effusion and rather vague discomfort without good localization.

TREATMENT. Treatment should be directed toward muscle rehabilitation, bracing (if necessary), and adjustment of activity.

Popliteal tendinitis

This is usually associated with running downhill and with conditions causing hyperpronation, such as running on banked surfaces. There will be localized tenderness just anterior to the fibular collateral ligament attachment to the femur.

TREATMENT. Treatment is the same as for the iliotibial band syndrome.

FOOT AND LOWER LEG INJURIES
Shin Splints

The pathogenesis of shin splints includes overuse of underdeveloped or untrained muscles, particularly the posterior tibial muscle. Small tears at the origin, belly, or musculotendinous junction of the involved muscle may occur with herniation of the muscle through the fascia. Shin splints may be associated with a periostitis, especially if the runner tries to run through the initial injury.

TREATMENT. Exclude ischemic compartment syndromes or stress fractures; then institute rest, stretching exercises prior to running, proper footwear (may need orthotics to prevent hyperpronation), and avoidance of running on hard surfaces.

Plantar Fasciitis
This generally follows excessive walking or running on a pronated foot, especially if there is a loose, poorly fitted heel counter in the shoe that

places undue tension on the plantar fascia. It is seen more commonly in people with a flattened longitudinal arch (flat feet). *Spur formation* results from traction of the plantar fascia on the periosteum of calcaneus.

TREATMENT. Raise the heel ¼ in, which removes tension placed on the calcaneus by the Achilles tendon and release tension of the fascia by plantar flexing the foot. Additional measures include heel cup, local injection (may require 2 to 3 injections for relief), and surgery to release plantar fascia.

References

1. Adelman, D. C., Saltiel, E., and Klinenberg, J. R. The neuropsychiatric manifestations of systemic lupus erythematosus: An overview. *Semin. Arthritis Rheum.* 15: 185, 1986.
2. Aho, K., Leirisalo-Repo, M., and Repo, H. Reactive arthritis. *Clin. Rheum. Dis.* 11: 25, 1985.
3. Appelboom, T., Boelpaepe, C. D., Ehrlich, G. E., and Famaey, J. P. Rubens and the question of antiquity of rheumatoid arthritis. *J.A.M.A.* 245: 483, 1984.
4. Austin, H. A., Klippel, J. H., Balow, J. E., et al. Therapy of lupus nephritis: Controlled trial of prednisone and cytotoxic drugs. *N. Engl. J. Med.* 314: 614, 1986.
5. Ayoub, W. T., Franklin, C. M., and Torretti, D. Polymyalgia rheumatica: Duration of therapy and long-term outcome. *Am. J. Med.* 79: 309, 1985.
6. Bayer, A. S., Chow, A. W., Louie, J. S., et al. Gram-negative bacillary septic arthritis: Clinical, radiographic, therapeutic, and prognostic features. *Semin. Arthritis Rheum.* 7: 123, 1977.
7. Berney, S., Goldstein, M., and Bishko, F. Clinical and diagnostic features of tuberculous arthritis. *Am. J. Med.* 53: 36, 1972.
8. Bohan, A., and Peter, J. B. Medical progress: Polymyositis and dermatomyositis. Part I. *N. Engl. J. Med.* 292: 344, 1975.
9. Bohan, A., and Peter, J. B. Medical progress: Polymyositis and dermatomyositis. Part II. *N. Engl. J. Med.* 292: 403, 1975.
10. Bohan, A., Peter, J. B., Boroman, R. L., et al. A computer-assisted analysis of 153 patients with polymyositis and dermatomyositis. *Medicine* 56: 255, 1977.
11. Boss, G. R., and Seegmiller, J. E. Hyperuricemia and gout: Classification, complications and management. *N. Engl. J. Med.* 300: 1459, 1979.
12. Bradley, W. G. Inflammatory Diseases of Muscle. In W. N. Kelley, E. D. Harris, Jr., S. Ruddy, and C. B. Sledge (Eds.), *Textbook of Rheumatology,* 2d Ed. Philadelphia: Saunders, 1985. Pp. 1225–1246.
13. Brandt, K. D. Osteoarthritis: Clinical Patterns. In W. N. Kelley, E. D. Harris, Jr., S. Ruddy, and C. B. Sledge (Eds.), *Textbook of Rheumatology,* 2d Ed. Philadelphia: Saunders, 1985. Pp. 1432–1448.
14. Brady, D. M. Running Injuries. CIBA Symp. 32:2, 1980.
15. Broy, S. B., and Schmid, F. R. A comparison of medical drainage (needle aspiration) and surgical drainage (arthrotomy or arthroscopy) in the initial treatment of infected joints. *Clin. Rheum. Dis.* 12: 501, 1986.
16. Calin, A., and Fries, J. F. An "experimental" epidemic of Reiter's syndrome revisited: Follow-up evidence on genetic and environmental factors. *Ann. Intern. Med.* 84: 564, 1976.
17. Calin, A., Porta, J., Fries, J. F., and Schurman,

D. J.   Clinical history as a screening test for ankylosing spondylitis. *J.A.M.A.* 237: 2613, 1977.

18. Calin, A.   HLA-B27: To type or not to type? *Ann. Intern. Med.* 92: 208, 1980.

19. Calin, A.   Ankylosing Spondylitis. In W. N. Kelley, E. D. Harris, Jr., S. Ruddy, and C. B. Sledge (Eds.), *Textbook of Rheumatology,* 2d Ed. Philadelphia: Saunders, 1985. Pp. 993–1005.

20. Calin, A.   Reiter's Syndrome. In W. N. Kelley, E. D. Harris, Jr., S. Ruddy, and C. B. Sledge (Eds.), *Textbook of Rheumatology,* 2d Ed. Philadelphia: Saunders, 1985. Pp. 1007–1020.

21. Campion, E. W., Glynn, R. J., and DeLabry, L. O.   Asymptomatic hyperuricemia: Risks and consequences in the normative aging population. *Am. J. Med.* 82: 421, 1987.

22. Chuang, T. Y., Hunder, G. G., Ilstrup, D. M., and Kurland, L. T.   Polymyalgia rheumatica: A 10-year epidemiologic and clinical study. *Ann. Intern. Med.* 97: 672, 1980.

23. Cupps, T. R., and Fauci, A. S.   *The Vasculitides.* Philadelphia: Saunders, 1981.

24. Daniels, T. E.   Labial salivary gland biopsy in Sjögren's syndrome. Assessment as a diagnostic criterion in 363 suspected cases. *Arthritis Rheum.* 27: 147, 1984.

25. Decker, J. L., Steinberg, A. D., Reinertsen, J. L., Plotz, P. H., Balow, J. E., and Klippel, J. H. Systemic lupus erythematosus: Evolving concepts. *Ann. Intern. Med.* 91: 587, 1979.

26. DeVere, R., and Bradley, W. G.   Polymyositis: Its presentation, morbidity and mortality. *Brain* 98: 637, 1975.

27. Dieppe, P. A., Jones, H. E., Scott, D. G., et al. Pyrophosphate arthropathy: A clinical and radiological study of 105 cases. *Ann. Rheum. Dis.* 41: 371, 1982.

28. Eisenstein, B. I., and Masi, A. T.   Disseminated gonococcal infection (DGI) and gonococcal arthritis (GCA): I. Bacteriology, epidemiology, host factors, pathogen factors, and pathology. *Semin. Arthritis Rheum.* 10: 155, 1981.

29. Fan, P. T., Davis, J. A., Somer, T., Kaplan, L., and Bluestone, R.   A clinical approach to systemic vasculitis. *Semin. Arthritis Rheum.* 9: 248, 1980.

30. Fauchald, P., Ryguold, O., and Oystese, B.   Temporal arteritis and polymyalgia rheumatica clinical and biopsy findings. *Ann. Intern. Med.* 77: 845, 1972.

31. Fauci, A. S., Haynes, B. F., and Katz, P.   The spectrum of vasculitis: Clinical, pathologic, immunologic, and therapeutic considerations. *Ann. Intern. Med.* 89: 660, 1978.

32. Fauci, A. S., Haynes, B. F., Katz, P., and Wolff, S. M.   Wegener's granulomatosis: Prospective clinical and therapeutic experience with 85 patients for 21 years. *Ann. Intern. Med.* 98: 76, 1983.

33. Feigenbaum, S. L., Masi, A. T., and Kaplan, S. B. Prognosis in rheumatoid arthritis: A longitudinal study of newly diagnosed younger adult patients. *Am. J. Med.* 66: 377, 1979.

34. Feinglass, E. J., Arnett, F. C., Dorsch, C. A., Zizic, T. M., and Stevens, M. B.   Neuropsychiatric manifestation of systemic lupus erythematosus: Diagnosis, clinical spectrum, and relationship to other features of the disease. *Medicine* 55: 323, 1976.

35. Fessel, W. J.   ANA-negative systemic lupus erythematosus. *Am. J. Med.* 64: 80, 1978.

36. Forrester, D. M., Brown, J. C., and Nesson, J. W. *The Radiology of Joint Disease.* Philadelphia: Saunders, 1978.

37. Fox, R., Calin, A., Gerber, R. C., and Gibson, D. The chronicity of symptoms and disability in Reiter's syndrome: An analysis of 131 consecutive patients. *Ann. Intern. Med.* 91: 190, 1979.

38. Gatter, R. A.   *A Practical Handbook of Joint Fluid Analysis.* Philadelphia: Lea and Febiger, 1984. Pp. 1–105.

39. Gilliam, J. N., and Smiley, J. D.   Cutaneous necrotizing vasculitis and related disorders. *Ann. Allergy* 37: 328, 1976.

40. Goldenberg, D. L., and Cohen, A. S.   Acute infectious arthritis: A review of patients with nongonococcal joint infections (with emphasis on therapy and prognosis). *Am. J. Med.* 60: 369, 1976.

41. Goldenberg, D. L., and Reed, J. I.   Bacterial arthritis. *N. Engl. J. Med.* 312: 764, 1985.

42. Gordon, D. A., Stein, J. L., and Broder, I.   The extra-articular features of rheumatoid arthritis: A systemic analysis of 127 cases. *Am. J. Med.* 54: 445, 1973.

43. Halverson, P. B., Cheung, H. S., McCarty, D. J., Garancis, J., and Mandel, N.   "Milwaukee shoulder": Association of microspheroids containing hydroxyapatite crystals, active collagenase, and neutral protease with rotator cuff defects: II. Synovial fluid studies. *Arthritis Rheum.* 24: 474, 1981.

44. Harmon, C. E.   Antinuclear antibodies in auto-

immune disease significance and pathogenicity. *Med. Clin. North Am.* 69: 547, 1985.

45. Harmon, C. E., and Portanova, J. P. Drug-induced lupus: Clinical and serological studies. *Clin. Rheum. Dis.* 8: 121, 1982.

46. Harris, E. P. Rheumatoid Arthritis: The Clinical Spectrum. In W. N. Kelley, E. D. Harris, Jr., S. Ruddy, and C. B. Sledge (Eds.), *Textbook of Rheumatology,* 2d Ed. Philadelphia: Saunders, 1985. Pp. 915–950.

47. Hawkins, R. A., Claman, H. N., Clark, R. A. F., and Steigerwald, J. C. Increased dermal mast cell populations in progressive systemic sclerosis: A link in chronic fibrosis? *Ann. Intern. Med.* 102: 182, 1985.

48. Haynes, D. C., and Gershwin, M. E. Immunopathology of progressive systemic sclerosis (PSS). *Semin. Arthritis Rheum.* 11: 331, 1982.

49. Healy, L. A., and Wilske, K. R. Polymyalgia rheumatica and giant-cell arteritis. *West. J. Med.* 141: 64, 1984.

50. Healy, L. A., and Wilske, K. R. Occult giant-cell arteritis. *Arthritis Rheum.* 23: 641, 1980.

51. Hunder, G. G., and McDuffie, F. C. Hypocomplementemia in rheumatoid arthritis. *Am. J. Med.* 54: 461, 1973.

52. Hochberg, M. C., Feldman, D., and Stevens, M. B. Adult-onset polymyositis dermatomyositis: An analysis of clinical and laboratory features and survival in 76 patients with a review of the literature. *Semin. Arthritis Rheum.* 15: 168, 1986.

53. Hoffman, B. I., and Katz, W. A. The gastrointestinal manifestation of systemic lupus erythematosus: A review of the literature. *Semin. Arthritis Rheum.* 9: 237, 1980.

54. Hollander, J. L. Introduction. In D. J. McCarty (Ed.), *Arthritis and Allied Conditions: A Textbook of Rheumatology,* 10th Ed. Philadelphia: Lea and Febiger, 1985. Pp. 3–8.

55. Holmes, E. W. Clinical Gout and the Pathogenesis of Hyperuricemia. In D. J. McCarty (Ed.), *Arthritis and Allied Conditions: A Textbook of Rheumatology,* 10th Ed. Philadelphia: Lea and Febiger, 1985. Pp. 1445–1480.

56. Hoppenfeld, S. *Physical Examination of the Spine and Extremities.* New York: Appleton-Century-Crofts, 1976.

57. Hochberg, M. C., Boyd, R. E., Ahearn, J. M., Arnett, F. C., Bias, W. B., Provost, T. T., and Stevens, M. B. Systemic lupus erythematosus: A review of clinicolaboratory features and immunogenetic markers in 150 patients with emphasis on demographic subsets. *Medicine* 64: 285, 1985.

58. Hurd, E. R. Extra-articular manifestations of rheumatoid arthritis. *Semin. Arthritis Rheum.* 8: 151, 1979.

59. Inman, R. D. Rheumatic manifestations of hepatitis B virus infection. *Semin. Arthritis Rheum.* 11: 406, 1982.

60. Kammer, G. M., Soter, N. A., Gibson, D. J., and Schur, P. H. Psoriatic arthritis: A clinical, immunologic and HLA study of 100 patients. *Semin. Arthritis Rheum.* 9: 75, 1979.

61. Kassan, S. S., and Gardy, M. Sjögren's syndrome: An update and overview. *Am. J. Med.* 64: 1037, 1978.

62. Keat, A. Medical progress: Reiter's syndrome and reactive arthritis in perspective. *N. Engl. J. Med.* 309: 1606, 1983.

63. Kelley, W. N. and Fox, J. H. Gout and related disorders of purine metabolism. In Kelley, W. N., Harris, E. D., Jr., Ruddy, S., and Sledge, C. B. (Eds.), *Textbook of Rheumatology,* 2d Ed. Philadelphia: Saunders, 1985. Pp. 1359–1398.

64. Kellgren, J. H., Lawrence, J. S., and Bier, F. Genetic factors in generalized osteoarthritis. *Ann. Rheum. Dis.* 22: 237, 1963.

65. Koffler, D. The immunology of rheumatoid diseases. *CIBA Symp.* 31: 1, 1979.

66. Lahita, R. G. Sex and age in systemic lupus erythematosus. In Lahita, R. G. (Ed.), *Systemic Lupus Erythematosus.* New York: Wiley, 1987. Pp. 523–539.

67. Leavitt, R. Y., and Fauci, A. S. State of art pulmonary vasculitis. *Am. Rev. Respir. Dis.* 134: 149, 1986.

68. Lee, P., Rooney, P. J., Sturrock, R. D., Kennedy, A. C., and Dick, W. C. The etiology and pathogenesis of osteoarthrosis: A review. *Semin. Arthritis Rheum.* 3: 189, 1974.

69. Liang, M. H., and Fries, J. F. Asymptomatic hyperuricemia: The case for conservative management. *Ann. Intern. Med.* 88: 666, 1978.

70. Lupi-Herrera, E., Sanchez-Torres, G., Marcushamer, J., Mispireta, J., Horowitz, S., and Vela, J. E. Takayasu's arteritis: Clinical study of 107 cases. *Am. Heart J.* 93: 94, 1977.

71. Masi, A. T., and Eisenstein, B. I. Disseminated gonococcal infection (DGI) and gonococcal arthritis (GCA): II. Clinical manifestations, diagno-

sis, complications, treatment, and prevention. *Semin. Arthritis Rheum.* 10: 173, 1981.

72. McCarty, D. J., and Halverson, P. Basic Calcium Phosphate (Apatite, Octacalcium Phosphate, Tricalcium Phosphate) Crystal Deposition Disease. In D. J. McCarty (Ed.), *Arthritis and Allied Conditions: A Textbook of Rheumatology,* 10th Ed. Philadelphia: Lea and Febiger, 1985. Pp. 1547–1564.

73. McCarty, D. J., Halverson, P. B., Carrera, G. F., Brewer, B. J., and Kozin, F. "Milwaukee shoulder": Association of microspheroids containing hydroxyapatite crystals, active collagenase, and neutral protease with rotator cuff defects: I. Clinical aspects. *Arthritis Rheum.* 24: 464, 1981.

74. McCarty, D. Heberden oration, 1982: Crystals, joints, and consternation. *Ann. Rheum. Dis.* 42: 243, 1983.

75. McCarty, D. J. Calcium pyrophosphate dihydrate crystal deposition disease—1975. *Arthritis Rheum.* 19: 275, 1976.

76. McKenna, F., and Wright, U. Clinical Manifestations. In P. D. Utsinger, N. J. Zvaifler, and G. E. Ehrlich (Eds.), *Rheumatoid Arthritis: Etiology, Diagnosis, Management.* Philadelphia: Lippincott, 1985. Pp. 283–307.

77. Medsger, T. A., Masi, A. T., Rodnan, G. P., et al. Survival with systemic sclerosis (scleroderma): A life-table analysis of clinical and demographic factors in 309 patients. *Ann. Intern. Med.* 75: 369, 1971.

78. Mitchell, D. Epidemiology. In P. D. Utsinger, N. J. Zvaifler, and G. E. Ehrlich (Eds.), *Rheumatoid Arthritis: Etiology, Diagnosis, Management.* Philadelphia: Lippincott, 1985. Pp. 133–150.

79. Moldofsky, H., Scarisbrick, P., England, B. S. R., and Smythe, H. Musculoskeletal symptoms and non-REM sleep disturbance in patients with "fibrositis syndrome" and healthy subjects. *Psychosom. Med.* 37: 341, 1975.

80. Moll, J. M. H. The clinical spectrum of psoriatic arthritis. *Clin. Orthop.* 143: 66, 1979.

81. Moll, J. M. H., and Wright, V. Psoriatic arthritis. *Semin. Arthritis Rheum.* 3: 55, 1973.

82. Moll, J. M. H., Haslock, I., Macrae, I. F., and Wright, V. Association between ankylosing spondylitis, psoriatic arthritis, Reiter's disease, the intestinal arthropathies, and Behcet's syndrome. *Medicine* 53: 343, 1974.

83. Nicholls, A. Histocompatibility antigens and the arthritis of chronic inflammatory bowel disease. *Clin. Rheum. Dis.* 3: 265, 1977.

84. Nimelstein, S. H., Brody, S., McShane, D., and Holman, H. R. Mixed connective-tissue disease: A subsequent evaluation of the original 25 patients. *Medicine* 59: 239, 1980.

85. Noer, H. R. An "experimental" epidemic of Reiter's syndrome. *J.A.M.A.* 197: 693, 1966.

86. O'Sullivan, J. B., and Cathcart, E. S. The prevalence of rheumatoid arthritis: Follow-up evaluation of the effect of criteria on rates in Sudbury, Massachusetts. *Ann. Intern. Med.* 76: 573, 1972.

87. Pagliano, F., and Jackson, J. W. Overuse syndrome in runners. *Runners World* 8: 42, 1980.

88. Peyron, J. G. Epidemiologic and etiologic approach of osteoarthritis. *Semin. Arthritis Rheum.* 8: 288, 1979.

89. Phillips, R. M., and Wasner, C. K. Scleroderma: Current understanding of pathogenesis and management. *Postgrad. Med. J.* 70: 153, 1981.

90. Pollak, V. E., and Kant, K. S. Systemic Lupus Erythematosus and the Kidney. In R. D. Lahita (Ed.), *Systemic Lupus Erythematosus.* New York: Wiley, 1987. Pp. 643–672.

91. Reeves, W. H., and Lahita, R. G. Clinical Presentation of Systemic Lupus Erythematosus in the Adult. In R. G. Lahita (Ed.), *Systemic Lupus Erythematosus.* New York: Wiley, 1987. Pp. 355–382.

92. Rocco, U. K., and Hurd, E. R. Scleroderma and scleroderma-like disorders. *Semin. Arthritis Rheum.* 16: 22, 1986.

93. Rodnan, G. P. Treatment of the gout and other forms of crystal-induced arthritis. *Bull. Rheum. Dis.* 32: 43, 1982.

94. Rodnan, G. P., and Medsger, T. A. The rheumatic manifestations of progressive systemic sclerosis (scleroderma). *Clin. Orthop.* 57: 81, 1968.

95. Rose, G. A., and Spencer, H. Polyarteritis nodosa. *Q. J. Med.* 26: 43, 1957.

96. Ryan, L. M., and McCarty, D. J. Calcium Pyrophosphate Crystal Deposition Disease, Pseudogout, Articular Condrocalcinosis. In D. J. McCarty (Ed.), *Arthritis and Allied Conditions: A Textbook of Rheumatology,* 10th Ed. Philadelphia: Lea and Febiger, 1985. Pp. 1515–1546.

97. Sergent, J. S., Lockshin, M. D., Christian, C. L., and Gocke, D. J. Vasculitis with hepatitis B antigenemia: Long-term observations in nine patients. *Medicine* 55: 1, 1976.

98. Shapiro, R., Weisner, K., McLaughlin, G. E., et al. Evaluation as a Prelude to Management:

Management of Patients. In P. D. Ulsinger, N. J. Zvaifler, and G. E. Ehrlich (Eds.), *Rheumatoid Arthritis: Etiology, Diagnosis, Management.* Philadelphia: Lippincott, 1987. Pp. 505–544.

99. Sharp, G. C., Irvin, W. S., Tan, E. M., Gould, R. G., and Holman, H. R. Mixed connective-tissue disease: An apparently distinct rheumatic disease syndrome association with a specific antibody to an extractable nuclear antigen (ENA). *Am. J. Med.* 52: 148, 1972.

100. Shearn, M. A. Sjögren's syndrome. *Semin. Arthritis Rheum.* 2: 165, 1972.

101. Shoen, R. P., Moskowitz, R. W., and Goldberg, U. M. *Soft-Tissue Rheumatic Pain: Recognition, Management, Prevention.* Philadelphia: Lea and Febiger, 1987.

102. Shoenfeld, Y., Antré-Schwartz, J., Stollar, B. D., and Schwartz, R. S. Anti-DNA Antibodies. In R. G. Lahita (Ed.), *Systemic Lupus Erythematosus.* New York: Wiley, 1987. Pp. 213–256.

103. Siegel, R. C. Scleroderma. *Med. Clin. North Am.* 61: 283, 1977.

104. Simkin, P. A. Management of gout. *Ann. Intern. Med.* 90: 812, 1979.

105. Simkin, P. A. The pathogenesis of podagra. *Ann. Intern. Med.* 86: 230, 1977.

106. Smythe, H. A. "Fibrositis" as a disorder of pain modulation. *Clin. Rheum. Dis.* 5: 823, 1979.

107. Soy, H. C., and Liang, M. H. The erythrocyte sedimentation rate guidelines for rational use. *Ann. Intern. Med.* 104: 515, 1986.

108. Stahl, N. I., Klippel, J. H., and Decker, J. L. Fever in systemic lupus erythematosus. *Am. J. Med.* 67: 935, 1979.

109. Steere, A. C., Malawista, S. E., Hardin, J. A., Ruddy, S., Askenase, P. W., and Andiman, W. A. Erythema chronicum migrans and Lyme arthritis: The enlarging clinical spectrum. *Ann. Intern. Med.* 86: 685, 1977.

110. Steere, A. C., Bartenhagen, N. H., Craft, J. E., et al. The early clinical manifestations of Lyme disease. *Ann. Intern. Med.* 99: 76, 1983.

111. Steere, A. C., Hutchinson, G. J., Rahn, D. W., et al. Treatment of the early manifestation of Lyme disease. *Ann. Intern. Med.* 99: 22, 1983.

112. Steere, A. C., and Malawista, S. E. Viral Arthritis. In D. J. McCarty (Ed.), *Arthritis and Allied Conditions: A Textbook of Rheumatology,* 10th Ed. Philadelphia: Lea and Febiger, 1987. Pp. 1697–1712.

113. Steinberg, A. D. Management of Systemic Lupus Erythematosus. In W. N. Kelly, E. D. Harris, Jr., S. Ruddy, and C. B. Sledge (Eds.), *Textbook of Rheumatology,* 2d Ed. Philadelphia: Saunders, 1985. Pp. 1098–1114.

114. Stevens, M. D. Systemic Lupus Erythematosus and the Cardiovascular System. In R. D. Lahita (Ed.), *Systemic Lupus Erythematosus.* New York: Wiley, 1987. Pp. 673–690.

115. Svejgaard, A., Plotz, P., Ryder, L. P., Nielsen, L. S., and Thomsen, M. HL-A and disease association: A survey. *Tranplant. Rev.* 22: 3, 1975.

116. Swezey, R. L. Dynamic factors in deformity of the rheumatoid arthritic hand. *Bull. Rheum. Dis.* 22: 649, 1971.

117. Tuffanelli, D. L., and Winkelmann, R. K. Systemic scleroderma: A clinical study of 727 cases. *Arch. Dermatol.* 84: 359, 1961.

118. Utsinger, P. D. and Roth, S. H. Nonsteroidal antiinflammatory drugs. In Utsinger, P. D., Zvaifler, N. J., and Ehrlich, G. E. (Eds.), *Rheumatoid Arthritis: Etiology, Diagnosis, Management.* Philadelphia: Lippincott, 1987. Pp. 545–547.

119. Ward, J. R., and Atcheson, S. G. Infectious arthritis. *Med. Clin. North Am.* 61: 313, 1977.

120. Wilke, W. S., and Machenzie, A. H. Proposed pathogenesis of fibrositis. *Cleve. Clin. Q.* 52: 147, 1985.

121. Wilkinson, M., and Bywaters, E. G. L. Clinical features and course of ankylosing spondylitis as seen in follow-up of 222 hospital referred cases. *Ann. Rheum. Dis.* 17: 209, 1958.

122. Winfield, J. B. Antilymphocyte Antibodies: Specificity and Relationship to Abnormal Cellular Function. In R. G. Lahita (Ed.), *Systemic Lupus Erythematosus.* New York: Wiley, 1987. Pp. 305–332.

123. Wyngaarden, J. B. Metabolic defects of primary hyperuricemia and gout. *Am. J. Med.* 56: 651, 1974.

124. Yunus, M., Masi, A. T., Calabro, J. J., et al. Primary fibromyalgia (fibrositis): Clinical study of 50 patients with matched normal controls. *Semin. Arthritis Rheum.* 11: 151, 1981.

9

Neurology

Michael P. Earnest*

Approach to the Neurologic Patient

The Clinical Process

The patient with a neurologic disorder presents three questions to the clinician: Where is it? What is it? and How urgent is it?

The first question asks the location of the lesion in the nervous system. The answer requires knowledge of neuroanatomy and nervous system function plus skills of neurologic examination to elicit the signs that localize the disease in a specific area of the nervous system. The answer to the second question requires both knowledge of the processes that affect the nervous system and skills to

elicit a neurologic history that explores the differential diagnosis.

The third question is answered by the history and selected signs on neurologic examination. Urgent processes require prompt intervention to prevent irreversible nervous system injury or death. Examples of such conditions are intracranial masses producing coma or increased intracranial pressure, tumors compressing the spinal cord, stroke causing progressively increasing deficit, and neuromuscular disorders producing respiratory failure [3, 46].

Cerebrovascular Diseases

Stroke and Transient Ischemic Attack

DEFINITIONS

Stroke is a generic term for a syndrome, caused by cerebrovascular disease, with acute onset of focal neurologic symptoms and signs that last more than 24 hours. It implies a locus of permanent damage in the central nervous system (CNS). *Cerebral thrombosis, cerebrovascular accident* (CVA), and *cerebral apoplexy* all refer to stroke.

Transient ischemic attack (TIA) applies to strokelike syndromes that persist less than 24

hours. Generally, a transient ischemic attack is not associated with a demonstrable brain lesion.

MECHANISMS

Stroke has two major mechanisms: failure of blood supply to a region of the central nervous system (ischemic infarction) and rupture of a blood vessel supplying the central nervous system (intracranial hemorrhage) (Table 9-1). Ischemic infarction may be due to thrombosis of a vessel, vascular occlusion by embolic material, hypoper-

*The author thanks Ms. Susan Padilla for her diligence in typing the manuscript and Jeffrey Cohen, M.D., for his helpful suggestions concerning the text.

Table 9–1. Cerebrovascular Mechanisms Causing Stroke

Brain infarction:
  Thrombosis
  Embolism
  Hypoperfusion
  Spasm (rare)
Intracranial hemorrhage:
  Subarachnoid
  Parenchymal
  Combined

fusion of a focal region of the central nervous system, or vascular spasm. The major causes of intracranial hemorrhage (ICH) are hypertensive cerebrovascular disease, congenital aneurysm, and arteriovenous malformation (AVM).

RISK FACTORS

Medical conditions that increase an individual's probability of having a stroke are risk factors. Major risk factors for stroke and transient ischemic attack are advanced age, hypertension, cardiac disease, atherosclerosis, diabetes mellitus, smoking, abnormal lipid metabolism, coagulation disorders, use of oral contraceptives, and illicit drug abuse. Treatment of these conditions may prevent future strokes [9, 66].

Ischemic Brain Infarction

THROMBOTIC BRAIN INFARCTION

Pathophysiology

Most thromboses occur at sites of atherosclerotic narrowing of the cerebrovascular system. However, blood hypercoagulability, thrombocytosis, vascular trauma, and vasculitis also may cause thrombotic occlusions. Hypertensive cerebrovascular disease selectively damages the small arterioles penetrating the base of the brain. Occlusion of one of those vessels causes a small, deep infarction (lacunar infarction or lacune) [31].

History

Ischemic infarction of the brain usually presents as a focal neurologic deficit with preservation of alertness. The patient may awaken with the full deficit or may experience the stepwise progression of symptoms over several hours. Headache, if present, is usually mild.

Physical Findings

The typical middle cerebral artery syndrome includes hemiparesis with hyperactive deep tendon reflexes in the weak limbs, a Babinski reflex in the weak foot, and depressed sensation on the paretic side of the body. The arm usually is weaker than the leg. If the dominant hemisphere, usually the left, is infarcted, aphasia is present.

Anterior cerebral artery infarctions produce weakness of one or both legs. A posterior cerebral distribution infarction causes hemianopia with mild or no hemiparesis. Infarction in the vertebrobasilar system produces depression of consciousness, impaired cranial nerve function, cerebellar signs, and bilateral motor, sensory, and reflex changes in the limbs. Certain clinical syndromes suggest lacunar infarctions, especially a pure motor hemiplegia, a pure sensory stroke, and dysarthria accompanied by a clumsy, weak hand [31].

Examination of the carotid arteries may disclose a diminished pulse or a bruit suggesting stenosis or occlusion.

Laboratory Findings

A reasonable selection of tests to search for occult risk factors includes complete blood count (CBC), urinalysis (UA), platelet count, prothrombin time (PT), partial thromboplastin time (PTT), serologic test for syphilis, erythrocyte sedimentation rate (ESR), and serum biochemical screen (SMA-12 or equivalent). An electrocardiogram (ECG) is done to exclude arrhythmias and other cardiac disease. Evaluation of younger patients with ischemic stroke includes serum lipid electrophoresis, serologic tests for vasculitis, blood and urine drug screens, and echocardiography. A lumbar puncture (LP) is indicated for most patients to exclude an inflammatory or infectious process. Noninvasive vascular studies of the carotid and periorbital arteries may help identify patients with stenotic internal carotid artery disease.

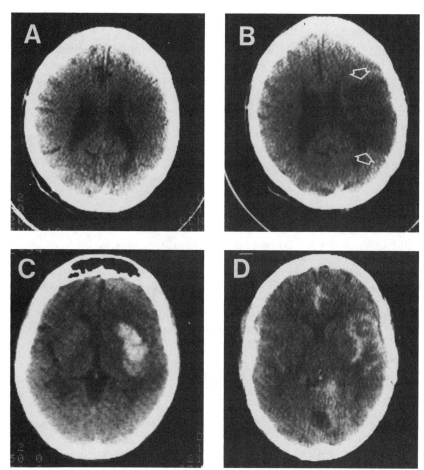

Figure 9–1. Head CT scan sections. (A) *Right cerebral brain infarct at 12 hours.* (B) *The same infarct at 11 days* (arrows). (C) *Hypertensive intraparenchymal hemorrhage.* (D) *Subarachnoid hemorrhage in both Sylvian fissures, the interhemispheric fissure, and under right occipital lobe.*

Radiologic Studies

A computer-assisted tomographic (CT) scan of the head will disclose any noncerebrovascular lesion that may masquerade as stroke. Brain tumor, cerebral abscess, subdural hematoma, and other nonvascular processes have been found by CT scan in 4 to 15 percent of large series of suspected strokes. The CT scan also indicates whether a brain infarction or intracranial hemorrhage has caused the stroke. Intracranial hemorrhage appears on CT as a high-density (white) lesion (Fig. 9-1). The typical CT scan of cerebral infarction is normal within the first 24 hours or has only subtle low-density changes in the white matter. The infarction evolves over the next several days as a progressively more sharply demarcated low-density lesion (Fig. 9-1). A magnetic resonance imaging (MRI) scan shows brain infarction within a few hours of onset. Cerebral arteriography (angiography) is indicated in some cases to look for surgically treatable atherosclerotic lesions of the carotid artery.

Acute Management
Brain infarction cannot be reversed once the ischemia has occurred. The goal of acute management is to protect the patient's brain from further injury by maintaining optimal blood glucose, ventilation, blood pressure, and cardiac rate and rhythm. For at least 24 hours the patient should be closely observed for worsening clinical signs. Progressing stroke often can be halted by immediate anticoagulation with heparin [51].

Chronic Management
Subsequent in-hospital management focuses on preventing and treating the complications of stroke—decubiti (bed sores), contractures, pneumonia, urinary tract infection, and depression. Early ambulation and institution of physical, occupational, and speech therapy will minimize complications and improve recovery. Treatment must be begun to reverse any risk factors. Anticoagulation is not routinely indicated.

Prognosis
About 15 percent of brain infarction patients die acutely, 45 percent cannot function independently after discharge, and 40 percent can live independently. Myocardial infarction is the major cause of late mortality. Control of hypertension is the best-documented measure for preventing future stroke and myocardial infarction.

EMBOLIC BRAIN INFARCTION
Pathophysiology
Emboli causing brain infarction usually are platelet-fibrin clumps that come from the heart or from an ulcerated atherosclerotic plaque at the origin of the internal carotid artery. Embolic infarctions initially are ischemic but often secondarily, 24 to 48 hours later, become hemorrhagic as damaged vessels leak blood into the infarcted area [14].

History
The historical feature most strongly indicative of embolic infarction is known heart disease, especially atrial fibrillation or a cardiac valve lesion.

Physical Examination
The general medical examination may disclose a cardiac murmur or arrhythmia, evidence for systemic emboli, or embolic material in a retinal vessel. The neurologic syndromes are generally the same as those from thrombotic infarction.

Laboratory Findings
An ultrasound examination of the heart (echocardiogram) may demonstrate valvular lesions, an atrial tumor (atrial myxoma), or intracardiac thrombus that produced the embolus.

Radiologic Studies
An embolic mechanism is suggested by presence of hemorrhagic infarction on CT or MRI scan.

Acute Management
Embolic infarction is managed as described for thrombotic infarction, except anticoagulation is indicated in most cases. Heparin is the drug of choice. Usually anticoagulation is delayed for 24 to 48 hours and the CT scan is repeated to ensure that the brain infarction has not become hemorrhagic [14].

Subsequent Management
Anticoagulation is continued after discharge using an oral drug, usually warfarin.

Prognosis
The risk of recurrent emboli is high with prosthetic valves, mitral stenosis, and cardiac ventricular aneurysm. However, most patients die from cardiac disease, not recurrent stroke.

Intracranial Hemorrhage
SUBARACHNOID HEMORRHAGE
Pathophysiology
Intracranial hemorrhage (ICH) occurs in two primary forms: subarachnoid hemorrhage (SAH) and parenchymal hemorrhage, often called intracerebral hemorrhage. An important mechanism of brain injury and a prominent cause of death in

intracranial hemorrhage is increased intracranial pressure. The most common nontraumatic cause of subarachnoid hemorrhage is rupture of a congenital (Berry) aneurysm of an intracranial vessel. An arteriovenous malformation is a less common source.

History

When subarachnoid hemorrhage occurs, the patient has a sudden severe headache. The pathognomonic description is "The worst headache of my life." Within a few hours the patient experiences a painful, stiff neck, photophobia, nausea, and vomiting because of meningeal irritation by blood in the cerebrospinal fluid (CSF).

Physical Findings

The patient is in obvious painful distress. Hypertension, sinus tachycardia, and tachypnea are common. The neck is stiff, and flexion causes pain. The neurologic examination usually shows depression of alertness, confusion, and occasionally hemorrhages in the retina and papilledema.

Laboratory Findings

A prothrombin time, partial thromboplastin time, and platelet count are required to exclude an occult hemorrhagic disorder. Lumbar puncture discloses an elevated opening pressure and bloody cerebrospinal fluid with xanthochromia, pleocytosis, and high protein. The cerebrospinal fluid glucose level usually is normal.

Radiologic Findings

The CT scan shows high-density blood in the cisterns at the base of the brain (see Fig. 9-1). The routine contrast-enhanced CT scan demonstrates most arteriovenous malformations, but will show only about 20 percent of aneurysms. Angiography definitively shows the site and anatomy of the aneurysm or arteriovenous malformation.

Acute Management

Life-support measures are often necessary. Once subarachnoid hemorrhage is proven, neurosurgical consultation and an angiogram are completed

as soon as possible. If an aneurysm is demonstrated, surgical clipping is done whenever possible [62].

Prognosis

About 50 percent of persons with a first aneurysmal subarachnoid hemorrhage die, and a high percentage of survivors have a recurrent hemorrhage within a month unless the aneurysm is surgically obliterated [62].

INTRAPARENCHYMAL HEMORRHAGE
Pathophysiology

Intraparenchymal hemorrhage (IPH) is caused by rupture of an abnormal blood vessel within the brain substance. Hypertensive cerebrovascular disease is the most common etiology, but an arteriovenous malformation or vasculitis also may be the cause [38, 61].

History and Physical Findings

The onset of illness is marked by a severe headache, then focal neurologic symptoms (a stroke syndrome), followed by depression of consciousness. The patient usually has hypertension, tachycardia, depression of consciousness, and prominent focal neurologic signs. The neurologic signs reflect the location of the hematoma.

Radiologic Studies

The CT scan shows a high-density mass within the brain compressing and distorting surrounding structures (see Fig. 9-1).

Management

Early management is the same as for subarachnoid hemorrhage. Brain herniation must be reversed, if present. Only occasionally is surgery necessary to remove the clot. Survivors often require prolonged nursing care and rehabilitation therapies.

Prognosis

About a third of patients die acutely. Survivors have major deficits, but few have recurrent hemorrhages if hypertension is controlled.

Transient Ischemic Attack

HISTORY

A transient ischemic attack usually is caused by a small embolus transiently occluding an intracranial vessel, leaving no infarction. However, transient ischemic attack syndromes may be caused by a small infarction or intraparenchymal hemorrhage, and, through uncertain mechanisms, a brain tumor or arteriovenous malformation. The symptoms are usually identical to those of a stroke but are distinguished by their brevity.

PHYSICAL FINDINGS

Symptoms and signs during a transient ischemic attack are the same as a stroke. The neurologic examination, by definition, is normal after the symptoms subside. A depressed carotid pulse or bruit may be present.

MANAGEMENT

Laboratory studies are obtained to evaluate stroke risk factors. If cardiac disease is suspected, an echocardiogram is indicated. Patients with recent-onset transient ischemic attacks in the vascular supply of a carotid artery should have noninvasive vascular studies or angiography. If a severely stenotic lesion is found, endarterectomy is indicated. Medical management usually includes oral anticoagulation for several months and then a change to drugs that suppress platelet coagulation functions (antiplatelet drugs) [13, 66].

PROGNOSIS

Over 20 percent of patients with a first transient ischemic attack will have a completed stroke within 3 years. However, the major cause of death is cardiac disease. Anticoagulation, antiplatelet drugs, and carotid endarterectomy probably reduce the incidence of future strokes [13, 66].

Seizures and Epilepsy

Definitions

A seizure is an episode of abnormal motor, sensory, psychological, or behavioral activity caused by abnormal electrical discharges within the brain. Epilepsy is recurrent seizures caused by a disorder of the brain [15, 22, 54]. The term *idiopathic epilepsy* generally refers to cases that have no definable cause other than disordered electrophysiology of the brain. *Seizure disorder* is equivalent to epilepsy.

The First Seizure

HISTORY

A single seizure or even a flurry of several seizures may be caused by many different nonepileptic conditions. General medical conditions that cause seizures include drug withdrawal (especially from alcohol and other central nervous system depressants), hypoglycemia, hypocalcemia, hyponatremia, hypoxia, uremia, hepatic encephalopathy, therapeutic drugs (e.g., aminophylline, lidocaine,

phenothiazines), illicit drugs (e.g., cocaine, amphetamines), and porphyria. A first seizure also may be the presenting event of an active brain disease such as meningitis, encephalitis, brain tumor, abscess, stroke, subdural hematoma, or arteriovenous malformation. An active central nervous system lesion is suggested by a history of head trauma, fever, severe headaches, focal neurological symptoms, or recent alteration of mental status.

PHYSICAL FINDINGS

The general medical and neurologic examinations are often normal interictally. If the patient is seen during the seizure, the seizure type may indicate a possible brain lesion—tonic deviation of the head or eyes to one side, predominance of motor activity on one side of the body, or a partial complex seizure (see below). The examination postictally also may show focal signs, ones that may resolve as the patient recovers—hemiparesis, asymmetry of deep tendon reflexes, a unilateral Babinski sign, or aphasia.

LABORATORY STUDIES

A battery of laboratory tests to disclose possible medical causes for the seizure includes determination of serum glucose, calcium, electrolytes; biochemical screen for renal and liver failure; arterial blood gases; and blood and urine toxicologic panels.

Every patient with a seizure whose general medical and toxicologic workup is negative requires an electroencephalogram (EEG). The electroencephalogram may show paroxysmal epileptic discharges, diagnosing epilepsy, or may show focal abnormalities, suggesting a structural brain lesion.

RADIOLOGIC STUDIES

A CT or MRI scan will disclose a focal brain lesion causing seizures [55].

ACUTE AND CHRONIC MANAGEMENT

If the patient is having recurrent seizures, the seizures are treated with an intravenous bolus of a benzodiazepine. Blood tests are drawn, and a glucose bolus (50 ml of 50% glucose in water) is given if there is any suspicion of hypoglycemia. The management is then dictated by the specific etiology.

Epilepsy

PATHOPHYSIOLOGY

A standard classification of the epilepsies is based on seizure type and electroencephalographic findings (Table 9-2) [15]. Generalized epilepsy is characterized by recurrent seizures with loss of consciousness. The electroencephalogram shows simultaneous involvement of the entire cortex of both cerebral hemispheres by the epileptic activity. A partial (focal) seizure has a focal onset clinically and on the electroencephalogram. Partial seizures may spread and become generalized (secondary generalization) [15, 22, 54].

Clinically, each seizure type has a characteristic

Table 9–2. *Classification of Epilepsy*

I. Generalized seizures.
A. Tonic, clonic, or tonic-clonic (grand mal)
B. Absence (petit mal)
C. Rare types: myoclonic, akinetic, and infantile epilepsies
II. Partial (focal) seizures:
A. Simple symptomatology:
1. Motor
2. Sensory
3. Autonomic
B. Complex (temporal lobe, psychomotor)
III. Partial seizures with secondary generalization

Source: Modified from Commission on Classification and Terminology of the International League Against Epilepsy. Proposal for revised clinical and electroencephalographic classification of epileptic seizures. *Epilepsia* 22: 489, 1981.

pattern. A generalized tonic-clonic (grand mal) seizure causes sudden loss of consciousness, tonic contraction of all muscles of the body, and then clonic jerking of the limbs and trunk for a period of seconds to several minutes, followed by limp unresponsiveness from which the patient slowly awakens. During the seizure the patient often bites his or her tongue and is incontinent of urine. Afterwards the patient is sleepy, confused, and has a headache and aching muscles.

A generalized absence (petit mal) seizure causes only a few seconds' lapse of consciousness, during which the person stares, smacks his or her lips, and has fluttering of the eyelids and twitching or other minor movements of the limbs. The patient immediately returns to full alertness, and the only residual is amnesia for events during the seizure. An electroencephalogram shows abrupt onset and cessation of rhythmic 3 per second spike-wave complexes time-locked to the clinical event. This type of epilepsy is most common in children and is uncommon in adults.

Partial focal seizures may have simple symptomatology, such as motor activity of one part of the body only, focal sensory symptoms, or special sensory symptoms (auditory, vertiginous, or olfactory). These partial simple seizures usually do not impair alertness. Partial complex seizures usually impair alertness and cause strange psychological experiences and bizarre behavioral episodes. A partial complex seizure often begins with the patient experiencing a warning symptom (aura), such as a sense of fear or a peculiar visceral sensation. An electroencephalogram during the seizure usually shows epileptic activity in one or both temporal lobes. Patients with partial epilepsy often have secondarily generalized (grand mal) seizures as well.

HISTORY

Diagnosis and management of epilepsy rely on a thorough analysis of the patient's history. Important details include age of onset of the epilepsy, precipitating illness or trauma, type and frequency of seizures, anticonvulsant drugs used (including efficacy and toxic effects), results of electroencephalograms, CT scans, and other laboratory tests, and family history of epilepsy. Important recent data are current medications and doses, toxic symptoms, most recent seizure, and how compliant the patient is with taking medications.

PHYSICAL FINDINGS

Focal neurologic signs may indicate a focal brain lesion.

LABORATORY STUDIES

The diagnostic test in epilepsy is the electroencephalogram. A single electroencephalogram will show paroxysmal epileptic activity in only about a third of epileptic patients. However, over half the patients will have some, albeit nondiagnostic, abnormality. Repeated electroencephalograms and studies with special procedures, such as prolonged sleep deprivation, drug-induced sleep, or nasopharyngeal or other special electrodes, may be required to demonstrate the pathognomonic activity.

RADIOLOGIC STUDIES

A CT or MRI scan will exclude a brain tumor or other structural lesion.

ACUTE MANAGEMENT

Patients and their family are instructed in care of the patient during a seizure. A person having a grand mal seizure should be protected from the injuries that may occur in a seizure, especially head trauma, burns, and drowning. Tongue lacerations may be prevented by a soft object placed between the teeth.

ANTICONVULSANT TREATMENT

An anticonvulsant is selected according to the seizure type [67]. Table 9-3 describes the commonly used anticonvulsants, their efficacy, typical daily doses, and range of therapeutic serum levels.

The general principles of anticonvulsant use are (1) use one drug in whatever dose is required to achieve a therapeutic blood level, (2) if seizures recur and the dose of the first drug cannot be increased, add a second drug, (3) then, if seizures are well-controlled, slowly withdraw the first drug, and (4) serum anticonvulsant levels are obtained whenever the patient has toxic symptoms or signs or has unexplained seizures and when the clinician changes the medications [67].

CHRONIC MANAGEMENT

Long-term management of the patient with epilepsy requires control of seizures, management of drug toxicity, and support of the psychosocial needs of the patient. These needs include vocational counseling and warning the patient against participating in activities during which a seizure would create immediate danger (e.g., swimming alone, hang-gliding, mountain climbing). Driving a motor vehicle is an important legal issue. Motor vehicle regulations in many states prohibit a patient from driving for 6 to 12 months following a seizure with loss of consciousness. Women with epilepsy need counseling about risks of pregnancy worsening epilepsy and about possible teratogenetic effects of anticonvulsants.

PROGNOSIS

About 80 percent of patients with epilepsy can be controlled with use of one anticonvulsant. If the patient has several years free of seizures, he or she

Table 9–3. *Commonly Prescribed Anticonvulsants*

Generic name	Trade name	Usual pills (mg)	Common daily adult dose (mg)	Efficacy (seizure type)	Serum Half-life (hours)	Therapeutic Blood Level (μg/ml)
Carbamazepine	Tegretol	200	600–1200	Grand mal, simple and complex partial, status epilepticus	12 ± 3	4–12
Ethosuximide	Zarontin	250	750–1500	Absence (petit mal)	40 ± 6	50–100
Phenobarbital	Luminal	30, 60, 100	60–180	Grand mal, simple and complex partial, status epilepticus	96 ± 12	15–35
Phenytoin	Dilantin	100	300–400	Grand mal, simple and complex partial, status epilepticus	24 ± 6	10–20
Primidone*	Mysoline	250	750–1500	Grand mal, simple and complex partial	6 ± 3	4–12
Valproic acid	Depakene, Depakote	250, 500	750–2000	Grand mal, absence	8 ± 2	50–100

*Much of the anticonvulsant effect is due to phenobarbital, a major metabolite.

often can be successfully withdrawn from medications. However, patients with a demonstrable brain lesion, mental retardation, epilepsy since infancy, multiple seizure types, or frequent seizures have a poor prognosis. They generally require lifelong anticonvulsants [54].

Status Epilepticus

HISTORY

Status epilepticus (SE) refers to frequently recurring seizures in a short period of time. Status epilepticus may occur with any type of seizure, but the most frequent and dangerous type is grand mal status epilepticus. Mortality in clinical series of grand mal status epilepticus is about 8 percent, but mortality is much higher if the status epilepticus cannot be stopped promptly. The most common setting for status epilepticus is the known epileptic patient who stops taking his or her medications.

ACUTE MANAGEMENT

The patient with grand mal status epilepticus usually is comatose between the seizures, and life-support measures, intravenous line, electrocardiographic monitoring, endotracheal intubation, and ventilation are required. Multiple laboratory studies are done in search of metabolic and toxic causes [67].

Recurring seizures are stopped by an intravenous bolus of 2 to 5 mg diazepam or 8 mg lorazepam. Then a loading dose of either intravenous phenytoin (15 mg/kg at 50 mg per minute) or phenobarbital (10 to 15 mg/kg divided in several boluses at 100 mg per minute) is infused. If seizures continue after a loading dose of the first drug, a serum level is obtained. Once the serum level of the first drug is therapeutic, then a loading dose of the second drug is given. If seizures continue after a second drug, general anesthesia usually is required. The goal of treatment is to stop the seizures within 2 hours.

Depression of Consciousness

Pathophysiology of Consciousness

Full alertness requires proper function of the reticular activating system (RAS), located in the rostral brainstem, and of the cortex of both cerebral hemispheres. Processes that impair these structures cause depression of consciousness [53]. The two types of processes that commonly depress alertness are toxic/metabolic disorders and focal structural brain lesions.

State (level) of consciousness connotes a spectrum of responsiveness ranging from full alertness to the deepest irreversible coma, brain death. A generally accepted definition of coma is eyes-closed unresponsiveness in which the patient makes no effort to speak and has no voluntary motor responses to painful stimuli.

A patient's state of consciousness is best understood by carefully observing the spontaneous activity and the responsiveness to stimuli [27]. Are the eyes open or closed? If closed, what stimulation is required to cause them to open. What is the best verbal response exhibited by the patient, and what stimulus is required? What is the best level of motor response, and what stimulus is required? The Glasgow Coma Scale represents this approach to defining level of consciousness (Table 9-4) [63].

The Clinical Evaluation of Coma

HISTORY

The first task when evaluating the comatose patient is to distinguish a focal brain lesion from a toxic or metabolic cause of coma [27, 53]. Structural lesions such as brain tumor, abscess, subdural hematoma (SDH), and intracranial hemorrhage (ICH) demand aggressive medical and surgical management to save the patient's life and preserve the brain.

Historical clues suggesting a structural lesion are the acute onset of loss of consciousness, recent trauma, severe headache, fever, focal neurologic symptoms, sinus, ear, or face infections, and a coagulation disorder or use of anticoagulants. A full medical and toxicologic history also is taken, searching for medical diseases, prescription or street drugs, or environmental toxins that may have caused the coma.

PHYSICAL EXAMINATION

Physical examination of the patient in coma due to a metabolic, drug, or toxic cause usually shows hypotension, depressed respirations, diminished muscular tone, absent or depressed deep tendon reflexes, but retained pupillary light reaction and symmetrical, nonfocal neurologic signs. Intracranial structural lesions usually damage the brain in an asymmetrical fashion and often cause increased intracranial pressure. Thus they produce an asymmetrical examination and excite tonic brainstem and spinal reflexes. The physical examination usually shows hypertension, tachypnea, increased muscular tone, and increased deep tendon reflexes. Asymmetrical movement of the limbs, asymmetrical tendon reflexes, or other focal neurologic signs commonly are prominent. Papilledema and retinal hemorrhages may be seen if the intracranial pressure is high.

Table 9–4. *The Glasgow Coma Scale*

Eye opening
  Spontaneous
  To voice
  To painful stimulus
  None
Best verbal response:
  Oriented
  Confused speech
  Inappropriate speech
  Incomprehensible sounds
  No response
Best motor response:
  Obeys commands
  Localizes painful stimulus
  Flexor posturing
  Extensor posturing
  No response to pain

Source: Modified from Teasdale, G., and Jennett, B. Assessment of coma and impaired consciousness: A practical scale. *Lancet* 2: 81, 1974.

The general medical examination can show important clues suggesting an intracranial mass as well. Signs of metastatic cancer, head trauma, a bleeding disorder, or purulent infection of the ear, face, or sinuses suggest an associated intracranial lesion.

LABORATORY STUDIES

General laboratory studies in a patient with coma of unknown etiology include a complete blood count, urinalysis, determinations of serum glucose, electrolytes, calcium, biochemical screen, blood and urine toxicologic screens, arterial blood gas determination, chest x-ray, and electrocardiogram. Other tests to be considered include coagulation studies, thyroid or other endocrine hormone levels, serum osmolality, carboxyhemoglobin or cyanide determination, quantitative blood levels of specific drugs (e.g., barbiturates, alcohol, tricyclic antidepressants), and blood cultures. A lumbar puncture may show blood or pleocytosis indicating central nervous system hemorrhage or infection [27].

RADIOLOGIC STUDIES

A CT scan is the best immediate study in any case of possible intracranial structural lesion. Supratentorial lesions are usually defined clearly by CT scan (see Fig. 9-2), but lesions within the brainstem and bilateral subdural hematomas that are isodense with the brain may be difficult to see.

ACUTE MANAGEMENT

Early management of a patient in coma is directed toward three goals: preserve the life, preserve the brain, and define and treat the cause. The first step is to treat significant abnormalities of cardiac rate and rhythm, hypotension, or respiratory insufficiency. Endotracheal intubation, mechanical ventilation, oxygen, and pressor agents may be required. An intravenous line is inserted, and a full battery of appropriate blood and urine tests is obtained; then a bolus of 50 ml 50% glucose in water is infused. A therapeutic trial of naloxone is given if narcotic overdose is suspected [27].

A decision must be made to do a lumbar punc-

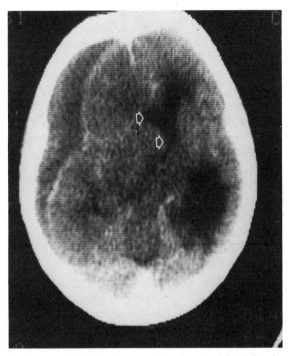

Figure 9–2. *Head CT scan section showing left subdural hematoma with transfalcine herniation of frontal horn of left lateral ventricle* (arrows). *There is hydrocephalus of the posterior right lateral ventricle* (dark oval) *due to obstruction of cerebrospinal fluid flow through the foramen of Monro.*

ture or a CT scan if a central nervous system infection or an intracranial mass lesion is suspected. The CT scan is done first if the history or physical findings indicate a possible intracranial mass.

Throughout this early management period the patient's level of consciousness and vital and neurologic signs must be observed at frequent intervals. Declining level of consciousness or increasing focal signs may indicate progressive brain injury or impending herniation that must be treated promptly. Deteriorating vital signs may presage cardiac or respiratory arrest.

CHRONIC MANAGEMENT

Patients in prolonged coma following trauma, cardiac arrest, stroke, or other severe brain injury require meticulous nursing and medical care to prevent decubiti, pneumonia, urinary tract infections, contractures, thrombophlebitis, malnutrition, and fluid imbalances. Mortality among patients in nontraumatic coma for 24 hours is 75 percent by 1 month [43].

Herniation of the Brain

Brain herniation denotes movement of a portion of brain from its normal position into another intracranial compartment (see Fig. 9-2). The cause usually is a focal mass lesion creating severely elevated pressure in that compartment. The most noteworthy herniations are the transtentorial ones, in which the mesial temporal lobe or the hypothalamus is forced medially and downward through the midline opening of the tentorium. The adjacent brainstem is compressed and often is damaged by secondary hemorrhages into the midbrain and pons. If the herniation process continues, permanent brainstem injury and irreversible coma result. The final event in progressive transtentorial herniation is brainstem infarction and cardiorespiratory arrest [53].

The general signs of impending herniation are deepening coma, deteriorating vital signs, and increasing focal signs. The most reliable specific sign of active herniation is a dilated, sluggishly reactive pupil due to compression of the oculomotor nerve. When the eye signs appear, immediate treatment begins with vigorous hyperventilation and boluses of dexamethasone (10 mg) and mannitol (1.0 gm/kg). The focal brain lesion must be removed whenever possible.

Brain Death

The diagnosis of brain death requires a judgment by the physician that there has occurred irreversible cessation of function of the entire brain, including the brainstem. This diagnosis should be made only by a physician trained and skilled in the neurologic evaluation of comatose patients. Confirmatory laboratory tests, such as an electroencephalogram, isotope brain scan, cerebral arteriography, or cerebral blood flow determination, may be useful. Current laws in most states permit the diagnosis of brain death and the removal of life-support devices once the diagnosis has been made. This diagnosis should never be made in the presence of hypothermia or central nervous system suppressing drugs [33].

Intracranial Tumors and Other Masses

Pathophysiology

Tumors and other intracranial masses cause brain dysfunction by several mechanisms. The primary lesion destroys tissue and compresses neighboring structures, causing focal dysfunction. Many lesions also cause edema within the adjacent brain. The mass of a primary lesion and surrounding edema often produce increased intracranial pressure (ICP) compromising the whole brain. Critically located masses also may obstruct cerebrospinal fluid flow and so lead to hydrocephalus. The consequences for the brain of the bulk of the tumor are called the *mass effect*. If the mass effect or hydrocephalus is severe, herniation of the brain may occur.

Processes included in the intracranial mass group are tumors, brain abscess, subdural hematoma, parenchymal hematoma, and obstructive hydrocephalus. Management must consider not only treatment of the specific process, but also therapy to reverse the secondary intracranial effects produced by the lesion.

Brain Tumors
VARIETIES OF TUMORS

Intracranial neoplasms may be malignant or benign. The common primary malignant tumors of the brain are glial-cell tumors. The secondary malignancies usually are metastases from solid tumors elsewhere, especially carcinoma of the lung and breast. Benign intracranial tumors usually are outside the brain, most commonly meningiomas [8, 68].

HISTORY

Tumors may present as a first seizure, as progressive dementia or subacute confusion, as slowly progressive focal symptoms and signs, as worsening headaches, or as a syndrome combining several of these features. The most characteristic history is the insidious onset and then progressive worsening of neurologic symptoms over several months. The malignant tumors generally have a more rapid course and more commonly have headaches and seizures.

PHYSICAL EXAMINATION

The general physical signs that suggest an intracranial tumor are presence of cachexia, signs of primary or metastatic neoplasm, or cutaneous neurofibromatosis. Patients with the latter disease have a high incidence of intracranial neoplasms. The neurologic signs typically are those of increased intracranial pressure and focal motor, sensory, and reflex changes. Depressed level of consciousness and an altered mental status may accompany large tumors and those causing hydrocephalus.

RADIOLOGIC STUDIES

The definitive test is a CT or MRI scan. Either test shows the location and size of the mass and indicates the probable histologic nature.

ACUTE MANAGEMENT

Once the location, size, and nature of the process are known, management includes a neurosurgical consultation to consider biopsy, total removal of the lesion, or ventricular shunting for hydrocephalus. A patient with signs of extensive brain swelling or impending herniation is given dexamethasone to reduce the intracranial pressure.

Benign intracranial tumors usually can be to-

tally removed. Primary or secondary brain malignancies often are biopsied and then given radiation therapy. Chemotherapy may be helpful in selected tumors.

PROGNOSIS

Outcome from a benign tumor is determined only by the patient's neurological condition following surgery. The tumor rarely recurs. Prognosis with primary malignant brain tumors is more limited. Most cause death within 3 years.

Brain Abscess

HISTORY

The pathogenesis and history of brain abscess are discussed more fully in Chapter 6. A brain abscess classically presents as a subacute illness with fever and headache followed by confusion, depression of consciousness, and focal symptoms. Focal and generalized seizures also may occur.

PHYSICAL EXAMINATION

The general medical examination may show fever and signs of medical conditions often associated with brain abscess—sinusitis, mastoiditis, systemic infection, cyanotic heart disease, or intravenous needle tracks suggesting drug abuse. The typical neurologic syndrome is one of depression of alertness, confusion, and focal signs.

LABORATORY STUDIES

The peripheral white blood cell count and erythrocyte sedimentation rate are usually elevated. The cerebrospinal fluid opening pressure, protein, and white blood cell count are usually elevated, but the glucose level is usually normal. However, lumbar puncture is contraindicated if increased intracranial pressure is suspected.

RADIOLOGIC STUDIES

The typical CT scan lesion is a single, rounded, contrast-enhancing ring with prominent edema in the surrounding white matter. Often the noncontrasted scan shows only the edema and concomitant mass effect. Magnetic resonance imaging (MRI) scans show a rounded lesion surrounded by extensive white matter edema. Multiple abscesses may be present.

Metastatic tumor, lymphoma, brain infarction, resolving parenchymal hematoma, and postoperative inflammation in the brain also can produce enhancing ring lesions. The clinical history and signs usually distinguish between abscess and the other possibilities.

ACUTE MANAGEMENT
The antibiotic management of bacterial brain abscess is presented in Chapter 6. If there is extensive brain swelling on the CT scan, dexamethasone may reduce the mass effect. When a brain abscess is large and is in an accessible location, surgical drainage is indicated. Small abscesses with little mass effect and multiple abscesses are probably best treated with antibiotics alone [11, 23].

If a bacterial abscess is suspected but other diagnoses are possible, surgical biopsy of the lesion is necessary to prove the etiology and guide specific therapy. In immunocompromised patients, biopsy of an abscess is especially important because of the high frequency of unusual organisms.

CHRONIC MANAGEMENT AND PROGNOSIS
Once an abscess has been fully treated by antibiotics alone or with surgery, it rarely recurs.

Subdural Hematoma
HISTORY
The usual subdural hematoma (SDH) of the acute variety is associated with severe head trauma. The patient with a chronic subdural hematoma often presents to medical attention as an elderly person with increasing confusion, unsteady walking, and minimal focal symptoms. Headaches are not prominent, and the history of trauma may be unimpressive. Anticoagulation treatment, bleeding

disorders, and alcoholism are risk factors for subdural hematoma [59].

PHYSICAL EXAMINATION
Signs of trauma or bruising may suggest recent falls and raise the suspicion of a subdural hematoma. The neurologic signs are depression of alertness, confusion, unsteady gait, a mild hemiparesis with reflex asymmetry, and a Babinski sign. Papilledema is uncommon.

LABORATORY STUDIES
The cerebrospinal fluid may show increased protein, red blood cells, and xanthochromia.

RADIOLOGIC STUDIES
The CT or MRI scan shows a collection of fluid between the brain and the skull, compressing the brain and often causing herniation (see Fig. 9-2). Bilateral subdural hematomas are common.

ACUTE MANAGEMENT
If a subdural hematoma is causing extensive mass effect, dexamethasone is indicated to reduce brain swelling and so reduce the risk of herniation. A large hematoma requires surgical drainage. A smaller one may be treated with corticosteroids for several weeks.

CHRONIC MANAGEMENT AND PROGNOSIS
A chronic subdural hematoma often reaccumulates. The patient should be examined frequently for several months, and a repeat CT or MRI scan should be done to evaluate the size of the lesion.

Obstructive Hydrocephalus
Obstructive hydrocephalus is dilatation of the cerebral ventricles caused by obstruction to normal cerebrospinal fluid flow out of the ventricles. It may be caused by a mass lesion blocking cerebrospinal fluid flow or by stenosis of the aqueduct of Sylvius. The patient usually has a history of months or years of headaches. The examination

often shows papilledema, depression of alertness, hyperactive tendon reflexes, and bilateral Babinski signs. Diagnosis is with a CT or MRI scan, and treatment is by neurosurgical placement of a ventricular shunt to drain the cerebrospinal fluid. A good prognosis depends on prompt ventricular drainage and then later treatment of the primary lesion [44].

Alteration of Mental Status

Definitions

The mental status of a patient includes all the person's cognitive and emotional functions. *Confusion* is a state of impaired cognitive functions. It implies an acute, reversible process. *Delirium* is an agitated confusion, usually with psychomotor and autonomic hyperactivity, often accompanied by hallucinations and delusions. *Dementia* is an acquired, irreversible loss of cognitive abilities. It may be static or progressive. *Mental retardation* is an abnormal reduction of cognitive functions since birth. The term *organic brain syndrome* (OBS) describes impairment of cognitive function caused by medical or neurologic disorders affecting the brain. *Acute organic brain syndrome* is equivalent to confusion, and *chronic organic brain syndrome* is equivalent to dementia [5].

The Dementias

A nonprogressive dementia may be due to brain damage from prior trauma, stroke, encephalitis, cardiac arrest, or other known cause. Dementia of the slowly progressive type usually is caused by Alzheimer's disease, cerebrovascular disease, or a combination of the two processes. However, treatable medical conditions must be sought in all cases. Important treatable etiologies are endocrine and metabolic disorders, toxins, medications, central nervous system infections, hydrocephalus, benign intracranial tumors, and chronic subdural hematomas. Severe depression also may present as apparent dementia (pseudodementia) which clears as the depression resolves.

Alzheimer's Disease

HISTORY

Alzheimer's disease (AD) is a disorder of unknown etiology that causes progressive injury and death of brain neurons. It typically affects persons over 60 years of age (senile dementia), but it may affect younger ages (presenile dementia). Among demented patients over 60 years of age, Alzheimer's disease is the etiology in more than 55 percent [64].

The first symptom usually is failing memory. This worsens over months or years and is joined by other impairments. The family often reports that the patient has been irritable and confused, has become socially withdrawn, has lost weight, and has had difficulty with shopping, driving, maintaining the checkbook, and other daily activities. Usually the spouse or other family member has assumed increasing responsibility to assist and supervise the patient.

PHYSICAL EXAMINATION

The general medical findings usually are normal. However, there may be signs of weight loss, poor grooming, dirt and food stains on clothes, and the ammonia-like smell associated with urinary incontinence. The mental status examination usually reveals a fully alert person who is somewhat defensive and has little insight into the problems related by the family, often denying them. Mental status testing shows disorientation, memory loss, hesitant, "empty" speech, impairment of calculations, difficulty following complex commands, and impaired ability demonstrating or mimicking performance of familiar tasks (apraxia), such as combing the hair, tying a tie, or putting on a coat [49]. There are no focal signs.

LABORATORY STUDIES

There is no specific laboratory abnormality associated with Alzheimer's disease. The search for treatable medical processes includes a complete blood count, urinalysis, serum serology for syphilis, serum electrolytes and biochemical screen, vitamin B_{12} level, and thyroid function tests. If a toxin is suspected, blood and urine toxicology studies are obtained. If an infection is suspected or the serologic test for syphilis is positive, a lumbar puncture is done to measure cerebrospinal fluid opening pressure, glucose, protein, cell count, VDRL, and cryptococcal antigen. An electroencephalogram usually is not helpful.

RADIOLOGIC STUDIES

A CT or MRI scan will exclude a focal intracranial lesion or hydrocephalus. The characteristic CT and MRI scan findings in Alzheimer's disease are widened cerebral sulci, enlarged ventricles, and prominent cerebrospinal fluid cisterns at the base of the brain.

MANAGEMENT

Once other causes of dementia have been excluded and a presumptive diagnosis of Alzheimer's disease has been made, the treatment is supportive care. The patient is maintained in the best possible medical and nutritional condition. Antihypertensive and other medications that may depress brain function are used in the lowest possible doses.

Patients who continue working, driving, and managing their own finances are advised when their impairment makes such activities financially or physically dangerous. The clinician also counsels the family about ensuring the patient's physical, emotional, and financial security.

Patients with a secondary depression may respond to antidepressants. The patient who is severely agitated or who is threatening and abusive to his or her family may require sedation with low doses of haloperidol or thioridazine. Nighttime often brings worsening symptoms and agitation ("sundowning"), which may respond to sedation at bedtime. Drugs reputed to cause vasodilation of cerebral vessels and central nervous system stimulants are not helpful. Recent studies have suggested that drugs that increase central nervous system acetylcholine activity may be helpful.

PROGNOSIS

Alzheimer's disease causes progressive disruption of mental function over several years, leading to death, usually from physical debilitation and systemic infection, in an average of 10 years from diagnosis.

Multi-Infarct Dementia

HISTORY

Multi-infarct dementia (MID) is caused by cerebrovascular disease. The most common form is the dementia that results from one or more clinically obvious strokes. However, some patients with a slowly progressive dementia have been found to have either multiple small infarcts or diffuse degeneration of the white matter in the periventricular region of both hemispheres. The historical features that may distinguish multi-infarct dementia from Alzheimer's disease are a history of hypertension, cardiac disease, prior clinical strokes, and a stepwise progression of dementia [34].

PHYSICAL EXAMINATION

The neurologic examination may be helpful to diagnose multi-infarct dementia by showing hemiparesis, asymmetry of tendon reflexes, or other focal signs. However, such signs also may indicate a subdural hematoma, brain tumor, or other structural lesions.

RADIOLOGIC STUDIES

The test of choice is a CT or MRI scan. The scan shows multiple, small, low-density defects in both cerebral hemispheres consistent with old infarctions. It often also shows a diffuse abnormality in the periventricular white matter [37].

MANAGEMENT

Management of the multi-infarct dementia patient is the same as for Alzheimer's disease. In addition, risk factors for stroke (discussed under Cerebrovascular Diseases) are treated in an effort to prevent further infarctions. Treatment of hypertension and cardiac disease is especially important.

PROGNOSIS

Patients with multi-infarct dementia, on average, have a shorter life expectancy than those with Alzheimer's disease. They usually die from cardiac disease.

Communicating (Normal-Pressure) Hydrocephalus

PATHOPHYSIOLOGY

Normal-pressure hydrocephalus (NPH) has been defined as a syndrome of progressive dementia due to communicating hydrocephalus but with a normal cerebrospinal fluid opening pressure on lumbar puncture [2]. Predisposing causes are prior head trauma, subarachnoid hemorrhage, and meningitis, but many cases are idiopathic. The pathologic substrate is obstruction of cerebrospinal fluid flow due to scarring and obliteration of the subarachnoid space at the base of the brain or over the convexities of the cerebral hemispheres.

HISTORY

The classic triad is progressive dementia, ataxia, and urinary incontinence [2]. Headache, seizures, weakness, and other neurologic symptoms are notably absent.

PHYSICAL EXAMINATION

The mental status signs are nonspecific, but the ataxia is a distinct one. The patient stands in a flexed position and then can only shuffle forward with irregular short steps, as if "stuck to the floor." However, similar gaits may be seen in multi-infarct dementia and Parkinson's disease.

RADIOLOGIC STUDIES

The CT or MRI scan shows prominent enlargement of all four ventricles and relative absence of sulci over the cerebral hemispheres. A radioisotope cisternogram may demonstrate reversal of cerebrospinal fluid flow with reflux into the ventricular system of the isotope that was injected into the lumbar subarachnoid space.

MANAGEMENT AND PROGNOSIS

Definitive treatment is a ventriculoperitoneal shunt. The best predictors of a good response to shunting are recent onset of symptoms, a known precipitating cause, and younger age [10].

Acute Confusional States

HISTORY

The patient often is brought to medical attention by a family member or other concerned person because there has been a recent change in behavior and mental status. Frequent causes of such a syndrome are street drugs, alcohol, prescribed medications, metabolic and electrolyte disorders, systemic or central nervous system infections, and structural brain lesions. The past medical history may provide valuable information about the specific cause [5].

PHYSICAL EXAMINATION

A complete physical examination is done to find occult medical processes. The neurologic examination includes a thorough mental status examination, as well as a search for focal signs that may indicate a structural brain lesion.

LABORATORY AND RADIOLOGIC STUDIES

A complete battery of medical, metabolic, toxicologic, and radiologic tests is required, similar to the tests done to evaluate coma of unknown cause. A lumbar puncture should be done if the patient is febrile. A CT scan is required if the history or examination suggests a focal brain lesion.

MANAGEMENT

Initially, the patient must be protected from harm resulting from confused or agitated behavior. Spe-cific therapy is given when the etiology of the confusion has been determined.

Multiple Sclerosis and Spinocerebellar Degeneration

Multiple Sclerosis

PATHOPHYSIOLOGY

Multiple sclerosis (MS) is a disease that selectively damages central nervous system white matter causing focal areas of demyelination (plaques). It affects white matter in the cerebral hemispheres, brainstem, cerebellum, spinal cord, and optic nerves alike. The cause is unknown, but clinical, laboratory, and epidemiologic studies implicate an early-life exposure to a viral or other environmental agent that later stimulates an immune response which causes the central nervous system lesions [17, 47].

HISTORY

The classic history of multiple sclerosis is one of "lesions disseminated in space and time." The usual disease runs a course of years of exacerbations and remissions of symptoms (dissemination in time) with signs of lesions in multiple locations in the central nervous system (dissemination in space). The onset commonly is between 20 and 40 years of age. Women are affected more often than men by about a 1.5:1 ratio.

The symptom patterns of multiple sclerosis are variable because the lesions may occur in any central nervous system location. Early symptoms commonly are numbness and paresthesias in one or more limbs, usually associated with weakness and clumsiness of the same limb. In younger patients, optic neuritis causing visual impairment in one or both eyes is a frequent presentation. In patients who are over age 40 at onset, especially men, a common syndrome is slowly progressive spastic ataxia.

The characteristic time course of an exacerbation of multiple sclerosis is for the symptoms to worsen over several days and then slowly resolve over several weeks. Early in the disease the symptoms usually totally resolve. However, later the resolution often is only partial and each attack leaves the patient with more overall neurologic deficit. Exacerbations are often brought on by infections, fever, excessive fatigue, and severe life stress. In the late stages of multiple sclerosis the patient may be incapacitated with dementia, often associated with an inappropriate euphoria, severe motor impairment of the limbs, dysphagia, dysarthria, and urinary incontinence. Optic nerve involvement may cause blindness.

PHYSICAL EXAMINATION

The general physical examination usually is normal until late in the disease, when the medical complications of chronic neurologic disease develop. The neurologic signs reflect the portions of the nervous system involved by the disease. The optic nerve heads (discs) often are pale and sharply demarcated, suggesting optic atrophy. Nystagmus, dysarthria, ataxic gait, limb motor and sensory signs, asymmetrical deep tendon reflexes, and Babinski signs are common. The characteristic pattern is that of physical signs indicating multiple central nervous system lesions.

LABORATORY STUDIES

The diagnostic laboratory findings are in the cerebrospinal fluid. During an acute exacerbation there may be a mild elevation of the cerebrospinal fluid white blood cell count and protein. The more diagnostic changes include elevation of the cerebrospinal fluid gamma globulin (IgG) as a percentage of total protein. An index comparing the cerebrospinal fluid IgG-albumin ratio with the serum IgG-albumin ratio is often elevated. Agarose electrophoresis of the cerebrospinal fluid shows abnormally migrating bands of IgG (oligoclonal bands) in 70 to 85 percent of patients, more frequently in patients with more advanced disease. Abnormalities of cerebrospinal fluid IgG and oligoclonal bands also occur in central nervous system infections and other inflammatory conditions, so the tests are diagnostic of multiple sclerosis only in the proper clinical setting and when other diseases can be excluded.

Electrophysiologic tests are valuable adjuncts to the clinical laboratory. Visual, brainstem auditory, and somatosensory evoked potentials are often abnormal.

RADIOLOGIC STUDIES

An MRI scan is the best radiologic test. It often demonstrates multiple lesions throughout the white matter of the cerebral hemispheres, most concentrated in the periventricular region (Fig. 9-3). Optic nerve, brainstem, cerebellar, and spinal cord lesions also may be shown.

A high-dose contrast-enhanced CT scan may demonstrate enhancing white matter lesions. However, the typical CT scan shows only mild ventricular dilatation and enlargement of cortical sulci.

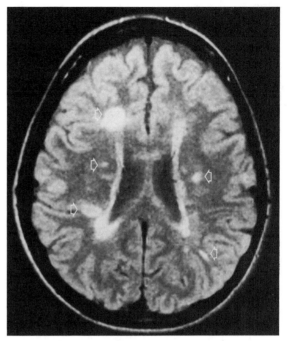

Figure 9–3. *Head MRI scan showing bilateral periventricular white matter abnormality (bright white rims) and multiple, rounded white matter plaques (arrows).*

ACUTE MANAGEMENT

Early in the course the most important task is to establish the diagnosis and to exclude other conditions. Important nondemyelinating diseases that can cause a clinical disease similar to multiple sclerosis are central nervous system syphilis, vasculitis, sarcoidosis, amyotrophic lateral sclerosis (ALS), cervical spondylosis, vitamin E deficiency, toxins (e.g., organic mercury), brainstem arteriovenous malformations, and spinocerebellar degeneration. The diagnosis of multiple sclerosis is founded on the typical clinical history and neurologic signs coupled with characteristic cerebrospinal fluid, evoked-potential, and MRI scan abnormalities [48].

When a patient with an established diagnosis of multiple sclerosis has an acute exacerbation, treatment with adrenocorticotropic hormone (ACTH) intramuscularly or intravenously for 10 to 14 days or oral corticosteroids daily or on alternate days for several weeks is indicated.

Treatment probably reduces the severity and duration of the attack, but there is no convincing evidence that it reduces long-term severity of disease. Acute exacerbations may be precipitated by urinary or other infections, so occult infection must be sought and treated.

CHRONIC MANAGEMENT

The tenets of chronic management of multiple sclerosis are to advise the patient about optimal rest and nutrition, to provide physical therapy and assistive devices (e.g., cane, crutches, wheelchair, braces), and to vigorously treat urinary, skin, or pulmonary complications. The clinician also counsels the patient and family about the disease and how to cope with its effects. Referral to the local multiple sclerosis society and multiple sclerosis support groups also may be helpful [48, 58].

Chronic treatment with immunosuppressive

drugs has been shown to slow progression and reduce the frequency of exacerbations in some studies. Such treatment is only indicated in selected patients under closely monitored supervision. There is no evidence that special diets, vitamin therapy, hyperbaric oxygen, cobra venom, or other unconventional therapies give any benefit.

PROGNOSIS

The average duration of disease has been extended to almost 35 years by improved management of infections, nutrition, and other complications of the chronic disease. Death usually is due to pneumonia or sepsis from infected urinary tract or decubiti. About half of multiple sclerosis patients are disabled from working within 10 years of diagnosis. Nonetheless, the disease has a highly variable pattern, and 20 percent of patients have a prolonged benign course [58].

Spinocerebellar Degenerations

The spinocerebellar degenerations (SCD) are a diverse group of diseases of unknown etiology that cause progressive neuronal death in the cerebellum, brainstem, and spinal cord and produce ataxia plus other neurologic symptoms and signs. They commonly are misidentified as multiple sclerosis. They usually are hereditary, and a thorough family history often documents as autosomal-dominant or autosomal-recessive neurologic disorder [35].

The typical course is one of gait ataxia slowly worsening over many years. Commonly associated neurologic symptoms are dysarthria, clumsy hands, and spastic legs. The CT and MRI scans show only ventricular dilatation and brain atrophy, often most severe in the cerebellum and brainstem. There are no specific treatments. Chronic management is similar to that for multiple sclerosis.

Movement Disorders

Pathophysiology

Movement disorders are neurologic conditions in which an abnormal involuntary movement is a prominent feature. The part of the central nervous system affected in these disorders is the extrapyramidal motor system, primarily in the basal ganglia. The clinical features of these conditions are involuntary movements plus abnormalities of voluntary movement, tone, and posture [29].

Parkinson's Disease

HISTORY

The prototype and best understood of the movement disorders is Parkinson's disease. Its major clinical features are tremor, rigidity, and paucity of spontaneous movements (hypokinesia or akinesia). Onset commonly is in the sixth or eighth decades. The patient and family often report that the first symptom was tremor of the hands and then, over months, the patient "slowed down," became less active, slower when moving, developed a stooped, shuffling walk, and lost dexterity in the hands. Stiffness, tightness, and aching of the muscles are also frequent complaints [29].

Most patients with the Parkinsonian symptom complex have idiopathic Parkinson's disease, a degeneration of the dopamine-containing pigmented neurons in the substantia nigra. Encephalitis, toxins such as methylphenyl tetrahydropyridine (MPTP), manganese, or carbon monoxide, multiple lacunar infarcts in the basal ganglia, and prescribed medications, especially phenothiazines, can cause identical symptoms and signs.

PHYSICAL EXAMINATION

The cardinal neurologic features are hypokinesia and slowness of movement (bradykinesia), tremor, postural muscle abnormalities, and increased muscle tone. The typical patient sits quietly, slightly bent forward, hands in his or her lap, and makes few or no spontaneous movements. Speech is likewise sparse and monotonous, and the voice has low volume. The face shows little emotional expression, and eye blinking is infrequent.

The classic tremor occurs with the hand at rest in the lap and is a 4 to 7 cycle per second rhythmic oscillation of the thumb and fingers suggesting "pill rolling." It typically goes away with complete relaxation of the hand and also with active use of the hand, such as reaching for an object. The tremor is thus called a "resting tremor."

Muscle tone is increased in all muscles, and the rigidity is present through the entire range of motion at the joint. A "cog wheeling" phenomenon may be felt by the examiner as a rhythmic, jerky relaxation of the muscle when it is stretched. When the patient walks, the trunk and neck are flexed forward, the arms are held flexed at the sides and do not swing, and the feet shuffle forward in short steps.

LABORATORY STUDIES
Routine laboratory studies and cerebrospinal fluid tests are normal, but the level of cerebrospinal fluid homovanillic acid, a metabolite of dopamine, is reduced.

RADIOLOGIC STUDIES
CT and MRI scans may be normal or may show mild cerebral atrophy. The main value of imaging tests is to exclude lacunar infarctions or other structural lesions causing the illness.

ACUTE MANAGEMENT
Pharmacologic therapy is based on the hypothesis that Parkinsonian symptoms are caused by a deficiency of basal ganglia dopamine and a relative excess of acetylcholine. Thus symptoms may be reduced by restoring dopamine, by blocking acetylcholine, or by doing both [25, 29].

Patients with early disease and minimally disabling symptoms probably are best treated first with an anticholinergic drug such as benztropine or trihexyphenidyl. Amantadine or a tricyclic antidepressant may be added when the first-choice drug has produced inadequate symptom relief. Dihydroxyphenylalanine (levodopa) is a synthetic amino acid that is converted in the brain to dopamine. It is given in combination with carbidopa, an enzyme inhibitor that prevents systemic degradation of the levodopa. The combination drug (Sinemet) is begun in low doses and slowly increased until symptoms are adequately reduced.

Bromocriptine, a dopamine agonist agent, may further reduce symptoms in patients on maximum doses of other drugs. Its use is limited by frequent side effects of confusion and nausea.

CHRONIC MANAGEMENT
Physical and occupational therapies are an important part of the continuing care. Therapy can improve walking and increase skills necessary for dressing, cooking, and performing other daily activities. An evaluation of the home by a physical or occupational therapist often produces valuable suggestions for improving the home environment and making living easier for the patient [25, 29].

PROGNOSIS
None of the drugs or other treatments retards progression of disease. However, the reduction of immobility and other symptoms significantly reduces morbidity and prolongs independent living.

Benign Essential Tremor
HISTORY
A condition often confused with Parkinson's disease is benign essential tremor, also called senile tremor. This condition appears in middle or late life as a rapid tremor of both hands that interferes with writing, causes spilling when the patient holds a cup, and impairs other fine-motor use of the hands. The patient often reports that anxiety and drinking coffee exacerbate the tremor, but drinking alcohol significantly reduces it. There frequently is a family history of similar tremors.

The tremor often is accompanied by tremors of the head and of the vocal muscles, causing an unusual quavering of the voice.

PHYSICAL EXAMINATION

The characteristic tremor is a rhythmic 8 to 10 cycle per second oscillation of the hands and fingers. It is present at rest but is exacerbated by movement and by holding the arms, hands, and fingers outstretched. The absence of bradykinesia, of increased muscle tone, and of postural gait abnormalities and exacerbation of the tremor by voluntary use of the hands distinguish benign tremor from Parkinson's disease.

LABORATORY AND RADIOLOGIC STUDIES

All routine tests, including CT and MRI scans, electroencephalograms, and cerebrospinal fluid studies, are normal.

MANAGEMENT

Suppression of the tremor can be attained by treatment with propranolol or a benzodiazepine tranquilizer. The patient may require only an occasional dose. The patient must avoid caffeine-containing beverages.

PROGNOSIS

The disease rarely progresses to disable the patient because the tremor usually can be controlled by medication.

Huntington's Disease

HISTORY

Huntington's disease (HD) or Huntington's chorea is an autosomal-dominant inherited disorder characterized by midlife onset of chorea and de-

mentia that progress to severe disability and death within the next two decades [45].

PHYSICAL EXAMINATION

The patient has multiple, irregular twitching movements of the limbs, trunk, neck, and face. The patient may try to cover up the movements by incorporating them into apparently purposeful movements. The patient also often is unkempt and depressed. Formal mental status examination may be normal initially, but dementia invariably appears as the disease progresses.

LABORATORY STUDIES

All routine studies, including those of the cerebrospinal fluid, are normal.

RADIOLOGIC STUDIES

An MRI or CT scan usually shows diffuse cerebral atrophy with enlargement of the ventricles and the cortical sulci. A specific finding that occurs only late in the disease is selective atrophy of the head of the caudate nuclei resulting in a characteristic deformity of the anterior horn of both lateral ventricles.

MANAGEMENT

There are no medical treatments to slow disease progression. Haloperidol, other neuroleptic agents, or reserpine will lessen the chorea. The major tasks in management are those of psychological and genetic counseling for the patient and family.

Peripheral and Cranial Nerve Disorders

Clinical Anatomy

Disorders of the peripheral nerves have two common syndromes: (1) distal symmetrical polyneuropathy, and (2) compression, entrapment neuropathy of a single nerve (mononeuropathy). The clinical pictures of the syndromes are distinct, and the etiologies differ.

Chronic Distal Polyneuropathy

HISTORY

The typical syndrome is one of sensory symptoms in the feet and hands that progressively worsen over months or years. The altered sensation usually has two aspects, numbness and paresthesias. Numbness is described as a sense of deadness and difficulty feeling things contacted by the hand or foot. Paresthesias usually are a spontaneous experience of "pins and needles" in the distal limbs. Some patients also have a burning, painful discomfort whenever the affected area is touched or rubbed (painful dysesthesia). In addition, the patient often experiences clumsiness and weakness of the hands [7, 26].

PHYSICAL EXAMINATION

The neurologic signs of polyneuropathy are diffusely hypoactive deep tendon reflexes, often with absent ankle jerks, and decreased sensation in the feet, hands, and distal limbs. In severe cases, weakness and muscle atrophy may occur in the hands, feet, and distal legs.

LABORATORY STUDIES

Use of laboratory tests is guided by knowledge of the diverse causes of distal peripheral neuropathy. The most common causes are diabetes mellitus and alcoholism, but other causes are chronic renal or hepatic failure, occult carcinoma, hypothyroidism, malnutrition, vitamin B_{12} deficiency, vasculitis, amyloidosis, porphyria, prescribed medications, heavy metals (lead, arsenic), and chronic vapor abuse (glue sniffing). Rarely, a neuropathy is hereditary.

The necessary blood tests include a complete blood count, glucose tolerance test, biochemical screen, erythrocyte sedimentation rate, thyroid function tests, and vitamin B_{12} level. If a heavy metal, other toxin, or a vasculitis is suspected, appropriate specimens are obtained.

The neuropathy is best documented by electrophysiologic nerve conduction velocity (NCV) studies, usually done in conjunction with an electromyogram (EMG) [6]. The nerve conduction velocity test stimulates and records the transmitted compound action and sensory potentials of various nerves. The electromyogram records the electrical activity of selected muscles. In a symmetrical peripheral neuropathy, the nerve conduction velocities of all distal nerves are below normal (slow). On electromyogram there may be signs of muscle denervation in all the distal limb muscles.

MANAGEMENT

Once an etiologic diagnosis has been made, appropriate treatment is begun. Good control of diabetes or other metabolic conditions may reverse or retard progression of the neuropathy. The patient should avoid alcohol and other toxins. If the neuropathy has caused chronically painful dysesthesias, a benzodiazepine, amitriptyline, carbamazepine, or phenytoin may reduce the discomfort.

PROGNOSIS

If a treatable etiology is not found, the neuropathy slowly worsens over the life of the patient.

Acute Polyneuropathy

HISTORY

The prototypical acute neuropathy is the Guillain-Barré syndrome (GBS). Guillain-Barré syndrome is an inflammatory polyneuropathy that typically begins with mild sensory symptoms in the feet and hands several weeks after a viral infection or an immunization. Over the next few days the feet and legs and then the hands and arms grow progressively weaker. Often the weakness progresses to cause total paralysis of the limbs and then failure of ventilation because of weakness of chest and abdominal muscles. The usual course is one of worsening symptoms and signs for 2 or 3 weeks and then slow recovery over several months. Acute toxic neuropathies from lead, arsenic, thallium, and porphyria may present in a similar fashion [7, 26].

PHYSICAL EXAMINATION
Weakness and absent deep tendon reflexes are the most striking findings. Sensory abnormalities vary, but they are usually mild. The presence of tachycardia and hypertension indicate involvement of the peripheral autonomic nervous system. Tachypnea or respiratory distress indicate chest-wall weakness and are ominous signs.

LABORATORY STUDIES
The diagnostic tests are the electromyogram and nerve conduction velocity studies. Nerve conduction velocities are slow, and after 2 weeks, denervation of distal muscles appears [6]. The cerebrospinal fluid in Guillain-Barré syndrome shows an "albuminocytologic dissociation" in which protein concentration is markedly increased but the white blood cell count is normal or only slightly elevated. Glucose level is normal. Other laboratory tests are not helpful unless studies for toxins or porphyria are indicated.

ACUTE MANAGEMENT
Patients with severe Guillain-Barré syndrome die from ventilatory failure. If the patient has respiratory distress or has significantly reduced vital capacity or minute volume, intubation and mechanical ventilation are instituted. Patients without respiratory distress are observed closely to detect early signs of ventilatory failure.

Management also requires intensive medical and nursing care for several weeks designed to maintain nutrition and fluid and electrolyte balance and prevent the complications of total paralysis. Compulsive ventilator and airway care are critically important. Corticosteroid treatment has been used in the acute stage, but this has not been shown to significantly affect the course or prognosis [39]. Plasmapheresis early in the course may reduce the severity and duration of weakness [16].

CHRONIC MANAGEMENT
As the patient recovers, physical therapy and several weeks in a rehabilitation unit are often required. Leg braces, wrist splints, and other assistive devices may be necessary.

PROGNOSIS
Acute mortality is low and is due to medical complications of protracted immobility. The acute neuropathies are self-limited diseases that resolve over several months. However, about 15 percent of patients have permanent deficits.

Nerve Entrapments and Mononeuropathies
HISTORY
A peripheral or cranial nerve may be injured by trauma, local compression, or vasculitis, among other conditions. The injury may be chronic, producing a slowly progressive syndrome, or acute, causing sudden onset of symptoms and signs [26].

The usual chronic mononeuropathies are those affecting the median and ulnar nerves. The median nerve is frequently compressed in the carpal tunnel at the wrist, causing numbness and paresthesias in the thumb and two adjacent fingers. Eventually, weakness and atrophy of the thenar muscles develop. Ulnar neuropathy causes paresthesias and numbness in the ulnar margin of the hand and ring and little fingers plus weakness and atrophy of the hand intrinsic muscles. The ulnar nerve typically is entrapped and compressed in the ulnar groove at the elbow. These entrapment neuropathies occur because of mechanical pressure on the nerve at one vulnerable location, but common predisposing conditions are diabetes mellitus, pregnancy, hypothyroidism, and arthritis.

Common acute mononeuropathies are those of the common peroneal nerve, femoral nerve, radial nerve, facial nerve, and oculomotor nerve. These neuropathies cause motor and sensory dysfunction in the specific nerve distribution. Trauma is a common cause, but nontraumatic etiologies are diabetes mellitus, pregnancy, and vasculitis. Acute facial nerve paralysis (Bell's palsy) also may follow viral infections [24]. Oculomotor nerve palsy may be caused by an expanding aneurysm of the posterior communicating artery.

PHYSICAL EXAMINATION
The physical signs reflect the particular nerve affected. An important sign indicating focal nerve injury is Tinel's sign. Percussion at the site of a nerve compression or traumatic injury produces brisk paresthesias in the distal sensory distribution of that nerve.

LABORATORY STUDIES
Tests for diabetes mellitus, hypothyroidism, pregnancy, and vasculitis are indicated. An electromyogram and nerve conduction velocity study will show the presence and location of the nerve entrapment.

MANAGEMENT
If a localized nerve entrapment is demonstrated, continuing injury of the nerve is prevented by advising the patient to avoid activities that traumatize the nerve and to use a protective pad or splint. Nonsteroidal anti-inflammatory agents may be useful if there is prominent tenderness or other signs of inflammation at the site of injury. If the symptoms and signs worsen, surgical decompression of the nerve is indicated. A 7- to 10-day course of oral corticosteroids may reduce the duration and severity of facial weakness from a Bell's palsy.

Neuromuscular Disorders

Muscular Dystrophy
HISTORY
Muscular dystrophy (MD) refers to a diverse group of hereditary diseases that cause progressive degeneration of skeletal muscle. The most widely known is Duchenne muscular dystrophy (DMD), an X-linked recessive genetic disorder. Onset is in infancy or early childhood and is marked by failure to achieve usual motor milestones in walking, running, or other motor activities. Over the next few years the boy becomes more severely weak in all muscle groups, especially in the pelvic girdle, and by his early teens, the patient is wheelchair-bound. Other forms of muscular dystrophy typically appear later in life, namely, the limb-girdle, oculopharyngeal, and facioscapulohumeral dystrophies. They primarily affect the muscles indicated by their names. Myotonic dystrophy has weakness, atrophy, and myotonia (failure of muscle relaxation after contraction). The family history usually includes relatives with a muscular disorder [12].

PHYSICAL EXAMINATION
Neurologic examination discloses muscle weakness, worse in proximal groups. The toe reflexes and sensory examination are normal.

LABORATORY STUDIES
Blood tests show elevation of the muscle-related enzymes creatine kinase (CK), lactate dehydrogenase, and aldolase. The most specific abnormality is a high muscle-origin creatine kinase fraction.

An electromyogram shows changes specific for muscle disease. The nerve conduction velocities are normal. Muscle biopsy shows specific myopathic changes.

MANAGEMENT
There are no specific treatments for muscular dystrophy. Management involves assistive devices, occupational and physical therapies, and careful medical management of pulmonary complications. Surgical tendon releases may prolong the

years of walking. The parents are counseled about the probability of having other affected children.

PROGNOSIS

Duchenne muscular dystrophy invariably causes death by respiratory complications in the second or early third decade. The other dystrophies progress at slower rates and have variable courses.

Nonhereditary Myopathies

HISTORY

Systemic medical conditions that can produce a slowly progressive disorder of muscle weakness and wasting (myopathy) include hyperthyroidism, corticosteroid therapy, chronic alcoholism, and occult carcinoma [12, 42]. Inflammatory myopathies include idiopathic polymyositis, a presumed autoimmune disorder, and sarcoidosis, toxoplasmosis, and trichinosis [20].

Weakness typically slowly progresses over months or a few years. The inflammatory myopathies often are accompanied by muscle aches and cramps.

PHYSICAL EXAMINATION

The main physical signs are proximal muscle weakness and wasting.

LABORATORY STUDIES

Blood tests, electromyography, and muscle biopsy are specific for a myopathy and are similar to those seen in the muscular dystrophies. The inflammatory myopathies usually have prominent inflammatory changes on biopsy.

MANAGEMENT

The myopathy resolves if a metabolic, toxic, or inflammatory disorder is discovered and treated [42]. Idiopathic polymyositis requires corticosteroids or other immunosuppressive drugs.

Myasthenia Gravis

HISTORY

Myasthenia gravis (MG) is a disorder of fluctuating weakness of somatic and brainstem-innervated musculature caused by impaired transmission of acetylcholine at the neuromuscular junction (NMJ). The basic defect is a circulating serum antibody to the acetylcholine receptor on the postsynaptic membrane of the neurosmuscular junction. The underlying cause is unclear, but it somehow relates to the thymus gland and thymus tumors [28].

The disease usually begins in the second to fourth decades and is more common in women. Symptoms include ptosis, diplopia, dysphagia, dysarthria, and limb weakness. These wax and wane, often being absent in the morning and then appearing late in the day.

PHYSICAL EXAMINATION

The neurologic signs are those of ptosis, dysarthria, dysphagia, bilateral facial weakness, and limb weakness. Tendon reflexes, toe reflexes, and sensory examination are normal.

LABORATORY STUDIES

A bedside test diagnostic of myasthenia gravis is the Tensilon test. Injection of edrophonium chloride (Tensilon), 10 mg IV, in increments will produce marked, but temporary, reversal of the symptoms and signs. The standard electromyogram and nerve conduction velocity tests are normal, but repetitive stimulation of a peripheral motor nerve at 2 to 5 stimuli per second shows a progressive decrement of the amplitude of the distal compound muscle action potential. Serum antibodies to acetylcholine receptor are detectable in about 85 percent of patients with generalized myasthenia. Thyroid function tests are necessary to rule out associated hyperthyroidism.

RADIOLOGIC STUDIES

A thymoma will be shown on chest x-ray in about 15 percent of patients with myasthenia gravis. CT and MRI scans of the mediastinum are both more sensitive for detecting small thymomas.

MANAGEMENT

Acetylcholinesterase inhibitors relieve symptoms by increasing available acetylcholine at the neuromuscular junction. Treatment of the primary autoimmune condition requires thymectomy and high-dose corticosteroids or other immunosuppressive drugs. Plasmapheresis is valuable for patients who are severely weak and are not responding to medications [16]. Drugs that may potentiate the underlying neuromuscular blockade should be avoided, especially aminoglycosides, polypeptide antibiotics, and possibly propranolol.

PROGNOSIS

About 60 percent of patients require no medications 5 years after thymectomy.

Motor Neuron Disease

HISTORY

Motor neuron disease (MND) is an idiopathic degenerative disorder of motor neurons in the anterior horn of the spinal cord and in the brain. The symptoms begin insidiously with clumsiness of the hands and legs. Then muscle weakness develops, usually in the hands, feet, and lower legs, and is associated with muscle fasciculations, cramps, and atrophy. Dysphagia and dysarthria are common because of involvement of bulbar motor neurons. The classic motor neuron disease is amyotrophic lateral sclerosis (ALS or Lou Gehrig's disease) [52].

PHYSICAL EXAMINATION

The neurologic signs are weakness and atrophy of distal muscles, brisk tendon reflexes, Babinski signs, and a normal sensory examination.

LABORATORY STUDIES

An electromyogram and muscle biopsy both show abnormalities diagnostic of diffuse denervation. The nerve conduction velocities are normal.

MANAGEMENT AND PROGNOSIS

The initial goal is to exclude a treatable condition that may masquerade as motor neuron disease [42]. Tests should include thyroid function tests, SMA-12, serum lead level, and a search for an occult malignancy.

If a diagnosis of idiopathic motor neuron disease is made, the subsequent management includes physical and occupational therapies, assistive devices, psychological counseling, and treatment of medical complications. In classic amyotrophic lateral sclerosis, death from pulmonary complications usually occurs within 5 years.

Disorders of the Spinal Cord

Cervical Spondylosis

HISTORY

Cervical spondylosis refers to severe osteoarthritis of the cervical spine compressing the cervical spinal nerve roots or the spinal cord. The classic symptom triad is chronic neck pain, then arm and shoulder pain from nerve root impingement, followed by progressive stiffness and weakness of the legs due to spinal cord compression. The patient usually is over 50 years old and more often male than female [1].

PHYSICAL EXAMINATION

The cervical spine has a limited range of motion, and movement causes pain. The pain may radiate into one or both arms. The neurologic signs in the arms are depressed tendon reflexes, weakness and wasting of the muscles, and sensory loss in a dermatomal pattern. The legs have increased tone, increased deep tendon reflexes, Babinski signs, and nondermatomal sensory abnormalities.

RADIOLOGIC STUDIES
Cervical spine x-ray studies show severe degenerative osteoarthritis. Myelography is necessary to prove the location and severity of spinal cord and nerve root compression. Conventional myelography requires instillation of radiopaque liquid contrast material into the subarachnoid space. Routine x-ray films or a CT scan show the dye inside the cervical spinal canal and demonstrate the abnormalities.

ACUTE MANAGEMENT
A cervical collar sufficient to limit neck movement and cervical traction may relieve pain and may slow progression of symptoms. Nonsteroidal anti-inflammatory drugs, analgesics, and local heat will reduce neck pain.

CHRONIC MANAGEMENT AND PROGNOSIS
Once a myelopathy develops, the symptoms and signs usually slowly worsen over years. If symptoms or signs progress, myelography and surgery are indicated.

Combined System Disease
HISTORY
Combined system disease (subacute combined degeneration) is a chronic, progressive myelopathy due to deficiency of vitamin B_{12}. Pathologically, it is characterized by degeneration of the white matter pathways of the dorsal and lateral columns of the spinal cord. Symptoms and signs suggest both spinal cord and peripheral nerve disease.

PHYSICAL EXAMINATION
The main signs on examination are severe loss of position and vibration sense in the feet and legs. The knee deep tendon reflexes are usually brisk, and Babinski signs are present, indicating the spinal cord involvement. However, the ankle-jerk reflexes often are depressed or absent, reflecting the peripheral neuropathy.

LABORATORY STUDIES
A macrocytic anemia may be present but often is not. The serum vitamin B_{12} (cobalamin) level is low. The intestinal absorption defect characteristic of pernicious anemia can be demonstrated by the two-stage Schilling test (see Chapter 5).

ACUTE AND CHRONIC MANAGEMENT
Treatment is with vitamin B_{12} (1000 μg IM) daily for several days and then monthly for the remainder of the patient's life.

Acute Myelopathy
HISTORY
Acute myelopathy is the syndrome of rapidly progressive symptoms and signs of spinal cord dysfunction, usually over several days. The most common cause is a malignant neoplasm in the spinal epidural space [57]. A benign tumor, epidural abscess, intraspinal hematoma, and idiopathic transverse myelitis are rare causes [18, 65].

The first symptom is pain in the spine at the level of the lesion and then pain extending in a radicular distribution around the trunk. The neurologic illness presents as progressive leg weakness and difficulty with urinary control.

PHYSICAL EXAMINATION
A prominent sign is back pain with focal tenderness over the lesion. Neurologic signs are those of spastic paraparesis with hyperreflexia, Babinski signs, and sensory loss below the level of the lesion. There may be urinary and fecal incontinence.

LABORATORY AND RADIOLOGIC STUDIES
Plain x-ray films of the painful area of the spine often show a bony abnormality indicating a tumor or abscess (Fig. 9-4). CT and MRI scans of the spine are even more sensitive. Conventional and CT scan myelography nicely demonstrate epidural lesions (see Fig. 9-4).

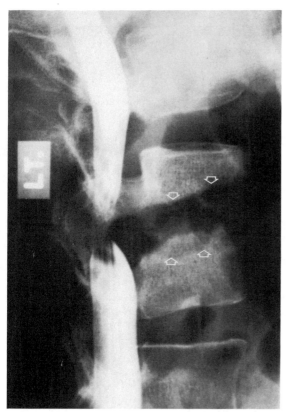

Figure 9–4. Conventional lumbar myelogram showing compression of dye column by epidural mass at site of partial destruction of two vertebral bodies by metastatic tumor (arrows).

ACUTE MANAGEMENT

Spinal cord compression from an epidural lesion is a critical emergency requiring immediate treatment to preserve spinal cord function. A suspected epidural abscess or hematoma is surgically drained. A malignant tumor is generally treated with radiotherapy plus high-dose intravenous dexamethasone [32].

PROGNOSIS

Prognosis depends on how promptly the offending lesion is treated. Once a patient with acute myelopathy can no longer walk, it is rare for him or her ever to walk again.

Headaches

Vascular Headaches: Migraine Type

HISTORY

Vascular headaches of the migraine type are headaches whose major characteristics are hemicranial throbbing pain accompanied by general malaise, nausea, and photophobia lasting several hours. Before the onset of pain there often is a sense of illness, and in the "classic" migraine, there is an aura of neurologic warning symptoms. The most typical aura is visual change, either bright flashing lights, wavering lines, or blind patches (scotomas) in the visual field. However, the more prevalent "common" migraine has no aura [21, 40, 41, 56].

The patient sometimes can relate headaches to precipitating events, including stress, alcohol use, or eating chocolate or other specific foods. Migraines tend to occur around the menstrual period, and oral contraceptive drugs often increase their frequency and severity.

A rare but potentially dangerous form of migraine is the "complicated" migraine, which is associated with prominent focal neurologic deficits. Hemiplegia, aphasia, or ophthalmoplegia may occur. Usually, the deficit resolves as the headache subsides, but sometimes it persists.

Migraine patients often have a family history of vascular headaches. Migraines commonly begin in adolescence or the third decade and subside in the fourth decade.

PHYSICAL EXAMINATION
The patient with a migraine headache looks ill and in pain, is often pale, and has a tachycardia. There may be prominence and tenderness of the superficial temporal artery on the symptomatic side. Unless it is a complicated migraine, there are no neurologic signs.

LABORATORY TESTS
Numerous abnormalities of platelet function, prostaglandins, and catecholamines have been described, but there are no diagnostic tests for migraine.

ACUTE MANAGEMENT
Mild migraine-type headaches may respond to aspirin, acetaminophen, or nonsteroidal anti-inflammatory drugs. However, the standard drug for more severe migraine is some form of ergotamine, a potent vasoconstrictor of extracranial vessels (Table 9-5). A patent drug combining isometheptene mucate, acetaminophen, and dichloralphenazone (Midrin) also may be effective. An especially severe or protracted migraine may be treated with intramuscular meperidine sedatives or intravenous metaclopramide or dihydroergotamine.

A patient with a migraine-like headache who has focal neurologic signs must have a CT or MRI scan to exclude a hemorrhage or other intracranial lesion.

CHRONIC MANAGEMENT
When a patient has more than two headaches per week, a regimen of daily administration of a preventive drug is indicated. Drugs that have been

Table 9–5. Medications Containing Ergotamine Tartrate

Trade name	Ergot	Other active agents	Administration route
Cafergot	1 mg	Caffeine	Oral
Cafergot PB	1 mg	Caffeine, pentobarbital, belladona	Oral
Cafergot suppository	2 mg	Caffeine	Rectal
Cafergot PB suppository	2 mg	Caffeine, pentobarbital, belladonna	Rectal
Ergomar	2 mg		Sublingual
Ergostat	2 mg		Sublingual
Migral	1 mg	Caffeine, cyclizine	Oral
Wigraine	1 mg	Caffeine, phenacetin, belladona	Oral
Wigraine suppositories	1 mg	Caffeine, phenacetin, belladona	Rectal

found effective include propranolol, amitriptyline, calcium-channel blocking agents, indomethacin, methysergide, phenytoin, cyproheptadine, and corticosteroids [19, 41, 56].

Patients should be advised to avoid stressful situations and foods, alcohol, or other known precipitants of their attacks. Women should discontinue the use of birth control pills.

Tension (Muscle-Contraction) Headaches
HISTORY
The typical headache has an onset with bifrontal or nuchal pressure which then extends to become a caplike or bandlike aching tightness over the entire head. It may be accompanied by nausea, but vomiting is rarely prominent. Visual symptoms are usually limited to mild blurring during the severe attacks. There are no focal neurologic symptoms. The headaches usually last 2 to 4 hours, but in severe cases they may last all day [21, 41, 56].

PHYSICAL EXAMINATION

There are no signs on physical examination other than apparent painful distress and frontal or nuchal muscle tenderness.

ACUTE MANAGEMENT

Aspirin, acetaminophen, or other nonsteroidal anti-inflammatory drugs often suffice. However, severe, protracted headaches may require acetaminophen with codeine or an analgesic plus mild sedation. Sleep usually cures the headache.

CHRONIC MANAGEMENT

Patients with severe tension-type headaches that frequently interfere with their activities of daily living often have significant psychological factors, commonly depression. These must be treated with counseling and antidepressant medications.

Combined Headaches

Many patients with frequent, severe headaches have attacks with features of both migraine and tension headaches. The examination is normal except for signs of pain during the headache. Treatment is selected according to the predominant symptoms.

Organic Headache

HISTORY

Intracranial tumor, infection, hematoma, hydrocephalus, and other dangerous processes often present with headaches. The features of the history suggesting an active central nervous system process are recent onset and increasing severity, strictly unilateral headaches, headaches awakening the patient at night, and focal neurologic symptoms. The patient with a sudden onset of "the worst headache of my life" often has had a subarachnoid hemorrhage. Older patients with recent onset of headaches may have temporal arteritis.

PHYSICAL EXAMINATION

A central nervous system process is suggested by fever, signs of a bleeding disorder, trauma, or tumor and focal neurologic signs. Temporal arteritis may cause tender, nodular superficial temporal arteries.

ACUTE MANAGEMENT

A CT or MRI scan of the head will exclude a mass, hydrocephalus, and subarachnoid hemorrhage. If the imaging study is negative, a lumbar puncture may yield cerebrospinal fluid with changes indicating an infection. The erythrocyte sedimentation rate is elevated in temporal arteritis. If temporal arteritis is suspected, an arteriogram and biopsy of the superficial temporal arteries are required.

Back Pain

Pathophysiology

Back pain is a common symptom and usually is due to benign musculoskeletal strain. However, it may be caused by more serious disorders such as herniated nucleus pulposus, intraspinal tumor, metastatic neoplasm, or vertebral compression fractures.

Low-Back Pain of Musculoskeletal Origin

HISTORY

Often the patient with low-back pain (LBP) describes the onset in association with lifting or some other physical exertion. The pain worsens over several hours after onset and is especially severe upon awakening the next morning. It is aggravated by bending and physical exertion and is only partially relieved by rest [4, 30].

PHYSICAL EXAMINATION

Palpation may show diffuse tenderness of the spine and adjacent tissues and prominent, tender paraspinous muscles (spasm). The range of motion of the lumbar spine is limited, especially in flexion, and movement increases the pain. The neurologic examination is normal.

LABORATORY AND RADIOLOGIC STUDIES

A complete blood count, erythrocyte sedimentation rate, and determinations of serum calcium, phosphorus, and alkaline phosphatase are indicated to look for occult medical diseases. Lumbosacral spine x-rays usually are normal, but they may show arthritis. Myelography is not indicated for typical low-back pain with no neurologic signs and normal lumbosacral spine x-ray studies.

ACUTE MANAGEMENT

The mainstay of early treatment is several days of bed rest with a firm mattress or bedboard. Minor analgesics, nonsteroidal anti-inflammatory agents, muscle relaxants, and heat to the back are helpful adjuncts.

CHRONIC MANAGEMENT

Once the worst pain, spasm, and limitation of motion have subsided, the patient may progressively resume full activities. Heavy physical exertion should be avoided until all symptoms have disappeared. An exercise program to strengthen the low-back muscles may prevent recurrent pain episodes.

PROGNOSIS

The patient with a single or occasional acute episode of back pain usually has no long-term disability. The patient with chronic severe pain, prominent depression, an industrial injury, a lawsuit in progress, or who has been disabled more than a year has a very low probability of returning to work or functioning normally in daily life.

Low-Back Pain and Herniated Disk

HISTORY

The paient with low-back pain from a herniated nucleus pulposus (HNP, ruptured disc) has a history of onset similar to that of the patient with musculoskeletal strain. However, features suggesting a herniated nucleus pulposus are pain radiating in a radicular band into one or both legs, numbness or tingling in a similar distribution, weakness of the leg or foot, and problems controlling urination [4, 30].

PHYSICAL EXAMINATION

Neurologic signs indicating a herniated nucleus pulposus are weakness in the painful leg, depression or absence of an ankle or knee reflex, and diminished sensation in a dermatomal distribution. Pain radiating into the leg when it is passively raised off the examining table (straight leg raising) suggests nerve root compression. The neurologic signs may be bilateral with a large herniated nucleus pulposus.

LABORATORY AND RADIOLOGIC STUDIES

Plain x-ray films of the lumbosacral spine may show narrowing of one intervertebral disk space, suggesting a herniated nucleus pulposus at that level. An electromyogram may indicate denervation of muscles supplied by the nerve root compressed by the herniation. The definitive test is a myelogram to outline the protruding disk.

ACUTE MANAGEMENT

If prominent neurologic signs or incontinence are present, hospital admission, early myelography, and surgery are indicated to preserve neurologic function [60]. Otherwise, a patient with a suspected herniated nucleus pulposus is managed as a musculoskeletal strain.

CHRONIC MANAGEMENT

Patients who have had surgery or who have recovered with conservative therapy require management as outlined for chronic musculoskeletal strain.

PROGNOSIS

The young patient with a herniated nucleus pulposus and mild signs usually recovers with bed rest alone. Of those requiring surgery, the majority have an excellent recovery and return to full activities [60]. Risk factors for poor outcome are the same as those for musculoskeletal low-back pain plus patients with a recurrent herniated nucleus pulposus after surgery.

References

1. Adams, C. Cervical Spondylotic Radiculopathy and Myelopathy. In P. J. Vinken and G. W. Bruyn (Eds.), *Handbook of Clinical Neurology: Injuries of the Spine and Spinal Cord,* vol. 26. New York: Elsevier, 1976. Pp. 97–112.

2. Adams, R. D., Fisher, C. M., Hakim, S., Ojemann, R. G., and Sweet, W. H. Symptomatic occult hydrocephalus with normal cerebrospinal fluid pressure: A treatable syndrome. *N. Engl. J. Med.* 273: 117, 1965.

3. Adams, R. D., and Victor, M. The Clinical Method of Neurology. In R. D. Adams and M. Victor (Eds.), *Principles of Neurology,* 3d Ed. New York: McGraw-Hill, 1985. Pp. 3–9.

4. Adams, R. D., and Victor, M. Pain in the Back, Neck, and Extremities. In R. D. Adams and M. Victor (Eds.), *Principles of Neurology,* 3d Ed. New York: McGraw-Hill, 1985. Pp. 149–172.

5. Adams, R. D., and Victor, M. Delirium and Other Confusional States. In R. D. Adams and M. Victor (Eds.), *Principles of Neurology,* 3d Ed. New York: McGraw-Hill, 1985. Pp. 301–310.

6. Aminoff, J. J. *Electrodiagnosis in Clinical Neurology.* New York: Churchill Livingstone, 1980.

7. Asbury, A. K. Disorders of Peripheral Nerve. In A. K. Asbury, G. M. McKhann, and W. I. McDonald (Eds.), *Diseases of the Nervous System,* vol. 1. Philadelphia: Saunders, 1986. Pp. 321–336.

8. Ausman, J. I., French, L. A., and Baker, A. B. Intracranial Neoplasms. In A. B. Baker and R. J. Joynt (Eds.), *Clinical Neurology,* vol. 2. Philadelphia: Harper and Row, 1985.

9. Barnett, H. J. M. Progress toward stroke prevention. *Neurology* 30: 1212, 1980.

10. Black, P. McL. Idiopathic normal-pressure hydrocephalus: Results of shunting in 62 patients. *J. Neurosurg.* 52: 371, 1980.

11. Boom, W. H., and Tuayon, C. U. Successful treatment of multiple brain abscesses with antibiotics alone. *Rev. Infect. Dis.* 7: 189, 1985.

12. Brooke, M. H. *A Clinician's View of Neuromuscular Disease,* 2d Ed. Baltimore: Williams and Wilkins, 1986.

13. Canadian Cooperative Study Group. Randomized trial of aspirin and sulfinpyrazone in threatened stroke. *N. Engl. J. Med.* 299: 53, 1978.

14. Cerebral Embolism Task Force. Cardiogenic brain embolism. *Arch. Neurol.* 43: 71, 1986.

15. Commission on Classification and Terminology of the International League Against Epilepsy. Proposal for revised clinical and electroencephalographic classification of epileptic seizures. *Epilepsia* 22: 489, 1981.

16. Consensus Conference. The utility of therapeutic plasmapheresis for neurological disorders. *J.A.M.A.* 256: 1333, 1986.

17. Cook, S. D., and Dowling, P. C. (Eds.). Multiple sclerosis update. *Neurology* 30 (part 2): 1, 1980.

18. Costabile, G., Husag, L., and Probst, C. Spinal epidural hematoma. *Surg. Neurol.* 21: 489, 1984.

19. Crouch, J. R., Ziegler, D. K., and Hassanein, R. Amitriptyline in the prophylaxis of migraine: Effectiveness and relationship of anti-migraine and antidepressant effects. *Neurology* 26: 121, 1976.

20. Currie, S. Polymyositis and Related Disorders. In J. N. Walton (Ed.), *Disorders of Voluntary Muscle,* 4th Ed. Edinburgh: Churchill Livingstone, 1981. Pp. 525–568.

21. Dalessio, D. J. (Ed.). *Wolff's Headache and Other Pain,* 4th Ed. Oxford: Oxford University Press, 1980.

22. Delgado-Escueta, A. V., Treiman, D. M., and Walsh, G. O. The treatable epilepsies. *N. Engl. J. Med.* 308: 1508, 1983.

23. DeLouvois, J. The bacteriology and chemotherapy of brain abscess. *J. Antimicrob. Chemother.* 4: 395, 1978.

24. Drachman, D. A. Bell's palsy: A neurological point of view. *Arch. Otolaryngol.* 89: 173, 1969.

25. Duvoisin, R. C. *Parkinson's Disease: A Guide for*

Patient and Family. New York: Raven Press, 1984.

26. Dyck, P. J., Thomas, P. K., and Lambert, E. H. *Peripheral Neuropathy,* 2d Ed. Philadelphia: Saunders, 1984.

27. Earnest, M. P., and Cantrill, S. V. Coma. In T. M. Bayless, M. C. Brain, and R. M. Cherniack (Eds.), *Current Therapy in Internal Medicine,* 2d Ed. Philadelphia: B. C. Decker, 1987. Pp. 1225–1228.

28. Engel, A. G. Myasthenia gravis and myasthenic syndromes. *Ann. Neurol.* 16: 519, 1984.

29. Fahn, S. The Extrapyramidal Disorders. In J. B. Wyngaarden and L. H. Smith (Eds.), *Cecil Textbook of Medicine,* 17th Ed. Philadelphia: Saunders, 1985. Pp. 2068–2079.

30. Finneson, B. E. *Low Back Pain,* 2d Ed. Philadelphia: Lippincott, 1980.

31. Fisher, C. M. Lacunar strokes and infarcts: A review. *Neurology* 32: 1, 1982.

32. Greenberg, H. S., Kim, J. H., and Posner, J. B. Epidural spinal cord compression from metastatic tumor: Results with a new treatment protocol. *Ann. Neurol.* 8: 361, 1980.

33. Guidelines for the determination of death: Report of the medical consultants on the diagnosis of death to the President's Commission for the Study of Ethical Problems in Medicine. *Neurology* 32: 395, 1982.

34. Hachinski, V. C., Iliff, L. D., Zilhka, E., DuBoulay, G. H., McAllister, V. L. et al. Cerebral blood flow in dementia. *Arch. Neurol.* 32: 632, 1975.

35. Harding, A. E. Hereditary Ataxias and Related Disorders. In A. K. Asbury, G. M. McKhann, and W. I. McDonald (Eds.), *Diseases of the Nervous System,* vol. 2. Philadelphia: Saunders, 1986. Pp. 1229–1238.

36. Hart, R. G., and Miller, V. T. Cerebral infarction in young adults. *Stroke* 14: 110, 1983.

37. Hershey, L. A., Modic, M. T., Greenough, P. G., and Jaffe, D. F. Magnetic resonance imaging in vascular dementia. *Neurology* 37: 29, 1987.

38. Hier, D. B., Davis, K. R., Richardson, E. P., and Mohr, J. P. Hypertensive putaminal hemorrhage. *Ann. Neurol.* 1: 152, 1977.

39. Hughes, R. A. C., Newsom-Davis, J. M., Perkin, G. D., and Pierce, J. M. Controlled trial of prednisolone in acute polyneuropathy. *Lancet* 2: 750, 1978.

40. Lance, J. W., and Anthony, M. Some clinical aspects of migraine: A prospective study of 500 cases. *Arch. Neurol.* 15: 356, 1966.

41. Lance, L. W. *The Mechanism and Management of Headache,* 4th Ed. London: Butterworths, 1982.

42. Layzer, R. B. *Neuromuscular Manifestations of Systemic Disease.* Philadelphia: F. A. Davis, 1985.

43. Levy, D. E., Bates, D., Caronna, J. J., Cartlidge, N. E. F., Knill-Jones, R. P., et al. Prognosis in non-traumatic coma. *Ann. Intern. Med.* 94: 293, 1981.

44. Lobato, R. D., Lamas, E., Cordobes, E., Munoz, M. J., and Roger, R. Chronic adult hydrocephalus due to uncommon causes. *Acta Neurochir (Wien)* 55: 85, 1980.

45. Martin, J. B. Huntington's disease: New approaches to an old problem. *Neurology* 34: 1059, 1984.

46. Martin, J. B. Approach to the Patient with Nervous System Disease. In E. Braunwald, K. J. Isselbacher, et al. (Eds.), *Harrison's Principles of Internal Medicine,* 11th Ed. New York: McGraw-Hill, 1987. Pp. 57–60.

47. McFarlin, D., and McFarland, H. Multiple sclerosis. *N. Engl. J. Med.* 307: 1183, 1982.

48. McFarlin, D. The treatment of multiple sclerosis. *N. Engl. J. Med.* 308: 215, 1983.

49. McKhann, G., Drachman, D., Folstein, M., Katzman, R., Price, D., and Stadlan, E. M. Clinical diagnosis of Alzheimer's disease: Report of the NINCDS-ADRDA work group. *Neurology* 34: 939, 1984.

50. Miller, J. R., Burke, A. M., and Bever, C. T. Occurrence of oligoclonal bands in multiple sclerosis and other CNS diseases. *Ann. Neurol.* 13: 53, 1983.

51. Millikan, C. H. Treatment of Occlusive Cerebrovascular Disease. In F. H. McDowell and L. R. Caplan (Eds.), *Cerebrovascular Survey Report—1985.* Washington: National Institute of Neurological and Communicative Disorders and Stroke, 1985. Pp. 149–188.

52. Mulder, D. W. (Ed.). *The Diagnosis and Treatment of Amyotrophic Lateral Sclerosis.* Boston: Houghton-Mifflin, 1980.

53. Plum, F., and Posner, J. B. *The Diagnosis of Stupor and Coma,* 3d Ed. Philadelphia: F. A. Davis, 1980.

54. Porter, R. J., and Morselli, P. L. *The Epilepsies.* London: Butterworths, 1985.

55. Ramirez-Lassepas, M., Cipolle, R. J., Morillo, L. R., and Gumnit, R. J. Value of computed tomographic scan in the evaluation of adult patients after their first seizure. *Ann. Neurol.* 15: 536, 1984.

56. Raskin, N. H., and Appenzeller, O. Headache. Monograph 19 in *Major Problems in Internal Medicine.* Philadelphia: Saunders, 1980.

57. Rodriquez, M., and DiNapoli, R. P. Spinal cord compression: With special reference to metastatic epidural tumors. *Mayo Clin. Proc.* 55: 442, 1980.

58. Scheinberg, L. C. (Ed.). *Multiple Sclerosis: A Guide for Patients and Their Families.* New York: Raven Press, 1983.

59. Sciarra, D. Head Injury. In L. P. Rowland (Ed.), *Merritt's Textbook of Neurology,* 7th Ed. Philadelphia: Lea and Febiger, 1984. Pp. 277–299.

60. Shannon, N., and Paul, E. A. L_{4-5}, L_5–S_1 disc protrusions: Analysis of 323 cases operated on over 12 years. *J. Neurol. Neurosurg. Psychiatry* 42: 804, 1979.

61. Stein, B., and Wolpert, S. Arteriovenous malformation of the brain. *Arch. Neurol.* 37: 1, 1980.

62. Sundt, T. M., and Whisnant, J. P. Subarachnoid hemorrhage from intracranial aneurysm: Surgical management and natural history of disease. *N. Engl. J. Med.* 299: 116, 1978.

63. Teasdale, G., and Jennett, B. Assessment of coma and impaired consciousness: A practical scale. *Lancet* 2: 81, 1974.

64. Terry, R. D., and Katzman, R. Senile dementia of the Alzheimer type. *Ann. Neurol.* 14: 497, 1983.

65. Verner, E. F., and Muscher, D. M. Spinal epidural abscess. *Med. Clin. North Am.* 69: 375, 1985.

66. Whisnant, J. P., Cartlidge, N. E. F., and Elveback L. R. Carotid and vertebral-basilar transient ischemic attacks: Effect of anticoagulants, hypertension, and cardiac disorders on survival and stroke occurrence: A population study. *Ann. Neurol.* 3: 107, 1978.

67. Wilder, B. J., and Bruni, J. *Seizure Disorders: A Pharmacological Approach to Treatment.* New York, Raven Press, 1981.

68. Wilson, C. B. Brain tumors. *N. Engl. J. Med.* 300: 1469, 1979.

Psychiatric Disorders

James H. Scully and
Steven L. Dubovsky

Organic Mental Syndromes

The term *organic mental syndrome* refers to any emotional and behavioral abnormalities caused by transient or permanent brain dysfunction. There are a wide variety of symptoms that may result from either the primary disturbance of brain function or the emotional reactions to cognitive deficits [6]. There are a number of formal categories of organic brain syndrome defined in the current nomenclature: *delirium, dementia, intoxication, and withdrawal* are discussed below [42]. *Amnestic syndrome* is characterized by prominent loss of memory but not clouding of consciousness caused by organic factors. Organically induced delusions, hallucinations, depressed or elevated mood, anxiety, and personality disturbances that are not accompanied by clouded sensorium or intellectual deteriorations are called respectively, *organic delusional syndrome, organic hallucinosis, organic mood syndrome, organic anxiety syndrome*, and *organic personality syndrome* [26].

Delirium

HISTORY AND PHYSICAL FINDINGS

Delirium is characterized by fluctuating clouding of awareness [25]. The onset is relatively rapid, usually in minutes to hours. Attention and short-term memory are impaired, and the patient is disoriented to time and place [52]. Illusions (misperceptions of actual stimuli) or hallucinations (sensory perceptions in the absence of an actual stimulus) may occur. Speech may be incoherent. The sleep-wake cycle is frequently abnormal. Patients may be hyperactive, restless, agitated, fearful, or assaultive or be stuporous and barely move at all. Activity may shift suddenly from one extreme to the other. Delirium may develop in association with any medical illness; elderly and demented patients who have diminished cerebral reserves, are more vulnerable [91].

The unpredictable fluctuation in mental state resulting from delirium causes some physicians to assume that the patient is in control of the symptoms when the patient appears clear (usually during the day). However, it is this very fluctuation that differentiates delirium from functional disturbances. As a syndrome of cerebral insufficiency, delirium can be compared to cardiac, renal, or pulmonary failure [78].

LABORATORY FINDINGS

The electroencephalogram (EEG) in delirium may show diffuse slowing, or it may be normal. Some common causes of delirium are listed in Table 10-1. Initial laboratory studies should include toxicology, renal and liver function studies, electrolytes, blood sugar, complete blood count (CBC), urinalysis, arterial blood gas determinations, electrocardiogram (ECG), and other studies indicated by suspected conditions that could directly or indirectly be affecting the brain [56]. Common laboratory abnormalities are listed in Table 10-2.

Table 10–1. Common Causes of Organic Mental Disorder

   I. Prescribed medications, especially sedative-hypnotics, tranquilizers, antipsychotic drugs, and anticholinergics. Almost any drug, e.g., anticonvulsants, digitalis, levodopa, penicillin, and steroids, can produce an organic brain syndrome.
  II. Alcohol and drug withdrawal
 III. Alcohol intoxication
 IV. Endocrine disorders:
    A. Pancreas (e.g., pulmonary embolus, pneumonia)
    B. Thyroid (e.g., hyperthyroidism, hypothyroidism)
    C. Parathyroid (e.g., hypocalcemia, hypercalcemia)
    D. Adrenal gland (e.g., Addison's disease, Cushing's disease)
    E. Pituitary gland (e.g., hypopituitarism, hyperpituitarism)
   V. Systemic diseases:
    A. Heart (e.g., congestive heart failure, arrhythmias)
    B. Kidney (e.g., uremia)
    C. Liver (e.g., liver failure)
    D. Blood (e.g., anemia, polycythemia)
  VI. Fluid, electrolyte, and acid-base disturbances:
    A. Water intoxication
    B. Disorders of Na^+, K^+, Ca^{2+}, and Mg^{2+} metabolism
    C. Acidemia and alkalemia
 VII. Diseases of the central nervous system:
    A. Infections
    B. Seizure disorders
    C. Vascular disease
    D. Tumors:
      1. Primary
      2. Metastatic
    E. Degenerative disease
    F. Trauma

Table 10–2. Common Laboratory Abnormalities in Organic Brain Syndrome

Anemia
Hyperthyroidism
Hypothyroidism
Uremia
Hyponatremia
Leukocytosis
Hypercalcemia
Hypocalcemia
Hypoxemia

TREATMENT

Treatment must ultimately be directed at the underlying medical condition that is causing delirium. Until the patient's mental state clears, he or she should be under constant observation. Excessive stimulation or sensory deprivation should be minimized. Unnecessary medications, especially central nervous system (CNS) depressants (e.g., tranquilizers), should be avoided because they may make delirium worse. The patient should be placed close to the nursing stations, and a night light, calendar, newspaper, and television should be provided to help orient the patient. Visits from family should be encouraged, since these may decrease the patient's anxiety, and the physician should frequently remind the patient who he or she is. When the patient is agitated or combative, a high-potency neuroleptic may control the patient. Low doses (e.g., 0.5 to 2 mg) of haloperidol two to four times per day are used, ideally coinciding with periods of agitation. Higher doses of intravenous haloperidol (up to 10 mg) also have been used to tranquilize severely agitated delirious patients.

General principles applicable to the treatment of all organic mental syndromes are summarized in Table 10-3.

PROGNOSIS

Delirium often lasts less than a week. If it persists for longer periods of time, it is likely to progress to dementia or death. If the underlying disorder is treated successfully, the patient generally has complete recovery from the delirium.

Dementia

HISTORY AND PHYSICAL FINDINGS

The primary feature of dementia (Table 10-4) is global loss of such intellectual functions as intellect, speech, foresight, social facility, memory, judgment, abstract thought, and other higher cortical functions. Changes in behavior, affect, and personality frequently accompany dementia. Dementias may be stable, remitting, or progressive,

Table 10–3. *General Treatment of Organic Mental Disorders*

1. Discontinue all nonessential drugs. They may worsen the problem and make diagnosis difficult.
2. Remind the patient frequently where he or she is and of the names of personnel who are treating him or her. This will correct the patient's forgetting where he or she is and assuming that his or her doctors, whom he or she does not recognize, wish to hurt him or her.
3. Provide a light at night. Symptoms are usually worse at night because of decreased cues for orientation ("sundowning").
4. Avoid putting the patient in a private room.
5. Place the patient near the nursing station.
6. Encourage frequent visits from family members and friends. Familiar stimuli orient the patient and decrease his or her anxiety.
7. Limit visits from strangers. Unfamiliar people may confuse and frighten the patient.
8. Avoid frequent changes of doctors and nurses.
9. Provide calendars, newspapers, television, and other orienting stimuli.
10. Restrain carefully for agitation. When necessary, use hydroxyzine or haloperidol.

Table 10–4. *Signs and Symptoms in Organic Brain Syndromes (OBS)*

Delirium	Dementia
Clouded consciousness	Loss of intellectual abilities
Fluctuating	Stable
Rapid onset	Variable onset
Duration—days	Duration—usually permanent
Attention deficit	Memory deficit
Disorientation	Loss of abstracting ability
Psychomotor activity and sleep cycle disturbed	Personality changes
Affect is labile and variable	Accentuate premorbid personality
	Affect is often depressed or withdrawn

depending on the etiology [83]. The most common cause of dementia (50 percent of cases) is Alzheimer's disease. The onset of Alzheimer's disease is usually insidious. Initially, there are problems with short-term recall [52]. The patient becomes less interested in the usual activities of life and becomes easily fatigued and less flexible psychologically. As the dementia progresses, the patient may become apathetic, depressed, emotionally labile, or suspicious. Dysphasia and perseverative speech are common. Whatever personality traits were present before the patient became ill tend to be exaggerated.

LABORATORY FINDINGS

Multi-infarct dementia, which accounts for roughly 10 percent of dementias, is caused by small cerebral occlusions, usually associated with chronic hypertension. While a single infarct seldom results in dementia, multiple small lesions cause a picture similar to Alzheimer's disease. Other irreversible causes of dementia include slow virus infections, head injury, and degenerative diseases such as Huntington's chorea [76]. Before ascribing dementia to one of these illnesses, it is essential to exclude potentially reversible causes such as normal-pressure hydrocephalus, brain tumors or cysts, drug toxicity, subdural hematomas, thyroid dysfunction, alcoholism, and central nervous system infections [13, 69]. Appropriate screening laboratory findings include computerized tomographic (CT) scans of the brain, review of all medications, information from the family about the patient's use of alcohol and nonprescription drugs, toxicology screens, thyroid tests, and serology for syphilis. Additional tests such as magnetic resonance imaging, blood sugar, vitamin B_{12} levels, heavy metal excretion, liver function tests, and lumbar puncture may be indicated by specific clinical findings [59].

Depression, especially in the elderly, may be indistinguishable from dementia. The patient with pseudodementia may have a past and family history of mood disturbance and may perform inconsistently on mental status testing (e.g., long-term memory more impaired than short-term memory) [35]. As many as 25 percent of primarily demented patients develop secondary depression that further impairs their cognitive function. A trial of an antidepressant is therefore indicated in every demented patient in whom the cause is not clear and in many with an identifiable etiology of their dementia [17].

TREATMENT

Although a centrally acting oral anticholinesterase has recently shown some initial promise in the treatment of symptoms of Alzheimer's disease, no medication has been definitively shown to reverse primary degenerative dementias [37]. The dihydrogenated ergot alkaloid Hydergine in a dose of 6 mg per day for 6 months, may improve depression and self-care in some demented patients. Meticulous attention to nutrition and hydration, elimination of all nonessential drugs, and treatment of intercurrent illness will reduce factors that can aggravate cognitive decline.

Demented patients who are agitated and cannot be controlled with the orienting measures described above are treated with low doses of nonsedating neuroleptics (e.g., haloperidol, 2 to 10 mg per day). Unpredictable assaultiveness may respond to propranolol in doses of 40 to 160 mg qid [42]. Observed or suspected depression in demented patients is treated with antidepressants that are low in sedating and anticholinergic potential such as desipramine and nortriptyline. In older patients, the starting dose should be low (e.g., 10 mg desipramine) and the dose should be increased very slowly to a final level that is about half that of younger patients (e.g., increase by 10 to 25 mg at a time to 75 mg per day desipramine). Treatment of the demented patient must involve the family and other social supports.

Amnestic Syndrome
HISTORY AND PHYSICAL FINDINGS
Amnestic syndrome consists of impaired short- and long-term memory with intact consciousness. The patient cannot learn new information or remember old information. The most common cause of amnestic syndrome is alcoholism (Korsakoff's syndrome). Other etiologies include head trauma, anoxia, cerebral infarcts, encephalitis, tumors, thiamine deficiency, lead poisoning, and seizures. Amnestic syndrome is associated with lesions of the limbic system, particularly the hippocampus, the amygdaloid nuclei, and the mamillary bodies. The patient may initially complain about being unable to remember, but later the patient may deny memory problems. Patients with amnestic syndrome are often long-winded and tangential and tend to confabulate (make up) information they have forgotten.

LABORATORY FINDINGS
A CT scan of the brain or other imaging techniques may demonstrate tumors or infarcts. The electroencephalogram may reveal epilepsy, and a lumbar puncture may suggest encephalitis [4]. Otherwise there are usually no specific laboratory findings. Psychogenic amnesia, fugue state, conversion reaction, malingering, and multiple personality also may produce amnestic symptoms. Psychiatric consultation should be requested to identify these conditions if an organic cause of amnesia is not found.

TREATMENT
Treatment depends on the primary etiology. With thiamine deficiency, early vitamin replacement usually ameliorates the condition. Most often, however, the goal is care rather than cure. There are no specific pharmacologic treatments. Good nursing care, orienting measures, and correction of memory lapses are crucial.

Organic Hallucinosis
In organic hallucinosis, recurrent hallucinations in the absence of delirium or dementia are caused by a specific biologic factor. This disorder is most commonly caused by chronic abuse of alcohol or hallucinogenic substances. Occasionally, hallucinosis may be caused by seizure foci in the

temporal or occipital lobes. The syndrome may appear transiently in response to sensory deprivation, blindness, or hearing loss. If it becomes chronic, organic hallucinosis must be differentiated from schizophrenia. Neuroleptics (e.g., haloperidol, 2 to 20 mg per day) may reduce symptoms, but there is no specific treatment.

Organic Affective Syndrome
DIFFERENTIAL DIAGNOSIS
Organic affective syndromes are manic or depressive states caused by organic factors but not associated with delirium or dementia. All central nervous system depressants, alcohol, antihypertensive medications (such as methyldopa and propranolol), reserpine, steroids, endocrine disturbances (particularly elevated or decreased thyroid or parathyroid function), viral syndromes, and occult tumors of the gastrointestinal tract (such as carcinoma of the pancreas) are among the more common causes of organically induced depression, whereas stimulants and corticosteroids may produce mania [54]. Organic affective syndromes may be indistinguishable from primary depression and mania [27].

LABORATORY FINDINGS
Careful neurologic examination, electroencephalogram, electrocardiogram, urinalysis, complete blood count, and blood chemistries, particularly endocrine studies, may uncover an undiagnosed medical cause of depression. Particularly careful attention should be paid to the patient's medication list and to the use of alcohol, nonprescription drugs, and drugs prescribed by other physicians.

TREATMENT
Treatment of organic affective syndrome should be directed at the underlying illness. If affective symptoms do not remit, or if the primary medical problem cannot be treated, antidepressants (e.g., imipramine, 25 to 50 mg tid) or antimanic (e.g., lithium, 300 mg tid) drugs are indicated [14].

Organic Personality Syndrome
HISTORY AND PHYSICAL FINDINGS
The most common changes in personality seen in patients with organic disease affecting the brain are emotional lability and impaired impulse control and social judgment. Patients with organic personality syndrome may explosively lose their temper or start crying suddenly. They may shoplift or expose their genitals in public. Others may become apathetic, indifferent, suspicious, or paranoid. The striking changes from premorbid behavior may initially be more obvious to the family than to the physician. Among the more common causes of organic personality syndrome are neoplasms, particularly in the frontal lobe, head trauma, and occasionally vascular disease. In addition, some patients with temporal lobe epilepsy, multiple sclerosis, or Huntington's chorea may develop personality changes in the absence of delirium or dementia.

LABORATORY FINDINGS AND TREATMENT
Laboratory evaluation should be dictated by careful medical and neurologic examination. A CT scan, electroencephalogram, urinalysis, complete blood count, and appropriate blood chemistries may be appropriate [4]. Treatment depends on the etiology.

Organic Delusional Syndrome
HISTORY AND PHYSICAL FINDINGS
Organic delusional syndrome is characterized by organically induced delusions, most commonly persecutory, in the absence of delirium or dementia. The patient may appear disheveled or eccentric and may have rambling, incoherent speech. The most common etiology is intoxication with drugs such as amphetamines, marijuana, or hallucinogens. Patients with temporal lobe epilepsy may suffer from an interictal organic delusional syndrome. Delusional syndrome also has been seen in patients with Huntington's chorea, vitamin B_{12} deficiency, systemic lupus erythematosus, encephalitis, head trauma, and brain tumors. Or-

ganic delusional syndrome must be differentiated from delirium, schizophrenia, mania, paranoia, and psychotic depression.

LABORATORY FINDINGS
A careful drug history and toxicology screen should be obtained. A complete blood count, uri-nalysis, serologic tests for syphilis, vitamin B_{12} levels, and CT scan may be appropriate.

TREATMENT
Treatment should be directed toward the under-lying condition. Neuroleptics may be useful in controlling psychotic symptoms and agitation.

Drug Withdrawal Syndromes

History and Physical Findings
Withdrawal from central nervous system (CNS) depressants, narcotics, and stimulants produces mental and physical disturbances in hospitalized patients when they are denied access to the drug. Withdrawal of all central nervous system depres-sants produce similar syndromes (Table 10-5). Shorter-acting compounds such as secobarbital, alprazolam, and lorazepam produce more severe disturbances that appear sooner after discontin-uation of the drug [11]. Longer-acting central nervous system depressants such as diazepam and chlordiazepoxide produce more attenuated syn-dromes that appear later. Alcohol abstinence syn-dromes (Table 10-6) are not substantially differ-ent from withdrawal from other central nervous system depressants [39, 45]. Subtle withdrawal symptoms have been reported as long as a year after discontinuation of benzodiazepines.

Narcotic withdrawal produces irritability, ab-dominal pain, lacrimation, and influenza-like symptoms. The syndrome is not life-threatening [57]. Abstinence from stimulants such as am-phetamines and cocaine can produce dangerous depression or violence.

Laboratory Findings
Blood levels of the offending medications are usually zero during an abstinence syndrome. A barbiturate tolerance test (see below) is used to diagnose central nervous system depressant with-drawal. Mean corpuscular volume is increased in chronic alcohol abuse [49, 50].

Treatment
Abstinence syndromes occur in patients who are tolerant to central nervous system depressants. Tolerance can be confirmed by the barbiturate tol-erance test: 200 mg pentobarbital or 60 mg phe-nobarbital is given orally. Significant intoxication (e.g., falling asleep) indicates that the patient is not tolerant and is not suffering an abstinence syndrome. Signs of moderate intoxication (e.g., nystagmus without sleepiness) indicates some tolerance. The absence of signs of intoxication in-dicates marked tolerance. For patients who ex-hibit tolerance, phenobarbital or pentobarbital are substituted for the suspected drug in sufficient dosages to suppress early signs of withdrawal. The dosage is then gradually reduced [89]. With-

Table 10–5. *Symptoms and Signs of Barbiturate Withdrawal or Withdrawal from Other CNS Depressants*

Early (6 to 8 hours after withdrawal)	Delayed (30 to 48 hours after withdrawal)	Late (4 to 7 days after withdrawal)
Anxiety, tremor, weakness, nausea, diaphoresis, hypertension, hyperactive reflexes, postural hypotension	Grand mal seizures	Delirium, disorientation, hallucinations

Table 10–6. *Alcohol Withdrawal Syndromes*

Name of syndrome	Signs and symptoms	Symptoms start	Syndrome lasts
Shakes	Tremor, mild diaphoresis, insomnia, mild organic brain syndrome, mild agitation	First day of withdrawal	2 days
Seizures	Generalized (grand mal)	5 to 30 hours, often within 6 hours after stopping alcohol	2 days
Delirium tremens (DTs)	DTs, prostration, fever, dehydration, tachycardia, profuse disphoresis, severe agitation	60 to 80 hours after stopping alcohol	5 days
Hallucinosis/paranoia	Persecutory auditory hallucinations with a clear sensorium	1 to 3 days after stopping alcohol	Days to weeks (may be chronic)

drawal from central nervous system depressants should only be attempted in a hospital, in consultation with a physician who is familiar with the appropriate techniques and medications.

If it is certain that other central nervous system depressants also are not being abused, uncomplicated alcohol abstinence syndromes are treated with rapidly decreasing doses of long-acting benzodiazepines such as diazepam (20 to 40 mg per day) and chlordiazepoxide (50 to 200 mg per day

to start). The discomfort of narcotic withdrawal may be averted by substituting methadone (no more than 50 mg per day in juice) for the narcotic and gradually reducing the dose over 5 to 7 days. Clonidine, an alpha$_2$ agonist that reduces many of the symptoms of opioid withdrawal, has been used for rapid detoxification from narcotics. Withdrawal from central nervous system stimulants is treated with imipramine or desipramine (50 mg tid) when symptoms are severe.

Depression

Differential Diagnosis

Depression is diagnosed when the following triad has been present for at least 2 weeks or when symptoms are severe: (1) a pervasive unhappy mood (irritability, anxiety, or apathy may be the presenting mood), (2) changes in perception of the self, the environment, and the future, including lowered self-esteem, guilt, hopelessness, suicidal thoughts, loss of interest in usual activities, and negative thinking, and (3) physiologic changes such as increased or decreased weight, sleep disturbance, diurnal mood swing (patient feels worse in the morning and better as the day progresses), loss of energy, decreased interest in sex, slowed thinking, constipation, and multiple somatic complaints [74]. Depressed mood may be

masked by unexplained physical symptoms, insomnia, personality change, substance abuse, or marital problems [42].

A number of medical illnesses and drugs can cause depression (Tables 10-7 and 10-8). Other conditions to be considered in the differential diagnosis of depression include grief, organic mental disorders, and primary anxiety disorders. Grief is a normal reaction to a significant loss. It is characterized by less prominent psychomotor retardation, guilt, and suicidal thinking than depression [48]. Anxiety and depression frequently accompany each other. Anxiety appearing for the first time after the age of 40 is more likely to be a symptom of depression or organic brain disease than a primary disorder [73].

Table 10–7. *Some Medical Illnesses that Can Produce Depression*

Hyperthyroidism
Hypothyroidism
Hyperparathyroidism
Hyperadrenalism
Hypoadrenalism
Porphyria
Pernicious anemia
Pancreatic carcinoma
Pheochromocytoma
Multiple sclerosis
Systemic lupus erythematosus
Hepatitis
Infectious mononucleosis
Pneumonia

Table 10–8. *Medications that Can Produce Depression*

Methyldopa
Reserpine
Beta blockers (e.g., propranolol)
Tranquilizers
Hypnotics
Narcotics
Clonazepam
Clonidine
Amantadine
Carbamazepine
Oral contraceptives
Alcohol
Withdrawal from stimulants

Laboratory Findings

Depression is associated with a number of neuroendocrine abnormalities [47]. About 50 percent of patients fail to suppress serum cortisol secretion below 5 gm/dl on the day following administration of 1 mg dexamethasone (dexamethasone suppression test, DST). A positive suppression test in the absence of a major medical illness, recent weight loss, recent hospitalization, or drugs that interfere with the metabolism of dexamethasone suggests depression, but a negative test does not rule out depression [28]. Because of many false-positive and false-negative results, the dexamethasone suppression test is not useful in screening for depression; however, failure of a positive test to revert to normal following symptomatic improvement may predict a high risk of relapse if treatment is discontinued. In 30 to 40 percent of depressed patients, the thyroid-stimulating hormone (TSH) response to an infusion of 500 mg thyrotropin-releasing hormone (TRH) is blunted (DTSH < 5 microunits/ml). This is not a practical diagnostic test in most cases.

The most reliable biologic test for depression is the sleep electroencephalogram. As many as 80 percent of depressed patients enter rapid eye movement (REM) sleep early and show other changes in sleep architecture. Identifying such decreased REM latency requires a specialized sleep laboratory [22].

Treatment

In double-blind controlled studies, a number of psychological therapies have been shown to be effective treatments for depression. Cognitive therapy systematically helps the patient to correct pervasive negative thinking by helping the patient monitor and change maladaptive cognitive patterns. Interpersonal therapy focus on distortions in important relationships that cause depression. Behavior therapy moves the patient toward more adaptive behaviors that are incompatible with depression by rewarding nondepressive behaviors such as becoming active and interacting with others while ignoring depressive behaviors such as lying in bed. These psychotherapies may be as effective as antidepressants in uncomplicated cases [66].

Antidepressants are indicated for severe depression, depression with vegetative signs, failure to respond to psychotherapy, past history of depression or response to an antidepressant, or family history of an affective disorder. Two broad classes of antidepressants are available. Cyclic antidepressants, with the exception of trazodone and bupropion, are generally administered in one bedtime dose. Therapy is initiated at a low dose (e.g., 25 mg imipramine), and the dosage is gradually increased to the therapeutic range. If the patient responds, the medication is continued for 4 to 12 months and then is withdrawn by 25 mg per month. The most common causes of failure to respond to an antidepressant are failure to prescribe an adequate dose, misdiagnosis, noncompliance, and presence of an illness, medication, or alcohol that aggravates depression or increases metabolism of the antidepressant. Common side effects of cyclic antidepressants include anticholinergic actions such as dry mouth, blurred vision, and urinary hesitancy and postural hypotension, sedation, irritability, and quinidine-like effects.

The second class of antidepressants is the monoamine oxidase inhibitors (MAOIs). These drugs may be effective when cyclic antidepressants are not helpful or cannot be tolerated. They may be superior to the cyclic antidepressant in cases of depression accompanied by severe anxiety, overeating, hypersomnia, fatigue, self-pity, histrionics, and personality problems. The major drawbacks of the monoamine oxidase inhibitors is that they can produce dangerous hypertensive reactions if tyramine-containing foods (e.g., aged cheese) or sympathomimetic amines are ingested. Monoamine oxidase inhibitors are usually administered in divided dose during the day.

The safest and most effective antidepressant therapy is electroconvulsive therapy (ECT) [19]. Its only absolute contraindications are space-occupying lesions and increased intracranial pressure. The major risk of electroconvulsive therapy is the risk of the brief general anesthesia used in the procedure. Electroconvulsive therapy produces a transient organic mental syndrome 50 percent of the time. There is no evidence that this therapy causes permanent brain dysfunction.

Mania

History and Findings
Mania is the behavioral and psychological opposite of depression. The majority of manic patients are also subject to bouts of depression, although only about 15 percent of depressed patients (about 1 percent of the general population) become manic. Mania tends to be recurrent, with recurrences occurring more frequently as the patient gets older. In 15 to 30 percent of patients, mania may become chronic.

Mania not severe enough to require hospitalization is referred to as *hypomania*. Hypomanic patients may be excessively cheerful, hyperenergetic, and engaging, but they also can be intrusive, irritable, and insensitive to the needs of others. Mania is easier to recognize, since it is characterized by rapid, pressured speech, flight of ideas, grandiosity, numerous impossible plans, spending too much money, a decreased need for sleep, and hypersexuality. Sleep deprivation may precipitate a manic attack the following day. The propensity to develop mania is inherited. Recently, an autosomal-dominant gene with about 60 percent penetrance was identified that leads to mania in a population of old order Amish people. In other groups the gene may be sex-linked. Hypomania may have a different genetic pattern than mania.

Laboratory Findings
Laboratory findings in mania are identical to those in depression, suggesting a psychobiologic unity between the two conditions. Nonsuppression on the dexamethasone suppression test and decreased REM latency on the sleep electroencephalogram may be useful in distinguishing manic from schizophrenic psychoses.

Treatment
About 70 percent of acutely manic patients respond to lithium (1200 to 2400 mg per day; blood level 0.6 to 1.2 mEq/liter). Patients who do not improve with lithium and those with frequent recurrences (rapid cycling) may have a better re-

sponse to carbamazepine (600 to 1200 mg per day). Alternative therapies include verapamil, clonazepam, and valproic acid, as well as electroconvulsive therapy. Because the response to antimanic agents is usually delayed 7 to 10 days, neuroleptics also are used for acute treatment. Some patients benefit from ongoing neuroleptic therapy. Psychotherapy is not effective for acute mania. Antimanic drugs should be continued for 6 to 12 months following a single acute episode and then should be gradually withdrawn [10]. Patients with frequent recurrences or very severe infrequent episodes require maintenance therapy. The maintenance dose of lithium is lower than for acute treatment (600 to 1200 mg per day; blood level 0.4 to 1 mEq/liter). Hypothyroidism and antidepressants can aggravate cycling between depression and mania.

Long-term use of lithium can cause a number of adverse effects. Hypothyroidism is generally not significant medically, but it may precipitate recurrences of mania and/or depression. Hyperparathyroidism occurs in the majority of patients taking lithium for more than 2 years, and parathyroid adenomas may develop. Although the data are still controversial, lithium may cause irreversible microscopic renal tubular and glomerular lesions of uncertain clinical significance.

Anxiety Disorders

Moderate amounts of anxiety with illness and stress are normal. Pathologic anxiety is classified in the current nomenclature as panic disorder or generalized anxiety [70].

Panic Attacks and Generalized Anxiety

Panic attacks are discrete episodes of intense unprovoked anxiety accompanied by dyspnea, palpitations, chest pains or discomfort, choking or smothering sensations, dizziness, vertigo or unsteady feelings, feelings of unreality, paresthesias, hot and/or cold flashes, nausea or abdominal distress, sweating, faintness, trembling or shaking, and fear of dying or going crazy [142]. Depression is a common complication in patients with a family history of depression. Substance abuse may develop as an attempt at self-treatment. There is excellent evidence in favor of a genetic contribution to panic disorder.

Generalized anxiety consists of diffuse nonspecific anxiety, often accompanied by such signs of arousal as motor tension, autonomic hyperactivity (sweating, palpitations), apprehensive expectations, worry, fear, hypervigilance, distractibility, and difficulty concentrating [79]. Generalized anxiety is more likely to be a maladaptive response to life stress than an endogenous syndrome like panic disorder [30, 34].

A number of medical illnesses may produce anxiety as the only symptom. Examples include thyroid disease, parathyroid disease, hypoglycemia, hyponatremia, paroxysmal tachycardias, and temporal lobe epilepsy [12, 21]. Anxiety can be produced by caffeine, stimulants, and central nervous system depressant withdrawal [27]. Motor restlessness (akathisia) associated with neuroleptics may mimic anxiety [24]. Medical causes of anxiety are summarized in Table 10-9.

LABORATORY FINDINGS

A panic attack can be provoked in patients with panic disorder but not in patients who do not suffer spontaneous panic attacks by the intravenous infusion of sodium lactate. This is not yet a practical clinical test, but it does illustrate the biologic nature of panic attacks [7].

Panic attacks are treated with cyclic antidepressants, monoamine oxidase inhibitors, alprazolam, or clonazepam. All antidepressants except bupropion and possibly trazodone ameliorate panic attacks completely in 90 percent of patients. Patients may remain symptom-free for some time after the drug is withdrawn, but eventual relapse

Table 10–9. *Medical Causes of Anxiety*

Acute asthma
Pulmonary embolus
Arrhythmias
Angina
Hyperdynamic beta-adrenergic circulatory state
Mitral valve prolapse syndrome
Hyperthyroidism
Hypoparathyroidism
Hyperparathyroidism
Pheochromocytoma
Caffeinism
Stimulant abuse
Withdrawal syndromes
Partial complex seizures
Menière's disease
Myocardial infarction
Reactive hypoglycemia
Transient cerebral ischemic attacks
Cushing's disease
Infections
Collagen-vascular disease

is common off of medication. Generalized anxiety is treated with benzodiazepines, which, with the exception of alprazolam, are largely ineffective for panic attacks. Benzodiazepines are most appropriately prescribed for patients who are acutely anxious in response to a time-limited stress who do not have a history of substance abuse. Buspirone (10 mg tid–qid) is a nonbenzodiazepine antianxiety drug that does not produce sedation, dependence, or significant interactions but also is not always effective. A month may be necessary for its clinical benefits to appear.

Taken acutely, propranolol (10 to 20 mg) is useful for stage fright. Atenolol and monoamine oxidase inhibitors have been used to treat social phobias. Beta blockers may attenuate signs of physiologic arousal associated with anxiety, but they are not particularly effective for panic anxiety or generalized anxiety [31].

All anxious patients benefit from behavioral techniques such as biofeedback, relaxation training, hypnosis, and stress reduction. Many patients with panic attacks develop phobias of being away from the house and other familiar places (agoraphobia) and of specific situations such as elevators and high places. Such phobic avoidance responds to systematic desensitization, a behavioral technique that teaches the patient to relax in situations that evoke anxiety [3].

Phobic Disorders
HISTORY AND PHYSICAL FINDINGS
Phobias are among the most common psychiatric disorders, although many phobic individuals do not seek treatment. All phobias involve compulsive avoidance of a feared situation despite awareness that the fear is irrational.

Simple phobia is characterized by a persistent irrational fear of a specific object or situation, such as heights, closed spaces, or certain animals. Phobias of a specific illness such as cancer or heart disease must be differentiated from hypochondriasis (conviction of having a specific illness), since the treatment is different.

Social phobia is characterized by fears of being out of control or humiliated in social situations. The social phobic avoids groups, public speaking, writing in the presence of others, and other situations involving exposure to public scrutiny.

Agoraphobia is the fear of being in any setting in which escape might be difficult or help might not be available if the patient became disabled or anxious. This results in progressive constriction of normal activities until most situations outside the home are avoided. Most cases of agoraphobia occur in patients with panic attacks.

TREATMENT
Simple phobias are treated with gradual exposure to the feared stimulus paired with a relaxation technique. Adjunctive antianxiety drugs may be used in the short term to decrease fearful reactions to the phobic object. Social phobias may respond to monoamine oxidase inhibitors and possibly to beta blockers. Adjunctive group therapy,

assertiveness training, or other behavioral techniques are also helpful. Agoraphobia usually improves when the underlying panic disorder responds to the appropriate medication. Systematic desensitization is utilized when medications alone do not resolve the phobia. Behavioral treatment of all phobias is more successful if it involves actual exposure to the phobic object or situation (in vivo exposure) in addition to exposure in fantasy in the doctor's office.

Posttraumatic Stress Disorder

HISTORY AND PHYSICAL FINDINGS

Posttraumatic stress disorder (PTSD) is an excessive, prolonged reaction to a stressful situation that is outside the normal range of experience, such as war, assault, or natural disaster. Symptoms include reexperiencing the trauma through intrusive and recurrent dreams, acting or feeling as if the trauma were recurring, numbing of responsiveness to the external world, constricted affect, hypervigilence, exaggerated startle response, sleep disturbance, guilt about survival or behavior required for survival, memory impairment, trouble concentrating, avoidance of activities that recall the traumatic event, and intensification of symptoms by exposure to events that symbolize the traumatic event [43]. Most cases of posttraumatic stress disorder begin shortly after the trauma and last less than 6 months. If symptoms last longer than 6 months, the prognosis is less favorable. Posttraumatic stress disorder is more severe when the trauma is manmade rather than natural. Depression and alcohol abuse are common complications of posttraumatic stress disorder.

TREATMENT

Psychotherapy of posttraumatic stress disorder is directed at helping the patient to relive and work through the stressful event. Tricyclic antidepressants and monoamine oxidase inhibitors may control anxiety symptoms associated with posttraumatic stress disorder.

Sleep Disorders

History and Physical Examination

At some time in their lives, 75 percent of people experience difficulty falling or staying asleep [18]. Insomnia is particularly common in medical patients, usually because of sleeping in a strange environment, the discomfort of medical illness, job stress, and marital discord. Alterations of sleep phase, which may occur spontaneously or with changes in work shift or time zone, may present as early morning awakening or sleeping late. Depression and chronic use of sedatives, antianxiety drugs, and alcohol are among the most common causes of insomnia. Difficulty initiating sleep, frequent awakenings, and decreased total time asleep are common in the elderly and do not necessarily require treatment unless the patient feels tired or depressed during the day.

Specific medical disorders can interrupt sleep without the patient being aware of the disturbance. Nocturnal myoclonus consists of sudden, repeated muscular contractions of the legs during sleep; the cause is unknown. In restless legs syndrome, dysesthesias or an urge to move the legs awakens the patient.

Sleep apnea is a condition in which breathing stops during sleep. Sleep apnea may be caused by momentary failure of the central respiratory drive or by intermittent airway obstruction. Obstructive sleep apnea may be associated with obesity or abnormalities of the oropharynx.

Laboratory Findings

Substance abuse as a cause of insomnia may be diagnosed by an unscheduled toxicology screen. Sleep laboratory evaluation, during which an electroencephalogram (EEG), electrooculogram (EOG), and electromyogram (EMG) are done, is useful in diagnosing unclear cases of depression, changes in sleep phase, sleep apnea, nocturnal myoclonus, and related conditions [33].

Treatment

Sleep disturbances caused by depression should be treated with antidepressants. Patients who chronically abuse tranquilizers and sleeping pills should be withdrawn gradually. Hospitalized medical patients should be asked if they anticipate trouble sleeping. If they desire a sleeping pill, they should be offered the opportunity to refuse the medication each night rather than being given the drug routinely.

Uncomplicated transient insomnia is treated with benzodiazepines [20]. Triazolam (0.125 to 0.25 mg), which has a very short half-life (3 hours), is most appropriate for patients who have difficulty falling asleep; however, it may produce rebound anxiety the next day. Temazepam (15 to 30 mg; half-life 6 hours) is prescribed for patients who find it difficult to stay asleep. Flurazepam (15 to 20 mg) is best for patients who wake up early and those who feel anxious during the day. The long half-life of flurazepam (40 hours or more) leads to drug accumulation in some patients, especially the elderly. Barbiturates, glutethimide, and ethchlorvynol should not be prescribed for insomnia. In addition to altering normal sleep, they are extremely difficult to withdraw and can be fatal in overdose.

Nocturnal myoclonus has been helped by muscle relaxation technique as well as clonazepam. Sleep apnea can be ameliorated by weight reduction when it is due to obesity; upper airway pathology may require pharyngopalatoplasty or tracheostomy. Apnea secondary to dysfunction in the central nervous system may respond to protriptyline, stimulants, or progesterone.

Schizophrenia

History and Physical Findings

Schizophrenia is a chronic illness characterized by intermittent or continuous psychotic symptoms (hallucinations, delusions, loss of reality testing) and deterioration in functioning. Genetic factors undoubtedly contribute to this major mental illness; environmental factors also exacerbate psychotic symptoms [61]. Schizophrenia is thought to be associated with dysregulation of dopaminergic systems in the brain, but the exact cause and pathophysiology remain unknown [68].

The manifestations of schizophrenia may be divided into positive and negative symptoms. Positive symptoms are characterized by their presence; hallucinations, delusions (fixed, false beliefs, not within cultural or religious norms), and agitation are the most common positive symptoms. Common schizophrenic delusions include convictions that everyday events (e.g., a television show) have a private meaning (e.g., a special message to the patient) or that some outside agency is withdrawing the patient's thoughts, imposing sensations on the patient, inserting thoughts into the patient's mind, or controlling the patient. Schizophrenic hallucinations are usually auditory; occasionally they are tactile, olfactory, or visual [75, 84]. Typical schizophrenic hallucinations include hearing voices speaking the patient's thoughts out loud, arguing about the patient, or commenting on the patient's activities [85].

Negative symptoms of schizophrenia are characterized by the absence of some important quality [2]. Examples include flattening or blunting of emotional expression (affect), poverty of speech, thought blocking, apathy, lack of motivation, inability to experience pleasure, loss of interest in work, hobbies, and sex, and decreased ability to feel intimate; there are few relationships with friends or peers. Negative symptoms, which also can be seen in other psychiatric illnesses such as depression, do not respond as well to antipsychotic medications as do positive symptoms.

Schizophrenia usually, but not always, begins

in late adolescence or early adulthood; a schizophreniform psychosis appearing for the first time after age 45 is likely to be due to organic brain disease or depression [81]. Deterioration of social and occupational functioning is the rule in schizophrenia [82]. Better outcome is associated with an acute onset, an episodic course, presence of confusion or depression, better premorbid history, and a family history of affective disorder [58]. Schizophrenia is associated with increased physical morbidity and mortality from suicide, poor self-care, and noncompliance with treatment for concurrent medical disease.

Differential Diagnosis

Organic mental disorders may mimic any or all the symptoms of schizophrenia. In most cases, mental status examination reveals a clouded sensorium, but some organic mental disorders, especially intoxication with stimulants, cocaine, and hallucinogens, alcoholic hallucinosis, and temporal lobe seizures, may produce schizophrenic symptoms in a clear sensorium [32]. Psychiatric illnesses that can be confused with schizophrenia include mania, psychotic depression, and brief reactive psychoses in patients with character disorders [65]. In schizoaffective disorder, patients exhibit symptoms of both manic-depressive illness and schizophrenia [46].

Laboratory Findings

Although positron emission tomographic (PET) scanning experiments have suggested decreased cerebral glucose utilization in frontal regions, there is no specific clinically useful laboratory test for schizophrenia. Initial investigations should be directed toward excluding drug intoxication and withdrawal and investigating possible causes of organic brain disease if this is suggested by mental status testing.

Treatment

Neuroleptics (antipsychotic drugs) are the cornerstone of the treatment of schizophrenia. There are currently four classes of antipsychotic drugs available in the United States: phenothiazines (e.g., chlorpromazine, trifluoperazine, butyrophenone, haloperidol), thioxanthenes (e.g., thiothixene), dihydroindolones (e.g., molindone), and dibenzoxazepine (loxapine). The specific choice of drug depends on past and family history and side-effect profile. Common acute side effects of neuroleptics include postural hypotension, anticholinergic effects, dystonia, akathisia, pseudoparkinsonism, and akinesia; the latter symptoms may mimic some of the negative symptoms of schizophrenia. Recent research suggests that lower doses of neuroleptics produce the same clinical benefit with fewer side effects. Tardive dyskinesia, a syndrome of involuntary movements of the mouth, lips, tongue, and extremities, occurs in 20 to 40 percent of patients taking neuroleptics for more than 6 months. Tardive dyskinesia may remit within 3 years if the medication is discontinued, but it is irreversible in 50 percent of cases. No treatment has been proven to be effective.

Psychosocial therapies are essential in the management of schizophrenia. The family should be helped to resolve guilt about the patient's illness and to avoid unrealistic expectations and expressions of intense emotion [23]. Periodic hospitalizations, group homes, sheltered workshops, and occupational therapy are useful in minimizing disability. Treatment of intercurrent depression, demoralization, family crises, and substance abuse also improves outcome, but expressive psychotherapy is not particularly useful.

Sexual Dysfunction

History and Physical Examination

Few patients volunteer that they are having sexual problems [36]. Most, however, will reveal such problems if they are asked about them directly. All patients therefore deserve a routine review of sexual functioning. The physician should ask an open-ended question, such as "How is your sex life?" How the question is asked is more important than what is asked. Concerns about sexuality should be addressed in more detail with patients with illnesses or treatments that affect physical appearance or sexual function or that cause pain or debilitation [41, 53, 72]. Examples include cardiac disease, hypertension, diabetes mellitus, spinal cord disease, depression, substance abuse, and Peyronie's disease [51].

Treatment

Most people who have had a myocardial infarction are concerned about how the heart condition will effect sexual performance. Unfortunately, a significant number of patients cease all sexual activity following a myocardial infarction for fear of damaging their heart further or of sudden death [60]. Usually this is due to ignorance on the part of the patient and failure of the physician to reassure the patient about the realities of stress on the heart caused by sexual activity. In general, if the patient can walk up two flights of stairs without symptoms, sexual intercourse should not be a problem. Even for those patients who experience moderate angina, sex after periods of rest (e.g., in the morning) may be appropriate [55]. Such patients should be counseled to try not to have sex after heavy food or alcohol ingestion. Some patients can use nitroglycerin or other cardiac dilators prophylactically prior to sexual activity.

An attempt should be made to change or reduce the dosages of medications that impair sexual functioning. Examples include beta blockers, guanethidine, methyldopa, low-potency neuroleptics, monoamine oxidase inhibitors, tranquilizers, and narcotics [67]. Alcohol should be discontinued. When sexual dysfunction is caused by depression, vigorous antidepressant therapy is indicated. Frank discussions of alternative means of sexual expression are necessary when patients have irreversible neurologic impairment of sexual function [86].

The partner should always be involved in the treatment of sexual dysfunction [44]. Reducing marital conflict improves many sexual problems. Primary physicians can treat a number of sexual disorders. Such conditions include problems due to ignorance about sexuality, uncomplicated premature ejaculation and impotence, miscommunication of sexual needs and preferences, and anorgasma. For example, women who have never had an orgasm frequently are able to become orgasmic when they learn sexual physiology and are instructed about effective sexual stimulation. This is practiced first through masturbation and then with the partner.

Many patients respond to reassurance and education. The physician can have a role in discussing with both partners ways in which they would like to have sex. Additional techniques include giving permission for the patient to discuss concerns about sexuality, educating about normal sexuality, and sensate focus therapy. In this therapy, the partners are given exercises to learn about each other's sexuality without intercourse. Intensive therapy for problem relationships and serious sexual inhibitions should be referred to a specialist.

The Dying Patient

Part of the mythology of being a doctor includes the fantasy that all illnesses can be cured. Many new physicians view terminal illness as a sign of personal defeat and react with anger, depression, and emotional distance from the dying patient [8]. Signs of these reactions in the doctor include not talking to the patient or the family, empty reassurances, forgetting to include the patient in rounds, inability to listen to the patient, moving the patient to a single room at the end of the hall, refusing to prescribe narcotic drugs for fear of addiction, and feeling uncomfortable without knowing why.

Our training has emphasized saving lives and sustaining and prolonging life. When this is no longer possible, then "there's nothing to be done." Indeed, there is much to be done [38]. It is important to remember that even when a patient cannot be cured, the doctor has an enormous amount to offer, especially a sense of hope that the patient can face death with dignity and free of pain and that the patient will not be alone.

In treating terminally ill patients, it is essential to prescribe analgesics in sufficient doses. Nonsteroidal anti-inflammatory drugs, antihistamines, and amphetamines can potentiate narcotic analgesia as well as reduce side effects. Narcotics should always be given on a regular schedule and never as needed (prn). Receiving medication and relief only when the patient is in severe pain leads to preoccupation with pain and increasing anxiety about whether pain will justify receiving a medication. Since anxiety increases the perception of pain, this schedule increases rather than decreases pain [16]. If the patient is kept out of pain by a regular analgesic schedule, anxiety is reduced and the total amount of pain medication required is also reduced. It is easier to keep patients from pain than it is to get them out of pain.

Separation from family and friends increases psychological and physical pain. To prevent this outcome, visiting hours should not be restricted. If family and friends are not emotionally available to the patient, the reasons should be explored by the physician. Reassurance that their own sadness will not upset the patient but rather will make him or her feel less abandoned often increases their availability.

Sometimes a dying patient's family becomes permanently unavailable for a variety of reasons. At these times, the doctor must be even more available to the patient and encourage the patient to express reactions to the illness. This sharing of intense emotional experiences decreases the patient's loneliness and ensures that even patients without families do not have to die alone. The doctor should not take on such an investment if he or she is unprepared emotionally for it. Talking about the experience with colleagues often is helpful to the doctor who is supporting a dying patient [90].

Hospice programs that specialize in the care of the dying patient and the family are continuing to develop throughout the nation. While not all dying patients are appropriate for treatment in a hospice program, physicians should be aware of what these programs offer.

Hospice care is most appropriate for patients with a life expectancy of 2 weeks to 6 months [63]. If death is imminent, transfer to a hospice program may be needless and disruptive to patient and family while not allowing the hospice staff adequate time to become involved. However, when the patient has a relatively long life expectance, hospice care can be too psychologically intense for patient and family [29].

Emergencies

A psychiatric emergency is an acute disturbance in behavior, feeling, or thinking which, if left unattended, could be harmful for the patient or others [71]. The emergency may be identified by the patient, by his or her friends or family, or only by the physician. In all cases, however, psychiatric emergencies occur when coping mechanisms fail because of the overwhelming nature of the stress or the inherent weakness of the patient's defense and resources, or both [62]. The stress may be external (e.g., loss of job, health, or a close friend or relative) or internal (e.g., psychological conflict or intoxication). Often several factors are present.

Suicide

In the United States, suicide is the eleventh leading cause of death in adults and the third leading cause in adolescents. Over half of all people who kill themselves visit their physician a month before they commit suicide, but only about one in six physicians uncovers the suicidal intent [88]. However, if asked directly, most patients will disclose their suicidal thoughts. The physician should therefore inquire directly about suicide in any patient who appears under stress [89]. Most suicides occur in patients who are depressed and/or alcoholic. Other psychiatric conditions that carry an increased risk of suicide include schizophrenia, organic brain syndromes, and narcotic abuse. A small minority of suicides have no psychiatric diagnosis. The best predictors of suicide risk are hopelessness and past history of a suicide attempt [5, 15]. Additional factors are listed in Table 10-10.

Patients hospitalized on medical floors occasionally attempt suicide [79]. These attempts are often impulsive and are associated with anger rather than depression [64, 80]. The patient often feels unsupported by the physician and staff. A good doctor-patient relationship, therefore, is an important preventive measure.

Table 10–10. Risk Factors for Suicide

Feelings of hopelessness

Past history of suicide attempts, especially multiple or serious attempts

Family history of suicide

Older age

Male

Caucasian

Divorced, widowed, or separated

Poor health in past 6 months (acute or chronic)

Loss of job (including retirement)

Psychosis

Communication of intent

Presence of depression, alcoholism, narcotic abuse, schizophrenia, and/or organic brain disease

TREATMENT

The first problem in the prevention of suicide is the identification of the suicidal patient. Although most patients do not volunteer suicidal ideas, they usually admit to them on direct questioning. All patients who are depressed, upset, chronically ill, or have made a suicide attempt should therefore be asked about suicidal thoughts. Patients with a specific plan that can be carried out or that nothing stops them from enacting should be hospitalized immediately on a medical or psychiatric ward and placed under continuous observation until psychiatric consultation can be arranged. Suicidal thoughts may be present for years, but the acute impulse usually lasts only a few hours or a day or two. Treatment of the precipitating crisis and of the underlying psychiatric disorder usually reverses suicidal thinking, even if the patient remains medically ill.

Threatening, Assaultive, or Homicidal Patient

Violent patients visit the physician in the hope of being stopped from acting on their impulses. Violent behavior usually arises in the context of an acute stress or exacerbation of a chronic psychosis or personality disorder. Substance abuse is a frequent aggravating factor.

If potential violence is suspected, the following procedures should be followed:

1. Do not see the patient alone.
2. Keep the examining room door open.
3. Allow unobstructed access to the door for both examiner and patient.
4. Do not see a patient if he or she is carrying a weapon.
5. Do not hesitate to call the police.
6. Do not argue or fight with the patient or challenge his or her self-esteem.
7. Do not threaten force unless the patient can be restrained without harm to anyone.
8. A physician should *never* engage in a physical struggle with a patient unless the physician's own safety is in immediate danger.

Usually patients who admit to violent plans want help, but they may not know how to get it. Negotiating with the patient is important. For instance, the patient may be persuaded to surrender any weapons and move out of the situation in which the danger of violence is greatest. Often the relationship that develops between doctor and patient will reassure the patient sufficiently to decrease the threat of violence. Hospitalization with immediate psychiatric consultation is mandatory if the patient has made a viable threat against a specific victim that can be carried out. Risk factors associated with homicide are listed in Table 10-11.

Discharge Against Medical Advice
Some patients who are ill often are frightened and confused about what is really wrong and attempt to leave the hospital in order to deny that they are sick. Other patients demand discharge because they feel misunderstood or humiliated by the physician. An optimistic, respectful, and kind listener can reassure many of these patients that the

Table 10–11. *Factors Associated with Increased Lethality in Homicide Evaluation*

Young male

History of poor impulse control, e.g., frequent fights and arrests

History of being involved in another's death, including in the military

Poor job, school, and military record

Disorganized life

Concrete plans or threats

Available weapons

Provocative victim

Drug or alcohol abuse

Psychosis

Organic brain syndrome

Antisocial personality

doctor will take good care of them, thus reducing their anxiety. A clear explanation of what is wrong and how long the patient will need to be hospitalized is often enough to encourage the patient to remain in the hospital. If not, the patient's family or friends should be asked to convince the patient to stay. Negotiating medication schedules and discharge date may give the patient a sufficient sense of control over the situation to feel comfortable delaying discharge until it is safe; however, sometimes an earlier discharge date turns out to be appropriate.

A rational person has the right to refuse treatment. Involuntary hospitalization is permissible if a disease (e.g., organic brain syndrome, schizophrenia, depression) prevents the patient from understanding the illness, recommended treatments, or the consequences of refusing treatment. The benefit of treating the patient involuntarily must outweigh the harm that is always inherent in restricting someone's liberty. In most states, physicians (not just psychiatrists) can obtain short-term emergency "mental health holds" that require the patient to remain in the hospital for treatment. Consultation with the hospital attorney is advisable.

The Agitated Patient

Patients with organic brain syndrome, especially delirium, may be agitated, hallucinating, frightened, or impulsive. Mental status examination usually reveals disorientation and a short-term memory deficit. The danger of assaultive behavior is high.

Functional disorders such as schizophrenia, psychotic depression, and mania also may produce agitation. If the patient is cooperative, mental status examination often reveals that memory and orientation are intact. Immediate psychiatric consultation should be obtained for psychotic patients, since they may exhibit impulsive and self-destructive behavior and further psychological decompensation.

Orienting measures, limit setting, and reassurance may help to quiet the agitated patient. Physical restraint is necessary in severe emergencies. This is accomplished by providing a sufficient number of people to allow the patient to submit without losing face. If the patient does not submit, one person restrains each extremity carefully, using leather arm and leg restraints. A fifth person should coordinate the restraint and watch the patient's head.

Emergency tranquilization is usually preferable to physical restraint. Intravenous haloperidol and/or lorazepam (e.g., 5 to 10 mg haloperidol with or without 1 to 5 mg lorazepam in the same syringe) has been found effective in a variety of organic and functional conditions. Drugs with marked hypotensive or central nervous system depressing effects (e.g., chlorpromazine, barbiturates, most benzodiazepines) should be avoided unless organic brain disease is excluded.

References

Recent

1. Anderson, D. J., Noyes, R., Jr., and Crowe, R. R. Panic disorder and generalized anxiety disorder: A comparison. *Am. J. Psychiatry* 141: 572, 1984.
2. Andreasen, N. C. Negative symptoms in schizophrenia: Definition and reliability. *Arch. Gen. Psychiatry* 39: 784, 1982.
3. Ballenger, J. C. Pharmacotherapy of the panic disorders. *J. Clin. Psychiatry* 47(Suppl.): 27, 1986.
4. Bear, D., and Fedio, P. Quantitative analysis of interictal behavior in temporal lobe epilepsy. *Arch. Neurol.* 34: 454, 1977.
5. Beck, A. T., Steer, R. A., Kovacs, M., et al. Hopelessness and eventual suicide: A 10-year prospective study of patients hospitalized with suicidal ideation. *Am. J. Psychiatry* 142: 5, 1985.
6. Bell, J. Organic Brain Syndromes. In J. Scully (Ed.), *Psychiatry* (The National Medical Series). Media, Pa.: Harwall, 1985. Pp. 65–69.
7. Carr, D. B., and Sheehan, D. V. Panic anxiety a new biological model. *J. Clin. Psychiatry* 45: 323, 1984.
8. Cassileth, B. R. The care of the patient, revisited. *Arch. Intern. Med.* 142: 1087, 1982.
9. Cleghorn, J. M., Bellissimo, A., Kaplan, R. D., et al. Insomnia: I. Classification, assessment and pharmaceutical treatment. *Can. J. Psychiatry* 28: 347, 1983.
10. Dubovsky, S. L. Calcium antagonist: A new class of psychiatric drug? *Psychiatr. Ann.* 16: 724, 1986.
11. Dubovsky, S. L. Abuse of Tranquilizers and Sleeping Pills. In J. Scully (Ed.), *Psychiatry.* Media, Pa.: Harwall, 1985. Pp. 107–108.
12. Dietch, J. T. Diagnosis of organic anxiety disorders. *Psychosomatics* 22: 661, 1981.
13. Endicott, J. Measurement of depression in patients with cancer. *Cancer* 53: 2243, 1984.
14. Falk, W. E., Mahnke, M. W., and Poskanzer, D. C. Lithium prophylaxis of corticotropic induced psychosis. *J.A.M.A.* 241: 1011, 1979.
15. Fawcett, J., Scheftner, W., Clark, D., et al. Clinical predictors of suicide in patients with major affective disorders: A controlled prospective study. *Am. J. Psychiatry* 144: 35, 1987.
16. Foley, K. M. The treatment of cancer pain. *N. Engl. J. Med.* 313: 84, 1985.
17. Glassman, A. H., Johnson, L. L., Giardina, E. G. V., et al. The use of imipramine in depressed patients with congestive heart failure. *J.A.M.A.* 250: 1997, 1983.

18. Hartmann, E. L.   Sleep Disorders. In H. I. Kaplan and B. J. Sadoch (Eds.), *Comprehensive Textbook of Psychiatry*, 4th Ed. Baltimore: Williams and Wilkins, 1985. P. 1247.

19. Homan, S., Lachenbrush, P., Winokur, G., et al. An efficacy study of electroconvulsive therapy and antidepressants in the treatment of primary depression. *Psychol. Med.* 12: 615, 1982.

20. Kales, A., and Kales, J. D.   Sleep disorders: Recent findings in the diagnosis and treatment of disturbed sleep. *N. Engl. J. Med.* 290: 121, 1983.

21. Klein, D. F., and Gorman, J. M.   Panic disorder and mitral prolapse. *J. Clin. Psychiatry Monogr.* 2: 14, 1984.

22. Kupfer, D. J., and Thase, M. E.   The use of the sleep laboratory in the diagnosis of affective disorder. *Psychiatr. Clin. North Am.* 6: 3, 1983.

23. Leff, J., Kuipers, L., Beckowitz, R., et al.   Life events, relative expressed emotion and maintenance neuroleptics in schizophrenic relapse. *Psychol. Med.* 13: 799, 1983.

24. Lesser, J. M., and Rubin, R. T.   Diagnostic considerations in panic disorder. *J. Clin. Psychiatry* 47(Suppl.): 4, 1986.

25. Lipowski, Z. J.   *Delirium: Acute Brain Failure in Man.* Springfield, Ill.: Charles C. Thomas, 1980.

26. Lipowski, Z. J.   Organic mental disorders: An American perspective. *Br. J. Psychiatry* 144: 542, 1984.

27. Mackenzie, T. B., and Poplin, M. K.   Organic anxiety syndrome. *Am. J. Psychiatry* 140: 342, 1983.

28. Meltzer, H. Y., Arora, R. C., Tricon, B. J., et al.   Serotonin uptake in blood platelets and the dexamethasone expression test in depressed patients. *Psychiatry Res.* 8: 41, 1983.

29. Mathew, L. M., Jahnigen, D. W., Scully, J. H., et al.   Attitudes of house officers toward a hospice on a medical service. *J. Med. Educ.* 58: 772, 1983.

30. Myers, J. K., Weissman, M. M., Tischler, G. L., et al.   Six month prevalence of psychiatric disorders in three communities: 1980–1982. *Arch. Gen. Psychiatry* 41: 959, 1984.

31. Noyes, R., Jr.   Beta-blocking drugs and anxiety. *Psychosomatics* 23: 155, 1982.

32. Reider, R. O., Mann, L. S., Weinberger, D. R., et al.   Computed tomographic scans in patients with schizophrenia, schizoaffective, and bipolar affective disorder. *Arch. Gen. Psychiatry* 40: 735, 1983.

33. Reynolds, C. F., Taska, L. S., Seivtch, D. E., et al.   Persistent psychophysiologic insomnia: Preliminary research diagnostic criteria and EEG sleep data. *Am. J. Psychiatry* 141: 804, 1984.

34. Robins, L. N., Helger, J. E., Weissman, M. W., et al.   Lifetime prevalence of psychiatric disorders in three sites. *Arch. Gen. Psychiatry* 41: 949, 1984.

35. Robins, P. V., Merchant, A., and Nastadt, G.   Criteria for diagnosing reversible dementia caused by depression. *Br. J. Psychiatry* 144: 488, 1984.

36. Scully, J. H.   Sexual Issues. In J. H. Scully (Ed.), *Psychiatry.* Media, Pa.: Harwall, 1986. Pp. 143–153.

37. Summers, W. K., Majovski, L. V., Mash, G. M., Tachiki, K., and King, A.   Oral tetrahydroaminoacridine in long-term treatment of senile dementia, Alzheimer's type. *N. Engl. J. Med.* 315: 1241, 1986.

38. Wanzer, S. H., Adelstein, J. S., Cranford, R. W., et al.   The physician's responsibility toward hopelessly ill patients. *N. Engl. J. Med.* 310: 955, 1984.

39. Weissman, M. M., Myers, J. K., Harding, P. S.   Prevalence and psychiatric heterogeneity of alcoholism in a United States urban community. *Q. J. Stud. Alcohol* 41: 672–681, 1980.

40. Yudofsky, S., Williams, D., Gorman, J.   Propranolol in the treatment of rage and violent behavior in patients with chronic brain syndromes. *Am. J. Psychiatry* 138: 218–220, 1981.

Review

41. Abram, H. S., Herta, L. R., Sheridan, W. F., et al.   Sexual functioning in patients with chronic renal failure. *J. New Ment. Dis.* 160: 220, 1975.

42. American Psychiatric Association Task Force on Nomenclature and Statistics.   *Diagnostic and Statistical Manual on Mental Disorders*, 3d Ed. Washington, D.C.: American Psychiatric Association, 1980.

43. Andreason, N. C.   Posttraumatic Stress Disorder. In H. I. Kaplan, A. N. Freedman, and B. J. Sadock (Eds.), *Comprehensive Textbook of Psychiatry*, 3d Ed. Baltimore: Williams and Williams, 1980. P. 1517.

44. Annon, J. S., and Robinson, C. H.   The Use of Vicarious Learning in the Treatment of Sexual Concerns. In J. G. Piccolo and L. L. Piccolo (Eds.), *Handbook of Sex Therapy.* New York: Plenum Press, 1978. Pp. 35–56.

45. Blum, E. M., and Blum, R. H.   *Alcoholism.* San Francisco: Jossey-Boss, 1969.

46. Carlson, G., and Goodwin, F.   The stages of mania. *Arch. Gen. Psychiatry* 28: 211, 1973.

47. Carroll, B., Curtis, G., and Mendels, J. Neuroendocrine regulation in depression: II. Discrimination of depressed from nondepressed patients. *Arch. Gen. Psychiatry* 135: 463, 1978.
48. Clayton, P. J., Herjami, M., Murphy, G. E., et al. Mourning and depression: Their similarities and differences. *J. Can. Psychiatr. Assoc.* 19: 309, 1974.
49. Colman, N., and Herbert, V. Hematological complication of alcoholism: Overview. *Semin. Hematol.* 17: 164, 1980.
50. Eckardt, M. J., Ryback, R. S., Rawlings, R. R., et al. Biochemical diagnosis of alcoholism: A test of the discriminating capabilities of gammaglutamyl transpeptidase and mean corpuscular volume. *J.A.M.A.* 246: 2707, 1981.
51. Ellenberger, M. Impotence in diabetes: The neurological factor. *Ann. Intern. Med.* 75: 213, 1971.
52. Folstein, M., Folstein, S., and McHugh, P. "Minimental state": A practical method of grading the cognitive state of patients for the clinician. *J. Psychiatr. Res.* 12: 189, 1975.
53. Frank, D., Dornbush, R. L., Webster, S. K., et al. Mastectomy and sexual behavior. *Sex. Dis.* 1: 16, 1978.
54. Hall, R. C. W., Gardner, E. R., Stickney, S. K., et al. Physical illness manifesting as psychiatric disease. *Arch. Gen. Psychiatry* 37: 989, 1980.
55. Jackson, R. W. Sexual intercourse and angina pectoris. *Br. Med. J.* 2: 16, 1978.
56. Jacobs, J. W., Berhard, M. R., Delgado, A., and Strain, J. J. Screening for organic mental syndromes in the medically ill. *Ann. Intern. Med.* 86: 40, 1977.
57. Jaffe, J. H. Opioids. In A. J. Frances and R. E. Hales (Eds.), *Psychiatry Update,* Vol. 5. Washington, D.C.: American Psychiatric Press, 1986. Pp. 145–146.
58. Kety, S. S., Rosenthal, D., Wender, P. H., et al. The Biologic and Adoptive Families of Adopted Individuals Who Become Schizophrenic: Prevalence of Mental Illness and Other Characteristics. In L. C. Wynne, R. L. Cromwell, and S. Matthysse (Eds.), *The Nature of Schizophrenia: New Approaches to Research and Treatment.* New York: Wiley, 1978.
59. Koranyi, E. K. Morbidity and rate of undiagnosed physical illness in a psychiatric clinic population. *Arch. Gen. Psychiatry* 36: 414, 1979.
60. Krop, H., Hall, D., and Mehta, J. Sexual concerns after myocardial infarction. *Sex. Dis.* 2: 91, 1979.
61. Leff, J. Schizophrenia and sensitivity to the family environment. *Schizophr. Bull.* 2: 566, 1976.
62. Levy, R. Suicide, Homicide, and Other Psychiatric Emergencies. In H. H. Goldman (Ed.), *Review of General Psychiatry,* Los Altos, Calif.: Lange, 1984. Pp. 660–661.
63. Mathew, L. M., and Scully, J. H. Hospice care. *Geriatr. Med.* 2: 617, 1986.
64. Reich, P., and Kelly, M. J. Suicide attempts by hospitalized medical and surgical patients. *N. Engl. J. Med.* 294: 298, 1976.
65. Robins, E., and Guze, S. B. Establishment of diagnostic validity in psychiatric illness: Its application to schizophrenia. *Am. J. Psychiatry* 126: 983, 1970.
66. Rush, A. J. *Short-Term Psychotherapies for Depression.* New York: Guilford Press, 1982.
67. Seagraves, R. T. Pharmacologic agents causing sexual dysfunction. *J. Sex. Marital Ther.* 3: 177, 1977.
68. Snyder, S. H. Neurotransmitters and CNS disease: Schizophrenia. *Lancet* 2: 970, 1982.
69. Tomlinson, B. E. The Pathology of Dementia. In C. E. Wells (Ed.), *Dementia,* 2d Ed. Philadelphia: F.A. Davis, 1977.
70. Uhde, T. W., Boelenger, J., and Vittone, B. J. Historical and Modern Concepts of Anxiety: A Focus on Adrenergic Function. In J. C. Ballenger (Ed.), *Biology of Agoraphobia.* Washington, D.C.: American Psychiatric Association, 1984. Pp. 1–26.
71. Weissberg, M. P., and Dubovsky, S. L. Assessment of psychiatric emergencies in medical practice. *Primary Care* 4: 651, 1977.
72. Wise, T. N. Sexuality in chronic illness. *Primary Care* 4: 199, 1977.

Classic

73. Akiskal, H. S., and McKinney, W. T., Jr. Depressive disorders: Towards a unified hypothesis. *Science* 183: 70, 1973.
74. Beck, A. T. *Depression: Causes and Treatment.* Philadelphia: University of Pennsylvania Press, 1967.
75. Bleuler, E. *Dementia Praecox or the Croup of Schizophrenics.* New York: International University Press, 1950.
76. Corsellis, J. The pathology of dementia. *Br. J. Hosp. Med.* 2: 695, 1969.
77. DaCosta, J. M. On irritable heart, a clinical form

of functional cardiac disorder and its consequences. *Am. J. Med. Sci.* 61: 17, 1971.

78. Engel, G., and Romano, J. Delirium: A syndrome of cerebral insufficiency. *J. Chronic Dis.* 9: 260, 1959.

79. Ettlinger, R. W., and Flordh, P. Attempted suicide: Experience of five hundred cases at a general hospital. *Acta. Psychiatr. Neurol. Scand. (Suppl.)* 103: 1, 1955.

80. Faberow, N. L., and McEvoy, T. L. Suicide among patients with diagnoses of anxiety reaction or depressive reaction in general medical and surgical hospitals. *J. Abnorm. Psychol.* 71: 287, 1966.

81. Feighner, J. P., Robins, E., Guze, S. B., et al. Diagnostic criteria for use in psychiatric research. *Arch. Gen. Psychiatry* 26: 57, 1972.

82. Goldberg, E. M., and Morrison, S. L. Schizophrenia and social class. *Br. J. Psychiatry* 109: 785, 1963.

83. Guze, S. B., and Cantwell, D. P. The prognosis in organic brain syndromes. *Am. J. Psychiatry* 120: 878, 1964.

84. Kraepelin, E. *Dementia Praecox and Paraphrenia.* Huntington, N.Y.: Robert Kreiger, 1971 (facsimile of 1919 edition).

85. Kraepelin, E. *Manic-Depressive Insanity and Paranoia.* Edinburgh: E & S Livingstone, 1921.

86. Masters, W. H., and Johnson, V. E. *Human Sexual Inadequacy.* Boston: Little, Brown, 1970.

87. Murphy, G. The physician's responsibility for suicide: I. An error of commission. *Ann. Intern. Med.* 82: 301, 1975.

88. Murphy, G. The physician's responsibility for suicide: II. Errors of omission. *Ann. Intern. Med.* 82: 305, 1975.

89. Smith, D. E., and Wesson, D. R. Phenobarbital technique for treatment of barbiturate dependence. *Arch. Gen. Psychiatry* 24: 56, 1971.

90. Weisman, A. D. Misgivings and misconceptions in the psychiatric care of terminal patients. *Psychiatry* 33: 67, 1970.

91. Wolff, H. G., and Curran, D. Nature of delirium and allied states: The dysergastic reaction. *Arch. Neurol. Psychiatry* 51: 378, 1935.

Dermatology

*Norman E. Wikner and
William L. Weston*

11

Bacterial and Fungal Infections of Skin

Impetigo

DIAGNOSIS

A preceding cut or skin abrasion that develops into a moist crust and spreads rapidly is characteristic of impetigo. Often, an upper respiratory illness or a history of exposure to others with skin infections can be obtained [81].

Erosions covered by moist, honey-colored crusts are suggestive of impetigo [34] (Fig. 11-1). Multiple lesions are present on the face, nasal orifices, and extremities. A border of clear blister may surround the crust in bullous impetigo. Invasion of the stratum corneum by *Streptococcus pyogenes* or *Staphylococcus aureus* produces the subcorneal blister and moist crust.

A Gram's stained smear of the blister contents will reveal gram-positive cocci, and bacterial cultures yield *S. aureus* or *S. pyogenes* [34].

TREATMENT AND PROGNOSIS

Oral antibiotics such as penicillin for streptococcal impetigo and dicloxacillin for staphylococcal disease are the treatment of choice [26]. Four 250-mg tablets daily for 10 days is recommended.

In areas endemic for streptococcal impetigo, treating all contacts with intramuscular penicillin is an effective strategy. Daily hand washing with a surgical soap may prevent new lesions.

Most patients with impetigo clear within 7 days of treatment [34]. If a nephritogenic strain of streptococcus is responsible for the impetigo, acute glomerulonephritis may occur. Prompt treatment will not prevent renal disease [34].

Acne

DIAGNOSIS

The common form of acne has its onset at puberty with whiteheads, pimples, or cysts restricted to those areas of skin which have abundant sebaceous follicles: the head, neck, and upper trunk [41]. New lesions appear weekly in contrast to drug-induced acne, where lesions all appear at the same time. A history of exposure to androgens, glucocorticosteroids, isoniazid, or hydantoin anticonvulsants may be obtained in drug induced acne [62].

In the common form of acne, a wide spectrum of lesions is present. Closed comedones (whiteheads) are 1- to 2-mm dome-shaped, white to skin-colored papules; red 1- to 3-mm papules and 1- to 4-mm yellow to white fluid-filled vesicles (pustules) also are seen [41]. Open comedones (blackheads) are 1- to 2-mm black, patulous follicular openings. Cysts are tender, 10- to 20-mm red nodules [41]. In drug-induced acne, all lesions are at the same stage at the same time. There are no diagnostic features [62].

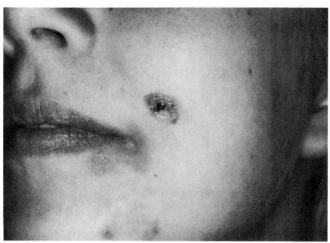

Figure 11–1. Impetigo: moist, honey-colored crust on cheek of patient with healing lesion at corner of mouth.

TREATMENT AND PROGNOSIS

For inflammatory (pustular) or cystic acne, overgrowth of bacteria in the obstructed sebaceous follicle is controlled by the use of oral antibiotics. Tetracycline or erythromycin (500 mg to 1 gm daily for 4 to 6 weeks) is given [44].

Topical keratolytic agents are the mainstay of therapy designed to clear the sebaceous channel which is obstructed by follicular cells [44]. Tretinoin 0.01 percent gel or benzoyl peroxide 5 percent gel are applied daily. In patients who have required oral antibiotics, topical antibiotics such as clindamycin phosphate 1 percent solution applied twice daily may be used [44]. In severe cystic acne resistant to standard management, isotretinoin tablets (40 mg twice daily for 4 months) are used [9]. Isotretinoin is teratogenic and should not be used in women without adequate contraception [9].

Acne may persist well into the fourth decade and require long-term therapy. Drug-induced acne may last 3 to 6 months after discontinuing the offending drug.

Bacterial Cellulitis

DIAGNOSIS

A skin puncture or penetrating wound that precedes the abrupt onset of fever, redness, and tenderness of the affected skin site is the usual history for bacterial cellulitis [84]. The area of redness enlarges within hours.

Tender, warm, red, swollen plaques with ill-defined borders are seen in this bacterial infection of the dermis and subcutaneous tissues. A red, macular linear streak may extend proximally from the plaque which represents lymphangiitis. Regional lymphadenopathy and fever are commonly observed [84].

Leukocytosis with neutrophilia and an increased number of bands is found [84]. Bacterial culture is technically difficult, but aspiration of the border of cellulitis may yield a positive culture [52]. Blood cultures also may be positive. *Streptococcus* and *S. aureus* are the two most common organisms recovered [52].

TREATMENT AND PROGNOSIS

Prompt administration of antibiotics is essential. Parenteral antibiotics are given if the patient is acutely ill or the face is involved. If localized to skin, then oral antibiotics to cover the common organisms can be used [33]. Chronic treatment is usually unnecessary.

With prompt therapy, the prognosis is excellent [33]. If treatment is delayed, the sequelae of septicemia may result [84]. These include acute bacterial endocarditis, osteomyelitis, brain abscess, or other serious internal infections.

Dermatophytoses

DIAGNOSIS

Itching and scaling are the usual complaints of dermatophytoses. The patient is often unable to describe the onset. Redness and blister formation and a thick, crumbly nail may be described [49].

Fungi responsible for dermatophytoses multiply between cells of the stratum corneum to produce superficial skin infections [38]. The most common site of involvement is the feet (tinea pedis) [49]. In adolescents, blisters and redness on the instep of both feet are observed. With increasing age, the findings evolve into diffuse scaling of the entire weight-bearing surface of the foot with a thickened, white great toenail. Scaling is particularly evident in the skin creases. Often, both feet and one hand are involved. Follicular pustules of the lower legs may be seen in severe infections.

Fungal infection of the groin (tinea cruris) produces symmetrical erythema and scaling also extending to the inner thighs. The satellite pustules of candidiasis and coral red fluorescence of the bacterial infection erythrasma on Wood's light examination will be absent [49].

Fungal infection of the nails (onychomycosis) often involves one to three nails which are thickened and white. The pitting and oil spots of psoriasis are absent [49].

Scraping of scales from the border of the skin lesion, dissolving them in potassium hydroxide, and examining them under the microscope will reveal hyphae and spores. A fungal culture will become positive in 5 to 14 days. *Trichophyton rubrum* and *Trichophyton mentagrophytes* are responsible for chronic tinea pedis, whereas *Epidermophyton floccosum* or *T. rubrum* are recovered from tinea cruris [49].

TREATMENT AND PROGNOSIS

Topical antifungal creams such as clotrimazole, miconazole, econazole, or ciclopirox applied b.i.d. for 3 weeks are the mainstays of therapy [49]. With nail involvement, oral griseofulvin (500 mg to 1.0 gm daily) may be required [38]. Many patients do not desire chronic oral therapy because 6 months to a year is required with a 30 percent cure. With follicular pustules or extensive skin involvement, griseofulvin may be required [49].

Fungi proliferate with heat and humidity; thus strategies to keep the feet or groin cool and dry are useful [47]. The use of powders and daily air drying are recommended.

Tinea pedis tends to be chronic and persistent despite therapy [47]. Tinea cruris responds well to antifungal strategies.

Candidiasis

DIAGNOSIS

The patient usually complains of itchy red skin, especially in intertriginous areas. A history of obesity, diabetes mellitus, or being restricted to bed is frequently obtained [60].

Intertriginous areas will reveal a poorly marginated, moist, red plaque with satellite red papules or pustules [77] (Fig. 11-2). Candidiasis is most common in the groin, but it will occur in axillary folds, inframammary folds, and interdigital webs. In patients who are bedridden, this fungal infection is commonly observed on the back [60]. In the oral cavity or vagina it appears as whitish plaques on a red mucosa sometimes with a creamy exudate [27].

Scales obtained from scrapings of satellite pustules or from mucosal sites will demonstrate budding yeast or yield a culture of *Candida albicans* [60].

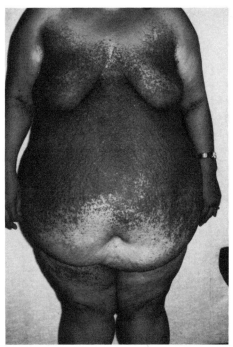

Figure 11–2. Candidosis: beefy-red erythema under breasts and on abdomen with satellite pustules.

TREATMENT AND PROGNOSIS

Miconazole, econazole, clotrimazole, or haloprogin creams applied twice daily for 2 to 3 weeks are effective [60]. Vaginal suppositories or throat lozenges of these agents are used for mucosal involvement [27, 77].

Strategies to relieve occlusion and keep the skin dry are useful.

Usually, clearing of the infection is prompt, but in immunosuppressed patients, the infection may persist [60].

Viral Infections of Skin

Warts

DIAGNOSIS

Patients will describe a growth beginning as a pinpoint spot that enlarges to become raised and rough on the surface. A history of frequent sexual contacts or of previous venereal diseases may be obtained in patients with condyloma [70].

The human papilloma virus (HPV) induces focal epithelial hyperplasia in a variety of patterns [46]. Common warts are 5- to 15-mm solitary papules with an irregular, rough surface. Flat warts (Fig. 11-3) are multiple, 1- to 4-mm, smooth-surfaced, skin-colored papules found on the face or extremities. Weight-bearing (plantar) warts are 3- to 10-mm, white, circumscribed papules with pinpoint dark spots. Venereal warts (condyloma) are multiple, 3- to 20-mm, grouped papules on genital mucosa and adjacent skin. Lesions of secondary syphilis (condylomata lata) mimic venereal warts but are moist [18].

A serologic test for syphilis should be obtained in a patient with condyloma. It is possible to identify human papilloma virus subtypes with DNA fingerprinting [46, 64] (Table 11-1).

TREATMENT AND PROGNOSIS

Cytodestructive therapy is the treatment of choice for warts. Cryotherapy is preferred for common warts [18]. Topical tretinoin cream is used daily for flat warts, 40 percent salicylic acid plasters are used for plantar warts, and podophyllin is used for condyloma. The podophyllin is washed off in 4 hours [18].

All forms of warts are due to persistent viral in-

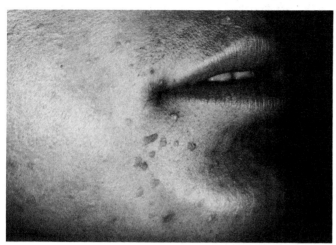

Figure 11–3. Flat warts: smooth-surfaced papules on chin.

Table 11–1. Wart types produced by papilloma viruses

Clinical wart	HPV subtype
Common	2,4,7
Flat	3
Plantar	1,4
Condyloma	6,11,16

fections with host immunity ineffective for 2 to 3 years [64]. Retreatment is frequently required.

Eventual clearing of warts is expected except in immunosuppressed patients [64].

Herpes Simplex

DIAGNOSIS

A history of recurrent localized skin lesions at or near the same skin site often is obtained, and this suggests an infection with herpes simplex virus (HSV). A history of precipitating events such as sunburn, illness with fever, sexual contact, or major psychological stress may be given. Pain may be described at the local site of blisters [97].

Grouped vesicles on a red base are the characteristic lesions of herpes simplex virus [24,

97, 101]. The most common skin sites of involvement are the lips, face, fingers, eyes, gingivae, and genital mucosa. Deep swelling may accompany the blisters and be confused with bacterial cellulitis. Tender regional lymphadenopathy may be found [24]. Usually, only a single group of vesicles is found, in contrast to several groups observed in zoster, but in immune-compromised patients, many groups or disseminated lesions, hemorrhagic blisters, or deep erosions are observed [24, 101]. Disseminated lesions are observed in patients with eczemas, burns, or malnutrition [101].

Viral culture of the vesicle fluid will yield herpes simplex virus within 72 hours. Wright's stained preparations of blister-content smears will reveal epidermal giant cells [24].

TREATMENT AND PROGNOSIS

In severe primary genital herpes or gingivostomatitis and in disseminated herpes simplex infection in an immune-compromised host, acyclovir given intravenously or as oral capsules (200 mg 5 times daily for 7 days) is recommended. For recurrent herpes simplex infection, no therapy is required [24].

Avoidance of precipitating factors such as sun exposure or the use of sunscreens may be preventive [97]. Use of condoms or a diaphragm with sexual partners is recommended [24, 101]. Prophylactic oral acyclovir has been beneficial for frequent recurrences [24].

Individual recurrent episodes last 5 to 10 days. Most patients have recurrences every 6 months, but some will have episodes every 2 to 3 weeks [97]. Recurrences will stop after 3 years in 50 percent [101]. In immune-compromised individuals, progressive herpes simplex infection may eventuate in encephalitis, pneumonitis, and death.

Herpes Zoster

DIAGNOSIS

Deep segmental pain that precedes the skin eruption by 3 to 5 days is described [80, 107]. The pain is so severe that it mimics angina pectoris, pleurisy, cholecystitis, renal colic, or migraine. Pain results in insomnia and an inability to function [80]. In some, an itching or burning sensation occurs [107].

Two to four groups of vesicles found over several adjacent dermatomes constitute the cardinal feature of zoster (Fig. 11-4). Each group is comprised of 5 to 20 vesicles. Hemorrhagic vesicles or pustules may occur.The dermatomal skin is ten-

der. Ophthalmic zoster may be accompanied by a red eye and keratitis. Vesicles on the pinna signify facial nerve involvement with facial palsy (the Hunt syndrome). Urinary or fecal retention may result from lumbosacral involvement. The varicella-zoster virus (VZV) is reactivated from a latent state in a nerve ganglion and inflammation of the nerve results [107].

Viral culture of the blister fluid will yield varicella-zoster virus in 2 to 6 days. Exfoliative cytology of blister contents will demonstrate epidermal giant cells [6].

TREATMENT AND PROGNOSIS

Oral acyclovir (800 mg five times daily for 10 days) will produce rapid healing, diminish viral shedding, and decrease the likelihood of postherpetic neuralgia [6]. Oral analgesics or narcotics may be required for pain control [107]. Long-term pain control may be required for neuralgia [107].

Untreated, lesions last 14 to 21 days and then heal, sometimes with scarring. About 5 percent of patients will disseminate after a transient viremic phase on day 4 or 5 after the onset of skin lesions. Rarely, the dissemination will result in encephalitis or pneumonia. Zoster may accompany malignancy such as lymphoma and in young males may be the presenting sign of acquired immune deficiency syndrome (AIDS) [107]. The elderly

Figure 11–4. *Herpes zoster: three groups of vesicles on right lower trunk; café-au-lait spot on left trunk.*

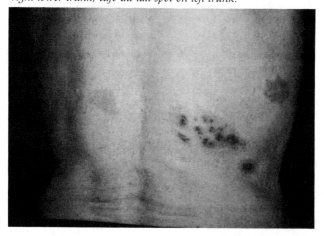

are most susceptible to postherpetic neuralgia with disabling pain for months.

Dermatitis

DIAGNOSIS

Inflammation of the skin that produces redness plus some feature of disruption of the skin surface is designated dermatitis (eczema) [50, 108]. Dermatitis is further subclassified as acute, subacute, or chronic depending on the intensity of the response. Acute dermatitis has blister formation with eventual oozing and crusting; a chronic dermatitis has epidermal thickening, scaling, and excoriations. Subacute dermatitis combines features of acute and chronic. Each of the six major types of dermatitis (allergic contact dermatitis, irritant contact dermatitis, dry skin dermatitis, atopic dermatitis, seborrheic dermatitis, and stasis dermatitis) may present as an acute, subacute, or chronic dermatitis [1, 30, 50, 89, 90, 100, 108].

Irritant contact dermatitis is often related to occupations where repeated exposures to irritating substances occur (scrub nurses, cement workers, industrial solvent users) [30, 89].

Allergic contact dermatitis is most commonly related to exposure to plants during outdoor activities (poison ivy, poison oak) or to metals containing nickle (watches, jewelry) [1, 100]. A detailed history of exposures, including cosmetic use, type of shoes worn, and work exposures, should be sought.

A family history of asthma, hay fever, or eczema and onset in childhood help in diagnosis of atopic dermatitis [67]. A history of frequent soaping of the skin or use of agents that dry the skin surface is obtained in xerosis [30, 89]. A history of oily skin of the face and scalp is obtained in seborrheic dermatitis [96]. A history of chronic swelling of the ankles and varicose veins is obtained in stasis dermatitis [48]. Itching may be a prominent feature of all six types of dermatitis.

The diagnostic features of dermatitis include redness of the skin plus disruption of the skin sur-

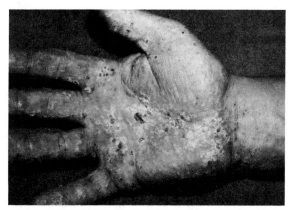

Figure 11–5. Hand dermatitis: erythema, scaling, excoriations of palm.

face (Fig. 11-5): blisters, oozing, crusts, fissures, excoriations, or scaling [30, 108]. Features of lichenification include epidermal thickening on palpation, exaggerated skin lines, and hyperpigmentation. Epicutaneous contact with chemicals is the only method known to induce dermatitis, and the distribution and arrangement of the dermatitis are clues to irritant or allergic contact dermatitis [89, 100]. Involvement of exposed areas such as the hands and face, including the upper eyelids, is seen. In contrast, in sun sensitivity, with involvement of sun-exposed skin, the upper eyelids are spared. Flexural involvement of the extremities is seen in atopic dermatitis, and greasy scales of the scalp and face are seen in seborrheic dermatitis [67, 96]. A dry, scaly skin surface is seen in dry skin dermatitis with fissured plates on the skin surface [89]. The elderly are particularly likely to develop dry skin dermatitis. Pinpoint areas of brown pigmentation of the legs and ankles plus signs of dermatitis are seen in stasis dermatitis [48].

Since dermatophyte infections and scabies can be red and scaly, skin scrapings should be obtained in search of mites and fungal hyphae. A skin biopsy should be obtained in any unresponsive dermatitis to exclude cutaneous T-cell lymphoma.

TREATMENT AND PROGNOSIS

Topical glucocorticosteroid creams or ointments are the mainstays of therapy [30, 89]. A moderate-potency preparation should be chosen, and treatment two or three times a day for 2 or 3 weeks should be started. If pustules, cellulitis, or regional lymphadenopathy are observed, bacterial infection secondary to scratching is likely and oral antibiotics effective against *S. aureus* for 10 to 14 days is indicated.

Avoidance of irritants or allergens, once identified, is useful strategy [1, 100]. Daily lubrication and hydration of the skin with moisturizers and emollients may be instituted for dry or sensitive skin. Elevation of the legs several times a day and the use of support stockings are useful in stasis dermatitis. Advise patients to stop use of proprietary creams that may aggravate the dermatitis [48].

Patients should be informed that many forms of dermatitis are chronic or recurrent and a good chronic management program will be required.

Scabies

DIAGNOSIS

Scabies presents with severe itching which is particularly intense at night. A close personal contact also may be experiencing itchy bumps [19, 68].

Many lesions seen in a patient with scabies are the result of scratching and rubbing itchy skin. S-shaped burrows are the diagnostic lesion, but they may be few in number and restricted to hands, wrists, fingers, and feet [19, 68]. The female mite requires 21 days to burrow into the outer layer of skin and lay her eggs within the stratum corneum [68]. Itching and redness are thought to be the result of mite feces or dying mites [19]. Lesions are found predominantly on the hands, feet, elbows, axillae, buttocks, breasts, and genitalia [19].

Microscopic identification of the eight-legged female mite, her feces, or eggs from skin scrapings is diagnostic [19, 68]. An unscratched burrow should be selected for scraping.

TREATMENT AND PROGNOSIS

Topical application of a scabicide to the patient and contacts is required. Gamma benzene hexachloride is applied for 6 hours from the neck down and then is washed off. This treatment should not be used in babies or pregnant women. Permethrin and 5 percent sulfur ointment are alternatives [103].

Patients will continue to itch 10 to 14 days after successful eradication of scabies mites. This is not an indication for retreatment. If new burrows appear, a second treatment may be indicated. There is no need for chronic use of a scabicide.

Untreated, scabies may persist for months to years. Complete clearing within 2 weeks of treatment is expected.

Papulosquamous Eruptions

Psoriasis

DIAGNOSIS

Gradual appearance of itchy, red, scaly patches on the skin or an area of severe dandruff is related by patients with psoriasis [31, 57]. Sixty percent of patients will have a family member with psoriasis. The patient may describe the appearance of psoriasis in a scratch, abrasion, or sunburn [31].

The epidermal hyperplasia characteristic of psoriasis results in red papules or plaques covered by a thick, silvery scale [31, 57] (Fig. 11-6). The entire cutaneous surface should be examined, since not all lesions are scaly, and clues to psoriasis may be found in the distribution [57]. Psoriasis has a predilection for the scalp, elbows, knees, gluteal cleft, genitalia, and nails. The fingernails will show distal yellowing with numerous pinpoint pits in the nail surface [31]. The isomorphic (Koebner) phenomenon is seen as linear papules at sites of scratches or other skin injury [57].

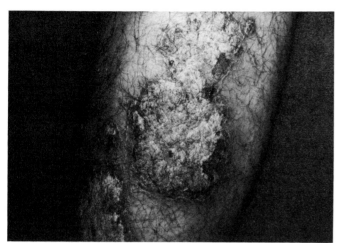

Figure 11–6. *Psoriasis: plaques on knee covered with thick, silvery scale.*

Scalp involvement is characterized by the presence of thick scales [31]. Pityriasis rosea, secondary syphilis, and drug eruptions can mimic psoriasis, but they do not have the nail changes or the thick scale found in psoriasis [57].

Objective signs of arthritis are found in 5 percent of psoriasis patients [79, 106]. Swelling and redness of one or more large joints, sausage-shaped swellings of the distal interphalangeal joints, spondylitis, or sacroiliitis may occur [79].

A few patients have a positive rheumatoid factor, and severe psoriasis may be accompanied by leukocytosis [79].

TREATMENT AND PROGNOSIS

Topical glucocorticoid creams and ointments applied twice daily for 7 to 14 days will improve psoriasis [57]. Ultraviolet light improves psoriasis, and sunbathing or sunlamp therapy is beneficial [57].

Anthralin or coal tar preparations may be applied to psoriatic lesions. Photochemotherapy may be used for resistant psoriasis [57]. The photosensitizing drug psoralen is given 2 hours before exposure to ultraviolet A (UVA) lamps (PUVA therapy). Treatment is three times weekly for 3 or 4 weeks until clearing, and then long-term maintenance therapy is required. Methotrexate (10 to 25 mg once weekly) is effective in resistant psoriasis [57].

Psoriasis is a lifelong, chronic disease with an unpredictable course, and the associated arthritis may be disabling [31].

Pityriasis Rosea

DIAGNOSIS

A large, pink, scaly spot which appears 1 to 14 days before the appearance of other lesions represents the herald patch [4]. Once multiple small spots appear on the trunk, itching occurs. Epidemics are well described, and a history of other affected persons may be obtained [69].

The herald patch is usually 10 to 30 mm in diameter, pink, and has a central scale [4]. It often clears in the center, thus mimicking tinea corporis. The other multiple lesions are oval, 3- to 8-mm, pink, and have central scales. They are symmetrically distributed over the trunk so that individual lesions are parallel to one another [4, 10]. Scales are thin, not thick as in psoriasis. In contrast to secondary syphilis, lymphadenopathy is absent and the palms and soles are not affected.

A serologic test for syphilis should be done.

Usually no treatment is required [10]. Oral anti-histamines may be given if itching is a problem. Sunbathing or ultraviolet B (UVB) phototherapy may clear the skin lesions [4]. Chronic management is not necessary.

Pityriasis rosea occurs in otherwise healthy young adults and may last 6 to 8 weeks. Recovery is complete.

Urticaria

DIAGNOSIS
A sudden onset of itchy spots that undergo rapid change is related to urticaria [74]. Some patients note hourly changes in shape and location of lesions. Deep swelling of the periorbital tissues, hands, feet, or lips may be described. A few patients are able to relate the onset to within a few minutes to hours of ingestion of a drug, an injection, eating a particular food, or inhaling an airborne substance. A preceding infection, particularly upper respiratory, may be described.

The diagnostic lesion is the wheal, a 2- to 5-mm, flat-topped, pink to red lesion with sharp borders [29, 74]. The tense edema produced by histamine release results in a dimpled surface [29]. Wheals are often multiple and evolve within minutes, either disappearing or enlarging to form large plaques with gyrate shapes (Fig. 11-7). Wheals disappear and reappear in 20 minutes to 3 hours [74]. Angioedema, which represents subcutaneous swelling, is a swollen area with indistinct borders. Angioedema of the eyelids, lips, and hands may accompany urticaria [74].

Eosinophilia is prominent in some patients, and antibody titers for specific infections or positive bacterial or viral cultures may be found [74].

TREATMENT AND PROGNOSIS
Epinephrine (1:1000 dilution) given subcutaneously at 0.01 to 0.05 ml/kg may be used for severe urticaria or angioedema [73]. Antihistamines are the mainstays of therapy, and hydroxyzine (25 mg) or diphenhydramine (50 mg) each given four times daily will be useful in control [73].

Withdrawal of suspected drugs, avoidance of suspected foods, and treatment of an associated infection are useful strategies. Chronic antihistamine administration may be required [73].

Most urticaria clears in 24 to 48 hours or recurs nightly for up to 3 weeks [74]. A few patients will experience urticaria for months.

Figure 11–7. Urticaria: gyrate erythema with flat-topped, tense edema of skin.

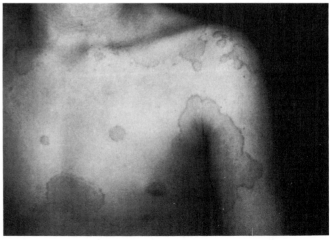

Skin Neoplasms

Benign Tumors and Cysts

There are many skin lesions that have no relationship to internal disease, are not malignant, and have only cosmetic importance to the patient. A patient will often be unaware that he or she has one or more of these lesions. Nevertheless, these lesions are frequently encountered in the physical examination of the skin and are in the differential diagnosis of other, more serious conditions. The physician will benefit from an awareness of the more common of these lesions. In the following discussion, the benign skin lesions have been classified according to their cell or tissue of origin.

KERATINOCYTES

Seborrheic Keratosis

DIAGNOSIS. One of the most common incidental findings in the examination of the skin is one or usually more seborrheic keratoses (SK) [16]. It is infrequent for a patient to come to a physician for the primary purpose of evaluating these lesions; when he or she does, it is usually because a lesion is on the face (and is therefore of cosmetic importance) or because it has become irritated through rubbing against a close-fitting article of clothing, such as a bra strap or elastic waistband. Seborrheic keratoses are usually asymptomatic. Most patients cannot recall the time of onset of these lesions. Furthermore, they are usually unaware of other such lesions that they may have in such inaccessible locations as the back. Not infrequently, a patient will notice an advanced lesion for the first time and erroneously report that it grew rapidly and suddenly. Thus the history may often be misleading. The onset of seborrheic keratoses is generally after the fourth decade. They tend to increase in number with advancing age. Patients may have a family history of such lesions [16]. The sign of Leser-Trélat refers to the sudden appearance of multiple seborrheic keratoses in association with various internal malignancies [92]. Whether this is a true entity is controversial. It should be noted that both seborrheic keratosis and internal malignancy are common in older people; thus their coincidence is to be expected [92].

The examination varies with the state of evolution of the lesion. Seborrheic keratoses usually begin as flat, yellow to brown patches less than 1 cm in diameter. They then enlarge upward, forming a flat-topped lesion with a rough (like sandpaper) surface and a very sharp margin. These features make it appear "stuck on" the skin. At this stage, the color is usually a light tan to brown. Close examination may reveal very small keratotic "plugs" in the surface. Lesions may be found anywhere except the palms and soles, but they have a predilection for the midtrunk and proximal extremities. They may be multiple (Fig. 11-9). They are usually distributed symmetrically. They usually remain sessile, but occasionally they become pedunculated. They occasionally attain a size of several centimeters. Physical trauma may cause a lesion to become inflamed, whereupon it will have a red background color.

Clinical examination is usually sufficient for making the diagnosis. In questionable cases, a biopsy of the lesion will reveal a characteristic histologic picture with hyperkeratosis, thickening of the epidermis, and papillomatosis.

TREATMENT AND PROGNOSIS. Patients often prefer to leave these lesions untreated. If the patient desires treatment, several modalities give good results. These include cryotherapy, electrodesiccation, curettage, and shave excision [16]. With any of these therapies, scarring is a possibility, as is recurrence.

Any new or recurrent lesions may be treated with the same methods used for acute management.

Long-term prognosis is nearly always benign. There have been a few case reports of basal cell or squamous cell carcinoma arising in a seborrheic keratosis [15]. A patient with multiple seborrheic keratoses is likely to develop more of them with increasing age.

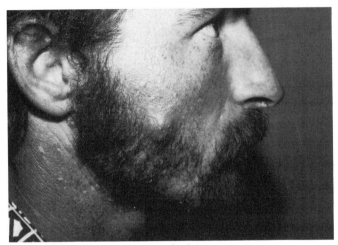

Figure 11–9. Epidermal cyst on cheek.

Epidermoid Inclusion Cyst

DIAGNOSIS. Epidermoid inclusion cysts or, more simply, epidermal cysts are the most common cysts of the skin. They sometimes result from traumatic implantation of epidermal cells into the dermis, but usually they seem to arise de novo. Usually, they are solitary, or there may be two or three lesions [58]. Occasionally, a patient will have multiple lesions. Finally, there is a dominantly inherited condition of multiple epidermal cysts, intestinal polyposis, and fibrous and/or muscular tumors (Gardner's syndrome) [58]. An epidermal cyst grows slowly and is usually asymptomatic unless it is located in an area of frequent trauma.

Examination will reveal one or more lesions consisting of movable cysts with a firm attachment to the overlying epidermis [58] (Fig. 11-8). At the time they are seen by the physician, lesions range in size from 0.5 cm to several centimeters in diameter. Often, by manipulating the lesion and observing carefully, the physician can appreciate a pore or punctum in the overlying epidermis that is the center of attachment of the cyst to the epidermis [58]. If the lesion has been traumatized or has had partial surgical manipulation in the past, it may be inflamed or bound down by

Figure 11–8. Seborrheic keratoses: multiple tan to brown "pasted on" papules on trunk.

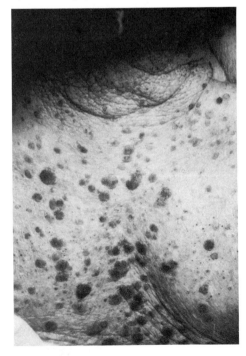

fibrosis. Biopsies of the skin will reveal a cyst within the dermis lined by true epidermis with the contents filled with stratum corneum.

TREATMENT AND PROGNOSIS. The only treatment for these lesions is excision. Incision and drainage are contraindicated because (1) this does not remove the cyst wall and the cyst will grow back, and (2) the procedure may allow the cyst contents to enter the dermis, causing an inflammatory reaction and subsequent scarring. If the lesions are small, they can be left untreated and followed for enlargement. Previously untreated lesions may be excised later if they enlarge. Scarring due to acute inflammation of the lesion may require subsequent surgical revision.

Following adequate excision, there is no recurrence. While some untreated lesions may continue to enlarge, others do not. Carcinoma has rarely been associated with epidermal cysts [95].

MELANOCYTES

Nevus

Strictly speaking, *nevus* refers to any new or abnormal growth, regardless of the tissue of origin. The word is commonly applied in a restricted sense, referring only to benign tumors of melanocytes or of melanocyte precursors [87]. Their importance lies in their relationship with (and frequent confusion with) malignant melanoma, a deadly cancer of these cells [102].

DIAGNOSIS. Nevi undergo a natural progression. They are absent at birth. They may begin to appear as early as 1 year of age, but they may appear later. They increase in number and size until the host is in his or her third or fourth decade of life and then they begin to regress [65]. The peak number of nevi in Caucasians ranges from 0 to several hundred; the average peak number seems to depend on sun exposure and sex (greater with higher sun exposure and in males) and ranges from 10 to 40 [65, 87].

Morphologically, there is also a progression of changes observed in nevi. Early lesions are 1- to 3-mm, sharply marginated, evenly pigmented macules [65]. Later they may enlarge and elevate to form pigmented papules, usually less than $\frac{1}{2}$ cm in diameter. During regression, they may lose their pigment and become fibrous, skin-colored papules. At an intermediate stage in this regression, the lesions may present as light-colored papules with flecks of darker pigment [65]. Throughout this evolution there may be considerable variation among individuals or between lesions in the degree of pigmentation, but individual lesions remain fairly evenly pigmented. Nevi may enlarge or become more darkly pigmented during pregnancy, puberty, and following sun exposure [87]. These changes may be sudden and cause alarm.

Several variants of nevi can be alarming because they resemble malignant melanoma. A blue nevus appears as a firm blue papule or nodule and consists of a focus of ectopic melanocytes in the dermis. A halo nevus appears as an ordinary nevus surrounded by a halo of depigmented skin [87]. Sometimes, either as a result of trauma or idiopathically, nevi become clinically inflamed, with a resulting erythematous border [87]. Finally, there is a variant known as the dysplastic nevus, which will be discussed in a separate section. Since these variants resemble some of the changes seen in melanoma, these lesions often must be biopsied.

Histologic examination can fairly reliably distinguish all forms of benign nevi from other pigmented lesions. A nevus will contain clusters or "nests" of round, uniformly sized cells with a central nucleus within the dermis, at the junction of the epidermis and the dermis, or both [87]. Clumps of brown pigment will be seen within the cells [87].

TREATMENT AND PROGNOSIS. The vast majority of nevi require no therapy. Nevi which (1) have sharp even margins, (2) are evenly pigmented, (3) are not inflamed, (4) have no foci of depigmentation, (5) are asymptomatic, and (6) are growing at a rate comparable to other nevi in the same individual can generally be presumed to be benign [65, 87, 102]. Removal of such a lesion is an elective cosmetic procedure that may be done at the discretion of the patient and the dermatologist or plastic surgeon. Atypical lesions need to be evaluated more carefully by an experienced practitioner; frequently, they should be biopsied. In the absence of a biopsy, even the most experienced physician can make both false-positive and false-negative diagnoses of melanoma [102]. Thus, in order to detect all melanomas, a significant number of benign lesions must be biopsied.

As new lesions arise they may, electively, be removed. Most untreated benign nevi will regress spontaneously [87, 102]. There is controversy over whether a malignant melanoma can arise within a benign nevus [102].

Lentigo

A common lentigo, or lentigo simplex, is a focal proliferation of melanocytes within the lower portion of the epidermis.

DIAGNOSIS. Unlike nevi, lentigines may be present at birth, although they also may be acquired. Because of confusion of these lesions with macular melanocytic nevi, little data are available about their natural history [55, 63]. The presence or numbers of lentigines is not related to sun exposure. Multiple congenital lentigines may be the presenting sign of several inherited disorders. Most notable among these is the Peutz-Jeghers syndrome, a rare autosomal-dominant condition of mucosal lentigines and (usually benign) intestinal polyposis [55, 63].

Clinically, lentigo simplex presents as a small (less than 5-mm), flat, uniformly pigmented dark brown to black macule with very sharp margination [55]. The border may be circular, oval, or slightly irregular. It can be quite difficult to distinguish clinically between a flat (junctional) nevus and a lentigo; only on biopsy can the two be distinguished.

The histologic features of lentigo simplex are characteristic and demonstrate elongated rete ridges with groups of pigmented melanocytes at the base of each rete ridge [55].

TREATMENT AND PROGNOSIS. No treatment is necessary. Excision may be electively performed.

No chronic management is indicated. Malignant transformation does not occur.

Solar Lentigo

Solar lentigines are a feature of chronically sun-damaged skin [21]. Thus they often occur on elderly individuals. For this reason, they have been called senile lentigines [51]. Younger individuals who have had excessive cumulative sun exposure, however, also may have these lesions. Thus the term *senile lentigo* seems inappropriate.

DIAGNOSIS. A history of long-term, repeated occupational or recreational sun exposure can usually be elicited [21, 51]. Careful questioning may be necessary; most people remain uneducated concerning the relationship between sun exposure, skin damage, and skin cancer and therefore will not realize that their own exposure has been excessive.

Solar lentigines occur on sun-exposed areas, usually on the face and backs of the hands (although any chronically exposed area may be affected) [21, 51]. They are usually multiple. The solar lentigo appears as a light to dark brown macule or patch with sharp but often irregular borders. Size is quite variable, ranging from a few millimeters to a few centimeters. The pigmentation is even throughout, and there is no induration or inflammation. These last features help distinguish it from lentigo maligna (a precancerous lesion), which has markedly variegated pigmentation [21, 51]. Occasionally, histologic examination may be necessary to differentiate between solar lentigo and lentigo maligna. Differentiation from lentigo simplex is relatively easy, since the latter is usually smaller, has more regular borders, is usually darker, and occurs on non-sun-exposed areas.

In questionable cases, a biopsy of solar lentigo yields a diagnostic histology of elongated, pigmented rete ridges which are club-shaped or show small but like extensions of basal epidermal cells. The epidermis in between the elongated rete ridges is often atrophic. Increased numbers of melanocytes are found within the elongated rete ridges [21].

TREATMENT AND PROGNOSIS. If the diagnosis has been *clearly established*, then it is possible to lighten the color of these lesions with light freezing. This alters the clinical course, however, and may lead to uncertainty if the alternate diagnosis of lentigo maligna is ever entertained. For this reason, it is usually best to leave these lesions untreated [88].

Periodic observation of these lesions at 1- to 2-year intervals (or sooner, if the patient notices a change) in order to confirm the diagnosis is warranted. Untreated solar lentigines persist indefinitely, and malignant transformation does not occur [21, 51].

Freckle

Freckles, also called ephelides, are small, light tan macules that occur in the sun-exposed skin of fair-skinned individuals [39]. Indeed, there may be a genetically determined propensity for forming these lesions in response to sun exposure [39]. They are relatively permanent, and there is no treatment.

DIAGNOSIS. Freckles may serve as a marker for individuals who are more susceptible than others to the damaging effects of sunlight [88, 102]. Thus affected individuals will often give a history of easy burning and no tanning (although they may mistakenly interpret their freckles as a tan). Freckles may occur in the first few years of life and increase in number and size with greater cumulative sun exposure [39]. In extreme cases they may become confluent, simulating a tan in an individual who otherwise does not tan. Freckles show an immediate darkening reaction, becoming more darkly pigmented within a few hours of sun exposure [39]. They fade during winter months.

Light brown macules, 1 mm to several millimeters in size are distributed over the sun-exposed areas of the skin, most notably the face and extensor surfaces of the extremities [39]. These lesions are rarely biopsied, but when they are,

they show larger and darker, but fewer, melanocytes in the epidermis [14].

TREATMENT AND PROGNOSIS. No treatment is indicated for acute management. Education regarding sun avoidance is of primary importance, since individuals with freckles are generally much more susceptible to sun-induced skin cancers. Freckles may fade with time and sun avoidance.

FIBROBLASTS
Dermatofibroma

DIAGNOSIS. Dermatofibroma is a very common tumor that usually arises in the dermis of the lower legs [16]. It tends to occur in young adults, is asymptomatic, and grows very slowly. Thus it often is not noted by the patient until it has attained its final size (about 1 cm) [16].

Dermatofibroma is a tumor of fibroblasts and endothelial cells, either of which may be predominant. In addition, some hyperproliferation and hyperpigmentation of the epidermis is often induced. Thus the tumor appears as a firm dermal nodule with indistinct borders that is either skin-colored or has varying degrees of purple or brown coloration [16].

Biopsy may be necessary to differentiate dermatofibroma from malignant dermatofibrosarcoma or malignant melanoma. Biopsy usually reveals a characteristic pathology of a proliferation of fibroblasts and young collagen within the dermis [16]. The dermis contains histocytes as well, and the overlying epidermis is thickened and contains increased pigment [16].

TREATMENT AND PROGNOSIS. No treatment is necessary. If desired, the lesion may be excised. Observation by the patient is sufficient chronic management. These lesions usually persist, although spontaneous regression is rarely reported [16].

Acrochordon

DIAGNOSIS. Acrochordons are commonly called skin tags. They usually appear in older individuals and may be more frequent in the obese [15, 104]. Younger patients may have them in association with acanthosis nigricans, with parturition, or with menopause [104]. They are asymptomatic unless inflamed.

Acrochordons appear as soft, sessile or pedunculated, skin-colored lesions [104]. They often occur as solitary lesions on the trunk, about 5 mm in size, or as multiple, thin projections of skin in the axilla or around the neck [104]. Biopsy will show loose connective tissue and prominent blood vessels within an outpouching of skin [104].

TREATMENT AND PROGNOSIS. No treatment is necessary. A common home remedy is to strangulate the lesion by tying a thread about the base. The physician may remove them by snipping at the base with scissors, by cryotherapy, or by electrodesiccation [104]. No chronic management is necessary. These lesions are entirely benign, and they persist indefinitely.

ENDOTHELIAL CELLS
Pyogenic Granuloma
Pyogenic granuloma is a complete misnomer, since the lesion is not a granuloma, nor is it of bacterial origin. Rather, it is a proliferation of new capillaries in a loose stroma. The cause of this lesion is unknown [109].

DIAGNOSIS. The lesion presents as a rapidly growing red nodule [109]. It has an increased frequency at sites of trauma. It is also seen more frequently in pregnancy.

A pyogenic granuloma appears as a single, dome-shaped, dull red, smooth-surfaced papule [2]. It is easily traumatized, however, and will then present an ulcerated surface. It may be difficult to distinguish from a hemangioma, glomus tumor, molluscum contagiosum, or a nodular amelanotic malignant melanoma [109].

The histologic appearance is distinctive, with a proliferation of capillaries within the dermis and thickening of the overlying epidermis with elongated rete ridges at the borders of the capillary proliferation [109].

TREATMENT AND PROGNOSIS. Because the differential diagnosis includes malignancy, and because this lesion will not resolve without treatment, excision in toto with histologic examination is al-

most mandatory [2]. This treatment is almost always curative; therefore, no chronic management is necessary. Lesions associated with pregnancy may involute spontaneously. Other lesions persist until removed. Removal will occasionally be accompanied by the appearance of multiple satellite pyogenic granulomas adjacent to the removal site [2]. Application of silver nitrate to these satellite lesions often will result in resolution [2].

Common Hemangiomas
DIAGNOSIS. The two most common hemangiomas are cherry angiomas and venous lakes [7, 8]. Both appear in middle-aged to elderly persons and may be present in large numbers. Venous lakes may be more common in those with sun-damaged skin [8].

Cherry angiomas appear as bright red papules, 0.1 to 2 mm in size, usually on the trunk [7]. Venous lakes are dark blue to purple papules, usually on the face and ears [8]. They are compressible and blanch when pressed with a glass tube or slide, only to refill when compression is stopped [7, 8].

The histologic features are unique. Cherry hemangiomas contain numerous dilated capillaries limited by flattened endothelial cells [12, 13]. Venous lakes show a solitary, greatly dilated vascular space filled with erythrocytes surrounded by a thin wall of fibrous tissue [12, 13].

TREATMENT AND PROGNOSIS. No treatment is necessary. For cosmetic purposes, the lesions may be electrodesiccated [7, 8]. No chronic management is necessary. Lesions usually persist and increase in size and number with age.

LIPOCYTES
Lipoma
DIAGNOSIS. A lipoma is a benign tumor of fat [36]. It is usually solitary, although multiple lipomas may occur around the neck and axillae [36]. It occurs most often on the trunk. It is asymptomatic, although a related lesion, the angiolipoma (composed of fat and blood vessels), can be tender. Angiolipomas are usually found on the upper arms of females.

A lipoma presents as a soft, compressible mass in the subcutaneous fat that is easily movable and not firmly fixed to the overlying epidermis. There is no color change [36]. Occasionally, a sarcoma may mimic a lipoma.

A biopsy shows the characteristic feature of a large collection of ordinary appearing fat cells surrounded by a thin connective-tissue capsule [36].

TREATMENT AND PROGNOSIS. Benign lipomas may be left untreated. Removal, if desired, is by excision [36]. No chronic management is necessary. Adequately excised lesions do not recur.

Premalignant Lesions

KERATINOCYTES

Solar Keratosis

DIAGNOSIS. Solar keratoses are also known as actinic keratoses. *Solar* and *actinic* refer to the induction of these lesions by sunlight [17, 82]. *Keratosis* means that the lesions are often hyperkeratotic, i.e., have excess keratin scale or horn on their surfaces. Solar keratosis may represent a mild form of epidermal squamous cell carcinoma in situ [17, 37].

Solar keratoses always occur in the setting of chronic, and usually high-intensity, sun exposure in a susceptible individual [17, 82]. The susceptibility of an individual correlates with his or her skin complexion. In general, red- or blond-haired people with light complexions are the most susceptible, while blacks are the least susceptible [82]. A stronger correlation exists with the history of acute reactions to sun exposure. Those who respond to 1 to 2 hours of midday summer sun exposure by always burning and never tanning are the most susceptible. Those who burn one or two times at the beginning of summer and then tan are somewhat less susceptible. Those who never burn and always tan are the least susceptible [17]. The most severely affected patients will have had long-term occupational (farmers, construction workers, surveyors, sailors) or recreational (surfers, swimmers, skiers, or sun bathers) sun exposure [17]. They will have taken few measures to protect themselves from sun exposure.

Patients will often complain of a lesion that appears to go away only to return in the same location. This is due to periodic shedding and regrowth of the overlying keratotic scale.

Solar keratoses are quite varied in appearance [17, 82]. The typical lesion is an irregularly shaped, flat, slightly erythematous macule or papule with indistinct borders and an overlying hard keratotic scale or horn. The erythema may be lacking, in which case the lesion is often more easily palpated than observed. The horn may be lacking, so that lesions appear as irregular red macules. If the lesions are numerous, they may be confluent. Because of other sun-induced changes in the skin (see below), they may be difficult to distinguish from the surrounding "normal" skin. The lesions are distributed exclusively on sun-exposed skin. The face and the backs of the hands are the most severely affected, followed by the ears, back of the neck, and extensor arms [82]. Often a peculiar pattern of sun exposure will be reflected in the distribution of lesions. For example, patients who habitually have dangled their left arm out a car window may have far more lesions on the left arm than on the right.

Solar keratoses often occur in the clinical setting of sun-damaged skin. Ultraviolet light produces a large number of nonmalignant changes. Damage to elastin and collagen produces wrinkling of the skin [82]. Hyperplasia of small capillaries together with this thinning produces multiple visible telangiectasias. A phenomenon known as solar elastosis, an accumulation of disorganized elastin in the upper dermis, may, if it is extensive enough, be visible grossly as yellowish papules [82]. Ultraviolet light also produces several types of melanocyte alterations and/or damage, visible grossly as irregular hyper- and hypopigmented macules [39, 87].

Solar keratoses have a sufficiently diverse morphology that their clinical diagnosis requires some experience. Nevertheless, most lesions can be diagnosed on clinical findings.

Skin biopsy will reveal a characteristic microscopic appearance with hyperkeratosis and large, atypical epidermal cells with a "disorganized" epidermis [17]. Biopsy may be necessary to distinguish a large or hypertrophic solar keratosis from a squamous cell carcinoma.

TREATMENT AND PROGNOSIS. Virtually any form of physical destruction is effective therapy for most actinic keratoses [17, 66]. The most convenient form of destruction is cryotherapy. Liquid nitrogen may be applied with a cotton applicator or with a spraying device, or copper rods cooled by liquid nitrogen may be applied to the lesions. Blistering usually results. If freezing is too deep, scarring may result.

When lesions are very extensive or confluent, and *after* any frank squamous cell or basal cell carcinomas have been removed, 5-fluorouracil may be applied as a topical cream to the affected areas. This selectively destroys neoplastic epidermal cells and will often reveal occult foci of solar keratosis. Two to 4 weeks of such therapy is usually required and must be monitored closely. Bacterial superinfection of eroded skin is a potential complication. There is often considerable discomfort for a long period; thus patients must be forewarned about this possibility.

Of course, the best therapy is prevention. Sun protection and sun avoidance are the key. In susceptible individuals, protection should begin in infancy and thus is a parental responsibility. Protection consists of avoiding all unnecessary exposure to sunlight, planning recreational activities so as not to coincide with periods of maximum ultraviolet flux (10 A.M. to 2 P.M.), wearing of protective clothing (hats, long-sleeved shirts), and using sunscreens on a regular basis. Inadequately treated lesions often recur, and the patient is also at risk for progression to skin cancer [37]. Some actinic keratosis appear to spontaneously regress [66], but most persist and actinic keratosis should be considered precancerous [17, 37].

Bowen's Disease

DIAGNOSIS. Bowen's disease is a peculiar form of squamous cell carcinoma in situ [11]. The patient complains of a gradually spreading "rash" or plaque that will not heal. Bowen's disease appears as a spreading red plaque with hyperkeratotic scale and distinct borders [11, 40]. It may attain several centimeters in size. Both sun-exposed and non-sun-exposed areas may be involved. The etiology of the non-sun-exposed lesions may be related to prior arsenic ingestion [40].

Biopsy shows characteristic large atypical epithelial cells scattered randomly throughout the epidermis and limited to the epidermis [40].

TREATMENT AND PROGNOSIS. Treatment is generally by excision, although electrodesiccation and curettage or adequate cryotherapy also are acceptable [40]. Patients must be observed for recurrence of the original lesion and for any new lesions associated with sun exposure or arsenic ingestion [40].

A significant percentage of such lesions transform into invasive squamous cell carcinoma. Such carcinomas are more aggressive than average. There is controversy over whether Bowen's disease is associated with an increased risk for internal malignancy [3, 40].

MELANOCYTES

Dysplastic Nevi

Dysplastic nevi are large, irregular nevi with a bizarre clinical and histologic appearance which, when they occur in families, are associated with an extremely high risk of melanoma [23, 43, 86]. The dysplastic nevus syndrome is the familial occurrence of multiple dysplastic nevi in an individual who also has a family history of dysplastic nevi and/or melanoma [23, 43, 86].

DIAGNOSIS. Dysplastic nevi occur in a range of clinical settings. In the most severe, a patient will complain of hundreds of large nevi, many of which have been present since early in childhood [43]. Many of the patient's family members also will have such lesions. The dysplastic nevus syndrome is defined as atypical nevi in a patient in which either the patient or one or more family members have already had a melanoma [43]. This syndrome is also said to exist if no melanomas have yet been detected. Some patients will have multiple dysplastic nevi, but no family history of dysplastic nevi or melanoma. Finally, the patient may have only one or a few dysplastic nevi and no family history. These last two circumstances are not called the dysplastic nevus syndrome.

Dysplastic nevi are generally larger than ordinary nevi (although this is not an absolute criterion). They can attain sizes of 1 to 2 cm and are usually elevated [23, 43]. The borders and the surface contour may be irregular. There may be erythema within or around part or all of the lesion [23, 43]. The lesions may be single or multiple and may occur anywhere on the body, although the face, palms, and soles are relatively spared. In the dysplastic nevus syndrome, hundreds of dysplastic nevi are present [43].

Dysplastic nevi have histologic features of "nests" of round pigmented cells in the dermis with "nests" of large nevus cells with hyperchromatic nuclei and individual large nevus cells at the junction of the epidermis and dermis [23, 43].

TREATMENT AND PROGNOSIS. Treatment is by excision. The entire lesion must be removed to allow histologic determination of both malignancy and adequacy of the surgical margins [23, 86]. Since melanoma may arise within these lesions, partial excision (such as a shave procedure) or destruction (such as electrofulguration or laser therapy) cannot be condoned. The question of which and how many lesions to excise is controversial. In cases of the dysplastic nevus syndrome, the risk of melanoma approaches 100 percent. Nevertheless, these patients may have hundreds of lesions, making excision of every lesion extremely impractical, expensive, and disfiguring.

Most physicians adopt a variant of the following strategy: (1) frequent (weekly) full-body self-examination by the patient, (2) physician examinations every 1 to 3 months with multiple photographs (multiple regional photographs plus close-ups of the more suspicious lesions), and (3) excision of any lesion that is symptomatic, which has changed in any way (by comparison with previous photographs or by patient history), or which on morphologic grounds is especially suspicious [43]. This strategy often results in several lesions being removed on each visit. Sun protec-

tion is absolutely essential, since there is compelling evidence that ultraviolet injury is a major factor in melanomas arising from dysplastic nevi [43, 54].

No reliable information is yet available on the prognosis of patients who have multiple dysplastic nevi but who have no family history either of dysplastic nevi or of melanoma. Ignorance breeds controversy; thus the treatment of such patients is even more controversial and is beyond the scope of this discussion [23, 43, 71].

Congenital Nevi

DIAGNOSIS. Congenital melanocytic nevi are those which are present at birth. They are of concern because of their potential for malignant transformation [53, 71, 86]. Some authorities project the likelihood of malignancy as 6 to 12 percent over a lifetime [86].

Most such lesions are less than 2 cm in diameter, but some are considerably larger, sometimes covering a whole limb or a large percentage of the trunk [42, 71]. They can be uniform in color and surface contour, or they can, especially in the case of the larger lesions, be quite varied, with patches of long, coarse hair within the lesion (hence the term *giant hairy nevus*) [71].

Histology shows characteristic patterns that differ from those seen in ordinary melanocytic nevi. Histology of congenital nevus reveals collections of numerous round, pigmented nevus cells throughout the full thickness of the dermis, often extending around hair structures. Small congenital nevi often have the histologic appearance of common acquired nevi [53, 71, 86].

TREATMENT AND PROGNOSIS. The treatment for these lesions is controversial [53, 85]. While the total removal of the large type of melanocytic nevus might seem wise on theoretical grounds (see below), in practice it is often quite difficult [71, 86]. The removal of all skin from a hand or from the entire bathing trunk area with subsequent engraftment of skin from another site is nearly impossible to achieve without complications, even when it is done in stages. The treatment of smaller congenital melanocytic nevi is even more controversial [53, 71, 86]. Malignant melanomas arise from small nevi beginning in the third decade of life [53]. Many dermatologists are willing to allow the infant to mature to adolescence before removing such lesions, so as to improve the cosmetic result of such a procedure.

If it is elected to leave such a lesion in place, it must be observed very carefully and frequently. The larger lesions ("large" is usually defined as 10 cm or greater) have a well-described increased risk of developing melanoma. The size of this increased risk is not well established. Such melanomas often develop early and are fatal. Whether this is because melanoma developing within such a lesion is not noted until it is well advanced or because such melanomas have intrinsically greater malignancy is unknown. There are no good data on whether the much more common small congenital melanocytic nevi have an increased malignant potential. The relative risk, if any, is small.

Lentigo Maligna

DIAGNOSIS. Lentigo maligna represents a type of malignant melanoma in situ [22, 25]. Its exclusive location in sun-exposed areas and correlation with a history of sun exposure establish the role of such exposure in its etiology [22, 25]. Thus, as in solar keratosis, the patient will always have a history of chronic ultraviolet exposure. Lentigo maligna starts as a small, usually dark brown macule and spreads very slowly over several years. Most lentigo maligna develop after age 20 [22, 25]. Since these lesions are usually on the face, the patient will often be aware of such growth.

Lentigo maligna appears as a dark brown patch of 1 cm to several centimeters in diameter. It is flat and nonpalpable. Any induration is probably a sign of progression to lentigo maligna melanoma [22, 25]. The pigmentation may be irregular, and the margins, although usually sharp, are also irregular. Inflammation, as evidenced by erythema, also may indicate progression to frank melanoma. These features are in contrast to solar lentigo, already described, with its even pigmentation, sharp margins, and no inflammation.

Biopsy of a suitable site within the lesion will reveal malignant melanocytic cells above the basement membrane without invasion into the dermis [25].

TREATMENT AND PROGNOSIS. Treatment is by complete excision of the lesion, although the lesions may be so large and so slowly progressive that in elderly, debilitated patients they may be left untreated [22]. Patients should be observed for the appearance of new sun-exposure-related neoplasms, as well as for recurrence of the lesion.

Prognosis for treated lesions is extremely good, since these lesions remain quite superficial and have a slow growth rate [22, 25]. If left untreated, a lesion will progress to lentigo maligna melanoma in almost all patients [25].

Malignant Lesions

KERATINOCYTES

Basal Cell Carcinoma

Basal cell carcinoma is considered a malignant epithelial tumor [45]. Its name derives from the resemblance of the cells to the basal layer of the epidermis, but its actual cell of origin is in dispute.

DIAGNOSIS. The history is usually that of a painless, slowly expanding lesion on the face, ears, or extensor upper extremities. The vast majority of basal cell carcinomas are caused by ultraviolet radiation [32, 98]. Only a few cases can be traced to other carcinogens, such as x-rays, burn scars, and arsenic, or to genetic predisposition [45]. The incidence of basal cell carcinoma varies with skin type and with sun exposure in a manner completely analogous to solar keratosis [17, 45]. Thus the typical patient is a fair-skinned individual who, either for occupational or recreational reasons, has had significant sun exposure. Not surprisingly, the incidence is higher in sunny areas, such as Albuquerque, than it is in cloudy, higher-latitude areas, such as Seattle [45]. For reasons unknown, the incidence is higher in males. In studies of basal cell carcinoma it has been estimated that a fair-skinned, sun-seeking male living to the age of 80 in Albuquerque can expect between two or three of such cancers [32].

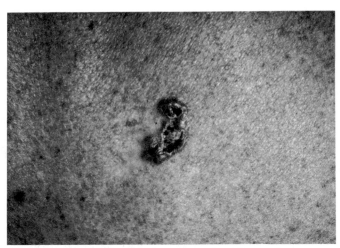

Figure 11–10. *Basal cell carcinoma: papule with central ulceration and pearly "rolled" borders.*

Basal cell carcinomas can have several different morphologies on physical examination. The most common one is the nodular basal cell carcinoma (Fig. 11-10). This presents as a dome-shaped papule with very sharp margination from the surrounding skin. The surface is very smooth and has been described as "pearly." Telangiectatic vessels are frequently seen overlying the lesion. In larger lesions the center may flatten or ulcerate, making clinical diagnosis slightly more difficult. Usually, however, the border will still be raised (a "rolled border") and possess the above-mentioned surface characteristics. These are sufficiently distinct that the diagnosis of this type of lesion can usually be made on visual inspection. Occasionally, the lesions may be pigmented, sometimes leading to confusion with malignant melanoma.

Other morphologies are more difficult to diagnose visually and usually require histologic confirmation. These include superficial basal cell carcinoma, which appears as a sharply marginated red plaque, usually on the trunk, and morpheaform basal cell carcinoma, which appears as a white to light yellow plaque with poor margins [45].

Basal cell carcinoma has a characteristic histo-logic appearance with an increased number of basal keratinocytes found in clusters within the dermis [45].

TREATMENT AND PROGNOSIS. The goal of treatment is the removal or destruction of all the malignant cells [45]. Numerous modes of treatment are all capable of accomplishing this goal. These range from microscopically controlled excision (Mohs' therapy [72]), simple excision, curettage with electrofulguration, cryotherapy, and x-irradiation. This is, however, not to say that a mode may be selected at random. Selection of the appropriate therapy depends on the size and location of the lesion, whether a primary or recurrent lesion is being treated, the skill and experience of the physician at a particular therapy, and cosmetic considerations. In certain areas on the face, Mohs' therapy is the only acceptable mode of therapy because of the relatively high risk and potentially dire consequences of recurrence in those areas [45, 72]. In other locations, one of the other modes may be used.

The chronic management of such lesions involves careful follow-up, both to monitor for recurrence of the treated lesion and to search for new lesions [45]. A patient who has a demonstrated susceptibility to basal cell carcinoma has a far higher risk for getting another. Once again, the most effective therapy is prevention. It has been estimated that 50 applications per summer of a sunscreen with a rated sun protection factor of 15 or greater from the age of 0 to 4 would produce a 50 percent reduction in the lifetime number of basal cell carcinomas and squamous cell carcinomas [98]. Such use through age 18 would produce an 83 percent reduction.

Basal cell carcinoma is a very unaggressive, slow-growing tumor that only rarely metastisizes, but its local growth is steady and relentless. In months to years, if untreated, it can invade bone, major blood vessels, the eye, or the brain [45]. Recurrences of treated basal cell carcinoma are unusual [45].

Squamous Cell Carcinoma

DIAGNOSIS. Patients with squamous cell carcinoma (SCC) may have differing backgrounds [35, 99]. Although the mechanisms of induction are not known, several environmental factors have been implicated in the induction of this skin cancer. Squamous cell carcinoma may arise from burn scars, in the margins of chronic ulcers, at sites of granulomatous inflammation, or rarely, at any site of chronic inflammation in the skin [99]. Infection with certain types of papilloma virus can lead to squamous cell carcinoma. X-irradiation of the skin [99] can lead to this carcinoma, sometimes decades later. Systemic exposure to certain carcinogens, especially arsenic, as well as topical exposure to organic agents, such as tars, oils, and chimney soot, also can lead to this variety of skin cancer [99].

By far the most important environmental factor, however, is ultraviolet light [35]. The association between squamous cell carcinoma and the combination of skin type and sun exposure is manifest to every practicing physician. It is also confirmed by numerous epidemiologic studies, which, although necessarily retrospective in nature, still show convincing elevated risk due to low latitude, fair or easily burned skin, sun worshiping, occupational sun exposure, and nonuse of sunscreens [32, 35]. These studies also show an increased risk in males over females which is

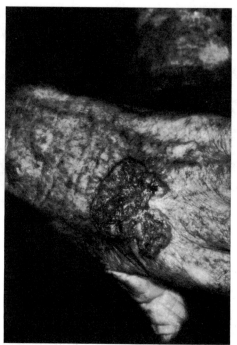

Figure 11–11. Squamous cell carcinoma: broad ulceration with indurated border arising in sun-damaged skin of hand.

unexplained. Thus a typical patient with squamous cell carcinoma presents with a persistent nonhealing lesion either in a sun-exposed area or at the site of one of the precursor lesions described above.

The morphology of squamous cell carcinoma is quite varied. Commonly it appears as a red to skin-colored papule surmounted by varying amounts of scale [99] (Fig. 11-11). The border with the surrounding skin can be obscure, especially if (as is often the case) the surrounding skin has many solar keratoses or is otherwise sun-damaged. The center may be ulcerated. The size can vary from a few millimeters to tens of centimeters, depending on the age of the lesion. Squamous cell carcinoma also can appear as a cutaneous horn, as an ulcer, or as a verrucous papule [99].

Often the diagnosis can be made only by biopsy. Histologically, the appearance is usually distinctive, with clusters of atypical keratoinocytes with hyperchromatic nuclei and spindle-shaped cytoplasm observed within the dermis [99].

TREATMENT AND PROGNOSIS. With few exceptions, therapy of squamous cell carcinoma is by excision with histologic examination of the margins [72, 99]. In cosmetically important areas, or in certain locations where the probability of deep invasion is high, Mohs' microscopically controlled excision is indicated [72]. Sun-induced squamous cell carcinoma on the limbs or trunk is sufficiently nonaggressive that curettage with electrofulguration may be elected in these areas.

Regular follow-up at 3- to 6-month intervals is necessary to check for recurrence or the appearance of new lesions [99]. In addition, chronic burn scars or other precursor lesions should be viewed with suspicion and followed regularly for the appearance of these skin cancers. Suspicious areas should be biopsied early. Sun protection is mandatory [32, 98].

With respect to prognosis, squamous cell carcinomas that arise from chronic inflammation, such as at burn sites and at the margins of chronic ulcers, are highly aggressive and metastasize early. The same is true when this skin cancer arises on the vermilion of the lip. In contrast, squamous cell carcinomas which arise on sun-exposed areas other than the lip are far less aggressive. Nevertheless, they grow relentlessly, are locally destructive, and do have the potential for metastasis [99]. The recurrence rate for excised squamous cell carcinoma is not insignificant.

Keratoacanthoma

DIAGNOSIS. Keratoacanthoma (KA) appears as a very rapidly growing, skin-colored to red, dome-shaped papule on sun-exposed areas [59, 94]. A keratoacanthoma can attain the size of 1 cm in 1 month. As it grows, it develops a central keratin plug. This clinical picture and history are virtually diagnostic [59, 94].

Histologically, keratoacanthoma strongly resembles a squamous cell carcinoma, and sometimes the distinction cannot be made, particularly if the lesion is incompletely excised [59, 94]. The entire epidermis is thickened with a homogeneous, "glossy" appearance at the base of the epidermis and a central crater filled with keratin [94].

TREATMENT AND PROGNOSIS. Acute treatment is by excision or by a unique "shelling out" procedure to which these lesions are amenable [99]. Injection of 5 fluorouracil into the base of the growth is an alternative therapy [78]. After acute treatment, patients should be observed at regular intervals (3 to 6 months) for recurrence and for any new sun-induced lesions.

Untreated lesions often resolve spontaneously, usually leaving a fairly significant scar [94]. Metastases are reported but are rare. Usually the treatment outlined above is curative. Recurrences do occur, however. Sometimes a ring of satellite lesions will develop around the site of a previous excision.

MELANOCYTES

Malignant Melanoma

Malignant melanoma (MM) is an extremely deadly cancer of melanocytes [20, 87, 90]. The incidence of melanoma is rising worldwide. Most countries are experiencing a doubling of the incidence every 10 to 14 years. The highest increases have occurred where large numbers of fair-skinned people live in very sunny climates [28]. The highest incidence is in Queensland, Australia; the second highest is in Tucson, Arizona.

The death rate from melanoma is also increasing, indicating that the increases in incidence are not just due to increased reporting. From 1971 to 1975, the rate was 16 per million for females and 26 per million for males [20]. However, the death rate for women is climbing faster than that for males [20].

The lifetime risk of developing melanoma also has been increasing. In the United States, someone born in 1930 has a 1 in 1500 lifetime risk. People born in 1950 have a 1 in 600 chance. Someone born in 1986 has about a 1 in 150 chance, and it is projected that someone born in 2000 will have a 1 percent lifetime risk [28].

DIAGNOSIS. Malignant melanoma is recognized as four types: lentigo maligna melanoma, acrolentiginous melanoma, superficial spreading melanoma, and nodular melanoma [90]. The classification is important because the presentation, course, and prognosis are different for the different types.

Lentigo maligna melanoma arises from lentigo maligna and is an extremely slowly growing tumor [22, 25]. It is caused by chronic ultraviolet exposure, as are basal cell and squamous cell carcinoma [25, 28]. Thus the typical patient with this kind of melanoma is a middle-aged to elderly person with a long history of a slowly growing pigmented patch, usually on the face.

Acrolentiginous malignant melanoma grows on the palms and soles, often in the web spaces or under a nail [90]. It has no relationship to sunlight. Especially if the lesion is on a foot, the patient may be unaware of it.

The relationship between nodular and superficial spreading melanomas and sun exposure is different from that between sun exposure and basal cell or squamous cell carcinoma or lentigo maligna melanoma [28]. Nevertheless, it is quite real and very important. These types of melanoma seem to be caused by brief, intense exposures. Thus a single blistering sunburn increases one's lifetime risk of melanoma by a factor of 2 [28]. Similarly, the people at highest risk are Caucasians who migrate to sunny climates or professionals who spend most of their time indoors but who take short vacations that involve sunbathing in tropical locations [20,28]. The increased incidence figures might be explained by the increased numbers of such vacations and migrations, together with clothing styles that expose more skin.

Many of the same host factors predisposing to squamous cell and basal cell carcinomas also predispose to the development of melanoma. Thus fair skin, easy burning, and poor tanning ability are all risk factors for melanoma [28]. One additional risk factor is the tendency to get benign nevi. The risk for melanoma correlates significantly with the number of countable nevi on a forearm [102].

Superficial spreading and nodular malignant melanoma are more rapidly growing [90]. The patient may notice a growing pigmented lesion that has changed size, shape, or color. The lesion may itch or hurt, and it may bleed or ulcerate [90].

Lentigo maligna melanoma differs from lentigo maligna in being raised, with a palpable surface [22, 25]. It also may have other features of malignant melanoma, such as more variation in pigmentation, "leakage" of pigment into the surrounding, otherwise normal appearing skin, depigmentation, or inflammation [25].

Acrolentiginous melanomas are rare. They appear as dark brown or black macules on the palms or soles [90]. They also may occur under the nails. If they involve the nail matrix (the specialized epithelium which manufactures nail), they will manifest as a brown or black longitudinal streak in the nail [90]. Such streaks are usually of benign origin in blacks or Orientals, but they must always be biopsied if they appear in Caucasians [90].

Superficial spreading melanoma is the most common type [90]. It presents as a raised lesion (much wider than it is high) that appears to be spreading by lateral extension. It has one or more of the following characteristics: uneven surface, uneven or indistinct borders, multicentric borders, leakage of pigment into the surrounding skin, or uneven pigment. One lesion may be mixtures of colors: white, tan, brown, black, red, or blue [90]. The white color reflects the loss of ability to make melanin by a clone of cells. The red color indicates inflammation. The blue color is due to seeing the pigment through several millimeters of collagen and the resulting scattering of blue light. Since this reflects deep invasion, it is a very poor prognostic sign [90].

Nodular melanoma presents as a hemispherical nodule [90] (Fig. 11-12). It may have any of the border or color characteristics of superficial spreading melanoma. In addition, it may have

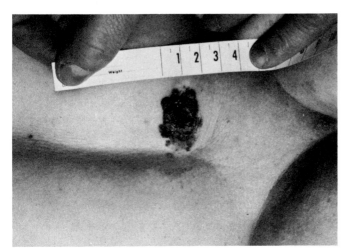

Figure 11–12. *Malignant melanoma: black nodule with irregular borders and shades of red, white, and blue within the lesion.*

satellite lesions, an indication of local metastasis.

Biopsy of the cutaneous lesions yields diagnostic pathology of a proliferation of pigmented cells with hyperchromatic nuclei and varied cytoplasmic shapes [90]. Dissection of local lymph nodes may reveal gross or microscopic evidence of metastasis. Metastasis to internal organs may be evidenced by conventional x-rays, NMR or CT scans, or nuclear medicine studies [90].

TREATMENT AND PROGNOSIS. The treatment of primary malignant melanoma is complete excision [90]. Because melanoma tends to spread laterally before invading, and because there can be histologic "skip" areas, with normal epidermis sandwiched between areas of involved epidermis, wide margins are usually taken. There is some disagreement and evolution in current thinking on how wide the margins should be. There is also disagreement over whether dissection of local lymph nodes is useful [90].

If there is clinical evidence for metastatic disease (e.g., palpable nodes, visible cutaneous metastasis), or if node dissection reveals involved nodes, noninvasive studies may be done to assess the extent of metastasis [90].

Patients who have had a primary melanoma excised should have regular follow-up for the purpose of detecting new primary melanomas or a recurrence of the original primary. Detecting metastatic disease is of secondary importance, since it will not affect the management of the patient [90].

The prognosis for metastatic melanoma is universally fatal regardless of treatment. Neither chemotherapy, radiation therapy, or immunotherapy have been shown to affect survival. The prognosis for primary melanoma with no clinical evidence of metastasis depends on two factors: the depth of the lesion and its location on the body [90]. Lesions less than 0.75 mm in depth are associated with a 7.5-year survival of 99 percent regardless of location [90]. At greater depths, survival depends on location. The location with the worst prognosis carries the acronym BANS, which stands for upper back, posteriolateral upper arms and neck, and scalp. Other areas of the body, in order of increasingly good prognosis, are hands and feet, non-BANS head and neck, non-BANS trunk, and non-BANS extremities (excluding the hands and feet) [90]. A primary melanoma in the BANS area greater than 3.64 mm deep with no evidence of metastasis at the time of excision still carries nearly a 100 percent mortality at 7.5 years.

Acrolentiginous malignant melanoma, because of its location, and both acrolentiginous and nodular malignant melanoma, because they invade deeply early, have poorer prognoses than the other types of melanoma. The type of melanoma, however, is not an independent risk factor over location and depth.

T-CELL MALIGNANCIES
Cutaneous T-Cell Lymphoma and Sezary Syndrome
Cutaneous T-cell lymphoma (CTCL) also has been known as mycosis fungoides [76]. The latter is a misleading name, and the former is to be preferred. As the name implies, it is a malignancy of small lymphocytes resembling T cells and bearing T-cell surface markers [56, 76]. These malignant cells have a strong tropism for the epidermis, and they localize and proliferate there [56, 76]. The percentage of malignant cells that are in the skin is so high that they often cannot be found anywhere else.

DIAGNOSIS. Cutaneous T-cell lymphoma usually appears in middle age, usually after age 40, although cases arising earlier are reported [76]. The incidence has been estimated at 2 per million. The disease characteristically has an extremely protracted and slow course and is difficult to diagnose in its early stages. Thus the patient usually presents with a puzzling persistent dermatosis and may have been to several previous doctors seeking a diagnosis [76]. Spontaneous remissions and exacerbations complicate the diagnosis [76]. More rarely, the patient presents with one of the advanced stages (see below).

During its course, the disease typically passes slowly through three stages which may overlap [76]. The first stage is called the eczematous or dermatitis-like stage. In this stage the patient presents with a variable and poorly defined dermatosis consisting of mild erythema, possibly with some fine scale [76]. The margins of the involved areas are poor and blend into the surrounding normal skin. The second stage is the plaque stage. The patient develops large (often several centimeters) plaques which are raised and flat-topped with a dull erythema [76]. The margins are better defined than in the previous stage. There may be some fine overlying scale. This stage also may last for several years.

Finally, the tumor stage ensues. Large, dome-shaped tumors develop either within the plaques or de novo. At this stage the disease may become quite extensive and may cover up to 100 percent of the body surface area [56]. The larger tumors often ulcerate [76].

The Sezary syndrome is a T-cell leukemia that can appear de novo or as a late stage of cutaneous T-cell lymphoma. The patient's entire skin surface is bright red, exfoliating, and sometimes weeping and crusted. It is extremely uncomfortable [76].

In the eczematous stage, the histologic appearance is as nonspecific as the clinical picture and only rarely shows lymphocytes that look definitely malignant [76]. Thus the patient may go undiagnosed for years. Even when the correct diagnosis is suspected, it can be exceedingly difficult to prove, often requiring multiple biopsies from various parts of the body and at successive monthly or even yearly intervals. Even in the second stage several biopsies may be required to make the diagnosis [56]. In the tumor stage, malignant cells may finally be detected in the skin, in the lymph nodes, and later, in multiple organs [76]. They also may be detectable in the peripheral blood [93]. In the Sezary syndrome, large numbers of malignant cells are detectable in the circulation [93].

TREATMENT AND PROGNOSIS. Acute management is directed toward making the diagnosis [76]. Attempts to provide symptomatic relief are often frustrating.

Treatment is by radiation and/or chemotherapy [76]. Immunotherapy is still in the experimental stage and has not yet produced clinically significant results. Three types of radiation therapy are electron beam, superficial x-ray, and PUVA (psoralen and ultraviolet A). All three have in common their superficial penetration. Thus they seek to exploit the epidermotropism of the disease and minimize systemic complications [76]. Topical chemotherapeutic agents, including nitrogen mustard and bischloroethyl nitrosourea (BCNU),

Table 11-2. Cutaneous Signs of Systemic Disease

General cutaneous signs	
Sign	Disease
Pruritus	Polycythemia vera, biliary cirrhosis, lymphomas, renal failure
Hyperpigmentation	Adrenal insufficiency, scleroderma, melanoma, lung cancer, hemochromatosis
Flushing	Pheochromocytoma, carcinoid tumor, mastocytosis
Hirsuitism	Adrenal virilizing syndromes, Stein-Leventhal syndrome, acromegaly, anorexia nervosa, porphyria cutanea tarda
Pyoderma gangrenosum	Crohn's disease, ulcerative colitis, myeloma, leukemia, rheumatoid arthritis
Erythema multiforme	Herpes simplex infection, drugs, histoplasmosis, coccidiomycosis, *Mycoplasma*
Erythema nodosum	Streptococcal infections; coccidiodomycosis; oral contraceptives; tuberculosis; leprosy; sarcoidosis

Specific cutaneous signs		
Skin finding	Other findings	Systemic disease
Angiofibromas of face	Ash-leaf white macules, shagreen patch, retardation	Tuberous sclerosis
Angiomas, spider	Palmar erythema	Cirrhosis
Blisters, erosions, scars on hands	Hirsutism	Porphyria cutanea tarda
Café-au-lait spots	Axillary freckling, soft skin nodules, scoliosis, retardation	Neurofibromatosis
"Chicken skin," i.e., loose skin of neck, axilla with linear rows of yellow papules	Angioid streaks in retina, cardiovascular disease	Pseudoxanthoma elasticum
Cysts, multiple on face and trunk	Colonic polyps	Gardner syndrome
Heliotrope, periorbital edema	Muscle weakness, photosensitivity, Gottron's papules	Dermatomyositis
Nevi of lips	Brown macules on nose, fingertips, buccal mucosa, small intestinal polyps	Peutz-Jegher syndrome
Necrobiosis lipoidica diabeticorum	Hyperglycemia	Diabetes mellitus
Pretibial myxedema	Exophthalmos	Hyperthyroidism
Palpable purpura	Arthralgias	Vasculitis
Pinch purpura	Waxy feel to skin, macroglossia	Amyloidosis
Pustular purpura	Arthritis	Gonococcemia
Telangiectasis of lips, face	Epistaxis, melena	Osler-Weber-Rendu syndrome
Xanthomas	Elevation of blood cholesterol, triglycerides	Hyperlipidemias

Fingernail signs	
Nail changes	Disease
White nails (Terry's nails)	Cirrhosis
Two parallel white bands (Muerhcke's nails)	Hypoalbuminemia
Blue nail lunula	Wilson's disease
Half and half nail (white proximal, brown distal)	Renal failure
Koilonychia (spoon nails)	Anemia

can be quite useful in ameliorating eczematous and even plaque-stage disease. Remissions are sometimes induced, but maintenance therapy is usually required. A dermatologist should be consulted for the exact indications for these therapies and for systemic chemotherapy [76].

While many of the preceding therapies provide visual and symptomatic improvement, there is no evidence that they prolong survival [76]. The disease course is so protracted, however, that patients often die of other causes before their disease has a chance to kill them. The ulcers that develop in the tumor stage do not heal and inevitably become superinfected with bacteria. Sepsis from this source is the most common terminal event [76]. The Sezary syndrome usually has a fulminant course with rapid demise of the patient [56].

ENDOTHELIAL CELLS

Kaposi's Sarcoma

Kaposi's sarcoma (KS) is a malignant tumor of endothelial cells [75]. It formerly was considered a fairly rare disease of elderly men. With the rise of the acquired immunodeficiency syndrome (AIDS), it has become far more common and warrants mention in this chapter [75, 105]. Kaposi's sarcoma is also seen in patients with other causes of immunosuppression. Only the immunodeficiency-related disease will be discussed.

DIAGNOSIS. Kaposi's sarcoma may be the presenting symptom in a new case of AIDS or it may arise later [105]. It is also seen in chronically immunosuppressed patients, such as renal transplant patients [75, 105]. It is usually asymptomatic and may first be detected by the physician, or the patient may note a growing nodule anywhere on his body.

Kaposi's sarcoma may involve any part of the skin, including the scalp, palms, and soles. It also may involve any part of the alimentary tract from mouth to rectum. Because of their endothelial origin, lesions arise in the dermis and, therefore, are hard to appreciate as early lesions [75, 105]. The lesions are quite varied in appearance. They begin as indistinct light red to purple to blue macules that grow to dermal papules and then nodules [75]. The lesions are usually multiple and seem to arise de novo at multiple sites. Less commonly, Kaposi's sarcoma may present as an enlarged lymph node [75, 105].

A biopsy is always needed for accurate diagnosis. The histologic findings are characteristic, with a proliferation of endothelial cells within the dermis or spindle cell formations containing vascular slots [75].

TREATMENT AND PROGNOSIS. Various systemic chemotherapies have been useful in obtaining brief remissions. Radiotherapy, which is useful in the more classic type of Kaposi's sarcoma, is less useful in immunodeficiency-related disease [105]. If a particular lesion is causing a functional problem, it may be excised. There is no good form of chronic therapy.

No treatment is curative. Brief remissions can be obtained with various chemotherapies, but relapse is rapid [105]. Also, such therapy markedly exacerbates the preexisting immunodeficiency and may lead to serious complications. The tumors may remain confined to the dermis or submucosa, or they may disseminate to multiple organs.

References

1. Adams, R. M., and Maibach, H.   A five-year study of cosmetic reactions. *J. Am. Acad. Dermatol.* 13: 1062, 1985.
2. Allen, R. K., and Rodman, O. G.   Pyogenic granuloma recurrent with satellite lesions. *J. Dermatol. Surg. Oncol.* 5: 490, 1979.
3. Arbesman, H., and Ransohoff, D. F.   Is Bowen's disease a predictor for the development of internal malignancy? A methodological critique of the literature. *J.A.M.A.* 257: 516, 1987.
4. Arndt, K. A., Paul, B. S., Stern, R. S., et al. Treatment of pityriasis rosea with UV radiation.

Arch. Dermatol. 119: 381, 1983.

5. Baer, R. L., Garcia, R. L., Partsalidou, V., et al. Papillated squamous cell carcinoma in situ arising in a seborrheic keratosis. *J. Am. Acad. Dermatol.* 5: 561, 1981.

6. Balfour, H. H., Jr. Acyclovir therapy for the herpes zoster: Advantages and adverse effects. *J.A.M.A.* 255: 387, 1986.

7. Bean, W. B. *Vascular Spiders and Related Lesions of the Skin.* Springfield, Ill.: Charles C. Thomas, 1958.

8. Bean, W. B., and Walsh, J. R. Venous lakes. *Arch. Dermatol.* 74: 459, 1956.

9. Benke, P. J. The isotretinoin teratogen syndrome. *J.A.M.A.* 251: 3267, 1984.

10. Bjornberg, A., and Hellgre, L. Pityriasis rosea: A statistical clinical and laboratory investigation of 826 patients and matched healthy controls. *Acta Dermatol. Venereol. (Suppl.)* 142: 1, 1962.

11. Bowen, J. T. Precancerous dermatosis: A study of two cases of chronic atypical epithelial proliferation. *J. Cutan. Dis.* 30: 241, 1912.

12. Braverman, I. M., and KenYen, A. Ultrastructure and three-dimensional reconstruction of several macular and papular telangiectases. *J. Invest. Dermatol.* 81: 489, 1983.

13. Braverman, M. S., and Braverman, I. M. Three-dimensional reconstructions of objects from serial sections using a microcomputer graphics system. *J. Invest. Dermatol.* 86: 290, 1986.

14. Breathnach, A. S. Melanocyte distribution in forearm epidermis of freckled human subjects. *J. Invest. Dermatol.* 29: 253, 1957.

15. Breckner, S. M. Fibroma molluscum gravidarum: A new clinical entity. *Am. J. Obstet.* 53: 191, 1906.

16. Brownstein, M. H. The benign acanthomas. *J. Cutan. Pathol.* 12: 172, 1985.

17. Brownstein, M. H., and Rabinowitz, A. D. The precursors of cutaneous squamous cell carcinoma. *Int. J. Dermatol.* 18: 1, 1979.

18. Bunney, M. H. Viral warts: A new look at an old problem. *Br. Med. J.* 293: 1045, 1986.

19. Burkhart, C. G. Scabies: An epidemiologic reassessment. *Ann. Intern. Med.* 98: 298, 1983.

20. Callen, J. P., Allegra, J. C. (Eds.). *Med. Clin. N. Am.* 70:3–94, 1986.

21. Cawley, E. P., and Curtis, A. C. Lentigo senilis. *Arch. Dermatol. Syphilol.* 62: 635, 1950.

22. Clark, W. H., Jr., and Mihm, M. C., Jr. Lentigo maligna and lentigo-maligna melanoma. *Am. J. Pathol.* 55: 39, 1969.

23. Clark, W. H., Jr., Reimer, R. R., Greene, M. H., et al. Origin of familial malignant melanoma from heritable melanocytic lesions: The "BK" mole syndrome. *Arch. Dermatol.* 114: 732, 1978.

24. Corey, L., and Spear, P. G. Infections with herpes simplex virus. *N. Engl. J. Med.* 314: 749, 1986.

25. Cramer, S. F., and Kiehn, C. L. Sequential histologic study of evolving lentigo maligna melanoma. *Arch. Pathol.* 106: 121, 1982.

26. Dillon, H. C., Jr. Topical and systemic therapy for pyoderma. *Int. J. Dermatol.* 19: 443, 1980.

27. Dreizen, S. Oral candidiasis. *Am. J. Med.* 77: 28, 1984.

28. Elwood, J. M., Gallagher, R. P., Davison, J., et al. Sunburn, suntan and the risk of cutaneous malignant melanoma: The Western Canada Melanoma Study. *Br. J. Cancer* 51: 543, 1985.

29. Emmelin, N., and Feldberg, W. The mechanism of the sting of the common nettle (*Urtica urens*). *J. Physiol.* 106: 440, 1947.

30. Epstein, E. Hand dermatitis: Practical management and current concepts. *J. Am. Acad. Dermatol.* 10: 395, 1984.

31. Farber, E. M., and Nall, M. L. The natural history of psoriasis in 5600 patients. *Dermatologica* 148: 1, 1974.

32. Fears, T. R., and Scotto, J. Estimating increases in skin cancer morbidity due to increases in UV radiation exposure. *Cancer Invest.* 1: 119, 1983.

33. Feingold, D. S., and Wagner, R. F., Jr. Antibacterial therapy. *J. Am. Acad. Dermatol.* 14: 535, 1986.

34. Ferrieri, P., Dajani, A. S., Wannamaker, L. W., et al. The natural history of impetigo. *J. Clin. Invest.* 51: 2851, 1972.

35. Findly, G. M. Ultraviolet light and skin cancer. *Lancet* 2: 1070, 1928.

36. From, L., and Assaad, D. Neoplasms, Pseudoneoplasms, Hyperplasias, and Mucinoses of Supporting Tissue Origin. In T. B. Fitzpatrick, et al. (Eds.), *Dermatology in General Medicine.* New York: McGraw-Hill, 1987. Pp. 1044–1045.

37. Fukamizu, H., Inoue, K., Matsumoto, K., et al. Metastatic squamous cell carcinomas derived from solar keratosis. *J. Dermatol. Surg. Oncol.* 11: 518, 1985.

38. Gentles, J. C. Experimental ringworm in guinea

pigs: Oral treatment with griseofulvin. *Nature* 182: 478, 1958.

39. Goldberg, L. H., and Altman, A. Benign skin changes associated with chronic sunlight exposure. *Cutis* 34: 33, 1984.

40. Graham, J. H., and Helwig, E. B. Bowen's disease and its relationship to systemic cancer. *Arch. Dermatol.* 80: 133, 1959.

41. Grant, R. R. The history of acne. *Proc. R. Soc. Med.* 44: 647, 1951.

42. Greeley, P. W., Middleton, A. G., and Curtain, J. W. Incidence of malignancy in giant pigmented nevi. *Plast. Reconstr. Surg.* 36: 22, 1965.

43. Greene, M. H., Clark, W. H., Jr., Tucker, M. A., et al. Acquired precursors of cutaneous malignant melanoma. The familial dysplastic nevus syndrome. *N. Engl. J. Med.* 312: 91, 1985.

44. Greenwood, R., Burke, B., and Cunliffe, W. J. Evaluation of therapeutic strategy for the treatment of acne vulgaris with conventional therapy. *Br. J. Dermatol.* 114: 353, 1986.

45. Grimwood, R. E., Siegle, R. J., Ferris, C. F., et al. The biology of basal cell carcinomas: A revisit and recent developments. *J. Dermatol. Surg. Oncol.* 12: 805, 1986.

46. Gross, G., Pfister, H., Hagedorn, M., et al. Correlation between human papillomavirus (HPV) type and histology of warts. *J. Invest. Dermatol.* 78: 160, 1982.

47. Hay, R. J., and Shennon, G. Chronic dermatophyte infections: II. Antibody and cell mediated immune responses. *Br. J. Dermatol.* 106: 191, 1982.

48. Hendrickson, W. M., and Swallow, R. T. Management of stasis leg ulcers with Unna's boots versus elastic support stockings. *J. Am. Acad. Dermatol.* 12: 90, 1985.

49. Hernandez, A. D. An approach to the diagnosis and therapy of dermatophytoses. *Int. J. Dermatol.* 19: 540, 1980.

50. Hill, L. W., and Sulzberger, M. B. Evolution of atopic dermatitis. *Arch. Dermatol.* 32: 451, 1935.

51. Hodgson, C. Senile lentigo. *Arch. Dermatol.* 87: 197, 1963.

52. Hook, E. W., III, Hooton, T. M., Horton, C. A., et al. Microbiological evaluation of cutaneous cellulitis in adults. *Arch. Intern. Med.* 146: 295, 1986.

53. Illig, L., Weidner, F., Hundeiker, M., et al. Congenital nevi less than or equal to 10 cm as precursors to melanoma: Fifty-two cases, a review, and

a new conception. *Arch. Dermatol.* 121: 1274, 1985.

54. Jung, E. G., Bohnert, E., and Boonen, H. Dysplastic nevus syndrome: Ultraviolet hypermutability confirmed in vitro by elevated sister chromatid exchanges. *Dermatologica* 173: 297, 1986.

55. Kamino, H., and Ackerman, A. B. A histologic atlas of some common benign pigmented lesions of the skin. *J. Dermatol. Surg. Oncol.* 5: 718, 1979.

56. Knobler, R. M., and Edelson, R. L. Cutaneous T cell lymphoma. *Med. Clin. North Am.* 70: 109, 1986.

57. Krueger, G. G., Bergstresser, P. R., Lowe, N. J., et al. Psoriasis. *J. Am. Acad. Dermatol.* 11: 937, 1984.

58. Lever, W. F., and Schaumburg-Lever, G. *Histopathology of the Skin*, 6th Ed. Philadelphia: Lippincott, 1983. Pp. 482–484.

59. Levy, E. J., Cahn, M. M., Shaffer, B., et al. Keratoacanthomna. *J.A.M.A.* 155: 562, 1954.

60. Lewis, G. M., and Hopper, M. E. Moniliasis, clinical forms. *N.Y. State J. Med.* 38: 859, 1938.

61. Lippman, S. M., Kessler, J. F., and Meyskens, F. L., Jr. Retinoids as preventive and therapeutic anticancer agents. Part I. *Cancer Treat. Rep.* 71: 391, 1987.

62. Lucky, A. W. Endocrine aspects of acne. *Pediatr. Clin. North Am.* 30: 395, 1983.

63. Lund, H. Z., and Kraus, J. M. Melanocytic Tumors of the Skin. In *Atlas of Tumor Pathology.* Washington, D.C.: Armed Forces Institute of Pathology, 1962. Sec. 1, fascicle 2.

64. Lutzner, M. A. The human papilloma viruses: A review. *Arch. Dermatol.* 119: 631, 1983.

65. MacKie, R. M., English, J., Aitchison, T. C., et al. The number and distribution of benign pigmented moles (melanocytic naevi) in a healthy British population. *Br. J. Dermatol.* 113: 167, 1985.

66. Marks, R., Foley, P., Goodman, G., et al. Spontaneous remission of solar keratoses: The case for conservative management. *Br. J. Dermatol.* 115: 649, 1986.

67. Marsh, D. G., Meyers, D. A., and Bias, W. B. The epidemiology and genetics of atopic allergy. *N. Engl. J. Med.* 305: 1551, 1981.

68. Mellanby, K. *Scabies.* London: Oxford University Press, 1943.

69. Messenger, A. G., Knox, E. G., Summerly, R., et al. Case clustering in pityriasis rosea: Support for

role of an infective agent. *Br. Med. J.* 284: 371, 1982.

70. Messing, A. M., and Epstein, W. L. Natural history of warts: A two year study. *Arch. Dermatol.* 87: 306, 1963.

71. Metcalf, J. S., and Maize, J. C. Melanocytic nevi and malignant melanoma. *Dermatol. Clin.* 3: 217, 1985.

72. Mohs, F. E. Chemosurgery for skin cancer: Fixed tissue and fresh tissue techniques. *Arch. Dermatol.* 112: 211, 1976.

73. Monroe, E. W. Treatment of urticaria. *Dermatol. Clin.* 3: 51, 1985.

74. Monroe, E. W. Urticaria. *Int. J. Dermatol.* 20: 32, 1981.

75. Muggia, F. M., and Lonberg, M. Kaposi's sarcoma and AIDS. *Med. Clin. North Am.* 70: 139, 1986.

76. Norris, D. A., and LeFeber, W. P. Mycosis Fungoides and the Sezary Syndrome. In B. H. Thiers and R. L. Dobson (Eds.), *Yearbook of Dermatology.* Chicago: Year Book Medical Publishers, 1982.

77. Odds, F. C. Genital candidosis. *Clin. Exp. Dermatol.* 7: 345, 1982.

78. Odom, R. B., and Goette, D. K. Treatment of keratoacanthomas with intralesional fluorouracil. *Arch. Dermatol.* 114: 1179, 1978.

79. Oriente, C. B., Scarpa, R., Pucino, A., et al. Prevalence of psoriatic arthritis in psoriatic patients. *Acta. Dermatol. Venerol. (Suppl.)* 113: 109, 1984.

80. Osler, W. *The Principles and Practice of Medicine.* New York: Appleton, 1892. P. 65.

81. Peter, G., and Smith, A. L. Group A streptococcal infections of skin and pharynx. *N. Engl. J. Med.* 297: 311, 1977.

82. Pinkus, H. Keratosis senilis. *Am. J. Clin. Pathol.* 29: 193, 1958.

83. Potter, M. Percivall Pott's contribution to cancer research. *Natl. Cancer Inst. Monogr.* 10: 1, 1963.

84. Rammelkamp, C. H., Jr. Epidemiology of streptococcal infections. *Harvey Lect.* 51: 113, 1957.

85. Reed, W. B., Becker, S. W., Sr., Becker, S. W., Jr., et al. Giant pigmented nevi, melanoma, and leptomeningeal melanocytosis: A clinical and histopathological study. *Arch. Dermatol.* 91: 100, 1965.

86. Rhodes, A. R. Melanocytic precursors of cutaneous melanoma: Estimated risks and guidelines for management. *Med. Clin. North Am.* 70: 3, 1986.

87. Rhodes, A. R. Neoplasms: Benign Neoplasias, Hyperplasias, and Dysplasias of Melanocytes. In T. B. Fitzpatrick, A. Z. Eisen, K. Wolfe, et al. (Eds.), *Dermatology in General Medicine,* 3d Ed. New York: McGraw-Hill, 1987. Pp. 877–889.

88. Rhodes, A. R., Harrist, T. J., and Momatz, T. K. The PUVA-induced pigmented macule: A lentiginous proliferation of large, sometimes cytologically atypical, melanocytes. *J. Am. Acad. Dermatol.* 9: 47, 1983.

89. Rietschel, R. L. Irritant contact dermatitis. *Dermatol. Clin.* 2: 545, 1984.

90. Rigel, D. S., and Friedman, R. J. (Eds.). Symposium on Melanoma and Pigmented Lesions. *Dermatol. Clin.* 3: 1, 1985.

91. Rios-Arizpe, S., and Ocampo-Candiani, J. Giant epidermoid cyst: Clinical aspect and surgical management. *J. Dermatol. Surg. Oncol.* 12: 734, 1986.

92. Ronchese, F. Keratoses, cancer and the sign of Leser-Trelat. *Cancer* 18: 1003, 1965.

93. Schechter, G. P., Sausville, E. A., Fischmann, A. B., et al. Evaluation of circulating malignant cells provides prognostic information in cutaneous T cell lymphoma. *Blood* 69: 841, 1987.

94. Schwartz, R. A. The keratoacanthoma: A review. *J. Surg. Oncol.* 12: 305, 1979.

95. Shelly, W. B., and Wood, M. G. Occult Bowen's disease in keratinous cysts. *Br. J. Dermatol.* 105: 105, 1981.

96. Soeprono, F. F., Schinella, R. A., Cockerell, C. J., et al. Seborrheic-like dermatitis of acquired immunodeficiency syndrome. *J. Am. Acad. Dermatol.* 14: 242, 1986.

97. Spruance, S. L., Overall, J. C., Jr., Kern, E. R., et al. The natural history of recurrent herpes simplex labialis. *N. Engl. J. Med.* 297: 69, 1977.

98. Stern, R. S., Weinstein, M. C., and Baker, S. G. Risk reduction for nonmelanoma skin cancer with childhood sunscreen use. *Arch. Dermatol.* 122: 537, 1986.

99. Stoll, H. K., and Schwartz, R. A. Squamous Cell Carcinoma. In T. B. Fitzpatrick et al. (Eds.), *Dermatology in General Medicine.* New York: McGraw-Hill, 1987. Pp. 746–758.

100. Stoner, J. G., and Rasmussen, J. E. Plant dermatitis. *J. Am. Acad. Dermatol.* 9: 1, 1983.

101. Strauss, S. E., Rooney, J. F., Sever, J. L., et al. Herpes simplex virus infection: Biology, treatment and prevention. *Ann. Intern. Med.* 103: 404, 1985.

102. Swerdlow, A. J., English, J., MacKie, R. M., et

al.   Benign melanocytic naevi as a risk factor for malignant melanoma. *Br. Med. J. (Clin. Res.)* 292: 1555, 1986.

103. Taplin, D., Rivera, A., Walker, J. G., et al.   A comparative trial of three treatment schedules for the eradication of scabies. *J. Am. Acad. Dermatol.* 9: 550, 1983.

104. Templeton, H. J.   Cutaneous tags of the neck. *Arch. Dermatol. Syphilol.* 33: 495, 1936.

105. Volberding, P. A.   Kaposi's sarcoma and the acquired immunodeficiency syndrome. *Med. Clin. North Am.* 70: 665, 1986.

106. Weinstein, G. D., McCullough, J. L., and Ross, P. A.   Cell kinetic basis for pathophysiology of psoriasis. *J. Invest. Dermatol.* 85: 579, 1985.

107. Weller, T. H.   Varicella and herpes zoster. Changing concepts of the natural history, control and importance of a not-so-benign virus. *N. Engl. J. Med.* 309: 1362, 1983.

108. Whitfield, A.   Some points on the aetiology of skin diseases. *Lancet* 2: 122, 1921.

109. Wolf, J. E., Jr., and Hubler, W. R., Jr.   Origin and evolution of pyogenic granuloma (Editorial). *Arch. Dermatol.* 110: 958, 1974.

Appendix

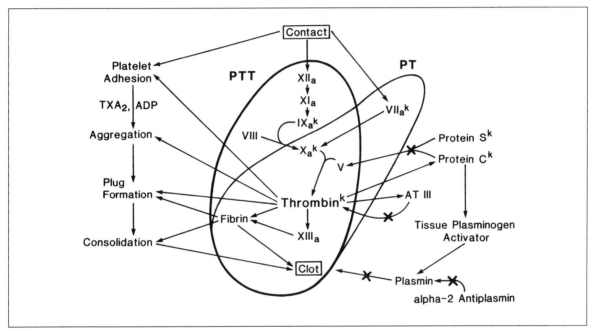

Figure 5–1. *Scheme of hemostasis. The platelet reactions are shown on the left; the soluble factors are to the right. The small k superscript denotes vitamin K-dependent factors. The dark x shows an inhibitory pathway. The circled factors starting with factor XII to the clot are the intrinsic pathway, measured by the partial thromboplastin time. The circled factors starting with factor VII to the clot are the extrinsic pathway, measured by the prothrombin time.*

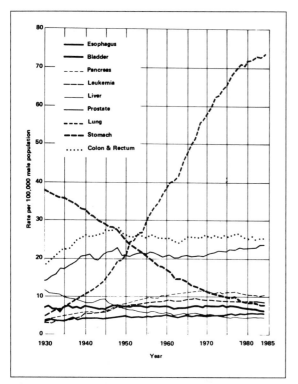

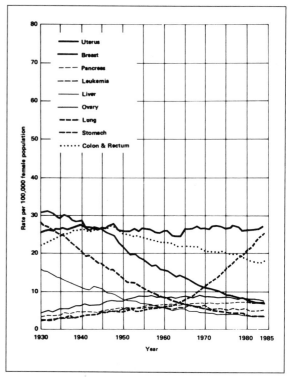

Figure 5–2. *Age-adjusted cancer death rates for selected sites, males, United States, 1930–1984. (From E. Silverberg, Cancer statistics, 1987. CA 37:10, 1987.)*

Figure 5–3. *Age-adjusted cancer death rates for selected sites, females, United States, 1930–1984. (From E. Silverberg, Cancer statistics, 1987. CA 37:11, 1987.)*

Index